NURSING CARE PLANS

Nursing Diagnoses in Planning Patient Care

Marilynn E. Doenges, B.S.N., M.A., R.N., C.S.

Clinical Specialist
Adult Psychiatric/Mental Health Nursing
Private Practice
Colorado Springs, Colorado

Mary F. Jeffries, B.S.N., M.S., R.N.

Major, US Army
Head Nurse, Surgical Section
Nursing Education and Training Consultant
Tripler Army Medical Center
Honolulu, Hawaii

Mary Frances Moorhouse, R.N., C.C.P.

Contract Practitioner
Critical Care
Colorado Springs, Colorado

F. A. DAVIS COMPANY ✹ **PHILADELPHIA**

S0-CFH-911

Copyright © 1984 by F.A. Davis Company

Second printing, June 1984
Third printing, July 1984
Fourth printing, December 1984
Fifth printing, January 1985

All rights reserved. This book is protected by copyright. No part of it may be reproduced, stored in a retrieval system, or transmitted in any form or by any means, electronic, mechanical, photocopying, recording, or otherwise, without written permission from the publisher.

Printed in the United States of America

The views expressed in this book are those of the authors and do not reflect the official policy or position of the Department of the Army, Department of Defense, or the US Government.

Library of Congress Cataloging in Publication Data

Doenges, Marilynn E., 1922-
   Nursing care plans.

   Includes bibliographies.
   1. Diagnosis. 2. Nursing. I. Jeffries, Mary F., 1944-   . II. Moorhouse, Mary Frances,
1947-   . III. Title. [DNLM: 1. Patient care planning. 2. Nursing process.   WY 100 D651h]
RT48.D64   1984   610.73   83-25211
ISBN 0-8036-2660-6

This book is dedicated to our families who have provided support and assistance in so many ways during this period. To the late Connie O'Neill of F. A. Davis, who had faith in the dream, and to Susan Taddei, formerly of F. A. Davis, who saw the dream and made it a reality and provided support when the going was difficult. To Adam Osborne, Tony Seran, and all the people at Academy Computers who brought us into the computer age and without whom the book would not have been completed. Lastly, to all our friends who were willing to listen when everything was impossible.

NOTE TO THE CLINICIAN

The care plans in this book focus on the adult medical-surgical patient wherever the patient is found, i.e., hospital, home, or long-term care facility. The book is designed to be a ready reference for the practicing nurse as well as a catalyst for thought in planning and evaluating nursing care. The use of nursing diagnosis within the framework of the medical diagnosis will assist you to give individualized patient care and to have an opportunity to use and define nursing diagnoses.

NOTE TO THE STUDENT

This book will help you in the learning environment to plan nursing care. It is not intended to be all-inclusive but rather to be a reminder of what the patient may need as a care plan is developed. Rationales are included to assist you to identify which interventions may apply to the individual patient and when modifications may be appropriate.

NOTE TO THE INSTRUCTOR

This book makes information available to students for use in learning to plan patient care. The instructor is responsible for guiding students in learning and developing their process skills. These care plans can be a useful tool in demonstrating the relevance of nursing diagnosis in a medical setting. Obviously, nursing care plans must always be designed for the particular patient. The care plans in this book are intended only as examples to help the student learn the process and structuring of individualized nursing care plans.

PREFACE

This book gives definition and direction to the development and use of individualized nursing care. The current state of the theory of Nursing Process, Diagnosis, and Intervention has been brought to the clinical setting to be implemented by the nurse. Therefore, this book is not an end in itself, but a beginning for the future growth and development of the profession.

The practicing nurse, as well as the nursing student, will welcome this text as a ready reference in clinical practice. It will serve as a catalyst for thought in planning and evaluating the care being rendered.

One of the marked differences in this book is the rationale, which not only states why an intervention is important but also gives a brief related pathophysiology, when applicable, to enhance the reader's understanding of the intervention.

One of the most significant advances in health care achieved during the last 20 years has been the emergence of the nurse as an active coordinator and initiator of patient care. The importance of the nurse within this system can no longer be denied or ignored. The transition from helpmate to health care professional has been painfully slow and is, of course, not yet complete. Each day brings advances in our struggle to understand the mysteries of normal body function. With this increased knowledge comes greater responsibility for the nurse. Today's nurse assesses and designs interventions that will move the total patient toward the goal of improved health.

Performance expectations of nurses by professional care standards, physicians, and patients will continue to increase. To meet this challenge competently, the nurse must have detailed, up-to-date knowledge of physical assessment skills and pathophysiologic concepts concerning the more common diseases presented on a general medical-surgical unit. This book is a tool, a means of attaining that competency.

In the past, care plans have been viewed principally as a learning tool for students, and seemed to have little relevance after graduation. As nursing has moved toward defining its professional status and accountability, the need for a written format to document and communicate individualized patient care has been recognized. In addition, governmental regulations and requirements of third party payers have created a need to validate the appropriateness of care given, as well as establish a framework for justifying patient care charges and staffing requirements.

Chapter 1 reviews the use of the nursing process to formulate plans of care and the nurse's role in the delivery of that care. The use of nursing diagnoses is discussed to provide the nurse with an understanding of their use in the nursing process. Chapter 2 discusses the use and adaptation of the care planning guides that are presented in this book.

The care plan guides are nursing-oriented and include information shared with the medical field. Each plan includes a nursing history, diagnostic evaluation, and physical examination termed the Patient Data Base. After the patient data base, nursing priorities are sifted from the information gathered to delineate the overall goals of care.

Each care plan is developed, identifying nursing diagnoses with supporting data that provide an explanation of potential patient problems. Outcomes are stated in behavioral terms that can be measured in specific ways. The interventions listed in each care plan are designed to assist with problem resolution. Rationales for the actions are designed to enable the nurse to decide whether the intervention applies to a particular patient.

The book has been designed for use in the acute medical-surgical setting and is organized according to systems for easy reference. Information is provided to assist the nurse in identifying and planning for discharge and rehabilitation as the patient progresses toward discharge. The nurse who uses this book will find it most helpful in planning the continuing care of the patient.

MED
MFJ
MFM

CONTRIBUTORS

Beam, Ida Marlene, RN
Major, Army Nurse Corps
Colorado Springs, Colorado
(Alzheimer's disease, psoriasis)

Blackwell, Suzan L., RN
Second Lt., U.S. Army Nurse Corps
Colorado Springs, Colorado
(thyroid, pituitary, adrenal)

Borup, Patricia, RN
Capt., Army Nurse Corps
Colorado Springs, Colorado
(cirrhosis)

Caylor, Anne Marie Sara, RN
Adult Nurse Practitioner
Capt., U.S. Army Nurse Corps
Ft. Carson, Colorado
(hiatal hernia, esophageal varices, Mallory-Weiss
   syndrome, achalasia, diabetes review)

Costantini, Sharon, RN, BSN, MS
Colorado Springs, Colorado (with Cooper,
Geraldine, RN, BS and Hagge, Elizabeth, RN, BS)
(ulcers)

Culver, Carla, RN, MSN
Cardiovascular Nurse Clinician
Cardiac Rehabilitation Unit
Penrose Hospital
Colorado Springs, Colorado
(valvular disease)

Davignon, Mary, RN, BSN, CCRN
Medical Intensive Care Unit
St. Mary's Hospital and Health Center
Tucson, Arizona
(myasthenia gravis)

Heath, Barbara, RN, BSN
Charge Nurse, General Surgical Unit with Urology
   Specialty

Penrose Hospital
Colorado Springs, Colorado
(ureterolithiasis, prostatic obstruction)

Heinrich, Pam, RN, BSN, MS, CCNA
Colorado Springs, Colorado
(fractures, casts, traction, amputation)

Hennings, Laurine, RN
Colorado Springs, Colorado
(radical neck surgery)

Hickey, Arlene, RN, BS
Patient Care Coordinator
Gorden S. Riegel Alcohol Treatment Center
Penrose Hospital
Colorado Springs, Colorado
(alcoholism)

Johnson, Laura Teigen, BSN, CNOR
Colorado Springs, Colorado
(surgical care)

Jones, Janet, RN, CCRN
Intensive Care Unit
Penrose Hospital
Colorado Springs, Colorado
(postoperative care of coronary artery bypass
   patient)

Knight, Anne, RN, BSN
First Lt., Army Nurse Corps
Honolulu, Hawaii
(increased intracranial pressure)

Lind, Patricia Trinosky, RN, MS
Instructor, Beth El School of Nursing
Memorial Hospital
Colorado Springs, Colorado
(diabetic ketoacidosis, HHNK)

McMahon, Cynthia L., RN, MS
Nursing Care Consultant

Colorado Springs, Colorado
(nursing diagnosis review, peritoneal dialysis and
hemodialysis, urinary tract infection, acute renal
failure)

McMinn, Cynthia, RN
First Lt., Army Nurse Corps
Colorado Springs, Colorado
(pneumonia, tuberculosis, degenerative joint
disease)

Mikkila, June A., RN
First Lt., Army Nurse Corps
Staff Nurse, Orthopedics
121st Evacuation Hospital
Seoul, South Korea
(rheumatoid arthritis)

Miller, Frieda, RN, ET, BSN
Penrose Hospital
Colorado Springs, Colorado
(fecal diversion [ostomy])

Murray, Rebecca F., RN
Colorado Springs, Colorado
(long term care)

Pietryka, Karen, RN, BA, BSN
Capt., Army Nurse Corps
121st Evacuation Hospital
Seoul, South Korea
(acute upper respiratory infection, strep throat,
acute epiglottitis, epistaxis)

Stephen, Marilyn, RN
Colorado Springs, Colorado
(herniated disk, laminectomy)

Tatkon-Coker, Andrea L., RN, MSN
Nurse Consultant
Pueblo-West, Colorado
(COPD, septicemia, mastectomy, paraplegia,
quadriplegia, chemical dependency,
hypoglycemia, total joint replacement)

Vernon, Joyce E., RN, BS
Burn Nurse Specialist
Critical Care/Burn Care Unit
Penrose Hospital
Colorado Springs, Colorado
(burns)

Watkins, Carolyn, RN, MSEd
Director, Aultman Hospital School of Nursing
Canton, Ohio
(guidelines chapter)

Wermers, Mary Ann, RN, MSN
Assistant Professor of Nursing
University of Southern Colorado
Pueblo, Colorado
(blood dyscrasias)

Wilson, Cathy Ave, RN, MSN, CCRN
Assistant Director of Training and Education
Penrose Hospital
Colorado Springs, Colorado
(ventricular aneurysm, cardiogenic shock,
digitalis toxicity, ARDS)

Woodhouse, Diana Kenney, RN, MS
Oncology Nurse Clinician
Woodland Park, Colorado
(cancer)

Woodling, Cynthia B., RN, BA, BSN
DeRidder, Louisiana
(osteomylitis)

Portions of the manuscript were reviewed by:
Alm, Albertine Lois Marie, RN, BSN
CCU and ACLS Certified
Tripler Army Medical Center
Honolulu, Hawaii

Vincent, Dale S., MD
Captain, Army Medical Corps
Chief Resident, Internal Medicine
Tripler Army Medical Center
Honolulu, Hawaii

ix

ABBREVIATIONS USED IN THIS BOOK

ABGs: arterial blood gases
AC: before meals
ACT: activated clotting time
ACTH: adrenocorticotropic hormone
ADH: antidiuretic hormone
ADL: activities of daily living
ASA: acetylsalicylic acid
ASO titre: antistreptolysin titre
A-V: atrioventricular

B & O: belladonna and opium
BFP: biological false positive
BSP: bromosulphalein
BUN: blood urea nitrogen

C & S: culture and sensitivities
Chol: cholesterol
CMV: cytomegalovirus
C/O: complains of
CPK: creatinine phosphokinase
Cr: creatinine
CRP: C-reactive protein
CT: computerized axial tomography
CTZ: chemoreceptor trigger zone
CVA: costovertebral angle; cerebrovascular accident

DIC: disseminated intravascular coagulation
DIP: distal interphalangeal
DPO: desired patient outcomes

EACA: e-aminocaproic acid
ESR: erythrocyte sedimentation rate

FIO$_2$: forced inspired oxygen

GF: glomerular filtrate
GFR: glomerular filtration rate
GU: genitourinary

HAA: hepatitis associated antigen
Hb & Hct: hemoglobin and hematocrit
H.S.: hour of sleep
HSV: herpes simplex virus

IABP: intraaortic balloon pump
IHSS: idiopathic hypertrophic subaortic stenosis
IMV: intermittent mandatory ventilation
IPPB: intermittent positive pressure breathing
IVP: intravenous pyelogram

JVD: jugular vein distention

KUB: kidney, ureter, bladder

LAP: leucine aminopeptidase/left atrial pressure
LDH: lactate dehydrogenase
LE cell: neutrophil
LOC: level of consciousness
LVEDP: left ventricular end-diastolic pressure

MAP: mean arterial pressure
M-mode: time-motion echocardiography
mOsm: milliosmol

NSU: nonspecific urethritis
N & V: nausea and vomiting

OTC: over-the-counter

PA: posterior anterior
PAP: pulmonary artery pressure
PAWP: pulmonary artery wedge pressure
PCWP: pulmonary capillary wedge pressure
PE: physical examination
PEEP: positive end-expiratory pressure
PIP: proximal interphalangeal
PMI: point of maximum impulse
PTH: parathyroid hormone
PTU: propylthiouracil
PVC: premature ventricular contraction
PWP: pulmonary wedge pressure

RAD: right axis deviation
RAI: radioactive iodine
RIA: radioimmunoassay
R/O: rule out

SGOT: serum glutamic oxaloacetic-acid-transaminase
SGPT: serum glutamic pyruvic transaminase
SIMV: synchronized intermittent mandatory ventilation.
SLE: systemic lupus erythematosus
SO: significant others
SOB: shortness of breath
SPF: sun protective factor
S/S: signs and symptoms

TCDB: turn, cough, deep breath
TIA: transient ischemic attack
TKO: to keep open
TRH: thyrotrophin releasing hormone
TUR: transurethral resection (of prostate)
TVC: true vomiting center

UA: urinalysis
UO: urinary output
URI: upper respiratory infection
UT: urinary tract
UTI: urinary tract infection

INDEX OF NURSING DIAGNOSES

appears on pages 695–696

CONTENTS

INDEX OF NURSING DIAGNOSES appears on pages 695–696

INDEX OF NURSING DIAGNOSES appears on pages 695–696

INDEX OF NURSING DIAGNOSES appears on pages 695–696

INDEX OF NURSING DIAGNOSES appears on pages 695–696

INDEX OF NURSING DIAGNOSES appears on pages 695–696

INDEX OF NURSING DIAGNOSES appears on pages 695–696

INDEX OF NURSING DIAGNOSES appears on pages 695–696

INDEX OF NURSING DIAGNOSES appears on pages 695–696

INDEX OF NURSING DIAGNOSES appears on pages 695–696

INDEX OF NURSING DIAGNOSES appears on pages 695–696

INDEX OF NURSING DIAGNOSES appears on pages 695–696

INDEX OF NURSING DIAGNOSES appears on pages 695–696

INDEX OF NURSING DIAGNOSES appears on pages 695–696

INDEX OF NURSING DIAGNOSES appears on pages 695–696

INDEX OF NURSING DIAGNOSES appears on pages 695–696

INDEX OF NURSING DIAGNOSES appears on pages 695–696

NURSING PROCESS AND CARE PLAN CONSTRUCTION

In using the nursing process in administering nursing care to patients, the nursing profession has identified a body of knowledge that contributes to the prevention of illness as well as the maintenance and/or restoration of the patient's health. The process is central to all nursing actions and is the essence of nursing; it can be applied in any health care or education setting, in any theoretical or conceptual framework, and within any nursing philosophy; the process is flexible and yet sufficiently structured so as to provide a base for the nurse's actions.

The nursing process uses observation and logical thinking to formulate and fulfil the goals of nursing. To use the process, the development of certain behaviors, including assessment, planning, intervention, and evaluation, is important so that the nurse's efforts will be more effective and the patient will receive quality care. Knowledge, attitudes, and abilities are fundamental to any nursing performance. Creativity, adaptability, commitment, trust, and leadership are behaviors that aid in using these fundamentals and in portraying appropriate attitudes in the performance of nursing actions.

The nurse is able to pursue goals and administer quality care, using vision and insight. Some elements of these goals may be recognized almost instantly, while others may require prolonged deliberation, research, and consultation to formulate a plan. This becomes an ongoing process. Adaptability suggests that the nurse is able to function in whatever situation is encountered. It suggests a plan in which perceptions of care are validated as the nurse plans with the patient. Adaptability suggests flexibility with enough structure to promote the process of nursing. A creative nurse initiates change as improvement is seen.

A successful nurse is committed. Patients are seen as individuals and respected for their humanity. To cope with the situation, whatever it may be (e.g., illness or trauma,), there needs to be mutual trust between the patient and nurse. With capable leadership qualities, the nurse initiates change, uses creativity, and performs as a role model to promote a sense of trust or a feeling of commitment, and to use adaptability in an effective way.

Use of the nursing process is a product of the nurse's efforts and thoughts. A supportive environment and the learning opportunities are crucial to this process. It is a time for group discussion and self-growth. The ultimate goal is quality health care. Only as this process is used, will there be an effective, viable, nursing care system that will be recognized and accepted as nursing's body of knowledge and shared with other health care professionals.

INFORMATION GATHERING

Interviewing: An interview defines a specific purpose. It is a specific set of data the nurse obtains from the patient and significant others through both observation and conversation. The interview may be called a multidimensional human contact interview, as the nonverbal communication is as important as the words expressed.

A creative interview permits an exchange of information to produce a level of understanding higher than either person could produce alone. More than data processing is sought; knowledge, understanding, and insight into the nature and behavior of the patient are important. The better prepared one is for the interview, the better the chances are of asking something new. The better listener one is, the better the chances are of hearing something new in the responses. The more perceptive one is, the better the chances are of seeing new and exciting connections among the data collected. The major medium used in the conversational exchange is the question. By stimulating the patient and/or significant others with the nurse's unique perceptions, expressed through the questions, their minds are encouraged to provide insights.

The system of the interview is made up of 10 anatomical parts: purpose, research, request, strategy, icebreaker, business, rapport, sensitivity, recovery, and conclusion. Having identified the parts of the system, let us explore each separately.

To be successful, the *purpose* of the interview needs to be stated specifically. All participants in the conversation need to know that the information to be gathered will be used in formulating the plan of care. This provides guidance in asking as well as answering questions, especially, when areas that appear to be unrelated to the current situation may be pursued.

Second, *research* needs to be conducted concerning the patient and the patient's family. Available resources, including previous admission records and other health team members can be used. During this information gathering process, notes can be made to identify key points. This research generates questions that should be written down so they are not lost. When the point of asking questions in the interview is reached, the information needed will be known. The end result of the interview is dependent upon what is put into it.

Third, the *request* for an interview with the patient and significant others can clearly promote a positive interaction. The nurse identifies oneself, explaining, precisely, the purpose of the data and how the data will be used. Together, a time is set for the interview. Give consideration to the needs of the patient and significant others for time to prepare for the interview. Your approach and attitude is important in selling the interview. "Mr. Jones, I would like to ask you some questions about yourself and your illness, so that together we may plan your care," is a much more positive approach than, "I need to know your history." The first approach not only sells the interview but stimulates the patient's thinking. The result of using these principles is a more productive interview.

Fourth, *strategy* is planned. Plan the details to be covered in the interview in accordance with the definition of purpose. Preparation and planning give a sense of security, a plan to fall back on if things go slowly or unexpectantly wrong. This also allows a comfortable departure from the plan when conversation takes an unexplored path into productive channels. A new twist and a refreshing insight are the gold nuggets of interviewing.

Fifth, within the first few minutes of the meeting, the nurse, patient, and/or significant others will make important decisions concerning the future of this relationship. How the *icebreakers* are used during these minutes may determine how the interview proceeds. During these minutes, the patient and/or significant others are making judgments of the nurse: sincere, trustworthy, sensitive, professionally competent? The icebreakers used at the beginning of the interview have vital importance in answering these questions. It is the first bond of human communication and trust in this new relationship. When the nurse sits down and appears relaxed and interested, this goal is more readily achieved.

Sixth, get to the *business* at hand. Here, the questions previously determined are asked. Listen then for answers and clues that will lead to other questions that have not been anticipated. The relaxed informality, which has been achieved before, continues through this phase. Don't expect insights immediately as they usually come with time, increased comfort level, and trust.

Seventh, as the interview progresses, *rapport* develops. Participants settle down as the conversation proceeds. Monitor the patient's and/or significant others' reactions to questions. Be careful not to bore them or intimidate them with embarrassing questions. It is important to know when to shift gears, speed up or slow down, or to ask more challenging questions.

Eighth, now you begin to involve questions of a somewhat threatening nature. Having laid the groundwork, proceed gently toward *sensitive* areas. You don't want to topple the tree and destroy the house, so cut down just a few feet at a time starting at the top. The same thing is done when the need is to approach a sensitive area of communication. Be alert to verbal/nonverbal cues that may indicate that the area of discussion is particularly sensitive for the patient. Ceasing exploration at this point demonstrates respect for the patient and the patient's privacy and can enhance the trust between nurse and patient.

Ninth, now *recover* the rapport. If the sensitive areas have been approached slowly, the recovery period should be fairly easy to accomplish. Warmth and caring evidenced by a smile and the touch of the hand are helpful.

Tenth, *conclude* the interview by summarizing the highlights of the interview and leaving the door open for further communication. An important way of doing this is to ask the patient and significant others if they have any questions to ask of you.

Whatever the technique of interviewing, be sure the purpose of the interview has been achieved. It should verify, clarify, and yield additional information. It gives the opportunity to see the patient and significant others, to use the nurse's perceptual abilities to obtain data, and to communicate concern, interest, and willingness to understand. It gives the opportunity to reinforce those behaviors conducive to wellness.

PATIENT DATA BASE

The data collected about the patient and/or significant others include a vast amount of information and many areas may be repetitious. In order to be useful, the nurse needs to organize the data in some concise systematic way. Initially, the nurse will be exposed to the total data and then with experience, the information collected will be individualized.

The purpose in developing a data base is to have a profile of the patient's health status. This is an intellectual process and will depend upon the:

1. knowledge base,
2. questions chosen to be asked,
3. method of asking questions,
4. ability to give meaning to responses,
5. ability to synthesize the data, and
6. ability to prioritize the data.

The philosophy and policies of the health care agency will also affect this process, as the data base must be valued, read, and used by all members of the health team.

When the gathered information is integrated, it becomes the patient data base (see Fig. 1). The information may be collected during one or more contact periods. Initially, determine the reason for the patient's presence and the severity of the patient's concern(s). As soon as possible, the total data base is collected and then updated as necessary. Information recorded in the medical history or elsewhere, if available, can be copied, avoiding repetition. Be aware that some repetition may have value for eliciting new/different information that may not have been recalled or volunteered previously.

NURSING HISTORY

Taking the data gathered in the interview and applying the data to the patient data base, forms the nursing history. The time devoted to obtaining a nursing history is well spent as it is a significant factor in saving time in any services or care given to patients and/or significant others. Failure to obtain data may create a climate of distrust and could add to the patient's cost and length of care.

In writing a history, the data collected from the interview are organized and recorded to assist in identifying problems. An understanding of the patient's holistic status is thus provided for oneself as well as for team members.

The history is more than writing information down. Review the data, organize and determine the relevance of each item, and document the facts. The quality of a history will increase with knowledge and experience.

The following are some principles that may be applied as the history is written. First, order is imperative. Develop a form that will facilitate finding information. The present illness needs to be presented in chronological order and include events from the past that are relevant. It is also useful to express topics in a uniform manner, such as, age 61 versus born in 1923.

Second, the amount of detail to be presented can be a problem. Enough material needs to be given so as total a picture as possible is presented, and yet not so much that it won't be read or used. Needed information includes all data (positive and negative) that are relevant to the situation. Some description is usually needed to make the data more meaningful; that is, cough versus cough: productive, yellow, large

FIGURE 1. Sample Form for Patient Data Base.

INITIAL NURSING DATA BASE

Admission Date _____
Admission Time _____
Mode of Admission _____
Admitted From: Home _____
           Nursing Home _____
               Other _____
Smoker _____ Nonsmoker _____
Language Barrier Yes _____ No _____
Describe _____
Cultural Factors _____
_____
Religion _____

Hearing Aid   _____
Dentures:
   upper   _____
   lower   _____
Glasses   _____
Contacts   _____
Prostheses   _____
Ambulatory
   Devices   _____
Other   _____

Familial Risk Factors:

Cancer   _____
Diabetes   _____
High Blood
   Pressure   _____
Strokes   _____
Heart Disease   _____
TB   _____
Kidney Disease   _____

Age _____
Sex _____
Ht. _____
Wt. _____
Temp. _____

BP _____ Rt. _____ Sitting _____ Lying _____ Standing
BP _____ Lf. _____ Sitting _____ Lying _____ Standing
P _____ Quality _____ Regularity _____
R _____ Quality _____

Reason for Hospitalization and History of Chief Complaint (In Patient's own words) _____
_____

Other Relevant Illnesses and/or Previous Hospitalizations (as patient recalls): _____
_____
_____

NURSING ASSESSMENT: SYMPTOMS (Check the appropriate blanks)

Neurologic: _____ None

_____ Fainting Spells/Dizziness
_____ Stroke (any residual effects?)
_____ Weakness (location?)
_____ Seizures (how controlled?)
_____ Tingling (location?)
_____ Numbness (location?)
_____ Other

Comments _____
_____
_____
_____
_____
_____

Gastrointestinal: _____ None

_____ Loss of Appetite/Taste
_____ Mastication problems
_____ Constipation (laxative used)
_____ Special Diet (type?)
_____ Nausea/Vomiting
_____ Diarrhea
_____ Heartburn (food intolerance)
_____ Last BM
_____ Character of Stool
_____ Changes in Weight
_____ Other

Comments _____
_____
_____

Urinary: _____ None

_____ Pain/Burning/Difficulty with Urination
_____ Incontinence
_____ Nocturia
_____ Character of Urine
_____ Other

Comments _____
_____
_____

Cardiovascular: _____ None

_____ High Blood Pressure
_____ Heart Trouble
_____ Ankle Edema
_____ Other

Comments _____
_____
_____

FIGURE 1. *Continued*

Eyes/ENT: _____ None

_____ Ears: _____ Hearing Loss
R ( ) L ( )
_____ Eyes: _____ Vision Loss
R ( ) L ( )
_____ Cataracts
_____ Glaucoma
_____ Nose: _____ Epistaxis
_____ Sense of smell
_____ Throat: _____ Sinus
_____ Swallowing

Comments _____
_____
_____

Respiratory: _____ None

Shortness of Breath (caused by?)   _____
Cough (productive?)   _____
Emphysema   _____
Bronchitis   _____
Other   _____

Comments _____
_____
_____
_____
_____
_____
_____

Skin: _____ None

_____ Rashes
_____ Sores
_____ Bruises
_____ Scars
_____ Changes in Moles
_____ Other

Comments _____
_____
_____

Musculoskeletal: _____ None

_____ Fractures/dislocations
_____ Arthritis/Unstable Joints
_____ Back Problem
_____ Other

Comments _____
_____
_____

Mark location of above on diagram.

Reproductive:

Last Menstrual Period _____
Do you practice breast self-exam?
Yes _____ No _____
Vaginal Discharge _____
Age at: Menarche _____
Menopause _____

_____ Penile Discharge
_____ Prostate, disorders of
_____ Vasectomy
_____ Do you practice breast
self-exam? Yes _____ No _____
_____ Do you practice testicular
self-exam? Yes _____ No _____

Allergies as Stated by Patient:

List   Reaction
_____   _____
_____   _____
_____   _____
_____   _____

Blood Transfusions: _____ Yes _____ No
When _____
Reaction: _____ Yes _____ No
What _____

Routine Medication as Stated by Patient:

Drug   Dose   Scheduled Time
of Last Dose
_____   _____   _____
_____   _____   _____
_____   _____   _____
_____   _____   _____
_____   _____   _____

Does Patient Take Medication Regularly:
_____ Yes _____ No

FIGURE 1. *Continued*

Activities of Daily Living:

_____ Independent in ADL
_____ Needs Assistance (specify):
     _____ Mobility
     _____ Feeding
     _____ Hygiene
     _____ Dressing
Usual Activities and Hobbies

_____
_____

Limitations Imposed by Illness

_____
_____
_____

Sleep:
_____ Hours
_____ Naps
_____ Aids
_____ Insomnia
Due to _____
_____
_____

Level of Education _____
_____
Occupation _____
_____
Alcohol _____
_____
_____
Tobacco _____

Nonprescription
     Drugs _____
_____

Comments _____
_____
_____
_____

Mental/Emotional:

Mental Status (check those that apply):
_____ Alert _____ Oriented
_____ Disoriented
     _____ Time
     _____ Place
     _____ Person
_____ Drowsy   _____ Listless
_____ Stuporous   _____ Forgetful
_____ Comatose   _____ Other
Specify _____
_____
_____
_____

Emotional Status (check those that apply):
_____ Calm   _____ Depressed
_____ Anxious   _____ Fearful
_____ Angry   _____ Restive
_____ Irritable   _____ Hysterical
_____ Other
Specify _____
_____
_____
Financial Concerns _____
Relationship Status _____

Patient's Perceptions and Expectations:
    What is your understanding of what will be done for you
    while you are in the hospital? _____
_____
_____
_____

Discharge Assessment:

    1. Do you anticipate changes in your living situation after discharge? _____ Yes _____ No

    (If answer is No omit the following questions)

    2. Areas that may require alteration (check those that apply):
_____ Food Preparation   _____ Physical layout of home   _____ Wound Care
_____ Shopping   _____ Additional help in home   _____ Medication
_____ Transportation   _____ Living facility other than home   _____ Treatments
_____ Ambulation   _____ Supplies

    3. Comments _____
_____
_____
_____

Information Obtained from: _____ Patient _____ Other (specify) _____
_____

Admitted By: _____
Reviewed By: _____

amount. Data not written are lost data. In contrast, data can be integrated into so much detail that it takes a persistent reader to find it.

Third, be as objective as possible. Identify only the patient's and/or significant others' contributions in this history and do not try to interpret the data. Record subjective data from the patient/significant others just as it was stated during the interview. Failure to do so will only confuse the issue.

Fourth, write legibly. This helps avoid lack of knowledge or misunderstood knowledge on the part of anyone reading the history. This can also save time and avoid inaccurate interpretation of the written data.

Fifth, write the history as soon as possible after gathering the information. This makes the data more accurate, for the longer one waits to record, the more the data and specific details will fade away. The following outline may be used (Fig. 1).

DIAGNOSTIC STUDIES

Laboratory examinations are included as part of the discussion of the nursing process, because this is part of the information gathering. Laboratory tests aid in the management, maintenance, and restoration of health. Some tests are used to diagnose disease, while others are useful in following the course of a disease or adjusting therapy. The origin of the test material does not always correlate to the organ or system; for example, a urine test for liver function. Many of the tests are useful in diagnosing diseases of more than one organ or system. In some cases, the relationship of the test to the pathologic physiology is clear while in others it is not. This is a result of the interrelationships between the various organs and systems of the body. In a few cases, the test is nonspecific, as it only indicates a disorder or abnormality and does not indicate where the problem is located, for example, sedimentation rate. Interpretation of these results by the physician involves careful integration with the history and physical findings that may be supplied by the nurse.

In evaluating laboratory tests, it is advisable to consider the drugs that are being administered to the patient. Drugs can cause erroneous interpretation of test results. This problem increases as more and more drugs are released for use. Thus, an important nursing role is to act as liason between the laboratory technician and the physician by indicating to the laboratory, the drugs the patient is receiving, and, in some cases, when the drug was administered.

There are also several mechanisms that may alter the laboratory results through the introduction of interfering materials. For example:

1. Food that gives a yellow color to serum will alter a bilirubin test.
2. Food or medication may contribute to the presence of substances in body fluids, such as iodine, which may mislead a diagnosis of hypothyroidism.
3. Drugs may elevate SGOT levels and confuse diagnosis of liver disease.

Knowledge of the preparation for the collection of the materials and interpretation of the results of the test is important as the plan of care is prepared and/or revised.

When ordering laboratory tests, the nurse needs to be aware of the requirements for individual tests. Some tests are done in a fasting state, others may require written consent as well as more detailed patient teaching. Knowledge of the individual is helpful to the nurse in tailoring the teaching. It is important to include information about the procedure and what will be expected of the patient following the testing. When patients are collecting a urine or feces sample for testing, it is important for them to know the proper collection procedures. This can be accomplished through explanation as well as by providing written materials for reinforcement, which can also enhance cooperation. The nurse needs to be aware of significant results that require reporting to the physician and/or initiation of specific nursing actions. A flow sheet may be used for noting trends/changes and aid in the assessment process.

PHYSICAL EXAMINATION

During this aspect of gathering information, exercise perceptual and observational skills to note the patient's expressions, posture, and dress. Be aware of physical limitations, such as deformities, failure to use an extremity properly, or absence of a part. Look for scars, discolorations, and lacerations. To facilitate these observations use the senses of sight, hearing, touch, and smell. Physical examination skills vary from the basic beginning practitioner to the advanced level of nurse practitioner/clinician. All levels will be discussed here.

Sight and hearing are used to elicit many responses in doing a head to toe examination. Touch can elicit data about muscle tension, moisture, and body temperature. Smell can elicit data about various body odors that may be significant in diagnosis or initiating certain nursing actions.

These abilities are combined into four methodologies commonly used during a physical examination. These are:

1. *Inspection,* which is a systematic observation. Sight is used to observe the skin for color, the lesion for drainage, or the respiratory pattern. Hearing is used to listen to the nature of a cough or the sound of a voice. Smell is used to detect a significant odor.
2. *Palpation* is the touching or pressing of a body surface with the fingers. Touch a surface to feel a lump or determine temperature. Press a surface to observe edema or pinch to observe skin turgor.
3. *Percussion* is direct or indirect tapping of a specific body surface to ascertain information about underlying tissues or organs. Tap the chest with the fingertips and listen for the sound indicating presence or absence of fluid, masses, or consolidation. Tap the knee with a percussion hammer and observe the presence or absence of lower leg movement.
4. *Auscultation* is listening for body sounds with the aid of a stethoscope and describing or interpreting them. This includes blood pressure as well as heart, lung, vascular, and bowel sounds.

The physical examination is done for purposes of gathering information and as a screening device. The nurse needs to know the normal physical and emotional characteristics sufficiently well enough to be able to recognize deviations from the normal. Approach the patient with a positive, sincere attitude in order to gain as much as possible from this procedure. This attitude portrays knowledge, interest, kindness, thoroughness, orderliness, and confidence. It is frightening when the nurse does not know what to do or is awkward in performing tasks. Give a clear explanation of the procedures to the patient. A skillful practitioner also demonstrates skill in verbal and nonverbal communication. These behaviors will yield the desired outcomes. The duration and length of any physical examination will depend on circumstances, such as condition of the patient and urgency of the situation.

When examining the skin use inspection and palpation. The patient is in a sitting, standing, or supine position. Inspect the skin for turgor, moisture, color, abnormalities, and evidence of lesions and scars. Palpate the skin for temperature, perspiration, dryness, and presence of lumps or masses. This is significant because the skin is a good indicator of the patient's general health status.

When examining the head and neck use inspection, palpation, and auscultation with the patient mostly in a sitting position. The skull is observed for size, shape, lesions, and pattern of hair growth. Observe the face for symmetry, placement of parts, and movement of facial structures. Inspect the neck for symmetry, deviations of the trachea and thyroid, range of motion (ROM), and visibility of neck vessels. Palpate for lymph nodes, size, shape, tenderness, and symmetry; size and shape of the thyroid; and carotid and temporal pulses. Auscultate for carotid bruits.

When examining the eye, look for the presence of external structures and for pupillary reaction to light, as well as coordination of movements and for accommodation. Visual acuity is tested through the use of an eye chart, visual fields by confrontation. Inspect the internal structures by using the ophthalmoscope. Observe the red reflex, the optic disc, and the macula retinae vessel for size, shape, and color. Observe for hemorrhages, exudates, A-V nicking, or arterial narrowing. The internal eye pressure may be measured with a tonometer and visual fields will give evidence of glaucoma.

Inspect the external ear for size, shape, symmetry, position, and the presence of lesions and exudate. Use an otoscope to examine the ear canal and the tympanic membrane. The use of a screening test can determine the patient's ability to hear.

Inspect the nose for patency and shape. Using a flashlight, examine the mucous membrane for color and the presence of exudate, lesions, and growths. Palpate and percuss the frontal and maxillary sinuses to determine sensitivity. Also, transilluminate sinuses in a completely dark room to ascertain membrane thickness or the presence of exudate within sinuses.

Examine the mouth by inspecting the lips, tongue, and mucous membrane for color, moisture, and presence of lesions and growths. With the aid of a tongue blade, inspect the pharynx for color, presence of exudate, edema, lesions, and growths. Also determine the size, movement, and position of the uvula and the presence and condition or the absence of tonsils. Determine patency of salivary glands by observing Wharton's and Stensen's ducts.

When examining the neuromusculoskeletal system, use inspection, palpation, and percussion. The patient is first sitting and then placed in a dorsal recumbent position. Palpation is used to determine the reactions to pain, vibration, and light touch. Test sensory function and reflexes through the use of a cotton swab, a safety pin, and a tuning fork. Test reflexes through the use of a percussion hammer. Observe for amputation, loss of function, or use of a prosethesis. Inspect the back and extremities for symmetry of contours, mobility, size, and coloration. The spine should have normal curvatures. Percuss for costoverte-bral angle tenderness at this time. Examine the joints for mobility, temperature, and edema. Determine muscle control when the patient performs regular activities of daily living.

To examine the thorax, inspect it for symmetry, shape, and respiratory movement while the patient is in a sitting position. Palpate to detect areas of tenderness and masses and note chest expansion and fremitus during respiratory excursion. Use percussion to detect movement of the diaphragm, lung or diaphragmatic excursion and the presence of air, and fluid or solids within the lung. Auscultate the lungs for the presence of normal and abnormal breath sounds as well as their duration, pitch, and intensity. If a cough is present, describe it in regard to expectorant (amount, color, and odor), duration, frequency, and tolerance. Also observe the use and handling of tissues. Note use of accessory muscles and level of respiratory effort.

Inspect for pulsation, heaves, bulges over the precordium and distentions of neck vessels. Palpate precordium for thrills and point of maximal impulse (PMI). Auscultate for heart sounds, evaluate their pitch, intensity, duration, and timing in the cardiac cycle. Auscultate for murmurs or other extra sounds. With patient at a 30 to 45° angle, palpate jugular veins and carotid arteries for fullness, pluse rate, rhythm, amplitude, and symmetry. Measure jugular venous pressure (JVP).

Inspection, auscultation, palpation, and percussion are the methods and order used to examine the abdomen as the patient is in a supine position. Inspect the abdomen for symmetry, distention, visible peristalsis, lesions, scars, position of the umbilicus, and effect of respiratory movement. Palpate the abdo-men to determine size, position, mobility, tenderness, and consistency of major organs, for example, liver, spleen, and kidneys, and for the presence of masses. Palpate the inguinal areas for hernias and lymph nodes. Use percussion to determine the presence of air or gas in the stomach and intestines and to determine the presence and size of organs and abnormal masses. Auscultate the abdomen for bowel and major blood vessel sounds or bruits.

With the patient in a Sims position, inspect the anal region for lesions, scars, edema, or drainage. Palpate the rectum for smoothness, edema, distortions, masses, and the presence of feces. If feces are present, a laboratory test for occult blood may be performed. In men, the prostate gland can be palpated for size, location, tenderness, and masses. In women, the uterus can be palpated for size, location, and masses.

Inspection and palpation are methods used in breast examination for both men and women. Inspect the breasts and nipples for symmetry, contour, lesions, dimpling, and nipple discharge. Palpate the breasts and axillary area for consistency, presence of lumps, and tenderness as well as lymph nodes. This may also provide the opportunity to do some health teaching on breast self-examination.

Inspection and palpation are used in examining the genitalia. In men, this is best done with the patient in a standing position. Inspect the penis for lesions, edema, erythema, discharge, and presence of circumcision. Inspect the scrotum for symmetry, edema, and lesions. Palpate the scrotum to determine size, shape, and consistency of testes, epididymis, and spermatic cords. Also test for inguinal hernias at this time. In women, this examination is best done in a lithotomy position. Inspect the external genitalia for size, color, lesions, masses, and discharge. Palpation of this area may detect edema or tenderness. An internal examination of the vagina, cervix, uterus, and adnexa may also be done at this time.

Following the examination, assist the patient as necessary. The patient may need assistance off the table for safety reasons, or assistance with dressing. Verification or clarification of communication associ-ated with the examination may also be needed.

As the physical examination is performed using knowledge and portraying attitudes and skills, gather the information in a thoughtful manner. Assume the ultimate responsibility for accuracy of the information gathered. Note patient responses to these interactions. Be sure to give explanations before and after the procedures are done as well as during. Offer emotional support and care where indicated.

Provide the patient with feedback as much as possible. Take advantage of any teaching opportunities. The health status profile you are providing is an important assessment tool.

Findings may be recorded according to the systems as they have been examined for easy reference.

NURSING DIAGNOSIS

Problem identification is not a new concept in nursing. Nurse educators and nurse practitioners have used the scientific method for a long time in the decision-making process of patient care management. The problem-oriented record is a more recent approach. The use of nursing diagnosis is an extension of this process. Nursing diagnosis is the definition of a standard nomenclature for describing health problems amenable to treatment by nurses.

A comparison of the scientific method, the problem-oriented record, and the nursing process follows:

Scientific Method	*Problem-Oriented Record*	*Nursing Process*
1. Problem identification: 　a. Recognize the problem 　b. Define the problem 　c. Recall data 　d. Add data	1. Data base	1. Assessment
2. Examine relevant data	2. Problem list	2. Analysis and problem statement(s)
3. Select relevant data	3. Initial care plan	3. Planning
4. Test data	4. Nursing orders	4. Implementation
5. Evaluate results	5. Nurses' notes	5. Evaluation

When using the nursing process, the nursing diagnosis list is the important result of all information gathered. It emerges after the data base is formulated and serves as a guide for the patient's plan of care. A nursing diagnosis may be defined as anything that requires nursing intervention and management; interferes with the quality of life the patient is used to or desires; and concerns the patient, significant others and/or the nurse. Each nursing diagnosis may be titled, numbered, and dated. As new diagnoses are identified and active diagnoses are resolved, nursing diagnoses may be added and/or already existing diagnoses can be changed. The following is a sample form:

Nursing Diagnosis List:

No.	Title	Date	Active	Inactive	Resolved Date
1.	Bowel elimination, alteration in, constipation.	month/day/year	x		
2.	Knowledge deficit, disease management.			x	month/day/year

The responsibility for establishing the nursing diagnosis list will vary with the theoretical framework of the nursing service organization; for example, functional method, team method, primary nursing, and case method. The nursing diagnosis list may contain a physical, sociologic, and/or psychologic finding and are listed in order of priority. Understanding of the diagnostic statement is dependent upon:

1. availability of data,
2. educational background of practitioner, and
3. practitioner's ability to analyze and synthesize data.

Psychosocial nursing diagnosis includes anything that pertains to, deals with, or affects the mind, intellect, and/or emotion; as well as those that pertain to the patient's life (e.g., alcoholic spouse; or unemployed, can't pay hospital bill) or relationships (e.g., retarded daughter). Demographic diagnosis statements include those that are hazardous to health (e.g., smoking).

After nursing diagnoses are written, they are numbered according to priority and are classified according to status: active, inactive, or resolved. Active diagnoses are those that require some form of action or intervention. Inactive diagnoses are those that may recur. Resolved diagnoses are those that no longer need action. These diagnoses may continue to have relevance to current problems as history of what has happened in the past. When the patient and/or significant others are unable to give all the data needed, the first diagnosis may need to be: incomplete data base.

The nursing diagnosis is the crux of the nursing care plan and the prime determinant of the style of nursing care to be administered. It focuses attention on certain areas. The affective tone of the nursing diagnosis can shape the expectations to the patient's response and the nurse's behavior toward the patient.

The nursing diagnosis is as precise as the data will allow. Seek, incorporate, and synthesize all relevant data available and make the statement meaningful so as to provide direction for nursing care. Compare these two diagnostic statements; "Constipated" versus "Bowel elimination, alteration in, constipation," with supporting data that states, "has daily bowel movement only with aid of laxative." The second statement is precise in identifying the interference with the activity of daily living involved and the nature of the coping deficit. It communicates the patient's situation at the present time.

The diagnostic process is one of defining the problem and involves both the patient and the nurse. The nurse is determining if the patient needs help in dealing with the interference or in seeking wellness. In general, but not necessarily, the patient needs to accept that a problem exists in order to have a successful outcome.

To adequately identify a diagnosis, the nurse needs a strong theoretical knowledge base in the biologic, physical, and behavioral sciences. Also, an understanding of the health care needs of the patient and family (significant others), the process of problem identification, and the individuality of the patient is important. The health care needs range from Maslow's human needs to the prevention of illness, maintenance, and/or restoration of health. Understanding the individuality of the patient requires recognizing the need for obtaining a personal, sociologic, psychologic, and medical history: performing a thorough physical examination and observing the test results plus integration of these data.

There are seven steps involved in the process of problem identification resulting in the writing of nursing diagnoses.

1. Collect a data base.
2. Analyze the data for discrepancies. Review the data to determine if there are any conflicts or differences in data that normally reinforce each other. Example; complains of pain RUQ, but doesn't flinch on abdominal examination. Further action is aimed at resolution of the conflict.
3. Synthesize the data. A thorough data base is lengthy as different parts of the data base are collected by different members of the health team. Thus, looking at all the data as a whole provides the nurse with a comprehensive picture of the patient in relation to the past, present, and future health status. The results of the synthesis of the data are written in a succinct, descriptive paragraph or concise, precise, diagnostic statements.
4. Analyze the data for relevant, positive, and negative findings. To adequately analyze wordy data into meaningful, organized, and pertinent information, the data need to be classified. Classifying data is the process of categorizing information according to established criteria. It is listing all positive findings (abnormalities) or relevant, negative findings (information expected to exist that does not).
5. Compare and contrast the relationships among the data. This step is crucial to the establishment of an adequate list of problem statements. Identify the meaning within each category of data and between each of the categories listed, based on an understanding of the patient and the nurse's knowledge of the biologic, physical, and behavioral sciences. After determining relationships and interrelationships, identify the causative factors within or between categories if they are known.
6. List the patient problems. Based on the data obtained from Steps 4 and 5, concisely and precisely write the nursing diagnosis.
7. Re-evaluate the problem list, being sure all areas of concern are identified.

Integrating these steps provides for a systematic approach to problem identification and the ultimate writing of nursing diagnoses.

DESIRED PATIENT OUTCOMES

When a nursing diagnosis is written, this implies that the past or present situation is not operational for either the patient or the nurse. Thus, a different outcome is desired, which becomes the outcome statement. While these outcomes may exist for either the nurse and/or the patient, it is important to remember that the desired outcome is what the *patient* will achieve, not the nurse. This topic can be approached by first looking at a process for writing an outcome statement.

First, write an outcome statement. Use whatever words are comfortable in jotting down ideas. Start by writing the objectives the patient and nurse want to achieve. Describe the objective in a comfortable, understandable way. Writing the statement provides direction for those involved. Identify whether the outcome is clearly defined. In doing so, state only the outcome and not the nursing intervention. To accomplish this, state only *what* is to be achieved and avoid saying *how* it will be done.

Second, identify the items someone will say or do that represent the outcome statement. To facilitate this, use only words or phrases. Don't write objectives as they represent how the goal is to be achieved. There are four strategies that may assist in writing outcome statements;

1. Answer the question: "What evidence is acceptable that the outcome has been achieved?" Write down everything without concern for duplication, completeness, relevance, and so forth.
2. Answer the question: "Given a team of patients, what criteria would determine who had achieved the outcome and who had not achieved the outcome?" Write down all information that is thought of.
3. Other nurses will be charged with the care of the patient. They will need to decide if the outcome is achieved. What instructions will be given? What can be looked for? Write all cues needed to answer these questions.
4. Think of some patient who has previously achieved this outcome. Write down the items that helped to determine that the outcome had been achieved.

Approach this from a positive aspect by writing down the items to observe that will determine that the outcome has been achieved. This is probably the most realistic approach. It might be helpful to list the items that would show the outcome has not been achieved.

Third, now that the items have been written down rework the list and sort out vagueness, duplication, and/or redundancies. Cross out any unwanted items. It will be shorter. The process is repeated until every item contributes toward achievement of the outcome.

Fourth, now go back to the original outcome, which was written down, and give it meaning. The outcome should be written so that it provides direction for planning the care that will be administered to the patient and significant others.

The statement, "to die with dignity" is too general. It could be used with several patients. It gives a general sense of direction with opportunity for different interpretations. A useful desired outcome needs to:

1. be realistic,
2. consider the patient's circumstances and desires,
3. set a direction,
4. specify an outcome, and
5. indicate a time dimension.

Thus, a desired outcome could be defined as specific and measurable, which may be achievable and which is desired by the patient and can be attained within a defined time period using the present situation and resources.

A desired outcome could be written as "promote maximal self-determination for remainder of life through participation in decision-making and performance of ADL." Desired outcomes written in association with the nursing process, emerge from the diagnostic statements. They will illustrate a relationship to specific coping deficits and the impact on the patient's lifestyle. These outcomes will focus on helping patients to use their own potential more effectively or to obtain more resources so they can function at a higher level. Where resources are not readily available or are inadequate, concentrating on modifying the activities of daily living and lifestyle through use of changed coping mechanisms and resources and the use of outside assistance may be necessary.

Balance of function

| Coping ability; resources (e.g., death, threatening signs, diagnosis, divorce, decreased mobility) | Activities of daily living, lifestyle (adjust to these in a satisfactory way) |

Having looked at ways of organizing outcome statements, we can now identify some principles that may be used in writing these statements:

1. Write in terms of the patient's behavior and outcome.
2. Write the statement concisely. Use only necessary, relevant words.
3. Use action verbs. When the patient is asked to perform an action, such as verbalize, anyone can determine if it has been met.
4. Use modifiers to add to the specificity. This indicates a style as to how the action is being done (e.g., ambulates with use of cane).
5. Identify a time element if it is needed.
6. Include the content area. It indicates what the person is to do specifically.

Outcomes involve different time spans. These may be long-term, intermediate, or short-term outcomes. They all are concerned with outcome behaviors but have different purposes. The *long-term outcomes* indicate the overall direction of behavior as a result of the use of the nursing process. The *intermediate outcomes* are shorter range so as to more specifically affect the nature of the interaction and activities of the patient and nurse. They will also create opportunity for motivation and set the pace for the occurrence of activities. They serve as indicators of progress toward achieving outcomes. The *short-term outcomes* are the specific guides to action for use in the nursing process. Thus, outcomes serve four purposes:

1. provide direction for nursing activities,
2. determine the pace of activities,
3. give a sense of achievement, and
4. serve as criteria for evaluation.

The nurse/patient outcomes are only part of the overall health care outcome(s). Each discipline involved in assisting the patient and significant others will have individual outcomes that contribute to the overall goal(s). These multidisciplinary outcomes must not conflict. The challenge is to write meaningful outcomes that can be understood and used by colleagues in health care and that will avoid conflicts.

NURSING INTERVENTION

The information is gathered, the problems are identified, and the outcomes are formulated. Now select the actions that can be expected to achieve the outcomes. This is called the nursing care plan with its basic unit known as the nursing intervention. A knowledge base is vital to this stage of development. The rationale for following the nursing intervention needs to be sound and feasible, whether it forms the basis for personal action or for actions of others. Actions that don't meet these criteria are headed for failure.

Nursing interventions are prescriptions for specific behaviors expected from nurses as well as other members of the health team. The expectation is that the prescribed behavior will benefit the patient and/or significant others in a predictable way related to the identified diagnosis and accepted outcome. These interventions have the intent of individualizing care and are geared toward meeting the individual patient's needs.

The medical plan of care is reviewed as nurses do implement these orders. So that patients do not suffer from neglect in nursing care as a result of the nurse believing the medical plan of care is also the nursing plan of care, it is important to recognize that there are two separate plans of care. The medical plan of care indicates the need for additional nursing actions so it can be fulfilled. These nursing actions could include:

1. Teaching, for example, instruction for wearing support hose to aid in prevention of blood clot formation.
2. Discussion of dietary supplements, for example, taking a diuretic with resulting potassium depletion.
3. Discussion of drugs that may be contraindicated, for example, aspirin when taking an anticoagulant drug.

When writing nursing interventions, the body of scientific knowledge that supports these interventions must be known. The nurse is accountable for being current and accurate and the interventions must be deliberate and purposeful.

There is a structure to writing these care plans. First, date them, then review the plans systematically in terms of the patient's response. Then decide if they are to be renewed, revised, updated, or discontinued. The time span for implementing this process is dependent upon the philosophy of the institution; that is, it will be done daily in acute care settings, while monthly may be adequate in long-term care settings. Dating also contributes to the continuity and momentum of care as well as evaluation.

Second, each nursing intervention begins with an action verb communicating a specific behavior. More specificity may be achieved by adding modifying words, such as demonstrate, tell, show, role play, and explain. For example, "Teach the patient _____" may be expressed as, "Demonstrate sterile technique."

Third, the content area deals with the "what" and the "place" of the intervention. "Show various injection sites to self-administer cortisone. Use rotation chart of injection sites." Content areas are important, especially when continuity and repetition are desired.

Fourth, the time element should indicate when, how often or how long the intervention is to be done. It may be a clock hour or it may be associated with a nursing action, a patient response, and so forth.

Fifth, the signature of the nurse must be present. The signature denotes accountability; it permits feedback, with the opportunity for clarification and/or exploring the rationale and choice of interventions.

Written nursing interventions are a means of guiding nursing care. Sound, scientific rationale are the basis for an effective plan of care. The nurse and the patient, when possible, are responsible and accountable for this care.

If the nursing interventions are to be successful, there needs to be a commitment to them. There is a growing awareness that nursing care is the key to survival, maintenance, rehabilitation, and preventive health care. Thus, there is a need for liability, accountability, and quality assurance. The nursing interventions need to be documented as to their quality and quantity as well as to their contribution to patient care.

Nursing interventions are a means of communicating the behavior to be done by the nurse to the rest of the nursing staff and health care members. Thus, clarity in verbalization is important. The following is a suggested form for communicating nursing interventions:

NURSING DIAGNOSIS:	**Knowledge deficit, disease management.**
SUPPORTING DATA:	**Patient needs to be self-sufficient in home setting.**
DESIRED PATIENT OUTCOMES:	**Administers cortisone to self, using correct technique, prior to discharge.**

Interventions	Rationale
Demonstrate sterile technique.	(May be used when helpful to the communication process.)

Show various injection sites to self-administer cortisone, using rotation chart of injection sites.

Have patient do two successful return demonstrations.

RATIONALE

With the "knowledge explosion," which began in the late 1950s, many disciplines have expanded their horizons. Nursing is no exception, having accepted the concept of total, individualized care of our patients as the basis for effective, therapeutic nursing care. Philosophically this has been termed a holistic approach to health care. In implementing the concept, nursing has identified the body of knowledge referred to as the "nursing process" as a means to administering effective, therapeutic nursing care.

If individualized care is to be accomplished, there must be an indication of the individual desires and needs of the patient. At first, nursing believed that no two patients were identical, thus, no two care plans could be identical. In implementing this thinking, an awareness began to occur that this approach was not practical, feasible, or cost effective. As a result, nursing today recognizes that although patients have many differences, they also have many common characteristics, needs, and problems. Thus, patients have some common responses, whether ill or well. Therefore, today's approach toward the use of the nursing process is to consider similarities as well as differences among patients. When this is accepted as a basic principle, rational and systematic plans of care can be developed.

The critical element for effective, therapeutic nursing care is the relevance of care based upon thorough, appropriately done assessments (first step of the nursing process). Because nursing recognizes the common elements as well as the differences among its patients, nursing care planning will reflect this. Standardized care plans may be used when similarities exist, and individualized when differences are identified. A standardized care plan is a method of responding to similar problems and needs and may be modified to meet the individual differences that have been identified. The written care plan communicates to the nurse, patient, and other members of the health care team, the past and present status of the care being given. It identifies problems solved and those yet to be solved; approaches that have been successful and those that were not successful; and patterns of patient's responses. It provides a mechanism for assuring continuity of care as the health team can be knowledgeable of the care being administered and progress in an orderly manner.

EVALUATION AND DISCHARGE PLANNING

How do nurses know when the patient is moving toward the outcomes chosen? How do they know the outcome has been achieved? How do patients know they are making progress toward achieving the outcomes? When these questions are asked, the evaluation process is beginning. This occurs as outcomes are being identified and written and continues through the nursing process. None of the components expressed are really isolated by definite beginnings and endings. They overlap and are continuous throughout the process.

Begin to think about evaluation as the use of the nursing process begins, but do not implement evaluation until after you have identified the outcome(s) and initiated some nursing interventions. In both assessment and evaluation, data are collected and judgments are made, but the sequence is different. In assessment, the data collection occurs first and leads toward formulation of outcomes. In evaluation, the outcome guides the data collection.

Evaluation consists of three sequential steps:

1. taking the previously stated "Desired Patient Outcomes" and denoting the appropriate question that can measure the outcome,
2. collecting data to answer the above questions, and
3. comparing evidence collected with the stated outcome and making a judgment on achievement or nonachievement.

Evaluation questions used to measure the outcome become operationalized. These indicate to the nurse what is to be collected, how it is to be collected, and the terms to be used in writing the description. Collect and report the relevant data in a systematic, consistent way that lends itself to the measurement of the achievement of the outcome.

Just as there are overlapping areas of responsibility for assessment and diagnosis among the health team members, so evaluation will involve shared territory of the involved disciplines. However, there is a valid basis in offering a primary focus to nursing care evaluation. This means the nurse will be the coordinator for evaluating the patient's responses to achieving the goals of daily living or Maslow's hierarchial needs, and so forth, as influenced by the patient's present health status.

It is important to chart the patient's responses to administered nursing interventions. Sometimes, the nurse is more concerned with charting what has been done and does very little with charting patient responses. These responses are very important to the evaluation process.

Evaluation and recording of patterns of nursing care together with patient responses are essential in the nursing component of health care. The skills of determining the criteria to be used, the data to be collected, and the recording system need to be well developed in order for this to be a useful tool. It is not difficult to add nursing's focus to the total evaluation of a patient's health care. It can fit with other disciplines and can serve to expand the total picture of the patient's response in coping with problems of health and the impact those problems have on daily living.

Discharge planning is crucial as it assures continuity of care and helps patients find the best solutions to their problems. Problem-solving techniques are used to: assess needs, identify problems, design a plan, test an action plan, and measure results.

Discharge planning begins with admission and is a means of providing for continuity of care. The question needing an answer here is, "Does the patient need continuation of care after the patient leaves the health care agency?" In many instances, the answer to this question is yes. The next question is, "What is involved in the care needs, plus how and where can these needs best be met?"

Planning for an alternative to present care is dependent on the answers to the above questions. The most common alternatives are: home care, board care, day-care center, skilled care, or a hospice setting.

Implementation begins with a commitment and can flow only with the health care agency philosophy and policies. It needs a team approach and the team needs an organized mechanism to accomplish the task.

All nurses need to be involved as their leadership is needed to ensure continuity of patient care. Concern for patients does not end when they leave the hospital. Two out of every three patients will probably still need instruction, equipment, treatment, or other care. They cannot be kept in the hospital until all their needs have been sufficiently met. This is far too costly, and beds are required for the acutely ill. In addition, patients normally improve faster in familiar home surroundings. If patients fail to master the home problems by themselves, do they return to the hospital? Again, while the cost of readmission is high, the possible appearance of physical and emotional regression needs to be considered. Are family members available for help or do they need an outside agency?

Who then is to take on the function of ensuring that patients do not endure needless pain, continued incapacity, and progressive demoralization, simply because no one initiated available aids? The nurse is in a key position to assume this responsibility. The nurse knows the patient's capacities, limitations, and what help they might need from others. The nurse talks with the physician, meets with significant others, learns the home situation, and knows what services are available outside the hospital from various community agencies, and therefore, can help patients and significant others plan the best ways to handle and/or prevent the patient's problems.

The assumption of this pivotal role in the total health team presents a vital opportunity and large responsibility to the nursing profession. Failure to fill this coordinating role, as a liaison-representative of the patient, leaves a tragic gap in our health care. Who will fill that role if the nurse declines?

The nurse is committed to planning continuity of care in all its aspects: between nursing shifts, between services within the hospital, and between the hospital and community. In the hospital, the nurse is responsible for initiating/cooperating in referrals to outside community services for all patients who need continued nursing or other help. In the community agencies, the nurse is responsible to periodically return to the hospital or educational center to learn the latest techniques in patient care and how they can be applied in the home or health care setting.

It is not enough to accept all this in principle or is it sensible for nurses to have to work out separately all the most efficient methods for this continuity of care. These guidelines are designed to help plan, with the patient, significant others, and health team members, the nursing and additional health services a patient may need after leaving the hospital. The guidelines suggest procedures in discharge planning: who does what, when, and how. The "why" is implicit in all needs of the patient, which this planning reveals.

What determines whether a patient will need a discharge plan? The optimum health care system today would evaluate every patient and draw up a plan to meet that patient's complete needs. Within the broader concept of total, integrated care, identify those patients who are most likely to require continuity of care from hospital to home or other health care facility.

Some alternatives to meet these identified needs include the following. Home health care as it exists today, is underused. It provides coordinated health care and supportive services to the ill or disabled person in that person's place of residence. It promotes and supports optimum health in the broadest sense. Home health care is provided by a multidisciplinary team under the direction of a physician and supervision of a professional nurse. This makes it possible for patients to be discharged while still needing the services of a professional staff.

Because a large proportion of patients in acute hospitals are elderly, there is an increasing number who need extended care in skilled nursing care facilities. Skilled care is usually necessary when a patient does not have family, when problems at discharge simply cannot be worked out for living at home, when medical problems are too great, or when family and community resources are too limited to provide any other alternative. Even here, the waiting time may be shortened by early discharge planning. The discharge plan includes the expected outcomes and needs at the skilled nursing facility and the possibility of eventual discharge to the community.

Hospice is an organized program of care for people going through the last stage of life. The whole family is considered the unit of care and this care extends through the mourning process. Emphasis is placed on pain control and palliative and supportive care for the patient and family before and after death. Hospice care is provided by an organized multidiscipline team available 24 hours a day, seven days a week.

The registered nurse is responsible for and accountable to the patient for the quality of nursing care. Thus, the nurse has a responsibility to plan for the continuity of the patient's care. Nursing administration is responsible for providing leadership, involvement, and, most importantly, budgeting time and money so that the staff nurse, team leader, or head nurse can fulfill responsibilities in this area.

Discharge planning is an integral part of daily care for the nursing staff. The nurse is giving direct care to patients and is in the best situation to assess their immediate and long-term needs. Patient care conferences and patient care plans are tools to communicate assessments and other information.

BIBLIOGRAPHY

Books and Other Individual Publications

BATES, B.: *A Guide to Physical Examination.* J. B Lippincott, Philadelphia, 1974.

FLYNN, P.A.R.: *Holistic Health The Art and Science of Care.* Robert J. Brady, Bowie, Maryland, 1980, p. 17.

LAMONICA, E.L.: *The Nursing Process,* Addison-Wesley, Menlo Park, California, 1979.

MAYERS, M.: *A Systematic Approach to the Nursing Care Plan.* Appleton-Century-Croft, New York, 1972.

SUNDEEN, S.J. ET. AL.: *Nurse Client Interaction, Implementing the Nursing Process,* ed. 2. C.V. Mosby, St. Louis, 1981, pp. 1–21.

Journal Articles

CHAMBERS, W.: *Nursing diagnosis.* AJN, 102–104, 1962.

KELLY, N.: *Nursing care plans.* Nursing Outlook, 61–64, 1966.

McCAIN, F.: *Nursing by assessment, not intuition.* AJN, 82–84, 1965.

POLAND, M.: *A system for assessing and meeting patient needs.* AJN, 1479–1482, 1970.

PRICE, M.R.: *Nursing diagnosis-making a concept come alive.* AJN, 668 +, April 1980.

SMELTER, C.: *Teaching the nursing process-practical method.* JONE, 31 +, November 1980.

WAGNER, B.M.: *Care plans-right, reasonable, reachable.* AJN, 986–990, May 1969.

CHAPTER 2
USE AND ADAPTATION OF CARE PLAN GUIDES

This book is intended for nurses who are working in the acute medical/surgical care setting. The nursing diagnosis is used to help nurses more accurately identify care needed by the individual. Given the state of the art of nursing diagnosis, the nurse is encouraged to investigate, learn, and fit the care plan to the individual patient. The care plan is a guide for the nurse to use in this process, rather than a standard plan that "fits all."

It is designed to give the nurse a sampling of information about the overall patient data base, identifying many factors that may or may not need to be given consideration when caring for any particular patient. Diagnoses and interventions are identified with rationale so the nurse can decide if this intervention is appropriate to this patient.

In writing this book, several basic assumptions have been made. One is the belief that the nurse has basic knowledge, abilities, and actions. Therefore, some interventions have been left to the nurse's discretion, such as notifying the physician, which is believed to be in the area of the nurse's professional decision. Supporting data are not intended to be complete but contain some ideas that can lead the nurse to further research if the information is not pertinent for this particular patient. Sufficient information is provided for the nurse to decide if the diagnosis is suited to the individual in the nurse's care.

An important aspect is involvement of patients' in their own care. Information is given at the level of their understanding and ability so they may participate in decisions about their care and its outcome. This negates the idea that health caregivers have control over patients lives.

Kim's Nursing Diagnosis List has been chosen because of the value it presents for identifying exactly what the problem is for any given patient. It may be helpful to create your own care plan using this process and decide what is most useful in your situation by using your own diagnoses and adding to and making the communication work in your setting with your patient.

In the patient data base, a variety of information has been included, but it is not an all inclusive list. Diagnostic studies include common tests and findings. In some places, common ranges for lab values have been stated, keeping in mind that different hospitals have different normals depending on the test procedures used. The physical examination sets out the most common findings anticipated in the disease/condition and the routine examination is expected to be done as indicated for the individual patient.

Nursing priorities have been identified and the nursing diagnoses follow in the same order. In general, these have been stated in measurable, observable terms that can be achieved by those involved. If your individual patient has different/additional priorities, they will need to be stated in your care plan. The progression of care is prioritized, recognizing that this may be an arbitrary decision in individual cases.

Interventions are designed to specify the action of the nurse and/or the patient and/or significant others. It is not an inclusive list and while such nursing actions as bathing have been left out, it is expected that these will be included in the patient care. In addition, the nurse is referred to the hospital procedure manual for interventions that are unfamiliar and to the drug manual for in depth discussion of pharmacologic concerns. Because this book speaks to all patient situations, the use of patient/they has been chosen to indicate an individual of either sex. The term significant others has been used instead of family, because it is recognized that for many individuals family may be a limiting term. Physiologic normals will need to be individualized to the specific patient. Sufficient rationale for most actions is provided to act on and spur the nurse to seek further information about why the actions will result in the desired result(s). This can be an exciting, challenging, and rewarding experience for the nurse and can open up new areas of learning and opportunity for growth. Sometimes, controversial issues have been included for information and because different treatments may be used in different parts of the country.

The medical management has been set out as a separate section. The nurse may identify what is in the province of the physician with resultant nursing actions versus what is nursing management of the whole patient and the patient's wellness. Nursing actions in regard to medical management have not necessarily been discussed, assuming the nurse will know these basic actions or be reminded to obtain further information.

Information for discharge planning has been included in two ways. While the care plans contain information throughout that will assist the nurse with discharge planning, a knowledge deficit diagnosis has been included in many of the care plans and serves as a reminder of some of the actions necessary to prepare the patient for discharge, home management, and rehabilitation.

Due to the organization of this book with patient data base, and the use of nursing diagnoses, supporting data, and desired patient outcomes with interventions and rationale, this format is compatible for use with the American Nurses' Association Standards of Care that are available and used in many institutions.

As often as possible, information has not been repeated, instead the nurse is referred to other care plans. However, where this did not seem feasible, the information has been repeated so it is readily available, avoiding the necessity of going from one care plan to another. Care plans that are general in nature are included in the "general section." These include the surgical care plan, which includes pre-intra- and postoperative care and allows the nurse to note information that may not be readily available elsewhere. A care plan on long-term care has been included, speaking to a belief that patients who are seen in the acute setting often come from, or are going to be discharged to, extended care facilities. It will also be helpful to nurses who have been working in an acute setting and now find themselves in the long-term care facility.

A plan addressed to psychosocial needs has been included with the belief that *all* patients experience problems in these areas when they are hospitalized. This care plan does not relate specifically to psychiatric patients, although they may have the same general needs. As with any patient, when you are dealing with the psychiatric patient, you are not dealing with a diagnosis but with the specific behavior being demonstrated.

Some factors involving the nurse's own self have been included because of a belief that you as, an individual, are an important part of the patient's care. Values and judgments are an integral part of each person and enter into the caregiver's interactions with the patient and/or significant others.

It is hoped that the nurse who uses this book will find it a guide to thinking about individual patients and their needs in specific situations and will spur further research and learning, which, in turn, will enhance quality patient care and result in an increased sense of self-esteem for the nurse.

BIBLIOGRAPHY

KIM, M AND MORITZ, D. (EDS.): *Classification of Nursing Diagnoses.* McGraw-Hill, New York, 1981.

CHAPTER 3
CARDIOVASCULAR

DIAGNOSIS: Hypertension

PATIENT DATA BASE

NURSING HISTORY

Patient may experience no symptoms.

History of headaches, migraines, especially in the morning, which resolve as the day progresses, and may be accompanied by stiff neck, dizziness, weakness, numbness and tingling in extremities, muscle cramps, visual disturbances, epistaxis, episodes of diaphoresis, dyspnea, palpitations, angina, fatigue, hemoptysis, metrorrhagia.

History of factors that may contribute to increased risk of hypertension: excess salt intake, use of birth control pills or other hormones, smoking, obesity, drug use, alcohol, sedentary versus active lifestyle, lipid abnormalities, diabetes mellitus, Afro-American heritage.

History of personality changes, memory deficits, anxiety, depression, periods of euphoria or chronic anger may indicate cerebral impairment. Outbursts of crying may be due to hypoxia.

Family/patient history of hypertension, atherosclerosis, heart disease, cerebrovascular disease may show familial predisposition for essential hypertension.

Assessment of strengths, coping mechanisms, and support system.

History of onset of symptoms, rapidity of disease progression, drug/regimen response; (behavioral changes may also be caused by antihypertensive therapy).

DIAGNOSTIC STUDIES

Thyroid studies: hyperthyroid may cause excessive stroke volume or pulse rate, which may lead to vasoconstriction and hypertension.

Serum cholesterol and triglycerides: elevated level may indicate predisposition for atheromatous plaquing.

Serum potassium: hypokalemia may indicate the presence of primary aldosteronism.

Chest x-ray: may demonstrate coarctation of, obstructing deposits in, and/or notching of aorta; cardiac enlargement.

Urine steroids: if elevated may indicate excessive serum catecholamines from hyperadrenalism, pheo-chromocytoma or pituitary dysfunction, Cushing's syndrome; renin levels may also be elevated. Hy-perglycemia may be associated with elevated catecholamine levels.

Fasting or two-hour postprandial blood glucose to check for diabetes mellitus.

Urinalysis, BUN, IVP: to rule out polycystic disease, chronic glomerular nephritis: proteinuria caused by toxemia, hematuria, renal parenchymal disease.

Uric acid: hyperuricemia has been implicated as a risk factor for the development of hypertension.

Urine VMA: catecholamine metabolite. If elevated, may indicate pheochromocytoma.

CT scan: to check for cerebral tumor, CVA, encephalopathy.

24-hour urine: for VMA if hypertension is intermittent, showing sporatic functioning of an adrenal tumor.

Renal vein renin level determination: to evaluate renin content of the blood.

ABGs: to check for pulmonary involvement, increased Pco_2.

Serum/urine aldosterone level: to check for primary aldosteronism.

Serum calcium: elevation may contribute to hypertension.

ECG: check heart size, conductiveness, strain.

PHYSICAL EXAMINATION

Vital signs: Blood pressure, pulses, heart sounds: Apical-radial pulse, femoral-radial pulse. Heart sounds to rule out valvular disease, congestive heart failure, aortic stenosis/regurgitation, murmur of coarcta-tion, AV fistulas, renal artery stenosis. Check for presence of normal S1 and S2 and abnormal S3 and S4. Location of point of maximum intensity (PMI): may be displaced laterally showing dilation of the heart.

Breath sounds: clear versus adventitious sounds present.

Check skin for signs of vessel inflammation: color, edema. May be indicative of polyarteritis nodosa, edema of congestive heart failure, toxemia, kidney disease.

Palpation of abdomen for mass (kidney enlargement caused by hydronephrosis or tumor); do not mas-sage unduly as this may increase blood pressure postexamination. Listen for abdominal bruit, which may indicate renal artery stenosis.

Height and weight may validate obesity, cachexia.

Neurologic examination to rule out cerebral tumor, neuropathy, hemiparesis. Hyperreflexia or positive Babinski may indicate cerebral pathologic changes.

Blood pressure supine and standing; arms and legs, blood pressure consistently elevated above 140/90 or 20 points above that considered normal for patient's age. May be systolic or diastolic elevation or both. Use equipment that is accurate; cuff bladder should be two-thirds diameter of the limb.

Fundoscopic examination to check for retinal changes/hemorrhage, papilledema, vessel tortuosity, silver/copper wiring of vessels.

NURSING PRIORITIES

1. Maintain blood pressure at acceptable levels.
2. Assist patient in learning of disease and treatment modalities.
3. Assist patient in recognizing and eliminating underlying causes or aggravating factors.

NURSING DIAGNOSIS:	Cardiac output, alteration in, decreased.
SUPPORTING DATA:	Hypertension increases the size of the capillary bed producing increased myocardial workload, which may cause failure and decreased cardiac output.
DESIRED PATIENT OUTCOMES:	Absence of signs of cardiac decompensation. No decrease of visual acuity.

INTERVENTIONS

Monitor blood pressure throughout day under same conditions. Take supine/sitting/standing and both arms. May be q.i.d. or more depending on vital signs and/or occurrence of side effects.

Assess time and frequency of angina, dyspnea, decreasing urine output.

Report visual changes, sensory/motor changes, severe headache, personality changes, nausea and vomiting. Take seizure precautions.

Encourage rest periodically during day and after meals.

Provide small meals and snacks.

MEDICAL MANAGEMENT

Low-sodium diet.

Antihypertensives.

RATIONALE

Allows more accurate comparisons by control of external influences.

Increased cardiac strain produces symptoms of congestive heart failure and fluid retention. Renal failure may result from a state of cardiac decompensation.

Narrowing of ocular vessels causes changes in visual acuity, which may be temporary or permanent. Hypertensive encephalopathy is a complication of extremely elevated blood pressure levels and is caused by reflex spasm of the cerebral vessels.

Decreases myocardial workload.

Requires less energy and reduces strain on cardiovascular system.

Decreases amount of intravascular fluid held by excess sodium, thereby, decreasing myocardial workload.

Drugs reduce hypertensive cause of headaches.

NURSING DIAGNOSIS:	Comfort, alteration in, headache.
SUPPORTING DATA:	Hypertension expands arterioles causing pressure on surrounding tissues resulting in pain. Excessive vascular pressure may cause vessels to dilate or rupture.

DESIRED PATIENT OUTCOMES:	Absence of discomfort. Dizziness/ epistaxis controlled.

INTERVENTIONS

Eliminate/minimize vasoconstricting activities that may aggravate headaches, including tobacco use.

Maintain bed rest or encourage limited activity.

Assist patient with ambulation as indicated.

Ice pack at back of neck, pressure over distal third of nose and leaning head forward may slow epistaxis.

Give soft foods or liquids and frequent mouth care when packing has been done.

MEDICAL MANAGEMENT

Analgesics.

Nasal packing.

Tranquilizers.

RATIONALE

Stress, smoking, or other secondary health problems may accentuate pain. Worsens increased blood pressure due to vasoconstrictive influence.

Avoids unnecessary stimulation.

Dizziness, headache is common with hypertensive states and hypotensive states associated with drug therapy.

Nasal capillaries may rupture; cold pressure compresses capillaries, which slows or halts bleeding.

Nasal packing may interfere with swallowing, require mouth-breathing, and lead to stagnant oral secretions.

Decreases pain, which may stimulate sympathetic nervous system causing increased blood pressure readings.

May be required if bleeding is severe or prolonged.

May aid in reduction of stress and discomfort.

NURSING DIAGNOSIS:	Nutrition, alteration in, more than body requirements.
SUPPORTING DATA:	Obesity plays a role in aggravation of hypertension and may predispose to exacerbation and possible severe complications, such as myocardial infarction and stroke.
DESIRED PATIENT OUTCOMES:	At or attaining desired weight.

INTERVENTIONS

Discuss necessity for decreased calorie intake. Encourage patient to minimize intake of salt, fats, and sugar.

RATIONALE

Excess calorie intake leads to deposition of adipose tissue. Faulty eating habits contribute to atherosclerosis and obesity, which predispose to hypertension and subsequent complications. Increased salt intake expands intravascular fluids and further aggravates hypertension.

Discuss with patient, the exercise program that will fit the patient's interests and physical condition.

Can assist in weight reduction, aid cardiovascular conditioning, and has the potential for improving mental outlook.

NURSING DIAGNOSIS: Fear, medication side effects and progression of disease.

SUPPORTING DATA: Situations viewed as beyond patient's control due to insidious nature of onset.

DESIRED PATIENT OUTCOMES: Behaviors within normal limits with fear and apprehension at manageable levels.

INTERVENTIONS

Be available for and encourage verbalization and questions.

Provide information about disease/prescribed regimen.

Emphasize that serious side effects can be controlled/eliminated.

Be alert to signs of denial and depression.

If not following prescribed regimen, discuss with patient.

RATIONALE

Can be helpful in decreasing vasoconstrictive response associated with stress, which may aggravate condition and worsen symptoms.

Will assist patient to make decisions and assume control over own health care.

Following prescribed regimen can minimize potential problems.

Are to be expected and need therapeutic intervention. (Refer to Care Plan: Psychosocial Aspects of Care in the Acute Setting.)

May reveal misunderstandings, concerns, or feelings related to restrictions of therapy, which need to be addressed.

MEDICAL MANAGEMENT

Tranquilizers and/or other prescribed drugs, p.r.n.

Patient may manifest tension and tremors that are intensified by symptoms and environmental stresses.

NURSING DIAGNOSIS: Knowledge deficit, disease/treatment.

SUPPORTING DATA: Hypertension may cause no observable symptoms for many years, but causes irreversible progressive damage to many organs, especially the eyes, kidneys, heart, and blood vessels. Many different drugs are used and produce a myriad of side effects and cautions.

DESIRED PATIENT OUTCOMES: **Verbalizes understanding of disease and role of drug therapy in its control. Identifies potential stressful situations and takes steps to avoid them. Verbalizes drug side effects and possible complications that necessitate medical attention. Blood pressure maintained within normal limits.**

INTERVENTIONS

Assess level of knowledge and provide additional information as desired.

Teach patient to take own blood pressure, record, and factors to be concerned about.

Stress importance of followup care.

Assist in identification of individual factors that produce stress and methods of handling.

Explore with patient lifetime changes that may be necessary.

Discuss drug actions/interactions/side effects.

Discuss potential of impotence in men.

Discuss replacing oral contraceptives with other birth control methods.

Provide information about the possibility of interactions with over-the-counter drugs, such as cough or cold medications.

Discuss general side effects of drugs; lightheadedness, lethargy, orthostatic hypotension. Teach patient to increase large muscle activity or lie down briefly if hypotensive effects occur.

Avoid standing still for any length of time, such as showering, shaving, standing in line.

Change positions slowly.

Avoid hot/steam baths, hot tubs, and saunas.

RATIONALE

Enables patient to make choices about lifestyle changes and adherence to medical regimen.

Knowledge of individual variations in blood pressure will enable the patient to exercise control in handling problems.

Monitors response to regimen, control of blood pressure and development of complications.

May accelerate disease process or exacerbate symptoms.

Identifying own stress/precipitating factors and ways of handling, allows patient to maintain feeling of control.

Adequate information enhances success of drug therapy.

Antihypertensive drugs affect autonomic nervous system, which plays a part in libidinal reactions. Change in drug or dosage may relieve signs/symptoms.

Oral contraceptives may increase renin production by the kidney and increase blood pressure.

May contain sympathetic nervous stimulants that may increase blood pressure or counteract antihypertensive effects.

Upright position produces decrease in venous return because of decreased blood pressure, decreased peripheral resistance, and decreased cardiac output.

Vasodilation of leg vessels causes blood pooling resulting in syncope or weakness. May be especially severe in the morning or within two hours after taking drug.

May cause sudden change in blood pressure.

Causes vasodilation and leads to decreased blood pressure.

If drowsiness occurs when taking drugs, caution about operation of mechanical equipment.

Common side effect that may slow reflexes and impair judgment.

Caution patient not to abruptly discontinue drug.

Causes rebound hypertension that may lead to severe complications.

ANTIHYPERTENSIVE THERAPY: (i.e., Apresoline).

Report promptly symptoms of chest pain, palpitations, dizziness, and headache.

Dilate vessels thereby decreasing peripheral flow and myocardial workload.

SYMPATHETIC INHIBITORS: (i.e., Methyldopa).

Not to be given to patients with history of psyschological depression; watch for depressive symptoms. Check for peptic ulcer and occurrence of ulcerative colitis. Caution patient that hot weather, alcohol intensify symptoms.

Central nervous system depressant.

Take with food.

May cause gastrointestinal upset, diarrhea.

Note quick weight gain, symptoms of congestive heart failure.

Aldomet may cause fluid and sodium retention. Myocardial decompensation may occur due to sympathetic blockage and depletion of tissue stores of norepinephrine.

Inform patient that effects take place slowly (especially with MAO inhibitors). Avoid foods containing tyramine (cheese, beer, wine, pickled herring, chicken liver).

Large intake of tyramine overrides drug effect to deplete tyramine and can result in hypertensive crisis.

Instruct patient to report occurrences of urinary retention or impotence.

Causes relaxation of smooth muscle.

Use cautiously in hypotensive patients.

Accentuates vasodilating action of narcotics and other agents that have relaxation effect on smooth muscle.

ORAL DIURETICS: (i.e., Diuril)

Warn of dry mouth, thirst, polyuria, weakness, drowsiness, lethargy, fatigue, and gastrointestinal disturbance, such as constipation.

Reduces the amount of water, sodium chloride in the body. May also cause electrolyte disturbances.

Discourage alcohol, barbiturate use concurrently.

May produce orthostatic hypotension due to cumulative effect.

(i.e., Lasix).

Check serum electrolyte balance and dehydration.

Causes diuresis by excess excretion of electrolytes.

POTASSIUM-SPARING DIURETICS: (i.e., Aldactone).

Do not give potassium supplement unless patient is losing potassium due to other means, such as with glucocorticoid therapy. Check serum sodium level.

Blocks effect of aldosterone resulting in potassium saving. Dyrenium may potentiate action of antihypertensive medications. Glucocorticoids promote sodium retention and potassium excretion.

Instruct patient to carry identification card giving name of drug, dosage, and so forth.

Gives needed information in case of emergency.

DIAGNOSIS: Congestive Heart Failure (CHF)

PATIENT DATA BASE

NURSING HISTORY

Complaints of chest heaviness or discomfort, anginal pattern, dyspnea on exertion, orthopnea, paroxysmal nocturnal dyspnea, nausea/vomiting, and fever.

Patient's description of onset of symptoms may include: clothes feel tighter, weight gain, acute onset versus chronic progressive disease, decreased urination, swelling of extremities, and sleeping on more than one pillow.

History of hypertension, angina, myocardial infarction, diabetes, open heart surgery, arrhythmias.

Note physical activities: sedentary versus active.

Dietary history: intake of fats, sugars, salt, liquor, caffeine, which may be associated with atherosclerosis.

Current medications: drug tolerance, cardiac suppressive drugs, use of steroids, large amounts of intravenous fluid or rapid administration, allergies.

Elimination pattern may suggest fluid retention secondary to CHF (nocturia).

Smoking habits: smoker, mode, packs/per day, how long, and whether patient inhales.

Posture, nervousness, anxiety may communicate discomfort.

History of asthma, obesity, pulmonary disease are factors that may increase myocardial workload and predispose to development of CHF.

DIAGNOSTIC STUDIES

Complete blood count may indicate severe anemia or polycythemia as cause of CHF.

White blood cell count: infection or leukocytosis consistent with acute myocardial infarction, pericarditis, and other inflammatory or infectious states.

Arterial blood gasses: assess degree of respiratory involvement.

Cholesterol/triglyceride level: elevation may increase risk for coronary artery disease with decreased perfusion.

Serum catecholamine levels to rule out adrenal disease.

Sedimentation rate may be elevated showing presence of acute inflammatory reaction as with myocardial infarction, pericarditis, and so forth.

Thyroid studies may disclose elevated thyroid activity.

Echocardiogram demonstrates valve incompetence/stenosis; also identified enlarged chambers, myocardial hypertrophy found in CHF.

Cardiac scan shows underperfused myocardium, which may contribute to decreased contractile capacity.

Chest x-ray may show enlarged heart shadow.

Cardiac catheterization demonstrates ejection fraction of ventricle.

ECG shows ventricular or atrial hypertrophy with axis deviation, ischemia and damage patterns, arrhythmias.

Liver studies, renal studies to show any adverse effects because of CHF.

PHYSICAL EXAMINATION

Evaluate overall cardiovascular status: height, weight, weakness, activity tolerance, color, edema, temperature, peripheral pulses, point of maximum intensity (PMI), blood pressure, and heart sounds. Pulses bisferiens (having 2 beats), S4 and early systolic murmur triad suggest obstructive cardiomyopathy, such as idiopathic hypertrophic subaortic stenosis (IHSS).

Presence of jugular venous pulse, pulsus alternans and laterally displaced PMI indicate myocardial decompensation.

Evaluate stress factors: insomnia, increased vital signs, highstrung or chronic worrier personality.

Palpate for hepatomegaly, due to fluid retention in CHF and may cause hepatic dysfunction and/or associated ascites.

Hepatojugular reflux may be elicited.

NURSING PRIORITIES

1. Decrease cardiac workload and improve myocardial contractility.
2. Assist in determination of underlying cause.
3. Provide information about disease/treatment/recurrences.
4. Provide support for psychosocial concerns.

NURSING DIAGNOSIS:	**Tissue perfusion, alteration in.**
SUPPORTING DATA:	**Damaged myocardium produces decreased cardiac output and is less capable of adapting to increased demands.**
DESIRED PATIENT OUTCOMES:	**Absence of signs of cardiac decompensation.**

INTERVENTIONS

Determine baseline ABGs, electrolytes, BUN and creatinine levels, accurate intake and output.

Monitor vital signs; take apical pulse.

Monitor/document arrhythmias.

Assess for hypotension, pulses alternans, tachycardia, regularity of pulse, decreased peripheral pulses and signs of decreased perfusion peripherally, such as cool skin, diaphoresis, and so forth.

RATIONALE

Decreased perfusion to lungs may be reflected in increased PCO_2. Increased sodium bicarbonate and decreased potassium and chloride reflect metabolic acidosis resulting from anaerobic metabolism, secondary to decreased tissue perfusion. Increase in BUN, creatinine and decreased urine output reflect decreased renal perfusion.

Decreased blood pressure, increased pulse/respirations may indicate worsening congestive failure.

Shows conduction alterations that often occur because of hypoxia. (Refer to Care Plan: Arrhythmias.)

Indicative of decreased and inadequate cardiac output.

Assess changes in sensorium.	May signify inadequate cerebral perfusion secondary to decreased cardiac output.
Initially keep on bed rest and eliminate activities eliciting a Valsalva response. Note response to activities.	Valsalva maneuvers increase heart demand abruptly; already stressed heart may be unable to respond adequately, cardiac output falls sharply and may cause a stroke or myocardial infarction.
Assess anxiety and maintain a quiet, relaxed environment with frequent rest periods.	Anxiety and restlessness increase myocardial workload. Rest allows for decreased myocardial workload and full rest of the body.
Institute measures to prevent thromboembolic phenomena. (Refer to Care Plan: Impaired Peripheral Vascular Function.)	Prolonged bed rest and increased circulation time predispose to formation of clots and emboli.
Give small, frequent feedings; frequent oral care.	Blood supply to digestive areas may be decreased leading to anorexia or nausea and abdominal distention with elevation of the diaphragm, which decreases lung capacity. Oral care removes stale secretions that may contribute to anorexia.
Give low-calorie diet, if indicated; observe for malnourishment.	Weight reduction decreases myocardial workload. Edema may mask hyponourishment.
Monitor serum digitalis levels periodically.	Liver congestion and decreased GFR may interfere with metabolization and excretion.
Monitor for side effects of drug therapy and signs of increased cardiac strain.	Drugs such as glycosides strengthen contractile force, increase myocardial oxygen requirements and therefore may compromise cardiac function.
Withhold digitalis preparation and notify physician if marked changes occur in cardiac rate and/or rhythm or signs of digitalis toxicity develop.	Incidence of toxicity is high because of narrow margin between therapeutic and toxic ranges. Toxicity produces arrhythmias similar to those being treated with digitalis therapy. (Refer to Care Plan: Digitalis Toxicity.)

MEDICAL MANAGEMENT

Serial ECGs and chest x-rays, as indicated.	ECG shows left ventricular strain; chest x-ray shows size of heart shadow. Serial reports document favorable/unfavorable changes.
Humidified oxygen.	Combats hypoxia, which further decreases myocardial contractility.
Give oxygen with meals.	Tissue oxygen needs are increased during digestion.
Cardiac glycosides.	Increase myocardial contractility and slow rate.
Inotropic and vasoactive drugs.	Decrease preload/afterload, reduce myocardial workload and improve cardiac output.
Tranquilizers, sedatives.	Decrease anxiety and restlessness.
Stool softeners, antiemetics, p.r.n.	Prevent activities that might elicit a Valsalva response.
Flow-directed catheter.	To monitor cardiac output and prevent fluid overload.
Insertion of left ventricular assist device, if needed.	(Refer to Care Plan: Cardiogenic Shock.)

NURSING DIAGNOSIS:	**Fluid volume, alteration in, excess, potential.**
SUPPORTING DATA:	**Ineffective pumping of the heart causes fluid backup into peripheral and pulmonary tissues; increased afterload and hypertrophy. Decreased glomerular filtration rate initiates water retention and vasoconstriction.**
DESIRED PATIENT OUTCOMES:	**Fluid volume is stabilized as shown by normal heart and breath sounds, respiratory rate, clearing lung fields, and absence of tissue edema.**

INTERVENTIONS	RATIONALE
Monitor blood pressure, pulse, CVP/PWP.	Increase reflects increased vascular fluid.
Monitor heart sounds as indicated. Palpate position of PMI.	Rub is sound of enlarged ventricles rubbing against pericardium. May become displaced to left and down indicating dilatation.
Evaluate breath sounds, noting decreased sounds and abnormalities, such as crackles, wheezes. Note appearance of increased amounts of sputum, dyspnea, tachypnea, orthopnea, paroxysmal nocturnal dyspnea, cough, increased fatigue.	Fluid in lungs may be result of left heart failure. Increased fluid in pulmonary system restricts blood oxygenation producing symptoms associated with hypoxia.
Observe for Cheyne Stokes respirations.	Often present, especially when patient is sedated; results from increased circulation, which affects the respiratory mechanism that controls rate and depth of breathing.
Palpate for hepatomegaly; note occurrence of nausea, vomiting, bloating, constipation; limit oral medications.	Liver becomes distended with excess fluid; signs of visceral congestion may also occur. Oral medications may not be adequately absorbed.
Weigh daily.	Gain in excess of four pounds/week constitutes a sudden weight gain that may represent fluid retention.
Observe for anasarca.	Increased vascular fluid resultant from decreased cardiac output, increased hydrostatic pressure and decreased colloidal holding pressure results in tissue edema. Decreased glomerular filtration rate stimulates renin-angiotensin-aldosterone system. Aldosterone is not adequately metabolized by the liver, so water and salt retention is accentuated.
Observe for cardiac arrhythmias.	Aminophylline/hypoxia produce arrhythmias.

Fluids may be limited. Give frequent mouth care, ice chips as part of fluid allotment, hard candy, gum.

Fluid restriction minimizes risk of fluid overload. Mouth care and ice chips moisten mouth and decrease dryness associated with decreased fluid intake.

Place in Fowler's or semi-Fowler's position.

Upright positions favor expansion of lungs by gravity and decrease abdominal organ pressure on diaphragm. Reclining position favors venous return, overloading already inefficient myocardium.

Limit gas-forming foods, such as legumes, some vegetables, fruits, carbonated beverages.

Abdominal distention places pressure against diaphragm limiting excursion of diaphragm and intake of tidal volume.

MEDICAL MANAGEMENT

Diuretics; note response.

Decrease extracellular fluid to decrease myocardial workload; if diuresis is not sufficient, other drugs, measures may be added to potentiate diuresis.

Aminophylline.

Bronchial dilation increases volume of gas delivered to alveoli, decreasing cardiac workload and increasing oxygenation.

Humidified oxygen under pressure.

Discourages serum transudation by exerting its pressure on pulmonary endothelium.

Thoracentesis, paracentesis, phlebotomy, rotating tourniquets.

May be used to decrease immediate vascular/body fluid load.

NURSING DIAGNOSIS:	**Fluid volume deficit, potential.**
SUPPORTING DATA:	**Diuretics are often used in CHF with side effects of excessive fluid and electrolyte depletion.**
DESIRED PATIENT OUTCOMES:	**Serum electrolytes maintained within normal limits.**

INTERVENTIONS

RATIONALE

Monitor diuretics. Inform patient of anticipated increase in urine output with diuretic use and the importance of observing for signs and symptoms of dehydration.

Decreased renal reabsorption of sodium results in water loss, which decreases vascular load.

Monitor serum electrolyte levels. Observe for signs and symptoms of low-serum potassium.

Potassium, sodium, chloride, calcium, hydrogen may be lost in excess with diuretics. Low-serum potassium may lead to digitalis toxicity, arrhythmias.

Refer to Care Plan: Fluid and Electrolyte Imbalances.

MEDICAL MANAGEMENT

Potassium supplements.

Replacement therapy may be necessary.

NURSING DIAGNOSIS:	**Skin integrity, impairment of, potential.**
SUPPORTING DATA:	**Required bedrest with decreased tissue perfusion and edema predispose to skin breakdown.**
DESIRED PATIENT OUTCOMES:	**Absence of reddened/ulcerated skin areas.**

INTERVENTIONS

Observe for reddened, excoriated areas.

Use eggcrate mattress pad, sheepskin, alternating pressure mattress, frequent massage, skin care, and position changes. Change linens when damp.

If redness, excoriations occur, initiate decubitus care.

RATIONALE

Allows for early treatment.

Edematous tissue is particularly vulnerable to trauma and pressure, which lead to necrosis. Moisture increases masceration and supports bacterial growth.

(Refer to Care Plan: Long-Term Care, Nursing Diagnosis: Skin integrity.)

NURSING DIAGNOSIS:	**Knowledge deficit, disease/treatment.**
SUPPORTING DATA:	**Misunderstandings of interrelatedness of cardiac function/disease/ stress, influence of risk factors, and necessary lifestyle modifications may lead to further episodes if not corrected.**
DESIRED PATIENT OUTCOMES:	**Verbalizes signs/symptoms of decompensation that require immediate intervention. Identifies stress factors and some techniques for handling. Identifies relationship of treatment regimen to recurring episodes/complications.**

INTERVENTIONS

Encourage patient/significant others to verbalize concerns, ask questions.

Discuss normal heart function.

RATIONALE

Information and sharing of fears can decrease anxiety.

Helpful in understanding of the disease process.

Discuss disease process, treatment regimen and need for followup care.	Knowledge of disease and expectations can facilitate adherence to prescribed regimen and prevent development of complications. Monitor response to therapy.
Discuss medications, purpose and side effects.	Prompt reporting of side effects can prevent occurrence of drug-related complications.
Discuss stress and risk factors that may influence state of compensation.	Identification of stressors and risk factors allows patient to plan for their avoidance or minimize their effects.
Discuss signs/symptoms that must be immediately reported to physician; shortness of breath, increased fatigue, weight gain, edema, cough.	Participation in health monitoring increases patient's responsibility in health maintenance by adherence to regimen.
Discuss sodium limitation, signs/symptoms of decreased/increased levels as part of treatment regimen. Give list of foods high in sodium.	Dietary intake of sodium above 3 grams daily will offset diuretic effect. Most common source of sodium is table salt and obviously salty foods.

Refer to Care Plan: Myocardial Infarction, Nursing Diagnosis: Knowledge deficit.

DIAGNOSIS: Digitalis Toxicity

PATIENT DATA BASE

NURSING HISTORY

History of therapeutic use of a digitalis preparation.

Awareness of type of preparation used and method of administration. Toxicity occurs more frequently when given parenterally and also when a long-acting preparation, such as digitoxin, is given orally.

Age is a factor in therapy; elderly patients are more sensitive to digitalis preparations than are younger patients due to the decrease in metabolic function that occurs with the aging process.

Analysis of medical diagnoses existing in conjunction with congestive heart failure or the reason for digitalis therapy. Hypoxia, associated with acute myocardial infarction of chronic/acute pulmonary disease, is known to aggravate digitalis intoxication as are the disease states, such as myxedema, hyperaldosteronism, and diabetic acidosis.

History of recent illness involving vomiting and/or diarrhea; both conditions are capable of altering serum digitalis levels.

Quinidine used in conjunction with digitalis preparations is known to cause an elevation of serum digitalis levels. Diuretic and corticosteroid therapy can alter serum electrolyte levels leading to conditions that aggravate digitalis toxicity.

DIAGNOSTIC STUDIES

Determination of serum digoxin/digitoxin levels, according to therapeutic regimen and preparation ordered.

Elevation of serum electrolyte status because the conditions of hypokalemia, hypomagnesmia, hypercalcemia, and hyponatremia are known to aggravate digitalis toxicity.

ECG: to display variety of arrhythmias associated with digitalis intoxication as listed in the nursing history.

PHYSICAL EXAMINATION

Auscultation for change in rhythm that might be indicative of frequent premature beats, bigeminy, the group beating of Wenckebach, tachyarrhythmias (both regular and irregular); a regular slow rhythm auscultated in the person who has previously been in atrial fibrillation might indicate atrial fibrillation with complete heart block.

Determine renal status: chronic condition versus acute azotemia because digitalis is excreted via the kidneys.

Manifestations of digitalis toxicity:

Common	Uncommon
Gastrointestinal: Anorexia, nausea, vomiting.	Abdominal pain, constipation, diarrhea, hemorrhage.
Cardiac; Worsening of CHF, ventricular premature contractions, atrial tachycardia with A-V block, non-paroxysmal A-V junctional tachycardia, varying degrees of A-V block (commonly Wenckebach phenomenon), sinus bradycardia and ventricular tachycardia.	Atrial fibrillation/flutter, ventricular fibrillation, sinus arrest, sinoatrial block, atrial premature contractions, junctional premature contractions.

Visual:
Color vision (green or yellow) with halos.

Blurring or shimmering vision, scotoma, micropsia or macropsia, amblyopia.

Neurologic:
Fatigue, headache, insomnia, malaise, confusion, vertigo, depression.

Neuralgia, convulsions, paresthesia, delirium, psychosis.

Nonspecific:

Allergic reaction, idiosyncrasy, thrombocytopenia, gynecomastia.

NURSING PRIORITIES

1. Document current digitalis therapy and patient usage upon admission and communicate to physician.
2. Monitor for arrhythmias/complications.
3. Educate patient, re: drug usage and signs/symptoms of developing toxicity.

NURSING DIAGNOSIS:	**Tissue perfusion, alteration in.**
SUPPORTING DATA:	**Certain disease states alter metabolism of digitalis preparations, which leads to elevated serum/tissue levels and digitalis toxicity. Electrolyte abnormalities intensify digitalis toxicity. The variety of arrhythmias associated with digitalis toxicity may lead to a decrease in cardiac output.**
DESIRED PATIENT OUTCOMES:	**Reduction in serum/tissue levels of digitalis to the therapeutic range and absence of induced arrhythmias.**

INTERVENTIONS

Monitor digitalis levels until within a therapeutic range.

Continuous ECG monitoring.

Assess hemodynamic parameters periodically.

RATIONALE

Withdrawal rather than reduction of the dosage is preferable because the therapeutic range is extremely individual; based on concurrent disease states, metabolic imbalances, and organ functions.

Provides early detection of arrhythmias. Several life-threatening arrhythmias are known to be associated with digitalis intoxication.

Bradyarrhythmias, tachyarrhythmias, and irregular rhythms may decrease perfusion and promote hypoxia, which worsens toxicity.

Evaluate status of congestive heart failure. (Refer to Care Plan: Congestive Heart Failure.)

Minimize physical and emotional stressors.

Promote rest through relaxation, and quiet environment.

Monitor serum potassium levels.

MEDICAL MANAGEMENT

IV line, rate at TKO.

Potassium, orally or slow IV infusion.

Dilantin, IV and oral maintenance. Give prophylactically prior to direct current shock.

Pronestyl (procainamide hydrochloride) and quinidine.

Xylocaine (lidocaine).

Magnesium sulfate, slow IV.

Direct current shock.

Artificial pacemaker.

Fab fragments.

Sedatives and hypnotics.

Toxicity has been found to be responsible for deterioration of preexisting congestive heart failure and/or the development of heart failure during digitalization.

Physical activity increases the oxygen demand in tissues and vital organs, which may lead to hypoxemia in the borderline congestive heart failure patient.

Emotional excitement stimulates the sympathetic nervous system producing cardiovascular effects.

Diuretics may be used for treatment of CHF.

Immediate IV access may be required for the treatment of life-threatening arrhythmias and resuscitation.

Potassium replacement may be useful when arrhythmia is related to depletion. Contraindicated in digitalis-induced A-V blocks without atrial tacharrhythmias unless the serum potassium is proved to be very low.

Effective agent in the treatment of digitalis-induced tachyarrhythmias, especially those ventricular in origin and is capable of preventing those arrhythmias induced by cardioversion.

May be effective in abolishing supraventricular and ventricular tachyarrhythmias induced by digitalis.

Raises the diastolic threshold of the ventricles to stimulation and may be preferred over Pronestyl for IV therapy because its effects are shorter and toxic effects can be minimized.

Has been demonstrated that hypomagnesemia predisposes to digitalis intoxication.

Not preferential treatment because it may induce more serious arrhythmias, such as ventricular tachycardia or fibrillation. If used, it is preferable to discontinue digitalis therapy prior to treatment. Discontinuation of short-acting preparations should precede the cardioversion by 24 to 48 hours.

Temporary ventricular pacing may be effective for increasing the rate component of cardiac output. (Pacing may prove dangerous because small electric stimuli may precipitate ventricular arrhythmias when digitalis intoxication is present.

Antidote for severe toxicity that is not controlled by reducing or withdrawing the medication.

May be necessary for rest.

NURSING DIAGNOSIS:	Comfort, alteration in.
SUPPORTING DATA:	Altered drug serum levels may be associated with uncomfortable or disconcerting side effects.
DESIRED PATIENT OUTCOMES:	Minimize discomforts related to toxic effects of digitalis toxicity.

INTERVENTIONS	RATIONALE
Provide darkened environment, place items close by, provide for safety and assistance when out of bed.	Visual disturbances may be present and place the patient in a very dependent, potentially anxiety-producing situation.

MEDICAL MANAGEMENT

Antiemetics.	Nausea and vomiting are considered to be central rather than gastric in origin.
IV therapy.	For dehydration.

NURSING DIAGNOSIS:	Knowledge deficit, disease process.
SUPPORTING DATA:	Lack of knowledge of disease and therapy/side effects may lead to failure to follow the prescribed regimen.
DESIRED PATIENT OUTCOMES:	Verbalize digitalis therapy instructions and signs/symptoms of digitalis intoxication.

INTERVENTIONS	RATIONALE
Discuss type of digitalis preparation and dosage.	Allows patient to assimilate and understand the information.
Provide essential information for the patient in writing as well as verbally.	Available for referral and minimizes personal interpretation and misinterpretation.
Discuss and devise a plan for taking medications.	Organization of prescription therapies may promote better adherence to the regimen and minimize duplication or deletion of pills.

DIAGNOSIS: Angina Pectoris

PATIENT DATA BASE

NURSING HISTORY

Sudden development of constricting/crushing, anterior/precordial/substernal chest pain that may radiate to other areas (arms, neck, jaw, back, epigastrium). Pain is usually related to physical exertion or great emotion, such as anger or sexual arousal. A poorer prognosis usually exists if pain occurs at rest or awakens patient from sleep. Pain may be associated with nausea, diaphoresis, dyspnea.

Description of pain as a new or on-going symptom, duration, precipitating cause, and relief mechanisms to help differentiate from other diseases that may produce chest pain.

Occupation: note physical stress and possible psychologic stresses.

Hobbies: indicate lifestyle, tension relieving/reducing activities.

Evaluate coronary risk factors: diabetes in patient/relative, high-serum cholesterol/triglyceride level, activity versus sedentary lifestyle, tobacco use, dietary intake of fats/sugars/caffeine/liquor/salt, history of hypertension, previous cardiac problems, such as myocardial infarction, congestive heart failure, valvular disease, and so forth. Weight compared with ideal weight.

Current medications: drug tolerance and treatment of concurrent disease conditions.

History of gastrointestinal problems, frequent indigestion, history of other disease that may cause epigastric discomfort or chest pain.

Family history of coronary artery disease or other vascular disease.

DIAGNOSTIC STUDIES

ECG: usually normal at rest: may show sagging S-T segment and flattened or inverted T wave during anginal attack or elicited by treadmill, and signifies ischemia. Arrhythmias may also be noted.

CBC, thyroid studies to rule out hyper/hypothyroidism and anemia as cause of angina, presence of infection that could involve cardiac valves and cause angina.

Cardiac isoenzymes are usually not elevated with angina.

Chest x-ray may show enlarged heart shadow indicating decompensation, left ventricular hypertrophy.

Echocardiogram shows valve excursion and size of chambers; abnormal valvular action may cause angina.

Serum cholesterol level: coronary artery disease (CAD) risk factor.

Myocardial scan to illustrate ischemic areas with exertion.

Left ventriculography to assess myocardial contractility and ejection fraction.

Cardiac catheterization, if indicated, to show coronary artery patency or demonstrate precise areas of occlusion; confirms valve competency.

PHYSICAL EXAMINATION

Investigate sleep patterns, type of personality ("A" or "B"), presence of anxiety.

Evaluate overall cardiac status: height, weight, fatigue, skin color and temperature, quality of respirations, activity tolerance, peripheral pulses, presence of edema, heart sounds, PMI, heart rhythm, blood pressure, body temperature.

Assess to rule out noncardiac causes of angina, such as esophagitis, costochondritis, gallbladder disease, ulcers, muscle strains, and so forth.

NURSING PRIORITIES

1. Relieve pain.
2. Assist patient in lifestyle modifications.
3. Provide information about disease/treatment/prevention.
4. Prepare for surgical intervention, if indicated.

NURSING DIAGNOSIS:	Comfort, alteration in, pain.
SUPPORTING DATA:	Myocardial ischemia produces severe pain. Atherosclerosis and spasms of coronary arteries reduce and/or temporarily stop blood flow to myocardium.
DESIRED PATIENT OUTCOMES:	Verbalizes relief of pain and tolerates increased activity without pain occurrence.

INTERVENTIONS	RATIONALE
Decrease physical activity during angina attack. Keep supine or in semi-Fowler's position.	Decreases demand on ischemic heart, thus alleviating pain.
Maintain quiet, comfortable environment. Avoid visitors who upset patient.	Mental/emotional stress may trigger sympathetic nervous system and increase myocardial workload.
Check vital signs immediately after giving pain medications and every 5 minutes for 20 minutes, or more frequently if unstable.	Hypotension may occur.
Monitor vital signs, CVP, heart sounds every two hours and note significant variations. (Refer to Care Plans: Congestive Heart Failure; Myocardial Infarction; Arrhythmias.)	Related conditions may be cause of or occur with chest pain.
Assess for occurrence of pain with verbal/ nonverbal cues (e.g., diaphoresis, restlessness).	Evaluate for progression to unstable angina.
Maintain patent IV line.	Keeps open route for administration of emergency drugs.
Provide for small, frequent, low- fat/salt meals.	Decreases demand for blood to digestive areas. Low-salt diet decreases retention of extracellular fluid, which could increase myocardial workload. Low-fat diet decreases serum cholesterol level.
Assist patient to identify pain precipitating events and discuss changes that may be necessary in daily activities.	Prevent angina attacks that may progress to myocardial damage.

MEDICAL MANAGEMENT

Vasodilators.

Nitrites and other specific drugs may decrease pain by increasing flow to myocardium by dilating coronary arteries and reducing preload/afterload, which decreases cardiac workload.

Aspirin/mild analagesics.

Cerebral vessels also dilate and may initiate headache.

Tranquilizers, antilipemics, barbiturates, beta blockers, antiarrhythmics, antihypertensives, diuretics, and so forth.

May be given to decrease myocardial workload.

Narcotics.

May be required if pain is unrelieved.

NURSING DIAGNOSIS: **Knowledge deficit, disease/treatment.**

SUPPORTING DATA: **Angina is symptomatic of progressive coronary artery disease.**

DESIRED PATIENT OUTCOMES: **Patient correlates symptoms with causative factors, makes necessary lifestyle changes, and cooperates with medical regimen.**

INTERVENTIONS

Discuss understanding of underlying disease process and purpose of treatment regimen.

Discuss symptoms that may occur due to disease and when to consult physician.

Discuss medication, actions/side effects and prophylactic use. Stress importance of checking with physician before using over-the-counter medications.

Discuss vasoconstricting effects of smoking.

Discuss dietary restrictions and provide sample menus.

RATIONALE

Anxiety increases myocardial workload through release of catecholamines. Knowledge can be helpful in decreasing anxiety and facilitating cooperation.

Knowledge of expectations can reduce concern for insignificant reasons. Changes may indicate need for alteration in treatment.

Various prescribed medications may be used to prevent angina. Dosage may need to be regulated if side effects occur/persist. The effect of these drugs may be potentiated or negated by OTC drugs.

Heart workload is increased when pumping against smaller vessel lumens and may produce myocardial ischemia. Increased levels of carbon monoxide from inhaled smoke decreases oxygen-carrying capacity of blood and may increase ischemia of myocardium causing angina.

Reduced body weight decreases cardiac workload. Decreased salt restricts amount of water held by body, which may expand vascular weight and increase myocardial workload.

Teach how to take pulse and what the acceptable limits are; discuss modification of activities.

Allows patient to identify how drugs and activities influence heart rate and may cause cardiac stress.

NURSING DIAGNOSIS:	**Coping, ineffective, individual.**
SUPPORTING DATA:	**Association of diagnosis with death. Loss of healthy body image and possible loss of place and influence in family structure.**
DESIRED PATIENT OUTCOMES:	**Discusses with staff/significant others impact of illness on self/lifestyle. Demonstrates effective coping behaviors.**

INTERVENTIONS

Observe signs of anxiety. Encourage communication with staff/significant others.

Allow expression of feelings of denial, depression, and anger and assure patient that these are normal reactions.

When appropriate, confront patient behaviors and assist in dealing with change in concept of body image.

Assess impact of illness of sexual needs and provide information, privacy, or consultation, as indicated.

Stress importance of followup care.

Refer to Care Plan: Psychosocial Aspects of Care in the Acute Setting.

RATIONALE

May be uncertain of how this diagnosis will affect the future and sharing worries/doubts can reduce tension and elicit support.

Recognizing and experiencing these feelings will enable patient to begin to deal with situation.

Reality checking allows for feelings of acceptance and establishing more adaptive behaviors. When patient is experiencing denial, confrontation may not be helpful and may result in suicidal gestures.

Patient may be afraid to have sexual intercourse because of fear of death and may see self as less masculine/feminine.

Provides ongoing assessment of disease progression and adequacy of treatment regimen.

DIAGNOSIS: Myocardial Infarction

PATIENT DATA BASE

NURSING HISTORY

Sudden but not instantaneous development of constricting/crushing, anterior/precordial/substernal chest pain, that may radiate to arms, face, jaw, neck, back, or epigastrium.

Pain may be associated with arrhythmias, hypotension, shock, nausea, vomiting, or cardiac failure, but does not change with exertion, position, or respirations.

Rarely painless, but may masquerade as acute congestive heart failure, syncopal episode, cerebral thrombosis, or unexplained shock, indigestion, or gall bladder attack.

Patient may display fever, shortness of breath, pallor, diaphoresis, symptoms of paroxysmal nocturnal dyspnea. May sleep on more than one pillow to avoid shortness of breath.

Description of conditions precipitating or aggravating pain help differentiate it from other conditions that may also cause chest pain.

Occupation may give insight into emotional stress level and physical exertion.

Note hobbies and tension-relieving activities.

Determine intake of saturated fats, sugar, caffeine, and liquor.

Elimination pattern may suggest fluid retention secondary to congestive heart failure.

Determine tobacco use; mode, how much, how long used.

Note communications suggesting pain: verbal, posture, nervousness, anxiety, restlessness.

Note past history of hypertension, angina, myocardial infarction, congestive heart failure, arrhythmias, cardiac surgery, and diabetes mellitus, which increase risk of myocardial infarction.

Determine current medications; note tolerance, dependence, illicit use, allergies, and treatment of concurrent illnesses.

Note history of insomnia, anxiousness, restlessness, "chronic worrier," and personality traits identified with Type "A."

Note family history of heart disease, hypertension, stroke, diabetes mellitus, peripheral vascular disease.

DIAGNOSTIC STUDIES

WBC: leukocytosis (10–20,000) usually appears on the second day post MI due to inflammation.

Sedimentation rate rises on second to third post MI day indicating inflammation.

Cardiac isoenzymes show typical damage pattern. Isoenzymes used to distinguish cardiac damage from other muscle damage.

BUN, creatinine clearance may indicate decreased glomerular filtration due to decreased cardiac output.

Arterial blood gases indicate tissue oxygenation or hypoxia.

Electrolyte battery to demonstrate abnormalities that may compromise contractility.

Serum cholesterol level, past and present elevation, triglyceride elevation increase risk of arteriosclerosis.

Blood cultures to rule out septicemia, which may involve cardiac tissue.

Drug levels for presence of toxic levels.

Electrocardiogram shows abnormal S-T wave elevation signifying ischemia, depressed or inverted T wave indicating injury and presence of abnormal Q waves signifying necrosis.

Chest x-ray may show an enlarged cardiac shadow suggesting dilatation secondary to congestive heart failure.

Myocardial imaging with radioactive isotopes illustrate ischemic or nonperfused areas.

Echocardiogram identifies abnormal cardiac structures and function.

PHYSICAL EXAMINATION

Note height, weight, lethargy, skin color, edema, temperature.

Determine quality of respirations, presence of rales or rhonchi.

Check activity tolerance, heart sounds, murmurs, friction rub, arrhythmias, PMI, blood pressure, jugular distention, hepatojugular reflux, clubbing of fingers, decreased mentation.

NURSING PRIORITIES

1. Relieve pain.
2. Reduce/correct factors contributing to coronary insufficiency, thus maintaining satisfactory cardiac output and tissue perfusion.
3. Prevent/detect and assist in treatment of life-threatening arrhythmias or complications.
4. Provide psychologic support.

NURSING DIAGNOSIS:	**Comfort, alteration in, pain.**
SUPPORTING DATA:	**Myocardial hypoxia may produce severe pain. Decreased pulmonary circulation because of low cardiac output leads to tissue hypoxia and dyspnea.**
DESIRED PATIENT OUTCOMES:	**Patient is relieved of pain and associated symptoms.**

INTERVENTIONS	RATIONALE
Monitor and document pain characteristics, shortness of breath, diaphoresis, restlessness as well as associated symptoms or factors.	Symptoms may help rule out other causes of chest pain. Recurrence of pain may indicate extension of infarct. If symptoms occur 1–3 weeks to 2–3 months after infarct, may indicate Dressler's syndrome.
Instruct patient to report pain to staff immediately.	Can assess and medicate quickly.
Administer drug before onset of extreme pain.	Pain may induce shock by stimulating sympathetic nervous system and increasing myocardial workload.
Check vital signs before and after drug administration and note response.	Narcotics are respiratory depressants.

Evaluate level of consciousness and note sensorium changes.

May be side effect of drug or decreased cerebral perfusion. Morphine is a vasodilator and may cause venous pooling and decreased cardiac output. Restlessness is often related to cerebral ischemia and increases metabolic demands on the heart.

Provide quiet environment and calm activity.

Can reassure patient and decrease anxiety, which may increase cardiac strain.

Give range-of-motion exercises to arms, especially left arm, after acute phase has passed, usually one week. Note tenderness or swelling.

Stiffness may occur and is usually treated symptomatically.

MEDICAL MANAGEMENT

Analgesics p.r.n., give IV in initial phase or if signs of shock are present.

Morphine is the drug of choice as it causes peripheral vasodilation and decreases myocardial workload. Intramuscular injections will not be well absorbed in underperfused tissue and will contribute to overdosage when blood pressure returns to normal and may also elevate enzyme levels.

Humidified oxygen continuously for the first one to two days with meals, for 30 minutes after meals and p.r.n.

When short of breath or has chest discomfort or pressure. May keep ischemic area from converting to infarcted tissue. Eating increases oxygen needs.

Streptokinase/urokinase via direct cardiac infusion.

May be given to help dissolve clot. Must be given within first few hours after infarct and is titrated directly into coronary artery per catheterization. May have limited use because of severe complications; newer techniques are currently being developed/tested.

NURSING DIAGNOSIS:	Tissue perfusion, alteration in.
SUPPORTING DATA:	Ischemia and damage result in decreased stroke volume and myocardial contraction. Arrhythmias decrease cardiac output. Circulation time increases because of decreased blood pressure and cardiac output. Emotional stress increases myocardial workload.
DESIRED PATIENT OUTCOMES:	Arrhythmias are controlled. Monitor shows normal or acceptable conduction pattern. Blood pressure and heart rate are maintained within normal range. Urinary output is adequate and signs of cardiac decompensation are absent.

45

INTERVENTIONS	RATIONALE
Monitor ECG continuously. Take 12 lead ECG daily × 3.	MCL1 and MCL6 are preferred leads and provide information about origination of arrhythmias. Greatest risk of death is arrhythmias. Serial ECGs note evolving pattern of damage and necrosis.
Record rhythm variations, take strips every 4 hours.	May decrease cardiac output and myocardial ischemia leading to myocardial irritability and ectopy.
Evaluate pulse every hour and as needed.	Pulse deficit may serve as rough parameter for detecting ectopy, as ectopics are frequently not peripherally conducted due to decreased stroke volume.
Evaluate for hypotension every hour and/or p.r.n.	Systolic blood pressure of 80mm or drop in systolic pressure 20mm below baseline pressure may indicate extensive myocardial damage and need for treatment of cardiogenic shock. Early recognition may prevent complications.
Evaluate heart sounds every hour.	Appearance of S3 and/or S4 indicate presence of congestive heart failure. Loss of definitive S1 and S2 with loud holosystolic murmur at left sternal border may indicate ventricular septal rupture. Friction rub may indicate pericardial effusion. Murmurs may indicate valve incompetence due to damage of supporting structures. (Refer to Care Plan: Valvular Heart Disease.)
Maintain fluid intake at 2000ml/24 hours to avoid over/under hydration.	Meets normal body fluid needs. May vary if dehydrated or overhydrated.
Maintain patent IV line at TKO rate.	Ready route for emergency drugs; fluid needs if unable to take orally.
Maintain bed rest, semi-Fowler's position.	Decreases energy expenditure, oxygen requirements, and myocardial workload and lowers venous return. Facilitates downward pull on diaphragm promoting better ventilation.
Avoid straining at stool.	Activities that require holding the breath and bearing down produce a valsalva maneuver leading to bradycardia, which temporarily decreases cardiac output. May cause rebound tachycardia and elevated blood pressure and result in cardiac arrest or cerebral infarct.
Avoid large meals, food in temperature extremes, rectal stimulation.	Increased myocardial workload may cause vagal stimulation causing bradycardia and ectopic escapes.
Provide bedside commode as alternative to bedpan.	Bedpan may be exhausting for the patient and commode uses less energy.
Limit visitors as indicated.	Some may engender feelings of stress, increasing myocardial workload.

Explain pattern of gradual activity return; up in chair when there is no pain and no exertion for one hour after meals. Take vital signs before and after activity; ECG strip.

Progressive activity increases demand on heart increasing strength and preventing overexertion. Digestion increases demand on heart.

Refer to Care Plan: Arrhythmias.

MEDICAL MANAGEMENT

Lidocaine/other antiarrhymics.

May be given prophylactically and as ordered for over 6 PVCs/minute, multifocal or coupled PVCs. PVCs demonstrate myocardial irritability, which may progress to life-threatening arrhythmias.

Digitalis.

For tachycardias and to increase cardiac contractility.

Pacemaker.

May be needed to maintain adequate rate.

Swan-Ganz catheter or arterial line.

To monitor blood pressure, PAP, PAWP, arterial blood gases.

NURSING DIAGNOSIS: **Fluid volume, alteration in, excess, potential.**

SUPPORTING DATA: **Heart decompensation may result from acute myocardial infarction. Maintenance of elevated stress level may contribute to decompensation.**

DESIRED PATIENT OUTCOMES: **Absence of cardiac decompensation and associated symptoms.**

INTERVENTIONS

Monitor for symptoms of fluid overload; abnormal CVP, PWP, edema. Weigh daily.

Monitor urine output; report if under 30ml/hour or if output is significantly less than intake.

Offer fluids, foods only as tolerated.

Encourage low-salt diet, avoidance of caffeine, alcohol.

Refer to Care Plan: Congestive Heart Failure.

RATIONALE

Edema and rapid weight gain are classic symptoms of cardiac decompensation and are helpful in documentation.

Decreased cardiac output with decreased kidney perfusion result in sodium and water retention with decreased urine output.

To decrease nausea that may be caused by sympathetic stimulation and underperfusion of gastro-intestinal tissues. Vomiting increases demand on heart by producing valsalva effect.

Salt increases fluid retention, which increases cardiac workload. Caffeine and alcohol are cardiac stimulants and may encourage ectopy and myocardial strain.

NURSING DIAGNOSIS:	Self-concept, disturbance in.
SUPPORTING DATA:	Loss of healthy body image because of temporary/permanent inability to perform previous role and resulting fear of rejection and feelings of worthlessness. Increased realization of mortality after coming close to dying.
DESIRED PATIENT OUTCOMES:	Verbalizes relief of anxiety and adaptation to altered body image.

INTERVENTIONS	RATIONALE
Support normalcy of grieving behavior.	Can provide reassurance that feelings are normal response to change in body image and will pass.
Provide privacy for patient and significant others.	Allows needed time for expression of feelings, relief of anxiety, and the establishing of more adaptive behaviors.
Limit number of staff caring for patient.	Increases continuity for the establishment of trust, sharing of thoughts and feelings.
Observe for verbal/nonverbal signs of anxiety and stay with patient. Intervene if patient displays destructive behavior.	Active listening, patient protection demonstrate worth of patient.
Accept but do not reinforce use of denial; avoid confronting the patient.	Denial can be beneficial in decreasing anxiety. Confrontation can increase depression and may increase use of denial or lead to suicidal gestures.
Encourage communication, especially with significant others.	Sharing information can relieve tension of unexpressed worries and doubts and elicits support.
Orient to routines and give information about expected changes.	Predictability and information can act to decrease anxiety.
Give care in calm manner. Coordinate schedules for treatments.	Anxiety is easily communicated and/or accelerated and results in vasoconstriction through stimulation of sympathetic pathways.
Allow for uninterrupted sleep time.	Allows thought organization and enhances available energy.
Encourage independence, self-care, and decision-making during recuperation.	Increased independence from staff promotes self-confidence and prevents feelings of abandonment with transfer/discharge from unit.

NURSING DIAGNOSIS:	Knowledge deficit, disease process.
SUPPORTING DATA:	Lack of knowledge of disease or therapies may lead to anxiety or failure to follow prescribed regimen.

DESIRED PATIENT OUTCOMES: Patient and/or significant others verbalize diet restriction, purpose of drugs and their side effects, necessity for followup care and symptoms that need immediate attention. Patient approaching ideal weight and on anti-smoking program if indicated.

INTERVENTIONS

Assess patient's/significant others' level of knowledge.

Reinforce explanations of disease, purpose of treatments and equipment as necessary.

Provide time for listening to patient's questions and concerns.

Discuss risk factors; weight reduction, discontinuation of use of tobacco, if applicable.

Discuss limitations; rest after meals or with temperature extremes, resumption of activities (including sex), and avoidance of fatigue.

Emphasize importance of contacting physician if chest pain, change in anginal pattern, or other symptoms recur.

RATIONALE

Verbalization identifies misunderstandings and allows for clarification.

Repeating information is helpful for retention and learning.

Establish rapport and clarify concerns.

Information helpful in providing opportunity for patient to assume control over disease progress and may enhance cooperation with medical recommendations.

Gradual increase in activity strengthens heart muscle and increases collateral circulation formation, decreasing myocardial workload during normal activity.

Knowledge of expectations in regard to disease and treatment is helpful to followup care.

DIAGNOSIS: Arrhythmias

PATIENT DATA BASE

NURSING HISTORY

Previous or concurrent conditions that may predispose to arrhythmias: congestive heart failure, myocardial infarction, drug (digitalis) intoxication, drug withdrawal, hypoxic episode, increased sympathetic stimulation, valvular abnormality, presence of infection (endocarditis), pulmonary disease, hypertension, recent weight loss, excessive nervousness, previous bouts of arrhythmias and treatment.

May complain of diaphoresis, fainting, palpitations or "skipped" beats, chest pain, shortness of breath, cool skin, mottling, decreased quality of peripheral pulses, nausea and vomiting, fatigue.

Precipitating factors: foods, especially those containing caffeine; drugs; activities; increased stress.

Occupations/hobbies: level of physical/mental stress, tension-relieving activities; sedentary versus active lifestyle.

Diet: intake of sugars, fats, caffeine, liquor may be cardiovascular risk factors/exogenous cause of arrhythmias.

May complain of nocturia, which may indicate fluid retention due to congestive failure pattern.

Smoking habits: mode, length of time, how much.

Review medical regimen: current use and understanding of medications may demonstrate drug tolerance, abuse.

Family history of cardiac problems, hypertension, stroke, diabetes, which may increase risk or indicate predisposition for atherosclerosis.

DIAGNOSTIC STUDIES

Serial isoenzymes of LDH, CPK to check for myocardial injury.

Twelve-lead ECG daily times three to demonstrate damage/ischemia/strain pattern, conduction aberrancy, axis deviation.

Chest x-ray may show enlarged cardiac shadow due to myocardial strain/failure.

Arterial blood gases to determine presence/level of hypoxia as cause/result of condition.

CBC to demonstrate anemia, active infectious process that may cause myocardial irritability and arrhythmias.

Myocardial imaging to demonstrate ischemic areas that may impede normal conduction/function.

Serum cholesterol level above 280 mg triglyceride level normal or elevated.

Serum catecholamine level: before and after injection of ACTH to check for catecholamine-producing cells.

Drug screen, if indicated. (Particularly cardiac drugs, such as digoxin, Pronestyl, quinidine.)

Thyroid studies: elevated serum thyroid levels may cause myocardial irritability.

Sedimentation rate: demonstrates active inflammatory process.

Electrolytes: elevated/decreased levels of potassium, decreased levels of calcium may cause cardiac irritability.

PHYSICAL EXAMINATION

Overall cardiac status: (Refer to Care Plan: Myocardial Infarction.)

Evidence of paroxysmal nocturnal dyspnea orthopnea, insomnia. (Refer to Care Plan: Congestive Heart Failure.)

Urine output pattern: frequency may indicate infectious process, diabetes.

NURSING PRIORITIES

1. Prevent/treat life-threatening arrhythmias.
2. Assist in identification of cause/precipitating factors.
3. Prevent further episodes/complications.
4. Assist patient/significant others with dealing with potentially life-threatening situation.

NURSING DIAGNOSIS:	**Tissue perfusion, alteration in.**
SUPPORTING DATA:	**Arrhythmias cause erratic cardiac filling and may lead to tissue ischemia/damage.**
DESIRED PATIENT OUTCOMES:	**Arrhythmias are minimized/controlled. Precipitating causes are identified/controlled/eliminated.**

INTERVENTIONS

Monitor pulse rate/rhythm continuously.

Note significant variations in vital signs, skin color, temperature, sensorium, decreased urine output, dyspnea.

Monitor electrolyte levels.

Assess for other possible causes of symptoms: e.g., congestive heart failure, valvular incompetence, myocardial infarction, hypovolemia, and drug toxicity.

Keep environment as quiet and relaxed as possible.

Observe for chest pain.

Determine/document type of arrhythmia and note response to treatment:

RATIONALE

ECG changes may herald arrhythmias necessitating change in treatment.

Indirect indicators of cardiac output and tissue perfusion.

Potassium abnormalities may cause cardiac irritability.

May need additional treatment.

Decreases release of catacholamines that lead to stimulation of the sympathetic nervous system, vasoconstriction and increase myocardial workload.

May indicate decreased myocardial perfusion or increased oxygen need due to arrhythmias.

Progressive and/or life-threatening arrhythmias require immediate intervention.

1. Non–life-threatening: atrial arrhythmias first and second degree heart block, functional arrhythmias, isolated and unifocal premature ventricular contractions occurring less than six per minute.

   Usually requires no immediate treatment.

2. Potentially life-threatening: tachy/bradycardias, progressing heart block.

   Usually require treatment if sustained for any period of time.

3. Life-threatening: ventricular arrhythmias, asystole; initiate resuscitative protocol; contact physician immediately. Initiate CPR. For asystole, administer precordial thump (refer to institution policy).

   Requires immediate interventions to assure cardiac output for perfusion of vital tissues.

MEDICAL MANAGEMENT

Humidified oxygen.

Decreases myocardial irritability caused by hypoxia.

Analgesic/narcotic.

For chest pain.

Sedatives.

Assist relaxation.

Digitalis, Pronestyl, quinidine, Inderal, Norpace, Verapamil.

Antiarrhythmic medications.

Pacemaker, cardioversion, carotid sinus massage.

Used for tachy/bradycardias, progressive heart block.

Lidocaine, Pronestyl, bolus/drip, bretylium tosylate by continuous drip.

Ventricular tach/flutter/fibrillation.

Epinephrine, calcium, IV.

Help stimulate myocardial contractility.

Defibrillate.

Initiates complete depolarization and encourages sinoatrial node to reestablish normal sinus rhythm.

Dilantin, IV.

May be given when arrhythmia is related to digitalis toxicity.

Potassium replacement.

Deficiency and potentiates digitalis effect. Prolongs or slows conduction.

IV glucose with insulin and/or $NaHCO_3$ (soda bicarbonate).

Emergency therapy to treat cardiac arrhythmias associated with hyperkalemia.

NURSING DIAGNOSIS:	Coping, ineffective, individual.
SUPPORTING DATA:	Former coping methods may not be adequate in life-threatening situations.
DESIRED PATIENT OUTCOMES:	Effective coping strategies are evident.

INTERVENTIONS	RATIONALE
Assess level of anxiety continuously.	May change with sequence of events.
Explain procedures/events.	Information can decrease anxiety and increase sense of control.
Stress positive body responses but do not negate the seriousness of the situation.	Honesty can increase patient trust.
Remain with patient/significant others. Tell them you will be with them and what will be done.	Provides reassurance that they will be taken care of as needed.
Encourage questions and allow verbalization of fears.	Can relieve tension and facilitate appropriate coping behaviors.
After acute phase, give additional information needed about events; cause, if known and potential course.	Help to elicit patient's/significant others' cooperation.
Increase activity slowly (avoiding those producing Valsalva effect) and note response.	Allows heart to adjust to increased demands; monitoring provides prompt recognition of cardiac stress.
During rehabilitative phase, teach patient/significant others to take daily pulse and report irregularities or rate changes. Give information about purposes/side effects of medications.	Increases sense of control and facilitates independence.

DIAGNOSIS: Cardiogenic Shock

PATIENT DATA BASE

NURSING HISTORY

Correlation of this condition with recent occurrence of disease states/conditions most known to be associated with cardiogenic shock: myocardial infarction, massive pulmonary embolism, post open heart surgery, acute cardiac tamponade.

DIAGNOSTIC STUDIES

Correlation of presenting symptomatology with classic clinical presentation of shock: hypotension; tachycadia; decrease in pulse pressure; tachypnea; cool, clammy skin; cyanosis; oliguria; anuria; abnormal temperature (patient is usually hypothermic in most shock situations except septic shock, which is associated with a temperature elevation); irritability; anxiety; mental obtundation.

Classic symptoms of cardiogenic shock versus other types of shock states:

Symptoms:	Cardiogenic	Hypovolemic	Neurogenic	Septic
CVP	Increased	Decreased	Decreased	Decreased
Cardiac output	Decreased	Decreased	Decreased	Increased
PAP/PCWP	Increased	Decreased	Decreased	Decreased
Heart rate (compensatory mechanisms)	Increased	Increased	Decreased	Increased

Hematocrit may be lower than normal depending on the amount of preexisting heart failure due to hemodilution.

Arterial blood gases demonstrate hypoxemia and respiratory alkalosis progressing to metabolic acidosis. The initial hyperventilation causing respiratory alkalosis is a compensatory mechanism for the hypoxemic state and increasing lactic acidemia. As shock progresses, metabolic acidemia/acidosis develops.

Hyperkalemia owing to oliguria and inadequate tissue perfusion.

Serum lactate elevation owing to anaerobic metabolism.

Elevation of BUN and creatinine related to diminished renal perfusion.

Serial cardiac isoenzymes elevation may correspond with acute myocardial infarction.

Drug levels, if any current medications may be involved, such as digitalis.

Chest x-ray: may demonstrate an enlarged cardiac shadow suggesting dilatation secondary to congestive heart failure and/or hypertension. May be normal if neither state previously existed. Acute myocardial infarction may produce pulmonary vascular congestion in the absence of cardiac enlargement.

Cardiac index via thermodilution flow-directed catheter less than 2.2 (normal = 2.5–4 liters/min/m2).

ECG: detection of life-threatening arrhythmias, changes associated with myocardial ischemia, changes associated with ventricular hypertrophy, changes characteristic of calcium and potassium imbalance, changes characteristic of drugs and their toxic effects.

PHYSICAL EXAMINATION

Cool, clammy skin; peripheral edema; cyanosis progressing to mottling of extremities; decreased quality of, irregular/absent peripheral pulses.

Jugular vein distention, hepatojugular reflux and hepatomegaly depending on preexisting CHF.

Tachypnea demonstrating increased work of breathing and presence of adventitious breath sounds.

Tachycardia with presense of S3, S4, or summation gallop, systolic murmur suggestive of papillary muscle or ventricular septal rupture.

Hypotension and abnormalities of pulses (pulsus alternans, paradoxical pulses associated with cardiac tamponade).

Decreased urine output.

Irritability and anxiety progressing to apathy, lethargy, and coma.

NURSING PRIORITIES

1. Maintain adequate oxygenation and tissue perfusion.
2. Reestablish/maintain cardiac function.
3. Provide for patient comfort and reduce anxiety.

NURSING DIAGNOSIS:	Tissue perfusion, alteration in.
SUPPORTING DATA:	Decreased tissue perfusion is associated with a variety of mechanisms related to cardiogenic shock, for example: 1) depressed ventricular function as may occur, post myocardial infarction or in association with hypoxia and acidosis; 2) decreased venous return because of hypovolemia or compensatory peripheral vasocontriction, which causes a redistribution of blood volume.
DESIRED PATIENT OUTCOMES:	Stable hemodynamic parameters with adequate perfusion.

INTERVENTIONS

Assess for signs/symptoms indicative of a decrease in tissue perfusion: color and temperature of skin, such as cool, pale, cyanotic, moist skin.

Monitor arterial blood gases, metabolic acidosis, and blood lactate levels.

RATIONALE

One of the body's first compensatory mechanisms for a sensed decrease in vital organ perfusion is peripheral vasoconstriction. This temporarily satisfies oxygenation and perfusion needs so that blood pressure and cardiac output do not initially decrease, but eventually this compensatory mechanism will fail. Therapeutic intervention may prove more effective when initiated at the first signs of cardiac decompensation.

Anaerobic metabolism owing to decreased tissue perfusion will lead to a rise in lactate levels and progressive metabolic acidosis.

Measure intake and output and evaluate total patient fluid status, including amount of fluid administered with medications, and injectate for cardiac output measurements.

Assess indices of renal function, urine output, BUN, creatinine.

A decrease in urine output is a fairly good indication of decreased renal perfusion that may be due to hypovolemia and/or decreased myocardial contractility.

Decreases in renal perfusion are reflected in deceases in urine output and possible increases in BUN and creatinine. Patients involved with counterpulsation are especially susceptible to decreased renal perfusion because the balloon's position in the descending aorta may physically impede flow to the renal arteries.

Observe for arrhythmias, signs/symptoms of congestive heart failure and its progression, myocardial infarction and/or extension.

Decreased coronary perfusion causes myocardial ischemia, which is a primary cause of arrhythmias, and can eventually cause an extension of the necrotic zone involved with the infarction. Decreased perfusion also decreases contractility that can cause congestive heart failure.

Observe for jugular distention.

As contractility decreases, blood is pumped less effectively from the ventricular chambers. Increased left heart pressure leads to pulmonary congestion and increases pressure in the right side of the heart, which is transmitted through the superior vena cava to the jugular vein where it becomes visible as jugular distention.

Palpate peripheral pulses for evidence of decreased quality and abnormalities (pulsus alternans/paradoxicus).

A peripheral pulse is a direct reflection of the contractility of the myocardium as well as its filling pressures.

Cardiac auscultation to determine heart rate abnormalities and evidence of atrial (S4), ventricular (S3), or summation gallops.

A ventricular gallop or S3 is physiologically related to the rapid ventricular filling phase in early diastole of the noncompliant ventricle. An atrial gallop or S4 is physiologically related to the atrial contraction or atrial kick that occurs at the end of diastole into the noncompliant ventricle. Summation gallop is the combination of S3 and S4 sounds in tachyarrhythmias.

Auscultate for harsh systolic murmurs.

A harsh systolic murmur suggests involvement or possible rupture of a papillary muscle or a ventricular septal defect.

Auscultate breath sounds, observe respiratory pattern, and note increased work of breathing.

Pulmonary congestion is associated with increased hydrostatic forces in the pulmonary vascular system, which can be associated clinically with crackles/wheezes. Tachypnea is most often associated with hypoxemia, indicative of atelectasis, bronchospasm, and pulmonary edema or may function as a compensatory mechanism in acidosis.

Observe for changes in mental status associated with decreased cerebral perfusion.

Cerebral perfusion is directly related to the aortic perfusion pressure. Decreases in perfusion lead to tissue hypoxia and changes in level of consciousness.

Maintain in supine position or with head of bed elevated.

Optimizes venous return, but must be evaluated considering the negative effects this position may have on spontaneous respirations if the patient is not being mechanically ventilated.

Maintain patent intravenous and hemodynamic lines.

Immediate IV access may be required for treatment of life-threatening arrhythmias and hypotension and resuscitation. Maintenance of hemodynamic lines ensures reliability of recorded parameters that guide therapy.

Assess effect of drug therapy and signs of toxicity.

Normal doses of medication may produce toxicity in the patient with decreased circulating volume and diminished renal and/or hepatic function.

Invasive monitoring and ventricular assist:

Monitor/assess hemodynamic parameters: blood pressure, mean arterial pressure, cardiac rate/rhythm/arrhythmias, PAP, mean PAP, PWP, CVP, cardiac output/cardiac index as indicated.

Continual readings are necessary to evaluate patient status and response to therapy. Blood pressure and mean arterial pressure reflect tissue perfusion. PAP and PWP reflect LVEDP, which directly relates to contractility of the heart. High-wedge readings may suggest ventricular failure.

Assess for presence of hypovolemia using flow-directed catheter readings, review of intake and output records, and analysis of daily weight recordings.

Low-circulating blood volume decreases venous return, and ventricular filling, which causes a decrease in LVEDP. (The PWP provides indirect readings of LVEDP.)

Monitor and record effects of fluid challenges on serial hemodynamic readings, changes in blood pressure, the rise in PAP (in particular PAEDP) and PWP, and effect on clinical signs of pulmonary congestion.

Serial hemodynamic readings after the bolus differentiate between ventricular failure and hypovolemia. Small elevations (less than 2mm Hg) in PWP with no change in blood pressure indicates low-fluid volume. Pulmonary congestion is directly related to PWP; increases in congestion indicate progressing ventricular failure.

Periodically assess the inflation/deflation indicators of IABP according to their intended effect on waveform and ECG. Make adjustments with changes in rate/rhythm if heart rate deviates by more than 7–10 beats per minute.

The balloon should deflate immediately prior to ventricular systole, thus decreasing afterload mechanically. The balloon should inflate during distole to promote coronary and cerebral perfusion via elevation of aortic perfusion pressure.

If machine failure occurs, manually inflate the balloon with half the amount of capacity every 2–3 minutes.

Prevents prolonged deflation of the catheter balloon with resultant clot formation and detrimental effects on cardiac output.

Monitor perfusion to cannulated leg; noting presence and quality of pulses, color, and warmth.

Vascular spasm around the catheter or clot formation on the catheter can impede blood flow to the affected extremity.

Restrict movement of the affected extremity. Do not raise head of the bed above 30° and instruct patient not to flex involved leg. (May need to reinforce with light restraints.)

In optimum position, the IABP catheter lies in the descending aorta. Flexion of the involved leg forces the catheter upward, which could either cause an aortic dissection or an intimal hematoma.

MEDICAL MANAGEMENT

Vasodilators, sodium nitroprusside (nitride).	Used to reduce afterload and oxygen consumption when excessive vasoconstriction is present.
Dopamine (dosage dependent) and dobutamine.	In low doses, dopamine promotes dilation of renal and mesenteric arteries. In higher doses, it is used for its inotropic effect to increase contractility and cardiac output, and its vasosconstrictive effects that increase peripheral resistance and blood pressure.
Isuprel, digoxin.	May increase the contractility of the heart, which may raise blood pressure or increase the heart rate.
Fluid challenges.	Will elevate PWP and PAEDP readings when the ventricle is unable to accommodate the extra fluid from venous return and therefore can be used to differentiate between hypovolemia and ventricular failure.
Diuretics (furosemide). Osmotic diuretics (mannitol).	Useful in situations related to sodium and fluid retention to 1) inhibit fluid/electrolyte reabsorption from the tubules, 2) block the effect of ADH or aldosterone, and 3) produce diuresis by hyperosmolarity.
Intraaortic balloon pump (IABP).	May decrease cardiac workload and increase coronary perfusion by diastolic augmentation.
Anticoagulants, low-dose heparin, dextran.	Patients who require counterpulsation are more prone to thrombus formation and thromboemboli related to possible dislodgement of atheromatous material during balloon insertion, turbulence of blood flowing around balloon, and RBC hemolysis with enhanced platelet-fibrin aggregation.
Antiarrhythmics.	Restore optimal rhythm and thereby maximize cardiac function.
Oxygen, high-flow rate, rebreathing mask.	High-flow rate and rebreathing masks are more controlled versions of oxygen low-flow systems.
Mechanical ventilation.	May be required if PO_2 remains low. More control of respiratory parameters and consequently the pulmonary status is possible with mechanical ventilation.

NURSING DIAGNOSIS:	**Comfort, alteration in, pain.**
SUPPORTING DATA:	**Tissue hypoxia due to decreased cardiac output may cause varying degrees of pain and discomfort.**
DESIRED PATIENT OUTCOMES:	**Pain absent/controlled.**

INTERVENTIONS

Assess verbal/nonverbal cues of pain; note location, quality, onset, and duration.

Monitor effect of pain medications on hemodynamic parameters.

Promote restful, quiet environment, planning care to allow maximum rest between activities. Use exercises and touch for relaxation.

Anticipate patient needs.

MEDICAL MANAGEMENT

Sedative/hypnotics.

Analgesics.

RATIONALE

Pain may be related to the hypoxia/hypoxemia state and may be an indilation of coronary insuffiiency (anginal). Abdominal pain may be associated with mesentery hypoxemia due to the hypotensive state. Peripheral pain may indicate thrombus/embolus problems.

Opiates must be particularly monitored for their respiratory depressant and hypotensive effects. Small, frequent doses of medication may be more beneficial to relief of pain while limiting hemodynamic effects.

Decreases the oxygen consumption of the myocardium and tissues. Rest is enhanced when anxiety is minimized.

Dependency on others for simple tasks may be anxiety-producing for the normally independent person.

May be necessary for rest.

Use as indicated when pain is not relieved by other measures.

NURSING DIAGNOSIS:	**Coping, ineffective, individual/ significant others.**
SUPPORTING DATA:	**Awareness of the seriousness of the situation and multiple activities/treatments create anxiety-producing situations in which the patient's/significant others' normal coping mechanisms may not be adequate.**
DESIRED PATIENT OUTCOMES:	**Level of anxiety is reduced, information and emotional support are provided.**

INTERVENTIONS

Assess level of anxiety on an ongoing basis.

Explain procedures in a simple concise manner.

RATIONALE

Treatment activities can create anxiety-producing situations.

Although patient may not appear alert, it is important to provide information that can be helpful in allaying anxiety.

Encourage verbaliztion of fears, concerns, and confrontation with death.

Communication can be helpful in reducing anxiety.

Provide significant others with frequent updates on patient's condition and opportunities to be with the patient.

Multiple therapies make it more difficult for SO to be close and provide emotional support. Frequent brief reports can keep them aware of prognosis and able to meet their own psychologic needs.

Determine need/desire for visit from a religious representative/counselor and make arrangements.

May provide patient/SO with emotional support and an opportunity to verablize in this crisis situation. Mortality associated with cardiogenic shock is considered to be 50–80%.

Refer to Care Plan: Psychosocial Aspects of Care in the Acute Setting.

DIAGNOSIS: Ventricular Aneurysm

PATIENT DATA BASE

NURSING HISTORY

History of myocardial infarction, most often associated with an occlusion of the left anterior descending coronary artery. Progression from infarction to scarring most often occurs within three months.

Recurrent episodes of left ventricular failure with accompanying dyspnea, fatigue, angina, edema, rales, gallop rhythm, and neck vein distention.

Continual problems with recurrent episodes of ventricular tachycardia (VT) and premature ventricular contractions (PVCs).

History of coronary insufficiency.

History of hypertension because there is a correlation between atherosclerosis, coronary heart disease, and hypertension.

Complaints of symptoms associated with decreased cardiac output, for example, syncope, weak extremities, decreased urinary output, decreased quality of peripheral pulses.

DIAGNOSTIC STUDIES

ECG: persistent ST-T segment elevation three weeks or more after the infarction; arrhythmias may be present.

Chest x-ray: normal if aneurysm is small or may cause abnormal contour (bulging) of left cardiac border. Ventricular dilatation when area of akinesis (20–25%) and pulmonary infiltrates when associated with congestive heart failure.

Electrolytes: dependent upon association with congestive heart failure and possible diuretic therapy.

BUN may be elevated indicating deceased renal blood flow.

HCT may be lower than normal due to preexisting heart failure and hemodilution.

Cardiac catheterization: ejection fraction less than normal (55%), increased left ventricular filling pressures, paradoxical movement demonstrated through left ventriculogram (left ventricular angiography) is required for definitive diagnosis and may reveal left ventricular enlargement with an area of dyskinesia (paradoxical movement) and/or akinesia (lack of movement) as well as diminished cardiac function. Noninvasive nuclear cardiology scanning may indicate the site of infarction and suggest the area of aneurysm.

PHYSICAL EXAMINATION

Signs/symptoms directly related to degree of congestive heart failure. Observe especially for hepatojugular reflux, jugular venous distention, visible systolic bulge in apical area.

Abnormal precordial pulsation medial or superior to cardiac apex; no abnormal precordial pulsations may be felt with inferior or posterior aneurysm. Diffuse PMI.

Abnormal heart sounds S3 and S4, presence of crackles and wheezes are directly related to the degree of heart failure.

NURSING PRIORITIES

1. Support medical therapy for adequate oxygenation of tissues and vital organs.
2. Promote hemodynamic and electrophysiologic stability.
3. Assist patient in acquiring knowledge about the disease and required therapy.

NURSING DIAGNOSIS:	Tissue perfusion, alteration in.
SUPPORTING DATA:	Because myocardial function is directly related to the amount of myocardial tissue involved in contraction, an aneurysm decreases the amount of functional tissue available resulting in decreased and/or paradoxical movement and diminished cardiac output. Decreased output decreases aortic perfusion pressure, which can compromise coronary perfusion.
DESIRED PATIENT OUTCOMES:	Cardiac output is sufficient to maintain adequate tissue perfusion. Signs of respiratory failure are absent or decreased.

INTERVENTIONS

Monitor/assess hemodynamic status: blood pressure and mean arterial pressure, cardiac rhythm, rate and presence of arrhythmias, PAP, mean PAP, PWP, CVP, cardiac output/index.

Calculate cardiac output/index injectate into intake and output; observe for signs of congestive heart failure.

Assess for cardiac decompensation:

skin: color, temperature, moistness;

jugular distention, increased work of breathing;

palpation of peripheral pulses for evidence of decreased quality or abnormalities (pulsus alternans, pulsus paradoxicus);

RATIONALE

Continual readings are necessary to evaluate patient status and response to therapy. Blood and mean arterial pressures reflect tissue perfusion. PAP and PWP reflect LVEDP, which directly relates to contractility of the heart. Low-wedge readings may suggest ventricular failure.

Injectate volume may vary according to type of cardiac output machine, but repeated calculations with the standard 10ml of injectate may promote fluid overload in the failing heart.

Vasoconstriction, an initial compensatory mechanism will produce cool skin, possible cyanosis and diaphoresis.

As contractility decreases, blood is pumped less effectively from the ventricular chambers and this produces increased pressures that are transmitted through the pulmonary circuit to the superior vena cava to the jugular vein where it can be visualized as jugular distention.

A direct reflection of the contractility of the myocardium as well as the filling pressures. Paradoxical pulses are associated with cardiac tamponade, pulsus alternans can be associated with a failing left ventricle.

cardiac auscultation to determine presence of atrial (S4), ventricular (S3), or summation gallops;

A ventricular gallop or S3 is directly related to a decrease in ventricular compliance in early diastole. An artial gallop or S4 is directly related to a decrease in ventricular compliance and is related to the atrial contraction that occurs at the end of diastole.

auscultation of increasing crackles/wheezes.

Pulmonary congestion is associated with increased hydrostatic pressures in the pulmonary vascular system.

Continuous ECG monitoring.

Promotes immediate diagnosis and treatment of arrhythmias. (Refer to Care Plan: Arrhythmias.)

MEDICAL MANAGEMENT

Vasodilator therapy; nitroprusside.

Vasodilator will decrease the afterload or pressure against which the malfunctioning ventricle must pump. Hypertension is often associated with the occurrence of a ventricular aneurysm because the pathologic origin for both disease states relates directly to atherosclerosis.

Inotropic agents: dopamine.

Increases the contractile ability of the myocardial tissue.

Antiarrhythmics.

Maximize cardiac function.

IABP (Refer to Care Plan: Cardiogenic Shock).

Counterpulsation has proved effective in the care of the ventricular aneurysm patient in crisis by decreasing afterload mechanically, thus allowing an increase in cardiac output.

Surgical excision.

Indications for aneurysmectomy are directly related to size of the aneurysm and its negative effects on cardiac output and its association with ventricular tachycardia, congestive heart failure, or problems with embolization. (Refer to Care Plan: Cardiac Surgery.)

NURSING DIAGNOSIS:	**Knowledge deficit, disease/ complications.**
SUPPORTING DATA:	**Prone to development of congestive heart failure caused by the increased strain on the malfunctioning myocardium and decreased muscle mass for contraction. Atrial flutter/fibrillation may predispose to clot formation.**
DESIRED PATIENT OUTCOMES:	**Symptoms of decompensation or associated complications are absent/treated.**

INTERVENTIONS

Discuss signs/symptoms of cardiac decompensation and how to recognize what is important to report to the physician.

Assist patient in learning the signs/symptoms of arterial emboli, the five "Ps" of diagnosis: pallor, polar, paresthesia, pulselessness, and pain.

Discuss anticoagulant therapy, signs/symptoms of complications, and the importance of followup studies.

RATIONALE

Early detection of and appropriate therapy for congestive heart failure decreases associated complications and enhances recovery.

Knowledge of possible complications and their symptoms will allow the patient to be more aware of the problem and the importance of early recognition.

Affects the clotting cascade to decrease the chances of further clot formation. Minor bleeding can become a major problem when on anticoagulants.

NURSING DIAGNOSIS:	**Comfort, alteration in, pain.**
SUPPORTING DATA:	**Decreased coronary artery perfusion resulting from decreased ejection fraction may cause angina.**
DESIRED PATIENT OUTCOMES:	**Pain is controlled with appropriate therapy for angina.**

INTERVENTIONS

Assess past experience with angina and knowledge of presenting symptoms. Discuss importance of reporting any change to physician.

Refer to Care Plans: Angina Pectoris; Myocardial Infarction.

RATIONALE

Left ventricular dysfunction related to the aneurysmal area in the myocardium decreases coronary perfusion and the patient is more susceptible to angina and occurrence of myocardial infarction.

DIAGNOSIS: Valvular Heart Disease (Aortic Stenosis/Insufficiency; Mitral Stenosis/Insufficiency)

PATIENT DATA BASE

NURSING HISTORY

Previous conditions that may predispose patient to symptomatic valvular disease: such as rheumatic fever, streptococcal infections, or heart disease.

Precipitating or aggravating conditions: physical exertion.

Note activity level: sedentary versus active; exercise: mode, amount; occupation; hobbies; lifestyle, which may be affected by illness.

Diet: caloric intake, fats, sugars, caffeine, and liquor have a relationship to development of cardiovascular disease.

Sleep pattern: nocturnal dyspnea and nocturia have a relationship to congestive heart failure and may interrupt normal rest and sleep patterns.

Current medications: drug tolerance, abuse, medical regimen.

History of heart murmur.

Family history of heart disease, streptococcal infections.

DIAGNOSTIC STUDIES

	Aortic stenosis	*Aortic insufficiency*
ECG:	left ventricular hypertrophy with strain pattern, conduction defects, first degree A-V block, left anterior hemiblock.	normal; may have septal Q wave in V5, V6, and left ventricular hypertrophy.
Arrhythmias:	atrial fibrillation.	present if congestive failure is severe.
X-ray:	cardiomegaly if severe CHF is present. Calcium in area of aortic valve.	left ventricular enlargement; cardiothoracic ratio of greater than 60 percent may be present; dilation of the ascending aorta.
Echocardiogram:	M-mode study will reveal increased echos and restricted movement of aortic valve.	will reveal enlargement of the aortic root, calcification or vegetation on the aortic valve. Leaflets or bicuspid valve configuration.
Cardiac catheterization:	usually not done.	regurgitant contrast media through aortic valve during diastole, evaluated left ventricular end diastolic pressure.

	Mitral stenosis	*Mitral insufficiency*
ECG:	may show notched broad A waves in I, II, III, and AVF and biphasic P wave with a prominent negative component in lead V1 and/or right ventricular hypertrophy.	normal; may show nonspecific S-T segment and T wave abnormalities, left ventricular hypertrophy, P wave abnormalities.

Arrhythmias:
  atrial fibrillation common.

premature atrial contractions, atrial fibrillation.

X-ray:
  enlarged right ventricle and left atrium; signs of pulmonary congestion/edema and increased vasculature.

may be normal, may show dilation of all cardiac chambers beginning with left atrium. May see increased vascularity in upper lung lobe with signs of pulmonary edema, calcification of mitral annulus.

Echocardiogram:
  left atrial enlargement, rigidity and calcification of mitral valve.

left atrial enlargement, left ventricular enlargement, prolapse of mitral valve leaflet.

Cardiac catheterization:
  pressure gradient in diastole between the left atrium and ventricle across mitral valve, decreased valve orifice (1.5 cm), elevated left atrial, pulmonary artery and right ventricular pressures.

regurgitation of contrast media through mitral valve during systole; elevated left atrial, pulmonary artery and wedge pressures. Elevation of "V" waves in pulmonary capillary wedge pressure.

PHYSICAL EXAMINATION

Aortic stenosis
Decreased pulse pressure (30–40mm Hg).

Carotid pulse contour is slow, small amplitude, gradual upstroke.

Apical heave during systole.

Harsh, high-pitched, crescendo-decrescendo systolic murmur heard over 2nd and 3rd intercostal spaces at right sternal border with radiation to neck.

Systolic ejection click.

S2 single, diminished, or absent.

Elevated left atrial and left ventricular end-diastolic pressure.

Aortic insufficiency
Widened pulse pressure. Visible arterial pulsations of neck, bounding with rapid rise and fall.

Forceful, sustained displaced apical impulse.

High-pitched diastolic murmur.

elevated left ventricular end-diastolic pressure.

Mitral stenosis
Apical impulse short and tapping quality.

S1 increased, decrescendo diastolic rumble heard at the apex, opening snap follows S2.

Elevated left atrial, pulmonary artery and right ventricular pressures.

Mitral insufficiency
Large, laterally placed apical impulse.

Apical systolic murmur, holosystolic. S1 diminished, S3 present.

Elevated left atrial, pulmonary artery and pulmonary wedge pressures.

SYMPTOMS

Aortic stenosis
Angina pectoris, syncope (during or immediately after exercise), left ventricular failure with exertional dyspnea, palpitations, fatigue, visual field defects, arrhythmias.

Aortic insufficiency
Dyspnea; excessive sweating; skin warm, flushed, and damp; head bobbing; lightheadedness; chest pain; left ventricular failure.

66

Mitral stenosis

Fatigue, orthopnea, paroxysmal nocturnal dyspnea, dyspnea on exertion, angina, palpitations, arrhythmias, hemoptysis, dry-nocturnal cough, left ventricular failure, systemic emboli.

Mitral insufficiency

Fatigue, dyspnea, palpitations, exercise intolerance, orthopnea, arrhythmias, systemic emboli, infective endocarditis.

NURSING PRIORITIES

1. Maintain optimum cardiac functioning.
2. Relieve/control pain.
3. Control arrhythmias.
4. Educate patient in prevention of complications.

NURSING DIAGNOSIS: **Tissue perfusion, alteration in.**

SUPPORTING DATA: **Valvular diseases may result in the failure of the heart to expell an adequate amount of blood necessary for the metabolic requirements of body organs and tissues. Congestive heart failure is a common complication of valvular disease.**

DESIRED PATIENT OUTCOMES: **Adequate cardiac output and tissue perfusion are maintained. Absence of signs and symptoms of decompensation.**

INTERVENTIONS

Assess presence/absence and equality of peripheral pulses, bilateral as indicated.

Assess lower extremities for color, warmth, texture, edema, and alterations daily and p.r.n.

Ongoing assessment of neurologic status.

Evaluate hemodynamic parameters (PAP, PCWP, CO, CVP), usually every 4 hours.

Measure and record intake and output (include fluids used to calculate cardiac output as part of intake measurement) every hour.

Auscultate heart sound every 4 hours.

RATIONALE

Provides indication of peripheral circulatory status. Diminished pulses suggest arterial insufficiency. Changes may be insidious or rapid.

Provides for differentiation of arterial or venous insufficiency. Vasoconstriction, an initial compensatory mechanism will produce cool, diaphoretic, and cyanotic skin.

Indication of decreased cerebral blood flow.

Indication of vascular tone, myocardial contractility, and fluid balance. Surgical management may be necessary if decreased cardiac output and tissue perfusion persist.

Decreased renal blood flow secondary to low cardiac output may result in lower glomerular filtration rate with fluid retention and vasocontriction.

Adventitious breath sounds may indicate developing congestive heart congestion.

Monitor blood pressure, temperature, respirations, and apical pulse every 4 hours and p.r.n.

Changes in respiratory pattern and heart rate reflect compensatory mechanisms for hypoxemia secondary to decreased cardiac output.

Provide for restful environment. Assist with planned, graduated levels of activity, allowing patient to rest between nursing activities.

Reduces myocardial workload by lessening the tissue demands for oxygen and eliminating factors that stimulate heart action.

Monitor patient continuously for arrhythmias.

Early detection and treatment of non–life-threatening atrial arrhythmias may prevent development of potentially life-threatening arrhythmias.

Document and determine type of arrhythmia present.

Arrhythmias are common in patients with valvular disease. Most common are atrial arrhythmias due to increased atrial pressures and volumes. Conduction abnormalities may occur with aortic valve disease.

MEDICAL MANAGEMENT

Cardiotonics.

Increase force and efficiency of cardiac contractions.

Diuretics.

Reduce blood volume to decrease ventricular volume and pressure.

Humidified oxygen.

Increases available oxygen for myocardial work.

NURSING DIAGNOSIS: **Comfort, alteration in, pain.**

SUPPORTING DATA: **Decreased cardiac output with diminution of coronary blood flow leading to increased cardiac work with accompanying increased myocardial oxygen demand. This results in angina.**

DESIRED PATIENT OUTCOMES: **Angina minimized/controlled.**

INTERVENTIONS

RATIONALE

Observe for verbal/nonverbal expressions of pain and discomfort.

Differentiation of symptoms are necessary to rule out other causes of pain.

Provide restful environment and decrease activities.

Activities that increase myocardial oxygen demands (sudden exertions, stress, heavy meals, cold exposure) may precipitate angina.

MEDICAL MANAGEMENT

Analgesics (morphine).

Induce mental and physical relaxation, relieve pain, and decrease cardiac workload.

Nitrates.

Decrease coronary vascular resistance and may increase coronary blood flow.

68

NURSING DIAGNOSIS:	Knowledge deficit, prevention of bacterial endocarditis.
SUPPORTING DATA:	Endocarditis is caused by the introduction of bacteria (streptococcus) into the blood stream. Preexisting valvular disease predisposes to invasion of valve leaflets with resultant scarring and distortion of valve.
DESIRED PATIENT OUTCOMES:	Verbalizes precautions to be taken to prevent endocarditis.

INTERVENTIONS

Discuss importance of reporting occurrence of signs/symptoms of infection: elevated temperature, malaise and anorexia, chills alternating with diaphoresis.

Discuss importance of consulting with the physician when conditions that predispose to endocarditis occur: dental or gum manipulation, genitourinary procedures, presence of skin boils, childbirth, and so forth.

Discuss maintenance of good oral hygiene program.

Reinforce need for followup care.

Refer to Care Plan: Pancarditis.

RATIONALE

Endocardial pathogens may enter the blood stream via the skin, respiratory, gastrointestinal, or genitourinary tracts. Patients with lowered resistance (congenital/rheumatic heart disease, or recovering from open heart valvular surgery) are most susceptible.

Preventive action can be taken.

Decrease need for dental procedures.

Identify progression of disease; assess patient response to therapy; and allow for early treatment of potential causes of complications.

DIAGNOSIS: Cardiac Surgery (Coronary Artery Bypass Graft; Valve Replacement), Postoperative Care

PATIENT DATA BASE

NURSING HISTORY

Coronary artery disease appears predominantly in persons over age 40; incidence is higher among urbanites; Type A behavioral patterns, harddriving and competitive, with high-stress levels; and appears to have some familial incidence.

Presentation of clinical manifestations of arteriosclerotic heart disease to include a history of angina, myocardial infarction, congestive heart failure, heart block, or gastrointestinal symptoms.

Predisposing factors: Hypertension, sustained blood pressure over 160/95 is a risk factor for the development of coronary artery disease (CAD); obesity, weight over 30 percent above ideal weight; intake of a diet high in saturated fats, sugar, caffeine, liquor, and calories; large amounts of nicotine absorbed into the blood stream, which may severely damage blood elements or the intima of the arteries.

History of cardiopulmonary illnesses: may predispose to postoperative complications, including bacterial endocarditis, pulmonary embolus, pneumonia, and abnormal bleeding.

History of diabetes mellitus, gout, or peripheral vascular disease.

History of congenital/acquired heart disease, rheumatic fever/viral infections; congestive heart failure secondary to valvular incompetence.

DIAGNOSTIC STUDIES

Baseline CBC, UA, ABGs, electrolytes, renal/hepatic function tests, and lipid profile.

ECG: evidence of ischemia, myocardial infarction, or heart block.

Hypercholesterolemia: total blood cholesterol above 250 mg/100 ml.

Baseline pulmonary function studies.

Myocardial scan: illustration of ischemic/nonperfused areas of the heart.

Cardiac catheterization and echocardiogram will demonstrate valvular incompetence.

Coronary arteriography: illustration of degree of occlusion in coronary arteries.

PHYSICAL EXAMINATION

Blood pressure: quality, presence of paradoxical pulse.

Apical pulse: rate, regularity, heart sounds, friction rub, pulse deficit, murmurs. PMI. Perphiral pulses: quality and equality.

Note skin color, temperature, and sensation.

Assess presence and degree of peripheral edema.

Assess respiration: rate, depth, rhythm; chest excursion, symmetry, splinting.

Presence of adventitous breath sounds, friction rub, resonant percussion.

Note level of consciousness; orientation to time, place, and person; pupillary response, size, reaction, equality; movement and sensation of all extremities, quality and equality; response to pain.

NURSING PRIORITIES

1. Promote adequate cardiovascular function, tissue perfusion, and stabilization of vital signs.
2. Maintain adequate ventilatory exchange.
3. Promote fluid/electrolyte balance and renal function.
4. Prevent and detect possible postoperative complications.
5. Assist patient/significant others in dealing with anxiety and promoting psychologic adjustment.

NURSING DIAGNOSIS:	Gas exchange, impaired.
SUPPORTING DATA:	Hypoventilation and atelectasis may result from any of the following: postoperative pain and splinting with difficulty in deep breathing and coughing; mediastinotomy with direct trauma to the chest wall, decreased compliance associated with interstitial edema and fibrosis.
	Ventilation/perfusion abnormalities may result from any of the following: postperfusion syndrome, atelectasis, microemboli, and residual intracardiac shunting.
DESIRED PATIENT OUTCOMES:	Adequate oxygenation and ventilation with arterial blood gases within normal limits. Lungs clear by auscultation and chest radiograph. Aeration equal and adequate bilaterally.

INTERVENTIONS

Refer to Care Plan: Ventilatory Assistance (Mechanical).

Turn every 1–2 hours using each side and semi-Fowler's position.

Suction as needed. Sigh with 100 percent oxygen before and after procedure.

Evaluate respiratory status every hour and p.r.n.:

    Presence of spontaneous respirations, depth of respirations and rate.

RATIONALE

Facilitates drainage of pulmonary secretions. Promotes optimal chest expansion.

Reduces retained secretions that may obstruct the airflow tracts and interfere with ventilation and perfusion.

Indicate recovery from anesthesia. May reflect pain or collection of secretions. Rapid rate may indicate airway obstruction, atelectasis, pain, fear, anoxia, excessive pulmonary secretions, acidosis, or gastric distention. Slow rate may indicate pain, CO_2 retention, or overmedication with narcotics.

Note respiratory effort, chest excursion, presence of dyspnea, intercostal retractions, bulging or use of accessory muscles.

Asymmetrical excursion may indicate pain, atelectasis, or obstruction of chest tubes. Dyspnea or retractions may result from retained secretions, airway obstruction, or acidosis. Bulging occurs with pulmonary air trapping.

Breath sounds:

Note presence of adventitious breath sounds.

Crackles (rales) are secondary to the delayed reopening of previously deflated small airways or alveoli. Wheezes (rhonchi) are due to partial obstruction to air flow in passages narrowed by secretions, mucosal edema, and so forth. Also associated with conditions of broncho-constriction and retained secretions. Pleural friction rubs occur when two inflammed pleural surfaces rub across each other during respiration.

Assess signs of central and peripheral cyanosis: color of nail beds, earlobes, and lips; or general duskiness.

May indicate the presence of hypoxia due to the presence of deoxygenated hemoglobin; may not be observed if anemia is present.

Monitor arterial blood gases.

Reveal the status of ventilation and perfusion.

NURSING DIAGNOSIS: **Breathing pattern, ineffective.**

SUPPORTING DATA: **Pneumo/hemothorax, pleural effusion will interfere with optimal lung expansion to a variable degree.**

DESIRED PATIENT OUTCOMES: **Fully expanded lungs on chest radiograph; clear breath sounds bilaterally. Resonant percussion of lung fields.**

INTERVENTIONS

Observe for decreased chest expansion.

RATIONALE

Air or fluid in the pleural space prevents complete expansion, thereby, decreasing air flow.

Listen for breath sounds.

Absence of air passage may indicate collapse of lung.

Percuss the lung fields for the presence of dullness or hyperresonance.

Hemothorax or pleural effusion will percuss dull over the affected area.

Maintain patency of chest tubes.

Allows for drainage and lung expansion.

MEDICAL MANAGEMENT

Chest radiograph daily.

Pneumo/hemothorax, or pleural effusion will be revealed.

Reposition or reinsert chest tube(s) as necessary.

To facilitate drainage that may be interfering with lung expansion.

NURSING DIAGNOSIS: Injury, potential for, emboli.

SUPPORTING DATA: Thromboemboli to the lungs will interfere with ventilation and perfusion. The radial artery is generally cannulated for arterial pressure readings leaving circulation to that extremity dependent on flow from the ulnar artery. Majority of grafts are from saphenous vein harvesting. Decreased cardiac output may result in formation of thrombi that may embolize. Cerebral emboli will interfere with cerebral blood flow, which results in cerebral hypoxia and edema.

DESIRED PATIENT OUTCOMES: Absence of symptoms indicative of peripheral thromboembolus. Maintenance of preoperative neuromuscular function.

INTERVENTIONS

Wrap aces on operative leg, tighter distally than proximally.

Assess peripheral pulses, especially radial, posterior tibial, and dorsalis pedis every hour and p.r.n.

Check the extremities for the presence and degree of edema and evidence of decreased tissue perfusion.

Encourage passive and active leg exercises.

Encourage early ambulation as tolerated.

Remove invasive lines as soon as possible or change the sites per hospital policy.

Observe for signs of phlebotic insertion sites of lines and sites of thrombus formation in deep leg veins: redness, pain, warmth over an area, increasing claudication, decrease in distal pulse.

RATIONALE

Improper fit constricts venous return.

Absence may indicate the presence of peripheral emboli obstructing blood flow in the extremity and/or inadequate collateral circulation.

Severe edema can hinder peripheral circulation by constricting the vessels. Poor tissue perfusion, if left untreated, will result in cellular destruction.

Muscular contraction aides in venous flow.

By preventing venous stasis and aiding venous return, thrombosis formation in the lower extremities can be decreased.

Any impediment to arterial or venous circulation predisposes to thrombophlebitis.

Thrombus may break away from the intima and embolize to the lungs.

Observe for signs and symptoms of pulmonary embolus: sudden onset of chest pain, cyanosis, respiratory distress, diaphoresis, hypoxia.

May result from thromboembolus related to imperfections in the cardiopulmonary bypass (CPB) machine, gas exchange membrane (release of lipids), fat from the sternotomy, or air.

Assess neurologic status:

Immediately postoperative as a control for further evaluations, then every two hours and p.r.n.: level of consciousness, pupillary response.

Failure to awaken from anesthesia may result from embolization of air, fat, or thromboembolic particles to the brain. Disorientation and restlessness may indicate anoxia or embolization to the brain. Changes denote increased intracranial pressure and may help localize the lesion. Pupils will dilate when blood contains excessive CO_2, or with narcotics.

Movement of extremities, quality and equality.

Orientation.

Hemiplegia or extreme weakness of an extremity may indicate embolization to the cerebellum.

Postpump psychosis may occur, causing disorientation, uncooperativeness, mild euphoria, forgetfulness.

MEDICAL MANAGEMENT

Antithromboembolic hose or Ace bandages to lower extremities.

May help to prevent venous stasis but this has not been proven.

Heparin.

May be necessary to minimize possibility of clot formation.

NURSING DIAGNOSIS: **Tissue perfusion, alteration in.**

SUPPORTING DATA: **Left ventricular failure resulting from intraoperative myocardial ischemia, recent or perioperative infarction or residual cardiac depression effects of anesthesia decreases myocardial contractility and, therefore, decreases cardiac output. Thrombus may form postoperatively and occlude the bypass graft. Hypertension may rupture bypass grafts at the anastomosis.**

DESIRED PATIENT OUTCOMES: **Adequate cardiac output for tissue perfusion. Absence of myocardial ischemia or infarction. Blood pressure within patient's normal limits. Decreased catacholamine release. Free of complications; tamponade, arrhythmias.**

INTERVENTIONS

Monitor blood pressure continuously through the use of arterial cannulation.

Allow for a slow, quiet recovery from anesthesia.

Maintain mean arterial pressure (MAP) between 70 and 90 mm/Hg.

Observe for signs and symptoms of myocardial ischemia or infarction: angina, restlessness, diaphoresis, ECG changes.

Observe for signs of decreased peripheral perfusion: cool, moist skin, decreased pulses peripherally.

Monitor cardiac rhythm continuously.

Maintain patency of chest tubes and milk or strip every 15 minutes for the first 4 hours postoperatively, then every hour until they are removed.

Record the amount and consistency of chest drainage hourly as indicated.

Observe for signs and symptoms of cardiac tamponade: hypotension, tachycardia, increased LAP and PCWP, narrowing pulse pressure, distant heart sounds, abrupt decrease in chest tube drainage, low voltage QRS on ECG, paradoxical pulse.

Monitor pulmonary artery pressure (PAP), pulmonary capillary wedge pressure (PCWP), and left atrial pressure (LAP) frequently as indicated, decreasing as patient stabilizes.

RATIONALE

Hypertension may be related to hypervolemia, delayed action of catacholamines stored in the capillaries during anesthesia, or continuing preoperative hypertension. Constant monitoring is essential to detect fluctuations in blood pressure that can occur suddenly.

The release of catacholamines will be more gradual and control of the blood pressure can be maintained.

Coronary flow is directly dependent upon the perfusion pressure (MAP). Too much elevation of MAP will rupture the graft at the anastomosis. Too low MAP will inadequately perfuse the myocardium.

May occur from CPB or thrombus formation in the bypass graft postoperatively. Severe ischemia will result in cellular necrosis.

Decrease in cardiac output decreases peripheral perfusion as blood is shunted to vital organs.

Depending upon the location of the coronary lesions, blood supply to the conduction system of the heart may have been disrupted, leading to rhythm disturbances. Tachycardias shorten diastole limiting coronary filling time and decreasing cardiac output. This increases cardiac workload and oxygen requirements.

Collection of drainage in the mediastinum increases pressure on the heart preventing it from filling properly and, thus, decreasing cardiac output.

Increasing chest drainage predisposes to cardiac tamponade, hypovolemia, while a sudden decrease may indicate fluid is collecting in the chest.

Without prompt treatment, cardiac arrest rapidly ensues.

Intramyocardial wall tension (preload) is determined by the pressure generated by the contracting muscle to eject the blood. (The greater the pressure, the greater the intramyocardial wall tension, the greater the oxygen consumption.) These pressures also give a direct reflection of left ventricular function, pulmonary hypertension, right and left heart failure.

Observe for signs and symptoms of left ventricular failure: hypotension, tachycardia, increased PCWP, LAP, pulmonary vascular congestion, decreased peripheral perfusion, ECG changes.

Decreases myocardial contractility and decreases cardiac output.

Observe for signs and symptoms of hypervolemia: hypertension, tachycardia, increased PAP, LAP, and CVP, increased urine output if heart function is adequate.

Determining the cause of hypertension will affect the type of treatment required.

Use caution when administering antihypertensive medications in the presence of hypovolemia.

The body tries to compensate for hypovolemia with increased peripheral vascular resistance. Administration of a vasodilator may abruptly lower the blood pressure to critical levels.

Monitor hematocrit and acid-base, hypoxia and electrolyte imbalances.

Low hematocrit decreases the oxygen-carrying capacity of the blood and predisposes to conditions that may decrease cardiac output.

Increased activity or temperature increases tissue oxygen requirements and myocardial workload.

Maintain on bedrest in early postop period. Monitor temperature every two hours.

Obtain daily weights.

Measure of fluid retention. With the use of CPB, the patient will receive approximately 1500ml additional fluid used to prime the pump as well as other sources of fluid that may be retained.

MEDICAL MANAGEMENT

Narcotics, analgesics.

To control pain that causes a sudden release of catacholamines into the blood stream, increasing muscle tension; blood pressure, especially systolic; and oxygen needs.

Antihypertensives.

Blood pressure tends to be quite labile in the early postop period because of intermittent release of catacholamines. Medications will need to be titrated accordingly to avoid drastic fluctuations.

Reduce sodium (Na) intake via IV and oral route.

Causes water retention predisposing to hyper/hypokalemia with metabolic alkalosis and irritable dysrhythmias.

Potassium.

Necessary to replace losses/maintain balance.

Transfusions.

To maintain adequate circulating volume and optimum O_2 carrying capacity.

Antiarrhythmics, catecholamines, digitalis, and diuretics.

Inotropic drugs increase cardiac output and renal blood flow.

Cardioversion.

Convert arrhythmias that compromise cardiac output and coronary blood flow.

Anticoagulants.

Minimize clot formation on prosthetic valves.

$NaHCO_3$.

Treat acidosis judiciously.

Pericardiocentesis.

May be necessary to remove fluid that may accumulate in the pericardium.

| NURSING DIAGNOSIS: | Injury, potential for, hypovolemia/hemorrhage. |

SUPPORTING DATA: Hypovolemia may result from the use of hypothermia during surgery, which produces high-peripheral resistance; with systemic rewarming, peripheral vasodilation occurs that may result in an inadequate circulating blood volume relative to vascular space. Hemorrhage may produce hypovolemia and may result from any one or a combination of the following: inadequate blood replacement, platelet destruction in CPB machine, blood replacement with old blood that is deficient in platelet and clotting factors, inadequate reversal of heparin given during CPB, diffuse intrathoracic oozing, or a missed bleeding vessel.

DESIRED PATIENT OUTCOMES: Normal coagulation profile and hemodynamic parameters within patient's normal limits.

INTERVENTIONS

Monitor hemodynamic parameters every 5–15 minutes for the first 4–6 hours; decrease to every hour as the patient stabilizes.

Rewarm patient gradually.

Monitor hematocrit levels, in the immediate postop period and repeating in approximately 6 hours.

Evaluate dressings every hour and chest drainage every 15 minutes to 1 hour for quantity, rate of drainage, and consistency.

Observe for signs of hemorrhage; chest drainage greater than 5ml/kg/hour, declining hematocrit, signs of hypovolemia.

RATIONALE

Stabilization following surgery usually indicates adequate cardiovascular function.

Too rapid rewarming causes peripheral vasodilation, increasing intravascular compartment, which can result in shock due to inadequate circulating volume.

Initial level used as a control for those drawn later but is an inaccurate measure of blood loss due to hemodilution.

Bright red drainage indicates active bleeding, lighter red drainage from chest tube is caused by dilution of the blood with the irrigation solution used to wash out the chest prior to closing. Clots will indicate adequate clotting factors.

Blood loss of 10 percent circulating volume can create a shock situation.

Observe for signs of coagulopathy: blood oozing from all entry sites, hematuria, bloody sputum, heme-positive nasogastric aspirates and stool.

Affects the entire vascular system with a disruption in the clotting mechanism.

MEDICAL MANAGEMENT

Activated clotting time (ACT).

Immediately postop or when "pump" blood has been completely infused. Evaluate the effectiveness of the protamine given to reverse the heparin used during CPB.

Protamine.

Additional may be needed to reverse anticoagulant effect.

PTT.

May also be used to evaluate the anticoagulation effect of heparin.

Coagulation profile.

To note delayed clotting, decrease in platelets, and the presence of fibrin split products indicating breakdown of existing clots.

Fresh blood (usually RBCs, platelets, or fresh frozen plasma) according to needs assessed by the profile.

Fresh blood contains all factors; used mainly to elevate the hematocrit. Platelets replace only platelets. Plasma contains fibrinogen and prothrombin factors.

IV fluids.

Replace fluid loss, especially before using any vasodilation therapy. Vasodilation in the presence of hypovolemia may result in an inadequate circulating blood volume relative to the vascular space.

Refer to Care Plan: Disseminated Intravascular Coagulation.

NURSING DIAGNOSIS:	**Fluid volume, deficit, potential.**
SUPPORTING DATA:	**Patient will be NPO for 24–30 hours; receive additional fluid (approximately 1500ml) with the use of CPB; metabolic acidosis/alkalosis; potassium shifts; hypokalemia/calcemia/natremia may occur and renal function may be impaired resulting in alterations in fluid and electrolyte balance.**
DESIRED PATIENT OUTCOMES:	**Fluid output is approximately two thirds of intake. Urine output equal to or greater than 30ml/hour. Laboratory studies are within patient's normals.**

INTERVENTIONS

Maintain accurate intake/output to include: IV/oral intake, nasogastric/chest drainage, urine output.

Correlate hemodynamic parameters with peripheral perfusion, urine output, and daily weight to determine adequacy of hydration and cardiac output.

Monitor serum electrolytes and observe for signs of imbalance: hyponatremia, hypo/hyperkalemia, and hypocalcemia.

Monitor BUN, creatinine, and urine electrolytes.

Observe for signs of dehydration: dry mucous membranes/lips, coated tongue, thirst, tachycardia, decreased blood pressure, PAP, PCWP, CVP, and LAP, low urine output, peripheral venous filling above five seconds.

Obtain urine specific gravity as indicated.

Observe for signs of paralytic ileus: abdominal distention, nausea/vomiting, hypoactive bowel sounds.

Start on clear liquids after NG tube is removed, progressing to solid foods as tolerated.

Monitor arterial blood gases and observe for signs of acid-base imbalances: metabolic and respiratory acidosis/alkalosis.

MEDICAL MANAGEMENT

IV fluids with D5W or lactated Ringer's injection.

Restrict parenteral/oral fluid intake to 2000ml/24 hours.

Electrolyte replacements as needed, particularly potassium, given slowly and with low concentrations (20 meq/hour in not less than 100 ml of solution).

RATIONALE

Balance needs to be maintained to prevent hypo/hypervolemia, and renal dysfunction.

Dehydration and hypovolemia will decrease cardiac output.

These imbalances may occur. (Refer to Care Plan: Fluid and Electrolyte Imbalances.)

In the presence of decreasing renal function, urine sodium differentiates between oliguria from dehydration versus acute tubular necrosis. In dehydration, the kidneys absorb almost all sodium from glomerular filtrate leaving no sodium in the urine; in acute tubular necrosis the tubules are unable to reabsorb sodium so that serum and urine sodium may almost be the same.

Represents a deficiency in electrolytes as well as water.

Dark urine with a high specific gravity may indicate hypovolemia or the presence of particulate matter, such as, RBCs; light urine with a low specific gravity may reflect effects of diuretics, hypervolemia, or developing renal failure.

May develop following any major surgery.

Return of bowel activity is necessary before intake is begun.

ABGs and serum electrolytes are tools by which acid-base states can be evaluated. (Refer to Care Plan: Fluid and Electrolyte Imbalances.)

Maintain fluid intake while NPO.

Overload of the circulatory system increases cardiac workload.

Left untreated, imbalances will lead to acid-base disturbances, arrhythmias, shock, convulsions, and death. Rapid replacement may result in arrhythmias and possible cardiac arrest.

2 gm sodium diet.	Restrict sodium intake, which could predispose to water retention.

NURSING DIAGNOSIS:	**Injury, potential for, infection.**
SUPPORTING DATA:	**These patients are prime candidates for infection in light of the multitude of invasive lines and catheters. Inadequate pulmonary hygiene and deficient ambulation contribute to the occurrence of pneumonia postop.**
DESIRED PATIENT OUTCOMES:	**Absence of infection.**

INTERVENTIONS

Maintain aseptic technique when administering IV fluids, medications and when changing IV bottles, and so forth.

Clean incisions daily with Betadine solution.

Check incisions, IV sites, and chest tube sites for signs of localized infection: redness, warmth, tenderness, edema, drainage.

Change the tubing and solutions connected to the invasive lines per hospital policy.

Remove lines and catheters as soon as possible.

Observe for signs and symptoms of sepsis: fever, chills, diaphoresis, altered level of consciousness, positive blood cultures.

Encourage early ambulation and vigorous pulmonary hygiene.

Observe for signs and symptoms of pulmonary infection: fever, changes in color, amount and consistency of sputum, atelectasis.

Observe for signs/symptoms of urinary tract infections: cloudy, foul-smelling urine, dysuria, flank pain, fever.

Observe for signs/symptoms of endocarditis: fever, positive cultures, petechiae of skin and mucous membranes, ECG changes including S-T elevation or depression.

RATIONALE

Prevent nosocomial infections and cross contamination.

A povidone-iodine solution effective against a variety of micro-organisms including Pseudomonas.

The skin itself harbors a variety of micro-organisms.

Many lines are kept patent with solutions containing dextrose, a prime media for bacterial growth.

Limit local irritation, and minimize opportunity for bacterial growth at the entry site.

Coronary bypass patients have a multitude of lines entering the blood stream.

Stagnant secretions are prime media for bacterial growth because of warm, dark, moist environment.

Inability to raise pulmonary secretions postoperatively predisposes to pneumonia.

Will have indwelling urinary catheters for 1–2 days depending upon the patient.

CVP, PAP, and LAP lines lie directly within the heart.

Observe for signs/symptoms of pericarditis: fever, chest pain with inspiration, pericardial friction rub, ECG changes including S-T elevation and T wave abnormalities.

Generally related to direct surgical manipulation.

MEDICAL MANAGEMENT

Antibiotics.

Usually ordered prophylactically.

Culture and sensitivities.

Identify organism.

Chest x-ray.

Visualize infiltrated areas.

NURSING DIAGNOSIS:	**Fear, heart surgery/death.**
SUPPORTING DATA:	**Severe depression frequently occurs in the postop open heart patient. Isolation in the intensive care unit, sensory deprivation/overload, sleep deprivation, fear/anxiety/depersonalization of the patient because of the staff's preoccupation with monitors and equipment may lead to states of confusion, hallucinations, and psychotic behavior.**
DESIRED PATIENT OUTCOMES:	**Anxiety reduced to a manageable level or eliminated. Patient is alert, oriented and depression and psychotic behavior are absent.**

INTERVENTIONS

Include significant others in the preoperative teaching.

Always address the patient by name and introduce yourself by name.

Frequently orient to date and time of day. If possible, place clock where patient can see it; place patient by window.

Schedule the patient's day so that periods of nursing care alternate with periods of rest and relaxation.

Involve the patient in planning for and carrying out care as much as possible.

RATIONALE

May decrease their anxiety associated with the unknown. Reducing the stress can enhance the support they offer to the patient during their visits.

Personalization reduces anxiety, establishes rapport.

Intensive care units are active and well-lighted 24 hours/day, which leads to time disorientation.

Sleep deprivation can easily occur with the intensive care demanded by these patients' conditions.

Will lessen the likelihood of depression and feelings of loss of control.

Extinguish as much unnecessary noise as possible.	Sensory overload encourages auditory and visual hallucinations, prevents restful sleep.
Provide meaningful conversation with the patient while performing the patient's care.	Helps eliminate sensory deprivation, restores personalization.
Explain procedures and events to take place.	To decrease fear and anxiety of unknown.
Provide an effective means of communication while the patient remains intubated.	Vital to the patient that needs and concerns be expressed.

NURSING DIAGNOSIS: **Knowledge deficit, specify.**

SUPPORTING DATA: **Problems necessitating cardiac surgery often are long-standing and progressive in nature. Convalescence and prevention may require continuing treatment as well as changes in lifestyle.**

DESIRED PATIENT OUTCOMES: **Verbalizes treatment regimen and altered lifestyle changes desirable for individual situation.**

INTERVENTIONS

RATIONALE

Instruct in differentiation between angina and postop pain.	Pain due to multiple incisions and wiring of sternum is normal but recurrence of angina may indicate problems with grafts.
Increase activities gradually, within specified limits; follow with short rest periods.	Programmed increase in activity level, within patient's ability, improves muscle tone and stimulates circulation.
Return to work requires physician approval on an individual basis; may start part-time and increase according to tolerance.	Somewhat dependent on type of work and physical activity involved, as well as extent of surgery and overall physical condition.
Driving is restricted until physician approval is given and long rides as a passenger are to be avoided.	Individual decision usually made at first postoperative checkup dependent on condition. Sitting for long periods of time may result in venous stasis and thrombophlebitis.
Discuss limiting weight of items lifted or carried.	May promote Valsalva effect and sternal incision may be weak.
Weigh every week, report significant gains and signs of edema, such as ankle swelling.	Gain of 3–4 lbs may indicate beginning CHF.
Discuss importance of limiting salt and cholesterol intake.	Sodium promotes water retention and cholesterol is limited in an attempt to avoid plaque deposition in bypass grafts.
Review drug therapy, potential side effects, and problems that are important to report.	Many patients remain on medications for different periods of time, some may be on medication indefinitely, such as warfarin for patients with prosthetic valves.

Discuss signs of infection at the incision sites that need to be reported to the physician.

Some soreness and redness is to be expected, however, persistent temperature, or fever above 101° F; swelling, redness, and purulent discharge at the incision need treatment.

Encourage patient to wear Medic Alert identification bracelet.

Notes type of cardiac problem and current drug therapy.

Discuss resumption of sexual activities.

Requires physician approval. Most patients have unexpressed concerns and fears and need opportunities for discussion. (Refer to Care Plan: Psychosocial Aspects of Care in the Acute Setting.)

Refer to Care Plan: Myocardial Infarction, knowledge deficit.

DIAGNOSIS: Pancarditis: Pericarditis, Myocarditis, Endocarditis

PATIENT DATA BASE

NURSING HISTORY

History of infections during the last four weeks, especially upper respiratory infection, recent childbirth, cystoscopy, TUR, dental work, or surgery.

May be nonspecific, developing after chest trauma or surgery, valve replacement, chest irradiation, myocardial infarction, connective tissue disorders.

Long-term intravenous therapy or indwelling catheter may produce site of organism entry.

Endocarditis is very common in drug abuse.

Known structural deviations of cardiac structures: valves, septa, patent ductus, aortic coarctation, and so forth; predisposing to endocarditis.

May complain of sharp chest or precordial pain aggravated by thoracic motion and deep inspiration and may be relieved by leaning forward.

History of recent fatigue, weight loss, dyspnea, palpitations, fever, chills, back pain, cough, arthralgias.

Symptoms may be aggravated by alcohol, myocardial toxic drugs, digitalis, or exertion.

History of immunosuppressive drugs, steroids predispose to microbial invasion.

DIAGNOSTIC STUDIES

Cardiac isoenzyme elevation indicates myocardial tissue damage.

Electrocardiogram may show indications of ischemia and strain (S-T changes and presence of Q waves), damage, conduction blocks, and arrhythmias.

Monitor to evaluate frequency and type of arrhythmias. ECG in pericarditis shows elevated S-T segment with flattened T waves that may progress to inversion. The absence of Q waves or decreasing R wave voltage in V leads differentiates from acute myocardial infarction.

PPD/ASO titers to show causative organism and rule out lupus, rheumatic fever, and sickle-cell disease.

Blood cultures to identify cause of infection and sensitivity to antibiotics. (Endocarditis most often caused by bacteria; myocarditis most often caused by virus.) May be drawn every week for six weeks to monitor for relapses.

Chest x-ray to show cardiac enlargement, pulmonary infiltrates.

CBC and differential to show acute or chronic infectious process; may also show anemia due to increased destruction of red blood cells by valves and splenomegaly.

Echocardiogram to show hypertrophy, valvular dysfunction, dilatation of heart chambers, presence of pericardial fluid or presence of valvular vegetation.

BUN to demonstrate kidney involvement due to decreased cardiac output.

ANA is associated with several autoimmune diseases, for example, lupus, and may be positive.

Positive rheumatoid factor may occur in endocarditis.

PHYSICAL EXAMINATION

Presence of congestive heart failure symptoms, signs of myocardial strain, injury, or decompensation.

Evaluate heart sounds, presence of friction rub, gallop.

Appearance of murmur or change in preexisting murmurs.

Presence of splenomegaly, neurologic deficits, hematuria, and petechiae, especially in mouth, neck, and distal part of extremities, are suspicious for embolization.

Roth spots on optic disks, Janeway lesions on palms and soles of feet, Osler's nodes at finger tips, splinter hemorrhages on fingers.

Elevated temperature and chills, appears fatigued and uncomfortable, prefers to sit up.

NURSING PRIORITIES

1. Decrease myocardial workload to prevent further heart strain or damage and complications.
2. Relieve pain.
3. Assist in treatment or alleviation of underlying infectious process.
4. Assist patient in understanding of disease etiology, prevention, and treatment.

NURSING DIAGNOSIS: Tissue perfusion, alteration in.

SUPPORTING DATA: Activity increases myocardial workload and further stresses heart. Cardiac decompensation and damage may result from inflammatory processes.

DESIRED PATIENT OUTCOMES: Arrhythmias absent or controlled with medications. Resolution of ECG changes. Negative blood cultures.

INTERVENTIONS

Evaluate vital signs, peripheral pulses, restlessness, friction rub, narrowing pulse pressure, decreased blood pressure, increased CVP, jugular distention, and paradoxical pulse.

If signs/symptoms of tamponade occur, place in Fowler's position, take vital signs every 5 minutes, and prepare for pericardiocentesis.

Monitor continuously.

Observe for signs/symptoms that may be indicative of developing failure, such as cough, palpitations, murmurs; assess for digitalis toxicity.

Take blood cultures during temperature spike and intermittently during the recovery phase.

Assure patency of IV lines.

RATIONALE

Indicators of tamponade that severely decreases cardiac output and leads to death if not treated.

Decreases cardiac pressure by increasing thoracic space while awaiting emergency procedure.

May show early signs/symptoms of myocardial irritability. Treatment can prevent life-threatening arrhythmias and other complications.

Watch for fluid overload in intravenous therapy. Worsening congestive heart failure may lead to myocardial damage. Many patients with myocarditis are sensitive to digitalis.

To identify organism and monitor drug adequacy.

Potent IV drugs may cause tissue sloughing if infiltrated.

Keep on bed rest until symptoms of cardiac stress have receded; evaluate response to activity.

Rest decreases myocardial workload and facilitates healing and resolution of infectious process; elevation of vital signs may indicate cardiac stress.

MEDICAL MANAGEMENT

Oxygen.

Increased oxygen to myocardium will promote aerobic metabolism. Anaerobic metabolism, caused by hypoxia, produces toxic byproducts causing pain and contributing to metabolic acidosis.

Digitalis preparations; diuretics.

Increase myocardial contractility and decrease myocardial workload by decreasing vascular fluid volume.

Titrated antiarrhythmics.

May show early signs and symptoms of myocardial irritability.

Antimicrobials IV.

Treat infecting organism.

Pericardiocentesis.

Decreases fluid pressure around the heart and causes dramatic improvement.

NURSING DIAGNOSIS:	**Comfort, alteration in, pain.**
SUPPORTING DATA:	**Chest pain, temperature elevation, diaphoresis, and chills occur with the diagnosis of pericarditis; may also occur with endocarditis.**
DESIRED PATIENT OUTCOMES:	**Patient comfortable and symptoms of diaphoresis, chills, and chest pain are absent.**

INTERVENTIONS

Observe verbal/nonverbal cues suggesting discomfort. Ask patient to report onset of symptoms.

Allow position of comfort.

Monitor temperature every four hours and as indicated. Observe for chills, diaphoresis/other signs of infection.

MEDICAL MANAGEMENT

Analgesics.

Antipyretics and nonsteroid anti-inflammatory drugs, such as aspirin.

Steroids, anti-inflammatory agents.

RATIONALE

Timing and characteristics help differentiate cardiac inflammatory process from other conditions that also cause chest pain.

May be more comfortable in upright position, leaning forward.

Indicates active inflammatory process.

Usually narcotics are required to relieve pain.

Decrease temperature and discomfort.

Decrease inflammation, temperature, effusion to decrease compromised function and chance of tamponade.

NURSING DIAGNOSIS:	Injury, potential for, venous or arterial embolization.
SUPPORTING DATA:	Presence of valvular vegetations, thrombi predispose to risk of venous/arterial emboli.
DESIRED PATIENT OUTCOMES:	Absence of symptoms of embolization.

INTERVENTIONS

Observe changes in all system areas, such as urine output, neurologic deficits, acute abdominal pain, blanching of extremities, and acute pain in extremities.

Observe for redness and swelling at IV site. Cover with antibiotic ointment and sterile dressing; change per hospital policy.

Provide for range of motion and frequent change of position.

Check for calf tenderness (Homans' sign), swelling, and redness.

MEDICAL MANAGEMENT

Anticoagulants.

Antiembolism hose.

RATIONALE

Embolization may occur, especially if valvular vegetations have been noted on echocardiogram. Splenomegaly may aggravate abdominal discomfort.

Long-term IV therapy, required with cardiac inflammation, predisposes to irritation or infection at infusion site.

Decrease risk of thrombosis formation.

Early identification of thrombus formation.

Decrease risk of thrombus formation. Contraindicated in pericarditis and/or tamponade.

Promote venous return.

NURSING DIAGNOSIS:	Knowledge deficit, disease process and management.
SUPPORTING DATA:	Cardiac infections are largely preventable. Patients with cardiac infections are predisposed to cardiac decompensation.
DESIRED PATIENT OUTCOMES:	Verbalizes symptoms of recurrence and complications to be immediately reported to physician. Cooperates with prescribed regimen.

INTERVENTIONS

Caution patient to report any episodes of temperature elevation or return of previous symptoms.

RATIONALE

May signify relapse.

Teach patient to note and report edema, palpitations, weight gain, fatigue, and cough.

Discuss relationship of predisposing factors to redevelopment of disease.

Discuss necessity of continued antibiotic therapy or prophylactic use before medical/dental procedures.

Discuss importance of maintaining physical activity within capability, avoiding stress beyond individual endurance.

Encourage activities requiring minimum exertion, such as reading, to combat boredom.

Stress importance of avoiding the use of alcohol and stimulants.

Awareness of signs/symptoms of cardiac decompensation allows for early intervention. Knowledge of what to expect can decrease anxiety.

Avoiding predisposing situations will help prevent recurrence.

Long-term therapy is required to eradicate organism. Prophylactic therapy treats bacteria that may invade blood stream during major/minor surgeries or manipulations.

Gradual increase in physical activity allows heart to adjust to increased demands. Pregnancies may not be advised.

Long-term hospitalization and/or bed rest may be necessary to allow for myocardial healing. Boredom may lead to disregard of restriction of activity.

Myocardial toxic agents, stimulants promote arrhythmias and retard healing.

DIAGNOSIS: Impaired Peripheral Vascular Function (Thrombophlebitis)

PATIENT DATA BASE

NURSING HISTORY

Male, under age 40 at onset of symptoms, heavy smoker (Buerger's disease).

Weakness, numbness, tingling, and pain in arms, dizziness.

Recent injury to extremity or vein caused by trauma or intravenous therapy that may have damaged vessel.

Leg/calf/foot/thigh/buttocks weakness, complaints of pain, cramping when walking or at night, heaviness/coldness/numbness/tingling/sexual impotence/tenderness along a vein, calf pain during dorsiflexion of foot, increased local/systemic temperature, pain in lower extremities may increase with activity and decrease with rest; color changes and ulceration may also be present.

Occupation/leisure activities indicate active versus sedentary lifestyle; high achiever, high stress, coronary artery disease risk factors.

History of hypertension, hypercholesterol levels, diabetes, renal disease, current medications, allergies, myocardial infarction.

Family history of cardiac problems, hypertension, stroke, diabetes, kidney problems, hypercholesterol/lipid levels.

History of cancer may produce hypercoagulability status.

DIAGNOSTIC STUDIES

Clotting studies: clotting defects, hypercoagulability may be associated with blood dyscrasias.

Blood cholesterol: 250 mg/100 ml or above suggests presence of atherosclerosis.

Blood glucose to test for diabetes mellitus.

Plasma electrophoresis: hyperlipidemia is considered a factor in atherosclerosis development.

12 lead ECG is examined for evidence of previous damage, present ischemia, or acute injury and conduction defects.

Peripheral arteriography is done to demonstrate narrowed or calcified areas in the vascular system leading to ischemic or blocked areas.

Lumbar sympathetic block may be done to evaluate leg peripheral circulation by means of temporary blocking of sympathetic ganglia (using local anesthetic), which produces blocking of vasomotor nerve fibers supplying ischemic limb. A decrease in limb pain and increase in skin temperature indicates sympathectomy may be of value to increase circulation to affected area.

Noninvasive vascular lab includes Doppler studies, phlebogram, oscillometry, exercise tolerance, skin temperature studies, plethysmography may help pinpoint partially or totally occluded vessels.

PHYSICAL EXAMINATION

Subclavian assessment: upper extremity pallor/cyanosis/coldness in one or both hands, clubbing of fingers, muscle atrophy, decreased/thready/absent radial or brachial pulsations. Brachial blood pressures may vary significantly (may indicate aortic coarctation or unilateral subclavian/brachial partial obstruction).

Aortic/common iliac/femoral/popliteal assessment: lower extremities may show pallor/cyanosis/coldness/ redness/increase of temperature/edema/loss of hair/atrophy, discolored/infected/loose/absent nails, diminished/absent pedal/popliteal/femoral pulses; skin ulcerations/gangrene.

Trendelenburg test for valvular incompetence.

General appearance: height, weight ratio, weakness, fatigue, color, response to activity.

Retinal assessment: arteriovenous nicking, silver or copper wiring of vessels, intraocular hemorrhage, papilledema.

NURSING PRIORITIES

1. Promote prescribed regimen to halt/slow disease progression.
2. Improve blood supply to severely ischemic areas, minimizing tissue damage, complications, and pain.
3. Assist patient in recognition/elimination of risk factors.
4. Provide psychosocial support.

NURSING DIAGNOSIS:	**Tissue perfusion, alteration in.**
SUPPORTING DATA:	**Reduction in vessel size, alteration of vessel structure caused by disease process may produce edema and increased circulation time.**
DESIRED PATIENT OUTCOMES:	**Patient recognizes causative factors and has altered lifestyle as indicated.**

INTERVENTIONS

Avoid smoking and vasosconstricting drugs.

Discuss avoiding exposure to cold and dressing warmly.

Encourage use of warm, moist packs, baths, and lamps by explaining correct use and safety procedures.

Avoid use of constricting clothing; long periods of standing/sitting; and discourage crossing of legs. Elevate legs when sitting or for rest periods during the day. Avoid sharp angulation of hip joint.

Provide restful, quiet environment.

Explain procedures, give information, allow patient to verbalize fears.

RATIONALE

Tobacco, specific drugs produce vasoconstriction and further impede circulation.

Wear socks and gloves; use cotton/flannel bed clothing, wear socks to bed. Natural fibers retain heat more efficiently.

Increases temperature and adds to patient comfort. With decreased sensation, careful safety measures must be used to prevent tissue damage.

Tight clothing (hose, girdles) has a tourniquet effect on circulation, inhibiting flow and may result in pooling of blood and edema of dependent tissues. Muscle action facilitates venous return.

Minimize stress that stimulates a vasoconstrictive response.

Information can decrease worry about the unknown.

Maintain bed rest. Avoid use of knee gatch and elevation of extremity above level of heart.

Reduces energy and oxygen requirements of tissues. If problem is arterial, gatching or excessive elevation may decrease or obstruct needed gravitational flow.

Increase activity as tolerated. Encourage active/passive range of exercises (Buerger and Buerger-Allen).

Promotes circulation and formation of collateral flow.

Elevate head of bed approximately 6 inches at night.

Increases gravitational blood flow.

Observe and record pallor, cyanosis, ulcerations, pulse deficits, bruits, temperature of the skin, and distention of vein.

Symptomatology is dependent on degree of ischemia/obstruction present. Pallor of foot on elevation indicates ischemia. After elevation, feet in dependent position should have normal color return in 10 seconds.

Monitor prothrombin time daily.

Maintain within the therapeutic range.

Monitor hematocrit/hemoglobin changes.

Anticoagulant therapy predisposes to bleeding tendencies.

Observe for epistaxis, ecchymosis, hematuria, black and tarry stools, hematemesis. Check injection sites for hematoma formation.

May need intervention to reverse anticoagulant effects.

Avoid use of salicylates, over-the-counter medications, excessive amounts of vitamins containing potassium, mineral oil, or alcoholic beverages.

May affect the anticoagulant actions.

Do not abruptly withdraw from anticoagulant therapy.

May cause rebound clotting to occur.

Give information about side effects of medications; headache, dizziness, tachycardia.

Irritation of the gastric mucosa; fall of blood pressure when patient rises abruptly; and stimulation of the parasympathetic nervous system may occur.

Encourage fluid intake, at least 2000 ml/24 hours unless contraindicated.

Avoids dehydration, which may lead to hypovolemia, increased stasis and viscosity predisposing to thrombus formation.

Check distal pulses, motion and sensation.

If patient has had recent femoral/popliteal or aortic/iliac graft to improve circulation, absence of pulse may indicate thrombosis of graft or obstruction by mechanical means. Paralysis after thoracic aortic surgery may signal occlusion of the spinal cord vessels.

MEDICAL MANAGEMENT

Tranquilizers, sedatives.

May be useful in providing relaxation and lessening anxiety.

Oscillating bed.

Provides passive assist to circulation.

Heparin, parenterally.

Inactivates thromboplastin, which increases clotting time and decreases formation of clots within the vascular system; decreases platelet agglutination.

Coumadin.	Depresses prothrombin and clotting factors; aids in preventing clot extension. Overlap when changing from parenteral to oral anticoagulants for maintenance, as Coumadin takes 2–3 days for onset of effect.
Protamine sulfate.	Antagonist for heparin, have available to reverse heparin effects if necessary.
Vitamin K.	Antagonist for Coumadin.
Whole blood.	May be needed to assist in reversing anticoagulant effects.
Vasodilators, orally for maintenance doses.	Increase available space in which blood circulates, thereby decreasing pressure in the vascular system and lowering blood pressure. May need to be given with food; antacids to reduce gastric irritation.
Sympathectomy.	May be done to eliminate vasospasm and improve peripheral blood supply.

NURSING DIAGNOSIS:	**Comfort, alteration in.**
SUPPORTING DATA:	**Ischemic tissues, distended, inflammed vessels cause discomfort. Ten percent of population has congenitally incompetent valves in lower extremities predisposing to venous distention.**
DESIRED PATIENT OUTCOMES:	**Patient is comfortable.**

INTERVENTIONS

Avoid vasoconstricting factors, such as smoking, activities that produce discomfort.

Note when discomfort occurs.

Provide diet high in protein, less than 300mg cholesterol and low in triglycerides. Arrange consult with dietitian if necessary.

Use alternate comfort measures; position changes, stretching, massage to other than involved areas.

Encourage diversional activities.

Observe for pain in hip, anterior thigh, and medial area of lower leg after lumbar sympathectomy; tell patient that pain is temporary.

RATIONALE

Leads to ischemic pain; increased demand of muscles for blood may cause claudication.

May indicate extent of disease and help define baseline for activity tolerance.

Provides essential nutrients for healing and retards tissue breakdown. Intake of antilipemics may decrease progression of atherosclerotic process, which aggravates symptoms. Hypercholesterolemia increases risk of heart attack three to four times.

Pain causes restlessness and increases tendency to overuse drug analgesics and other measures can reduce need for medication.

Decrease concentration on awareness of discomfort.

Neuritis may occur up to two weeks and will spontaneously remit.

MEDICAL MANAGEMENT

Analgesics.

May be needed after sympathectomy and when pain is not relieved by other measures.

Papaverine.

Relief of vessel spasms.

Antilipemics, may give with food, but do not give with other drugs.

Lower serum cholesterol, phospholipids; block synthesis of lipids. Other drugs may adversely affect action.

Neostigmine, rectal tube.

Relieves abdominal distention; decreased peristalsis may occur with sympathectomy because of interruption of intestinal nerve fibers.

NURSING DIAGNOSIS: Injury, potential for.

SUPPORTING DATA: Ischemic, atrophic skin is more susceptible to decreased sensation, which may predispose to injury.

DESIRED PATIENT OUTCOMES: Identifies potential sources of injury and takes measures to avoid them.

INTERVENTIONS

Discuss care of dependent limbs, body hygiene, application of emolients, wearing shoes and socks. May need referral to podiatrist for foot care. Do not use strong antiseptics/potions on skin.

Use paper instead of adhesive tape.

Protect affected extremity with bed cradle, use of heel guards, sheepskin, or foam mattress.

Exercise caution in the use of hot water bottles or heating pads.

RATIONALE

May have decreased level of sensation and minimal trauma can result in a significant infection. Stasis ulcers, gangrene, and even the loss of a limb are possible outcomes. Removal of callouses, corns, and so forth is best done by an expert.

Less sticky and less likely to cause skin breaks when removed.

Pressure increases discomfort and may lead to extension or development of new ulcerations.

Artificially applied heat may cause burns to tissues with decreased sensitivity due to ischemia. Heat also increases the metabolic demands of already compromised tissues.

NURSING DIAGNOSIS: Gas exchange, impaired.

SUPPORTING DATA: Thrombophlebitis often leads to pulmonary embolism.

DESIRED PATIENT OUTCOMES: Exhibits no symptoms of pulmonary embolization.

INTERVENTIONS

Maintain bed rest. Assist patient on and off bedpan; encourage adequate fluids and roughage in diet.

Do not massage legs; discuss thoroughly with patient/significant others.

Auscultate chest for breath sounds each shift and p.r.n.; note level of consciousness, occurrence of chest pain dyspnea, or unexplained restlessness.

RATIONALE

Decrease/prevent activities that cause strenuous muscle contractions that may dislodge and propel clots.

May dislodge clot and cause pulmonary embolization.

Documents early changes that may signify pulmonary embolization. (Refer to Care Plan: Pulmonary Embolism.)

MEDICAL MANAGEMENT

Stool softeners.

Apply antiembolism stockings.

Assist in prevention of straining at stool.

Compresses peripheral vessels to increase deep vein flow and decrease stasis and clot predisposition.

NURSING DIAGNOSIS:	**Self-concept, disturbance in.**
SUPPORTING DATA:	**Disease management requires changes of lifestyle; long-term prognosis is uncertain.**
DESIRED PATIENT OUTCOMES:	**Verbalizes acceptance of self as someone with a chronic progressive disease.**

INTERVENTIONS

Assist patient in incorporating disease management regimen into activities of daily living.

Encourage verbalization of personal and work conflicts that may arise.

Assess patient's level of adaptation and progress.

Provide opportunities for listening to concerns and questions and provide information as needed.

Discuss referrals to biofeedback clinic, or other resources for help with stopping smoking and/or learning relaxation skills.

RATIONALE

Lifelong treatment process is more easily managed on a daily basis.

May have concerns about employment, financial insecurity, or the risk of being a burden to the family.

Rapidly progressing disease can result in uncertainty and instability for the patient/significant others and they can become discouraged and depressed.

Can offer encouragement, support and give patient a sense of value and self-worth.

Smoking may be used to relieve tension. Important to learn other methods for relieving tension.

NURSING DIAGNOSIS:	Skin integrity, impairment of, actual.
SUPPORTING DATA:	Progression of disease; increased metabolic demands; borderline circulation; decreased sensation; and required bed rest may be factors in skin breakdown.
DESIRED PATIENT OUTCOMES:	Skin breakdown is treated/prevented.

INTERVENTIONS

Note location of skin breakdown. Take decubitus precautions.

Cleanse wound with sterile saline, hydrogen peroxide.

Compression bandage, warm, moist, sterile packs may be applied intermittently to elevated leg.

Refer to Care Plan: Long-Term Care, Nursing Diagnosis: Skin integrity.

RATIONALE

Early treatment minimizes size of breakdown area and limits complications. Ulceration may occur after phlebitis episode but may also occur after trauma to extremity.

Rids area of necrotic tissue that may harbor bacteria and allows healing to take place.

Encourages circulation, protects against further trauma to area and decreases edema formation.

NURSING DIAGNOSIS:	Knowledge deficit, disease process and treatment.
SUPPORTING DATA:	Interrelatedness of the symptoms of thrombophlebitis with atherosclerosis and its risk factors, is important to understand, as they predispose to pulmonary embolism.
DESIRED PATIENT OUTCOMES:	Verbalizes cause/treatment of disease as it manifests itself individually.

INTERVENTIONS

Discuss need for rest of affected extremity.

Instruct in active/passive range of motion exercises to unaffected extremity.

Encourage walking, rather than sitting or standing.

RATIONALE

Rest allows vessel to heal, absorb clot and limits embolization.

Maintain muscle tone.

Activity discourages venous stasis caused by dependency.

Plan for teaching of foot and skin care.

Instruct patient in symptoms to report to physician; pain in lower extremity, chest pain, or dyspnea.

Discuss importance of followup visits and laboratory studies.

In Beurger's disease, needs to avoid rye.

Discuss factors that adversely affect the progression of atherosclerosis.

Discuss possibility of surgical interventions if medical management is unsatisfactory.

Minimize skin breakdown.

Signs of thrombophlebitis and pulmonary embolus.

Monitors patient progress, drug effects, and provides opportunity for questions and further health teaching.

By-products produce vasoconstriction.

Incidence and severity is significantly increased in patients having one or more of the modifiable risk factors (hypertension, stressful living, obesity, hyperlipidemia, smoking, sedentary living).

Sympathectomy is helpful in relieving symptoms due to ischemia. Necessity for amputation is lessened if treatment is begun early.

DIAGNOSIS: Vein Ligation and Stripping

PATIENT DATA BASE

Refer to Care Plan: Impaired Peripheral Vascular Function.

NURSING DIAGNOSIS:	Tissue perfusion, alteration in, potential.
SUPPORTING DATA:	Edema of tissues, irritation, immobility of extremities, and inadequate venous return. Application of circular bandage.
DESIRED PATIENT OUTCOMES:	No evidence of compromised circulation of involved extremity.

INTERVENTIONS

Elevate extremities approximately 30 degrees (unless patient also has arterial insufficiency). Do not gatch knees.

Remove and rewrap Ace bandages from toes to groin as necessary to keep snug and avoid constrictive discomfort. Note normal distal sensation, motion, and color.

Check involved part for edema, complaints of heaviness, dilation of leg veins, complaints of leg cramps when standing. Tell patient that these symptoms are normal.

Encourage activity and elevation of the limb.

Observe for ulcerations, symptoms of thrombophlebitis. (Refer to Care Plan: Impaired Peripheral Vascular Function.)

RATIONALE

Elevation augments gravitational venous flow to decrease edema. Gatching creates pressure and impedes popliteal flow.

Bandages may constrict proper blood flow.

Vein stripping removes enlarged, unsightly vessels allowing tissues to be drained by smaller veins that may enlarge somewhat to accommodate increased venous flow. During this time, some symptoms of engorgement may be expected.

Decreases engorgement, edema, and stasis.

May occur due to poor circulation to tissues and stasis.

NURSING DIAGNOSIS:	Skin integrity, impairment of, actual.
SUPPORTING DATA:	Surgical incisions.
DESIRED PATIENT OUTCOMES:	Healing surgical incisions without evidence of infections.

INTERVENTIONS

Check dressings for bleeding; reinforce change as necessary.

Check temperature four times daily.

RATIONALE

Drainage should be minimal; freely bleeding areas should be called to the attention of the physician for evaluation.

May indicate systemic reaction to infection.

NURSING DIAGNOSIS:	Comfort, alteration in, pain.
SUPPORTING DATA:	Surgical incisions.
DESIRED PATIENT OUTCOMES:	Patient comfortable.

INTERVENTIONS

Assess pain and circulation to toes and loosen Ace wrap as indicated.

MEDICAL MANAGEMENT

Analgesics.

RATIONALE

Pain may be surgical in origin or secondary to tight dressings with inadequate circulation.

Pain medication relieves discomfort associated with surgical trauma.

Refer to Care Plans: Surgical Intervention; Impaired Peripheral Vascular Function.

NURSING DIAGNOSIS:	Knowledge deficit, recurrence.
SUPPORTING DATA:	Varicosities tend to recur.
DESIRED PATIENT OUTCOMES:	Verbalizes development of varicosities and takes steps to avoid or minimize occurrence.

INTERVENTIONS

Discuss the importance of measures to minimize venous stasis and to maximize venous return.

RATIONALE

Blood carried by removed veins is now carried by other vessels, which may become varicosities with time.

Refer to Care Plan: Impaired Peripheral Vascular Function.

DIAGNOSIS: Raynaud's Disease

PATIENT DATA BASE

NURSING HISTORY

History of sensitivity to cold.

History of pain in chest and arms; use of vasoconstricting drugs, smoking habit, injury to chest/arms.

On exposure to cold or during emotional upset, fingers/toes/ear lobes/nose/cheeks/chin blanch and become numb, turn cyanotic, purple, deep red, then return to normal color as warming ensues; involvement is symmetrical.

History of insomnia, hobbies, sedentary versus active living habits gives insight into stress-coping strategies.

DIAGNOSTIC STUDIES

Peripheral vascular evaluation with Doppler.

Observation of typical signs and symptoms of Raynaud's disease on exposure to cold.

PHYSICAL EXAMINATION

Posture, position convey anxiety.

Peripheral pulses present/absent in all extremities.

Intermittent changes in skin color of fingers/toes observed.

Presence of thrombosis, skin atrophy, nail deformity, areas of gangrene.

NURSING PRIORITIES

1. Maintain tissue perfusion to extremities.
2. Provide information and support to enable necessary lifestyle changes.

NURSING DIAGNOSIS:	**Tissue perfusion, alteration in.**
SUPPORTING DATA:	**Loss of normal color and sensation of affected areas because of vascular spasm.**
DESIRED PATIENT OUTCOMES:	**Attacks have decreased in frequency. Patient has stopped smoking and demonstrates tension-reducing behaviors. Verbalizes side effects of vasodilators, symptoms of thrombosis/gangrene, and when to contact physician.**

INTERVENTIONS

Avoid exposure to cold. Protect susceptible areas with clothing, gloves and promote overall warmth with additional clothing and increased room temperature.

To assist in rewarming, part may be submerged in lukewarm water, put in dependent position.

Observe for degenerative skin changes, such as ulceration, gangrene.

During attack, caution patient to cease activity and protect affected part until normal sensations return.

Discuss avoidance of use of tobacco, if patient is still smoking.

RATIONALE

Cold produces typical vasoconstriction and may lead to tissue damage from prolonged or repeated ischemia, which causes thickening of the arterial wall and may lead to occlusion and gangrene.

Slow rewarming is less harmful to the tissues.

Signify compromised tissue circulation and may require further interventions.

Prevent further damage.

Tobacco is a vasoconstrictor.

MEDICAL MANAGEMENT

Vasodilators; reserpine, Cyclospasmol, and so forth.

Sympathectomy or nerve block.

Increase flow to deprived areas, prevent vasoconstrictive response.

Block is temporary, sympathectomy is permanent causing specific vessels to dilate, preventing spasm.

BIBLIOGRAPHY

Books and Other Individual Publications

BAINBRIDGE, M.V.: *Postoperative Cardiac Intensive Care.* Blackwell Scientific, Boston, 1981.

BEYERS, M. AND DUDAS, S: *The Clinical Practice of Medical-Surgical Nursing.* Little, Brown & Co., Boston, 1977.

BRUNNER, L.S. AND SUDDARTH, D.S.: *The Lippincott Manual of Nursing Practice,* ed. 2. J.B. Lippincott, Philadelphia, 1980.

BUDASSI, S.H. AND BARBER, J.M.: *Emergency Nursing: Principles and Practice.* C.V. Mosby, St. Louis, 1981.

DAVIES, H. AND NELSON, W.: *Understanding Cardiology.* Butterworth's Group, 1978.

GOLDBERGER, E.: *Treatment of Cardiac Emergencies,* ed. 3. C.V. Mosby, St. Louis, 1982.

GOLDBERGER, E.: *Textbook of Clinical Cardiography.* C.V. Mosby, St. Louis, 1982.

HART, L.K. ET AL.: *Concepts Common to Acute Illness: Identification and Management.* C.V. Mosby, St. Louis, 1981.

HURST, J.W.: *The Heart,* ed. 5. McGraw-Hill, New York, 1982.

JOHANSON, B.C. ET AL: *Standards for Critical Care.* C. V. Mosby, St. Louis, 1981.

KIM, M. AND MORITZ, D. (EDS.): *Classification of Nursing Diagnosis.* McGraw-Hill, New York, 1981.

LUCKMAN, J, AND SORENSON, K.C.: *Medical-Surgical Nursing,* ed. 2. W. B. Saunders, Philadelphia, 1980.

MCGURN, W.C.: *People with Cardiac Problems, Nursing Concepts.* J. B. Lippincott, Philadelphia, 1981.

PHIPPS, W. J., LONG, B. C., AND WOODS, N. F.: *Medical-Surgical Nursing.* C. V. Mosby, St. Louis, 1979.

RAPAPORT, E.: (ED.): *Current Controversies in Cardiovascular Diseases.* W. B. Saunders, Philadelphia, 1980.

RAREY, K.P. AND YOUTSEY, J.W.: *Respiratory Patient Care.* Prentiss-Hall, Englewood Cliffs, New Jersey, 1981.

TILKIAN, S. M., CONOVER, M. B., AND TILKIAN, A.G.: *Clinical Implications of Laboratory Tests.* C. V. Mosby, St. Louis, 1979.

WENGER, N.K. ET AL.: *Cardiology for Nursing.* McGraw-Hill, New York, 1980.

WILKINS, R. W. AND LEVINSKY, N.G. (ED.): *Medicine, Essentials of Clinical Practice.* Little, Brown & Co., Boston, 1978.

Journal Articles

ADELUS, S.: *Subacute bacterial endocarditis.* Nursing Times, Vol. 77 No. 35, 1497–1500, Aug./Sep. 1981.

ALEXY, B.: *Monitoring cardiovascular status with noninvasive techniques.* Cardiac Care Symposium, The Nursing Clinics of North America, Vol. 13 No. 3, 423–436, Sep. 1978.

BROWN, A.J.: *Your 'heat of the moment' guide to emergency drugs.* RN, 45:26–31, 1982.

BUDASSI, S.: *Chest trauma.* Cardiac Care Symposium, The Nursing Clinics of North America, Vol. 13, No. 3, 533–541, Sep. 1978.

CHRZANOWSKI, A.: *Intra-aortic balloon pumping: Concepts and patient care.* Cardiac Care Symposium, The Nursing Clinics of North America, Vol. 13, No. 3, 513–532, Sep. 1978.

DE TOLEDO, L.W.: *How vasodilators backfire (and when to expect it).* RN, 45:40–45, 1982.

Drugs used in the care of the cardiac patient. Cardiac Care Symposium, The Nursing Clinics of North America, Vol. 13, No. 3, 473–498, Sep. 1978.

HATHAWAY, R.: *The Swan-Ganz catheter.* The Nursing Clinics of North America, Vol. 13, No. 3, 389–408, Sep. 1978.

KINNEBREW, M.N.: *Add paradoxical pulse to your assessment routine.* RN, 44:32–33, 1981.

MEADOR, B.: *Cardiogenic shock: Help break the vicious circle.* RN, 45:38–42, 1982.

MICHAELSON, C.R.: *Bedside assessment and diagnosis of acute left ventricular failure.* CCQ, 4:1–11, 1981.

RYAN, J.L.: *Dobutamine vs dopamine.* CCN, 1:18–19 +, 1980.

SOLOMAN-HAST, A.: *Anxiety in the coronary care unit: Assessment and intervention.* CCQ, 4:75–82, 1981.

TYLER, M.: *Basic cardiopulmonary resuscitation.* Cardiac Care Symposium, The Nursing Clinics of North America, Vol. 13, No. 3, 499–512, Sep. 1978.

YOUNG, L.C.: *Coronary artery bypass surgery: Commonplace yet complicated.* CCN, 1:15–24, 1981.

DIAGNOSIS: Chronic Obstructive Pulmonary Disease (COPD)

PATIENT DATA BASE

NURSING HISTORY

May have emphysema. Early in syndrome; complains of sudden dyspnea after rising, often associated with violent coughing with small amounts of mucoid sputum brought up. With disease progression, dyspnea with exhaustion is present throughout the day with evident fatigue. Prolonged expiration, breathlessness occurs with basic activities of daily living (ADL).

In asthma, attack is sudden, with shortness of breath, feelings of suffocation, dyspnea, wheezing that improves slightly with positioning.

In bronchitis, may be insidious onset, often associated with other diseases, persistent productive cough, dyspnea, infection, history of smoking or working in a polluted environment.

Note smoking habits: type, how much, how long, and if the patient inhales.

Note dietary habits: may use warm liquids to raise tenacious secretions; may be anorexic due to shortness of breath; how much and what kind of fluid intake.

May have history of coughing: severe, relieved with warm liquids, hacking cough, sputum.

Occupation: note hazards of pollution and/or respiratory irritants.

May have history of chronic coughing, infections, aspiration, tumors, exacerbation during winter months may be response to cold air inhalation.

Note current medications, drug tolerance, allergies, concurrent disease.

What hobbies and activities can the patient do without distress?

Note patient's description of conditions precipitating symptoms.

How long has respiratory difficulty existed?

Family history of emphysema, chronic bronchitis, asthma, bronchiectasis. May have familial predisposition associated with α_1-antitrypsin deficiency.

DIAGNOSTIC STUDIES

Pulmonary function studies: total vital capacity may be normal but one second vital capacity is decreased.

Sputum cultures may be positive for bacteria, pneumococcus, or staphylococcus in chronic bronchitis.

Leukocytosis may be present due to infection.

ABGs: decreased PO_2, frequently increased CO_2.

Chest x-ray to rule out other disease. In bronchiectasis, may reveal areas of bronchi dilatation and atelectasis.

Bronschoscopy shows mucopurulent secretions present in and around involved areas.

Bronchogram maps out areas of bronchial dilation.

PHYSICAL EXAMINATION

Note speech pattern, posture, anxiety, restlessness.

Chronic hyperexpansion, increased anteroposterior diameter of chest is present and associated with kyphosis in emphysema.

During inspiration, there is elevation of the shoulder girdle and retraction of the subclavicular fossae.

There are prolonged expirations, presence/absence of cyanosis, hyperresonance with diminished heart tones, upper hepatic dullness, and minimal movement of the diaphragm.

On auscultation, breath sounds are diminished in intensity with a prolonged expiratory phase; breath holding is reduced, presence of bronchospasms. Wheezing, scattered crackles (rales) may be present.

Pulse and respiration are elevated.

Neck veins may be distended, may complain of pain in the right upper quadrant due to cardiac failure and hepatic congestion.

Abdominal muscles may be used during expiration.

Note presence of sputum, amount, color, consistency.

Altered sensorium may indicate developing hypoxia.

Clubbing of fingers is not usually present unless there is underlying cardiac disease.

NURSING PRIORITIES

1. Maintain patency of bronchial airways and facilitate CO_2/O_2 exchange.
2. Assist patient in dealing with long-term aspects of disease.

NURSING DIAGNOSIS:	**Airway clearance, ineffective.**
SUPPORTING DATA:	**Retained secretions produce chronic obstruction leading to dyspnea and dysfunctional exchange and produce an excellent medium for bacterial growth. Decreased rate of expiration does not produce enough force to properly expectorate secretions.**

DESIRED PATIENT OUTCOMES:	Optimal ventilation through proper expectoration of excessive secretions.

INTERVENTIONS

Discuss avoidance of smoke, dust, pollen, dander.

Assess breath sounds and note use of bronchodilators.

Increase fluid intake to 2000 ml/daily within level of cardiac reserve.

Give warm liquids rather than cold.

Monitor hematocrit and hemoglobin levels.

Elevate head of bed, give postural drainage and percussion to all but asthmatic patient.

Encourage deep breathing.

Observe for signs/symptoms of infection: fever, dyspnea, change in sputum color, amount or character. Obtain sputum for culture and sensitivity.

Observe for decrease in symptoms and side effects of drugs.

Monitor serial chest x-rays.

Provide opportunities for rest; keep activities to a minimum.

RATIONALE

Irritating factors leading to increased sputum production.

Nearly all patients have some degree of spasm. Increase in breath sounds, decreased adventitious sounds demonstrate opened airways.

Help liquify secretions and decrease their viscosity so they can be more easily expectorated.

Facilitate expectoration of secretions and decrease spasms.

Provide indication of hydration.

Facilitates ventilations; clears all lung areas of secretions, especially lower and midlung lobes in COPD.

Opens airways and helps to prevent atelectasis caused by blockage.

Early signs of infections. Worsening of symptoms after period of remission may demonstrate presence of superinfection.

Signs of improvement. Tremors, tachycardia, diaphoresis may accompany bronchodilator use. Steroids may cause gastric irritation.

For resolving areas of infiltration if condition improving.

In acute stage of illness. Increase in activity increases oxygen requirements.

MEDICAL MANAGEMENT

Bronchodilators.

Expectorants, ultrasonic nebulization.

Antimicrobials, steroids.

Antacids.

Bronchoscopy.

Decrease mucosal edema and smooth muscle contraction by stimulation of the sympathetic nervous system.

Liquify secretions.

Control infection, inflammation.

For gastric irritation.

May be indicated to remove secretions that patient is unable to expectorate.

105

NURSING DIAGNOSIS:	Gas exchange, impaired.
SUPPORTING DATA:	Disease process causes narrowed airways, air trapping, and hyperinflation of chest leading to poor gas exchange.
DESIRED PATIENT OUTCOMES:	Arterial blood gases within normal range for patient. Absence of other symptoms associated with respiratory distress.

INTERVENTIONS

Monitor ABGs, document level of O_2/CO_2. Decrease in level of consciousness, presence of headache, visual disturbances.

Elevate head of bed; remove restrictive clothes.

Monitor vital signs, use of accessory muscles. Auscultate breath sounds every eight hours and p.r.n.

Observe for cyanosis.

Avoid sedatives, tranquilizers.

MEDICAL MANAGEMENT

Oxygen, low flow rate (2L/min) in emphysema; higher with other conditions.

May require compressed air for IPPB treatment.

Intubation and ventilatory assist.

Refer to Care Plan: Ventilatory Assistance (Mechanical).

RATIONALE

CO_2 may be low at first because of compensatory hyperventilation and relatively better diffusability of CO_2. Symptoms of CO_2 narcosis may occur.

Decreases tension on respiratory structures and work of breathing.

Indicate signs of stress, hypoxia, increased respiratory effort.

Late sign of hypoxia due to deoxygenated hemoglobin.

Masks symptoms of hypercapnia.

Lessens hypoxemia effects and decreases right ventricular strain. Higher O_2 flow rates will decrease hypoxia, which is only respiratory stimulant in long-term COPD patient.

Patient who retains CO_2 may lose hypoxic drive to breathe if O_2 is used.

If patient is too "weak" to breathe or secretions too difficult to manage.

NURSING DIAGNOSIS:	Nutrition, alteration in, less than body requirements.
SUPPORTING DATA:	Medications, sputum, fatigue, shortness of breath, distention may cause anorexia, nausea, and vomiting. Increased work of breathing uses more calories.

DESIRED PATIENT OUTCOMES:	Approaching normal weight.

INTERVENTIONS

Assess dietary habits and needs.

Provide high-protein diet, frequent feedings in well-ventilated environment.

Avoid gas-producing foods and carbonated beverages.

Avoid very hot/cold foods.

Record amount of food intake.

Consult dietitian as indicated.

Give frequent oral care; remove expectorated secretions promptly; provide specific container for disposal of tissues and sputum.

Weigh weekly.

RATIONALE

Can be helpful to individualize the diet when appetite is poor.

Diet may have been protein deficient because it takes more energy to eat. Frequent feedings lessen fatigue.

Limit excursion of diaphragm and hamper abdominal breathing.

Extremes may increase coughing spasms.

Gives information regarding calorie intake.

To plan attractive, nutritious food when intake is insufficient.

Stale/visible secretions may cause loss of appetite.

Gives estimate of adequacy of nutrional plan intake.

MEDICAL MANAGEMENT

Oxygen.

Vitamin supplements.

Give while eating. Decreases dyspnea and increases energy for eating.

May be necessary.

NURSING DIAGNOSIS:	Injury, potential for, infection.
SUPPORTING DATA:	**Patient with COPD is usually prone to upper respiratory infections, and perhaps systemic infections, if in a debilitated state. Each acute upper respiratory infection increases pulmonary tissue damage, decreasing patient's ability to compensate.**
DESIRED PATIENT OUTCOMES:	**Absence of evidence of acute infection.**

INTERVENTIONS

Collect sputum for culture and sensitivity.

RATIONALE

Identifies causative organism and susceptibility to various antibiotics.

Monitor temperature.	Indication of infectious process.
Monitor visitors for colds and so forth.	Protect from exposure.

MEDICAL MANAGEMENT

Antimicrobial therapy.	May be prescribed prophylactically, especially, during times of increased risk.
Postural drainage and percussion.	Drains bronchioles of secretions that may provide medium for bacterial growth.
Vaporizer, humidifier.	Increases humidity to help liquify secretions. May be controversial in some areas/contraindicated in some disease conditions.
Bronchoscopy, segmental resection.	Drains blocked airways; removes diseased portions of lung.

NURSING DIAGNOSIS:	**Knowledge deficit, disease and complications.**
SUPPORTING DATA:	**Lack of knowledge about disease and treatments may lead to anxiety and/or failure to follow prescribed regimen.**
DESIRED PATIENT OUTCOMES:	**Verbalizes and follows medical regimen. Avoids activities that aggravate condition, increase risk of upper respiratory infection, or predispose to complications.**

INTERVENTIONS

RATIONALE

Reinforce explanation of disease, medications, and equipment.	Knowledge can decrease anxiety and lead to better cooperation.
Encourage patient/significant others to ask questions.	Questions, comments can provide opportunity for clarification of misunderstandings.
Discuss drugs, side effects, followup care, and symptoms to report to the physician.	Allows patient to participate in own health care. May avoid serious complications.
Discuss use and misuse of different types of inhalers.	While they can be helpful under proper supervision, they can be harmful when misused.
Stress importance of proper oral hygiene, regular dental care.	Decrease oral bacterial growth.
Discuss importance of avoiding people with active respiratory infections.	Decrease incidence of acute upper respiratory infections.
Discuss factors that may aggravate condition: excessive dryness, temperature changes, pollen, tobacco smoke, pollution irritants.	May induce bronchial irritation/spasm leading to further production of secretions and airway blockage.

If patient is a smoker, provide assistance with stopping. Refer to support groups as indicated.

Even when patient wants to stop smoking, it is often difficult to do by oneself.

Stress importance of periodic sputum cultures and examinations.

Test for presence of infection and causative organism.

Provide information about limitations of activities, occupation and environment requirements, such as adjusting activities to fatigue patterns.

Knowledge of activities and occupations that increase symptoms, patient can make decisions regarding change.

Develop exercise program, breathing pattern exercises and use of pursed lips.

Increases general sense of well-being and helps increase activity tolerance. Strengthens accessory muscles and helps minimize collapse of airways.

Discuss ways of managing frequent rest periods.

Avoids overwhelming fatigue, which can be a factor in dyspnea. May decrease ability to expectorate excess secretions.

NURSING DIAGNOSIS:	Self-concept, disturbance in.
SUPPORTING DATA:	Multiple issues of decreased independence, body image, chronic illness, and sexual limitations can interfere with an individual's self-image.
DESIRED PATIENT OUTCOMES:	Maintains positive self-image despite limitations and changes in lifestyle.

INTERVENTIONS

RATIONALE

Assess level of patient's knowledge and anxiety.

Beginning at patient's level of knowledge is more helpful in assisting patient to deal with necessary changes. Level of anxiety can interfere with learning process.

Provide information as patient desires.

Will hear only what patient is ready to accept. Accurate information will help in making decisions.

Refer to Care Plan: Psychosocial Aspects of Care in the Acute Setting.

DIAGNOSIS: Bacterial Pneumonia

PATIENT DATA BASE

NURSING HISTORY

History of recent upper respiratory infection (URI).

Complains of dyspnea, pleuritic chest pain, fever, chills, hemoptysis, productive cough with rusty or purulent sputum.

Check nutritional status; indication of susceptibility to infection.

Determine allergies; may help differentiate cause or aggravating factors.

Activity level may favor pooling of secretions.

Note age and sex: three times more common in middle-aged men.

Determine occupation: may be exposed to pollutants.

Determine smoking, alcohol, and drug habits.

History of general health decline, concomitant diseases, or conditions that might lower resistance to infection, such as chronic respiratory infections and disorders, influenza, smoking, fibrocystic diseases, malnutrition, cardiac failure, tracheotomy, immunosuppressive therapy, depression of cerebral function, impaired ciliary/phagocytic action, and aspiration.

DIAGNOSTIC STUDIES

Culture of sputum and blood: bacteria must be recovered and identified for adequate treatment. More than one type of organism may be present. Most common is Diplococcus pneumoniae. May be Staphylococcus aureus, group A hemolytic streptococcus, Escherichia coli, Hemophilus influenzae, Klebsiella-Enterobacter-Serratia group, Francisella tularensis, Proteus, Pseudomonas.

CBC, electrolytes: leukocytosis usually present, low-sodium and chloride levels, increased bilirubin and sedimentation rate.

Chest x-ray usually shows scattered or localized infiltration, which assists in identifying structural distribution (lobar, bronchial).

ECG: tachycardia may or may not be present in response to fever, hypoxemia.

ABGs: abnormalities may or may not be present, depending on the progression of the disease.

PHYSICAL EXAMINATION

Lung evaluation: breath sounds may be diminished or absent over involved area; coarse inspiratory crackles (rales) may also be heard. Resonance may be decreased over areas of infiltration and tactile fremitus may be initially decreased and gradually increase with consolidation. Pneumonia is the most common reason for bronchial breath sounds. This is the opposite of decreased breath sounds, although both are possible in this condition.

Skin is usually pale, dry with poor turgor; herpes simplex is not uncommon.

Movement of chest wall is guarded over involved lung; patient commonly lies on affected side to restrict movement.

Observe for nostril flaring, cyanosis; use of accessory muscles.

Abdomen may be distended, with increased bowel sounds due to nausea and vomiting.

Temperature is usually elevated, sometimes to extremes, pulse elevated, respirations rapid with increased effort, blood pressure may or may not be outside normal range.

NURSING PRIORITIES

1. Maintain adequate oxygenation of tissues.
2. Increase patient comfort.
3. Increase patient's/significant others' knowledge regarding spread of infection, prevention of disease and complications.

NURSING DIAGNOSIS:	**Airway clearance, ineffective.**
SUPPORTING DATA:	**Incessant, painful cough with production of increased amounts of sticky, rusty-pink sputum. Splinting of affected hemothorax during respiration/coughing discourages adequate expectoration.**
DESIRED PATIENT OUTCOMES:	**Adequate expectoration of secretions from airways.**

INTERVENTIONS

Assist in frequent coughing and deep breathing exercises.

Assess respiratory movements.

Encourage fluids frequently.

Assist with nebulizer treatments and respiratory physiotherapy.

Demonstrate effective coughing; splint chest for comfort.

Teach necessity of raising secretions and expectoration versus swallowing to provide suitable means of disposing of expectorations.

Suction p.r.n.

Monitor for symptoms of CHF.

Assess for symptoms of electrolyte imbalances.

RATIONALE

Coughing is a natural self-cleaning mechanism of the airway and a major means of assisting the airway cilia in maintaining patent airways.

Splinting decreases movement of secretions.

Adequate hydration keeps secretions watery and easier to expectorate.

Nebulizer with saline helps keep mucous membranes moist and thins secretions, making them less adherent.

Ineffective coughing tires patient.

Patient may find expectoration offensive and will attempt to limit or avoid it.

To stimulate cough and mechanically clear airway.

Cardiac function may be compromised with hypoxia.

Loss of fluid is accompanied by loss of electrolytes.

MEDICAL MANAGEMENT

Expectorants.

Usually given later in course of illness to clear lung of exudates and secretions.

IV fluids, electrolytes.	May require additional fluids due to increased loss from profuse diaphoresis, increased temperature, diarrhea, vomiting.
Bronchoscopy.	May be indicated to remove mucous plugs and prevent/treat atelectasis.

NURSING DIAGNOSIS: Gas exchange, impaired.

SUPPORTING DATA: Rapid, shallow respirations decrease oxygen intake and eventually compromise adequate oxygenation of tissues.

DESIRED PATIENT OUTCOMES: Improved ventilation and adequate oxygenation of tissues.

INTERVENTIONS

Monitor vital signs every four hours, using rectal temperature.

Observe for signs of shock and pulmonary edema.

Maintain bed rest, assist with personal hygiene, place necessary items within easy reach, and minimize verbalizations.

Gradually increase activity after temperature has been normal for 2–5 days.

Evaluate response to therapy and activity.

Evaluate anxiety and restlessness.

RATIONALE

Mouth is frequently open and may not give accurate temperature. Air hunger, dyspnea, tachycardia, increased cardiac output, increased systolic blood pressure, elevated temperature, headache, disorientation, and cyanosis can all be related to inadequate oxygenation.

Need immediate action as these are the most common causes of death in pneumonia.

Rest decreases tissue demand for oxygen, thereby decreasing dyspnea and work of breathing.

Extreme fatigue, elevation of temperature, dyspnea indicate patient is not ready for that level of activity.

Resolving leukocytosis, normal ABGs, stable vital signs are indicators of positive response.

May be uncomfortable or hypoxic. Anxiety may be due to dyspnea, expectoration of bloody sputum, or pain.

MEDICAL MANAGEMENT

Aminophylline IV.	May help relieve bronchospasm and increase oxygen to lung areas for exchange.
Sputum culture and sensitivities.	To choose appropriate antibiotic therapy.
Antibiotics.	Pneumococci almost uniformly susceptible to penicillin, erythromycin.
Analgesics.	Helpful to ensure rest.

Humidified oxygen, IPPB.	Oxygen therapy may help patient breathe and rest more easily. Restoration of normal oxygen tension is of major importance. Any gas delivered under pressure is extremely drying to the mucous membranes, and moisture helps prevent mucosal irritation as well as loosen secretions. IPPB stimulates deeper inspiration.
Endotracheal intubation.	May be necessary to ensure patent airway and assist with adequate oxygenation.

NURSING DIAGNOSIS: Comfort, alteration in, pain.

SUPPORTING DATA: Inflammation may involve nerve endings causing pleuritic pain, which is increased on respiration and coughing.

DESIRED PATIENT OUTCOMES: Comfort is increased.

INTERVENTIONS

RATIONALE

Change damp linen immediately and avoid exposing patient during skin care and bath.	Chilling is uncomfortable and fatiguing.
Provide mouth and nose care every 3–4 hours.	Helps prevent breath odors, unpleasant taste, accumulation of thickened mucus that in turn helps prevent complications, such as rhinitis, parotitis, lung abcess. May be mouth breather or have herpes simplex lesions and mouth care increases comfort.
Assess change in character and location of pain.	Cardiac complications, such as pericarditis, endocarditis, or myocarditis, may occur.

MEDICAL MANAGEMENT

Analgesics and sedatives.	Relief of pleuritic pain and mild sedation promote freer breathing, allow for coughing effectively, and relieve anxiety.
Antipyretics.	Fever increases metabolic requirements and the demand for pulmonary ventilation, increasing work of breathing.

NURSING DIAGNOSIS: Nutrition, alteration in, less than body requirements.

SUPPORTING DATA: Appetite is often very poor, result of fever, dyspnea, fatigue, and fear of coughing. Increased metabolic need increases calorie requirements in order to maintain weight.

113

| DESIRED PATIENT OUTCOMES: | Maintenance of desired body weight. |

INTERVENTIONS

Offer small feedings of soft/liquid nutritious foods at frequent intervals, allowing patient to assist with choices.

RATIONALE

Need foods that are easily swallowed and provide adequate nutrient intake to promote optimum healing.

NURSING DIAGNOSIS:	Knowledge deficit, recurrence.
SUPPORTING DATA:	Misinformation or lack of knowledge of the disease may lead to spreading of infection to others and/or exacerbation of present condition.
DESIRED PATIENT OUTCOMES:	Infection is controlled.

INTERVENTIONS

Institute isolation techniques according to hospital policy and causative organism.

Teach proper handwashing techniques and provide masks as necessary.

Discuss increasing activity, respiratory exercises, and continuation of medications.

Encourage patient to give up smoking.

Reinforce need for followup care.

RATIONALE

Pneumococcal pneumonia is not highly communicable, but can be transmitted to others by contact with host or airborne droplets.

Reduce spread of infection.

As lung tissue heals, overexertion buildup of secretion or discontinuance of medications may halt healing and bring about relapse. Fatigue and weakness may be expected for several weeks post pneumonia.

Irritates mucosal lining, increases secretions, damages ciliary cleaning action, and inhibits macrophage action.

Demonstrate clearing lung fields and rule out complications.

DIAGNOSIS: Pleurisy

PATIENT DATA BASE

NURSING HISTORY

May complain of pain aggravated by respiratory motion or by any activity requiring work by the thoracic muscles. Pain is sharp, usually in upper portion of thorax and may be localized or may radiate to abdomen or neck.

History of recent URI, congestive heart failure, chest trauma, infection, or hypertension.

History of pleural effusion, inflammation, pulmonary emboli, cancer, heart failure.

Complains of fever or chilliness, irritating nonproductive cough, dyspnea; onset of pain may be sudden.

DIAGNOSTIC STUDIES

Chest x-ray may show classic density higher laterally than medially and sweeping upward. If fluid level is horizontal, air and gas have entered pleural space. When patient lies on side of effusion, liquid gravitates to lateral chest wall.

ABGs are usually normal; unless underlying disease has altered them.

WBC may be increased.

Culture and sensitivities, blood and sputum, may note underlying bacterial infection or other underlying cause as pleural inflammation.

ECG is usually normal.

Lung scan is normal.

Thoracentesis for effusion is sent for cytologic exam, culture and sensitivity to identify invading organism.

PHYSICAL EXAMINATION

Pain usually occurs on inspiration; absent when breath is held.

Dullness to percussion, decreased fremitus and breath sounds over affected area. Effusion may shift mediastinal structures away from affected side.

Pleural friction rub, loss of breath sounds on affected side may occur due to effusion.

Pulse elevated because of pain; respiration rapid and shallow, splinted on affected side to control pain.

Color pale; patient appears anxious.

Temperature may be present, with nonproductive cough.

NURSING PRIORITIES

1. Reduce pain.
2. Maintain tissue oxygenation.
3. Prevent/minimize complications.
4. Provide information to prevent recurrence.

NURSING DIAGNOSIS:	Gas exchange, impaired.
SUPPORTING DATA:	Pain at site of infiltrate, anxiety, dyspnea may decrease respiratory effort. Hemo/pneumothorax may occur post-thoracentesis, shock may alter blood oxygenation.
DESIRED PATIENT OUTCOMES:	Tissue oxygenation is maintained.

INTERVENTIONS

RATIONALE

INTERVENTIONS	RATIONALE
Place in upright position.	Permits greater lung expansion to improve aeration.
Take vital signs every 15 minutes until stable.	After thoracentesis, increased pulse, respiration, and blood pressure may be normal responses or may signal pneumothorax, hypoxemia, or cardiac decompensation.
Assess breath sounds, pain, and chest expansion post-thoracentesis and every four hours p.r.n.	Alterations may signal hemo/pneumothorax.
Provide a calm atmosphere.	Can reduce anxiety and anticipatory pain.
Splint chest when coughing.	Reduces pain while allowing greater chest expansion and deeper cough.
Apply heat or cold to area.	Provides symptomatic relief.
Assess patient for signs of pleural effusion.	Can be a complication of pleurisy.

MEDICAL MANAGEMENT

Analgesics.	Medication inhibits conduction of motor response, produce sedative effects, alter patient mood or sense of pain.
Oxygen.	Per nasal cannula. Increases available oxygen to tissues decreasing ischemia and dyspnea.
Antitussives.	Decreases exhaustive coughing and reduces excess irritation to the pleura.
Nerve block or subcutaneous injections.	Procaine HCl may be injected subcutaneously at area of greatest discomfort. Paravertebral infiltration with anesthetic agent may be used to block area of intercostal nerves.
Thoracentesis.	Removal of effusion may decrease or increase pain, relieve dyspnea by allowing greater expansion of lung on affected side.
Antibiotics, if indicated.	Treatment of underlying disease entity often allows the pleurisy to resolve.

NURSING DIAGNOSIS:	Injury, potential for, infection.
SUPPORTING DATA:	Often patients with pleurisy have infections as the primary underlying cause of the pleurisy.
DESIRED PATIENT OUTCOMES:	Absence of active infection.

INTERVENTIONS

Assess patient for chills/fever.

Encourage patient to cough/deep breath every 2–4 hours with splinting of affected area.

Encourage adequate dietary intake.

RATIONALE

Signs of infection or reinfection.

Increases expectoration of secretions.

Nitrogen and protein homeostasis allows body to fight infection more effectively and increases resistance to infections.

MEDICAL MANAGEMENT

Steam vaporizer.

Blood/sputum cultures and sensitivities.

Antibiotic therapy.

Breaks up secretions and facilitates expectoration.

Identify the causative bacterial agent, if applicable, and treat with the most appropriate antibiotic.

Decreases bacterial pool that may cause pneumonia.

NURSING DIAGNOSIS:	Knowledge deficit, disease and complications.
SUPPORTING DATA:	Lack of knowledge about disease/treatment may lead to anxiety and/or failure to follow prescribed medical regimen.
DESIRED PATIENT OUTCOMES:	Verbalizes and follows medical regimen.

INTERVENTIONS

Discuss ways of preventing URI, if applicable.

Discuss medication routine, type, purpose, and dose.

Provide information about signs/symptoms of primary disease if underlying the current condition and the importance of consulting medical attention.

RATIONALE

Can predispose to pneumonia/pleurisy.

Knowing what to expect of the medication regimen can help the patient to follow through.

Early detection and treatment of primary disease can prevent a recurrence.

DIAGNOSIS: Pulmonary Embolism

PATIENT DATA BASE

NURSING HISTORY

May have history of recent immobilization, such as a hospitalization, surgery, fracture, trauma to lower extremities.

History of heart disease or condition that causes blood stasis or clotting.

Prior history of calf tenderness, deep vein thrombosis, obesity.

May complain of shortness of breath, difficulty breathing, syncope, hemoptysis, sudden chest and shoulder pain, or confusion.

History of oral contraceptive usage.

DIAGNOSTIC STUDIES

Blood enzymes show increased LDH, SGOT, and CPK. Isoenzymes necessary to rule out MI.

Chest x-ray may be normal or show elevation of diaphragm on affected side, wedge-shaped opacity, decreased vascularity, dilated pulmonary arteries.

Pulmonary angiograms: most effective diagnostic tool showing filling defects of the pulmonary arterial system.

ABGs: may show decreased PaO_2, decreased PCO_2, severe respiratory alkalosis (massive PE).

Lung scan shows underperfused areas (sometimes known as a ventricular/perfusion scan).

Increased serum leukocytes.

ECG: may show acute right heart strain, which is associated with pulmonary embolism; inverted T waves in V1 and V4, transient right bundle branch block, right axis deviation, right ventricular hypertrophy, tall P waves in leads 2,3, AVF. PVCs may be associated with hypoxia or electrolyte imbalance.

PHYSICAL EXAMINATION

May display rapid and shallow or gasping respirations.

Tachypnea, tachycardia, hemoptysis, friction rub may be heard, hypotension, and shock. (Paroxysmal supraventricular tachycardia may be the sole sign.)

May have temperature elevation.

In acute episode, may have pulmonary hypertension secondary to pulmonary arterial pressure after massive embolization and acute right ventricular failure.

Decreased activity tolerance, dyspnea, decreased breath sounds.

Increased pulmonic component of S2, abnormal splitting of S2, right ventricular heave and presence of S3 and S4.

Systemic hypotension secondary to increased pulmonary vascular resistance and decreased cardiac output.

Evidence of venous thrombus or a history of unilateral swelling or pain in the extremities.

Appears anxious, restless, may progress to confusion; grimacing related to discomfort.

Distended neck veins.

NURSING PRIORITIES

1. Relieve pain/anxiety.
2. Minimize potential for decreased tissue perfusion.
3. Minimize complications/prevent recurrence.
4. Increase patient's knowledge of disease/treatment/prevention.

NURSING DIAGNOSIS:	Comfort, alteration in, pain.
SUPPORTING DATA:	Pulmonary embolism causes decreased pulmonary circulation leading to hypoxia and ischemia causing pain.
DESIRED PATIENT OUTCOMES:	Pain is reduced to a functional level.

INTERVENTIONS

Position in semi- or high-Fowler's.

Stay with patient.

Refrain from performing nonessential procedures. Encourage rest.

Explain procedures to patient/significant others.

Evaluate respirations and pain relief.

RATIONALE

Upright position favors better lung expansion.

Provides support and can reduce anxiety.

Restricting activity decreases oxygen usage and dyspnea.

Knowledge can decrease emotional stress that may increase metabolic demands on an already compromised system.

Relief must be noted in order to evaluate therapy.

MEDICAL MANAGEMENT

Medication/sedatives. Meperidine and morphine in minimal effective doses.

Oxygen.

Allows patient to rest and reduces anxiety by relaxation. Opiates can cause a decrease in blood pressure/respiratory depression.

May increase perfusion into the tissues, decrease ischemia, which may result in pain relief.

NURSING DIAGNOSIS:	Tissue perfusion, alteration in.
SUPPORTING DATA:	Other thrombi may be present and become emboli.
DESIRED PATIENT OUTCOMES:	Absence of further thrombus formation.

119

INTERVENTIONS

Evaluate dyspnea, restlessness, vital signs, and associated symptoms.

Monitor blood gases; baseline on admission and periodically.

Assess lower extremities for evidence of phlebitis. If found, do not handle or massage. Elevate extremity.

Observe for increased bleeding/bruising, and hematuria.

Monitor activated partial thromboplastin time.

Observe for abrupt pain, pallor, and pulselessness of extremity.

Instruct patient not to massage legs or gatch knees.

MEDICAL MANAGEMENT

Antiembolic stockings.

Anticoagulants; heparin, Coumadin.

Thrombolytic therapy (streptokinase, urokinase).

Surgery.

Refer to Care Plan: Surgical Intervention.

RATIONALE

Rule out other causes of chest pain. Recurrent pain may indicate extension of emboli. Abnormal vital signs may indicate increased heart strain or shock that requires increased interventions to support cardiopulmonary systems and prevent complications.

Determine effectiveness of, or need for, alteration of therapy.

Most common areas of thrombophlebitis formation that may lead to pulmonary embolization.

Treatment predisposes patient to bleeding tendencies.

Therapeutic APTT level is approximately 47 seconds but may have varying effects on different patients.

Patient on heparin is prone to arterial emboli due to platelet aggregation.

May dislodge thrombi. Gatching knees can cause circulatory stasis.

Increase circulation and decrease stasis in the deep vessels.

Decrease formation of new clots.

Lysis of existing thrombus.

Venacaval ligation, filtering, or embolectomy may be performed to prevent further pulmonary embolization or extract the present major pulmonary embolus.

NURSING DIAGNOSIS:	**Gas exchange impaired.**
SUPPORTING DATA:	**Pulmonary embolisms can cause ventilation perfusion imbalance causing hypoxia.**
DESIRED PATIENT OUTCOMES:	**Adequate tissue oxygenation maintained.**

INTERVENTIONS

Monitor arterial blood gases.

Assess level of consciousness.

Measure intake and output.

Maintain fluid level.

Deep breath q 2–4 hours during the stabilized period.

Observe for bleeding.

Avoid strain and constipation.

RATIONALE

Provide a method of assessing tissue perfusion. Treatment can be adjusted depending on results.

Irritability, restlessness, and so forth can be early indicators of hypoxia, hypercapnia.

To assess fluid equilibrium.

Fluid equilibrium is needed for proper cell functioning.

Increases CO_2–O_2 exchange and increases arterial O_2 concentrations.

Anticoagulants can cause bleeding and need to be monitored closely when used.

Can cause an increase in cardiac and pulmonary pressures and decrease tissue perfusion.

MEDICAL MANAGEMENT

Oxygen.

Sedation.

Cardiac monitor.

Invasive pressure monitoring.

Cardiotonics, antiarrythmics, diuretics.

Maximize amount available to the tissues.

To slow respiratory rate and decrease body oxygen requirements.

Arrhythmias frequently occur with pulmonary embolus and may require intervention.

Assess intercardiac pressure measurements and need for intervention.

Assist in maintaining cardiovascular integrity.

NURSING DIAGNOSIS:	Knowledge deficit, disease and prevention.
SUPPORTING DATA:	Often patients with pulmonary emboli disregarded symptoms of thrombi.
DESIRED PATIENT OUTCOMES:	Verbalizes and follows medical regimen, which decreases risk of emboli.

INTERVENTIONS

Instruct in importance of avoiding behaviors, such as wearing restrictive clothing, standing/sitting for prolonged periods, that cause circulatory stasis.

RATIONALE

Predisposes to thrombus and embolus formation.

Discuss and plan an individualized exercise program.

Will be more likely to follow through with program when patient is involved in the planning.

Discuss rationale and importance of stopping smoking and assist in setting up a program for quitting.

May already have information and discussion will help patient in making decisions.

Discuss symptoms that are important to report to the physician.

Deep leg pain, increased tenderness, sharp chest pain. Early identification will increase chance of recovery.

Have patient identify medication routine; reason for taking, dosage, and side effects.

Knowledge/understanding allows patient to participate/cooperate in drug therapy management.

Instruct patient which symptoms to note if on anticoagulant therapy.

Increased risk of bleeding.

DIAGNOSIS: Lung Cancer: Surgical Intervention; Resection, Lobectomy, Pneumonectomy

PATIENT DATA BASE

NURSING HISTORY

Usually occurs in middle to late years with peak incidence between 55 and 60.

Usually occurs more frequently in men than women, though there is a marked increase noted in women who smoke.

Occupation: may expose patient to irritation pollutants, industrial dusts, radioactive materials.

Cigarette smoking: elicit number of years smoked, number of cigarettes per day, if patient inhales smoke. Lung cancer is fairly rare in the nonsmoker.

Alcohol intake: there is a marked correlation between smoking, drinking, and cancer.

History of a cold that has been present more than three weeks; check time cough occurs during the day, amount of sputum produced and description. May be frank blood in sputum indicating involvement of the blood vessels of the lung. Chest pain, anxiety, and fatigue may be present.

Review level of preventive health care received in maintenance of general well-being.

Dietary habits: if weight loss is reported, assess food intake and appetite.

Family history of cancer, especially lung cancer.

Activity level: lassitude, weakness usually appear in advanced stages only.

Chest pain: rarely associated with early lung cancer and not always associated with more advanced stages. Usually occurs when metastasis has extended into pleura or chest wall.

Lungs are the most frequent sites of metastasis from primary lesions elsewhere because tumor cells entering the blood stream in any organ must go through the capillaries of the lungs.

Ninety-eight percent of all primary lung tumors are malignant.

DIAGNOSTIC STUDIES

Chest x-ray may indicate presence of a lesion, a mass in the hilar region, pleural effusion, atelectasis, erosion of ribs or vertebrae. Most cases of early lung cancer are detected from routine chest x-rays. Higher incidence of right lung cancer is seen probably because it is larger, the right bronchus is shorter, wider, and straighter, allowing freer passage of pollutants.

Cytologic examination: aspiration of pleural fluid, pleural biopsy, lymph node biopsy. Sputum is also collected for examination of abnormal cells.

Bronchoscopy: a large percentage of bronchogenic malignancies may be seen through bronchoscopy; therefore, the procedure is essential and presents little risk to the patient.

Lung scan permits demonstration of ischemic areas, all of which block the diffusion of radioactive dye.

PHYSICAL EXAMINATION

Obstruction of bronchus leads to most of the signs/symptoms observed clinically, although there may be no absolute or reliable findings.

The chest may be normal or there may be changes in dullness on percussion over a large tumor mass. There may be increased breath sounds, increased tactile fremitus and bronchial breath sounds. Physical signs vary according to the location of the lesion. If air entry is impaired, brief crackles and wheezes may be heard on inspiration or expiration. A space-occupying lesion may be indicated by tracheal shift or persistent crackles and wheezes.

May guard affected side and reduced chest excursion may be noted. (Pain is rare in early stages.)

Dyspnea, aggravated by exertion may be present.

May appear thin and apprehensive. Extreme emaciation, malnutrition, and wasting (cachexia) may appear only in the late stages of wide spread disease.

Palpation of lymph nodes may indicate metastatic spread of disease.

Extension of the lung lesion can affect the pleural cavity; tumor located near pleura may cause pleuritic pain; near the diaphragm may irritate the phrenic nerve causing referred shoulder pain and perhaps dyspnea; involving bronchial plexus causes arm pain; in the mediastinal area may invade or exert pressure on esophagus causing bleeding and/or dysphagia; pressure on superior vena cava causes jugular distention; pressure against trachea may involve laryngeal nerve causing hoarseness or vocal cord paralysis. Bronchogenic carcinoma may produce ACTH causing adrenocortical hyperplasia.

NURSING PRIORITIES

1. Monitor/maintain respiratory function.
2. Provide information about disease process/treatment/prognosis to enable patient to make decisions appropriate to the individual.

Refer to Care Plans: Surgical Intervention; Cancer for other priorities and interventions.

NURSING DIAGNOSIS:	Gas exchange, impaired.
SUPPORTING DATA:	Invasion of the lung tissue or pleura by tumor cells may result in areas of effusion, obstruction resulting in atelectasis, or compression/invasion of other pulmonary tissues and structures of the mediastinum. Surgical resection of tumor may further decrease amount of functional lung.
DESIRED PATIENT OUTCOMES:	Decrease work of breathing and increase gas exchange.

INTERVENTIONS	RATIONALE
Auscultate lungs and note rate, depth, and pattern of respirations.	Assess changes, such as atelectasis, failure, hemo/pneumothorax.
Assess restlessness.	May indicate increased hypoxia.
Monitor ABGs/pH.	Assess effectiveness of respiratory system. Decreasing PO_2 may indicate need for mechanical support.

Administer pain medications with caution.

Postop pain may restrict chest movement resulting in decreased ventilation but oversedation may decrease respiratory effort resulting in the same effect.

Maintain patency of chest drainage system. (Refer to Care Plan: Pneumothorax.)

Assess and/or prevent complications, such as hemorrhage, mediastinal shift, cardiac tamponade.

Reposition every hour including Fowler's position. (Lobectomy patient should not be positioned on unaffected side.)

Maximize lung expansion.
Can restrict ventilation of unaffected lung.

Monitor for sudden onset of dyspnea, tachypnea, irregular pulse, anxiety, restlessness.

Indicators of mediastinal shift, complication of pneumonectomy.

MEDICAL MANAGEMENT

Humidified oxygen.

Promote maximum oxygenation. Maintain arterial PO_2 at desired level.

Arterial line.

To facilitate collection of arterial blood to assess ABGs.

Chest tubes.

Re-expansion of remaining lung tissue by draining fluid/air from pleural/mediastinal cavity.

NG tube.

May be needed to decompress stomach in presence of gastric distention that can impinge upon thoracic cavity and reduce respiratory excursion.

NURSING DIAGNOSIS: **Airway clearance, ineffective.**

SUPPORTING DATA: **Increased viscosity of secretions combined with restriction of chest movement secondary to postop pain and diminished cough reflex.**

DESIRED PATIENT OUTCOMES: **Secretions are removed and airway patency is maintained.**

INTERVENTIONS

Routine turn, cough, deep breathe, and suction.

Adequate hydration and room humidifier.

Splint incision to cough.

Postural drainage.

RATIONALE

Mobilize secretions. Suctioning may be necessary if patient can not clear secretions by coughing.

To liquify/loosen secretions.

Allows for deeper inspiration and increase force in cough with decreased pain.

Assists in drainage of secretions.

MEDICAL MANAGEMENT

Incentive spirometer or blow bottles.

Encourages deep breathing.

Ultrasonic nebulizer.

Increases inspired humidity and loosens secretions.

Bronchodilators.

Relieve bronchospasm.

IPPB.

May have questionable use if patient is at risk for pneumothorax.

Bronchoscopy.

To clear mucous plugs and prevent atelectasis if other measures fail.

NURSING DIAGNOSIS: **Comfort, alteration in, pain.**

SUPPORTING DATA: **Pain is compounded by anxiety. Involvement of the pleura is painful and surgical pain may last for some time.**

DESIRED PATIENT OUTCOMES: **Patient is comfortable and anxiety/ fear are reduced.**

INTERVENTIONS

RATIONALE

Assess anxiety level and encourage discussion of fears.

Patient's tolerance for pain may be lowered by anxiety and fear and interfere with ability to cope.

Involve in treatment planning, providing factual information.

Allows for feeling of control in dealing with illness, treatment, and prognosis and may decrease anxiety.

Involve significant others in care planning as much as possible.

Can foster independence and provide support for patient in a difficult period.

Evaluate symptoms associated with tumor development.

Location of pain may indicate area of growth.

MEDICAL MANAGEMENT

Analgesics.

Medication required will depend on level of pain.

Sedatives, including Valium.

Promote rest and relaxation.

NURSING DIAGNOSIS: **Knowledge deficit, disease management.**

SUPPORTING DATA: **Seriousness of disease and necessity for followup care require cooperation of patient/significant others. Accurate knowledge is helpful to disease management.**

DESIRED PATIENT OUTCOMES:

Verbalizes required treatment and cooperates in care.

INTERVENTIONS

Encourage deep breathing/cough routine. Continue arm/shoulder exercises.

Use local heat in addition to oral medication.

Avoid lifting activities until cleared by physician.

Avoid exposure to smoke, air pollution.

Schedule alternate periods of activity/rest.

Encourage annual influenza vaccinations.

RATIONALE

Expand lung capacity and prevent atelectasis. Avoid ankylosis of affected shoulder.

To control pain.

Chest muscles will be weak for 3–6 months.

Irritate the lungs.

Generalized fatigue and weakness are usual in the first few weeks.

Necessary in pneumonectomies to decrease risk of infection.

DIAGNOSIS: Pneumothorax

PATIENT DATA BASE

NURSING HISTORY

If pneumothorax is spontaneous, there is unilateral pain followed by difficulty in breathing.

Symptoms may appear while coughing or straining.

Patient is often male and between ages 30 and 40.

History of lung biopsy.

History of prior chest trauma, spontaneous pneumothorax, COPD.

DIAGNOSTIC STUDIES

Chest x-ray can confirm gas in pleural space. X-rays are taken at inspiration and expiration to show extent of pneumothorax.

Arterial blood gases show decreased PO_2, perhaps decreased PCO_2 due to hyperventilation.

PHYSICAL EXAMINATION

On the affected side, decreased chest excursion, fremitus is decreased or absent, breath sounds are absent or decreased.

Tracheal deviation away from affected side showing mediastinal shift.

Respiratory distress, cyanosis, use of accessory muscles for respirations.

Depression of the diaphragm.

Tachycardia, decreased blood pressure.

May have sucking chest wound.

Patient very anxious.

NURSING PRIORITIES

1. Prevent impaired gas exchange.
2. Relieve pain and anxiety.
3. Educate patient about disease and treatment.

NURSING DIAGNOSIS:	**Gas exchange, impaired.**
SUPPORTING DATA:	**Air entering pleural space eliminates normal negative pressure that keeps lung expanded. Increased air pressure in pleural space forces collapse of part or all of lung, and decreases available surface for gas exchange. Pressure on one side of chest can cause pressure on mediastinal structures, decrease cardiac output, and lead to restricted expansion of unaffected side.**

DESIRED PATIENT OUTCOMES:	Promote normal chest pressures to ensure normal lung functioning.

INTERVENTIONS

If present, cover sucking chest wound.

Keep patient in upright reclining position, turned on affected side, or slightly sitting Fowler's.

Provide for complete bed rest and a quiet environment.

Take vital signs every 5–15 minutes. Note respiratory rate, rhythm, symmetry, expansion, breath and voice sounds, and wheezes. Monitor BP, rate, rhythm, and volume of pulse, notation of pain, cyanosis, and shock.

Note position of trachea.

Take vital signs and assess breath sounds q 15 minutes after thoracentesis until patient stable, q 4 hours.

Monitor for cardiac arrhythmias.

Do central venous or wedge pressures every hour, if available.

Note alterations in level of consciousness.

Milk or strip chest tubes every 15 minutes for one hour then every hour p.r.n. Avoid kinking tubing, tape all tubing connections, and make sure water covers drainage tubing at prescribed level.

Monitor for fluctuation of drainage in tubing, if underwater seal chamber is present.

Monitor chest drainage and report if > 100 ml in first hour.

Encourage coughing and deep breathing.

Assist in a graduated exercise program avoiding exhaustion.

Change puncture site dressing and assess redness, healing, drainage, and swelling.

RATIONALE

Prevents further air from entering pleural space to increase pneumothorax.

Favors better lung expansion, decreases pressure of abdominal organs on diaphragm allowing freer movement, and less energy is used to support self in sitting position.

Reduces O_2 demands and anxiety until lung can be reexpanded.

Increased pulse, respirations, decreased blood pressure are signs of increasing shock due to hypoxia, stress, pain. Atelectic area will have no breath sounds and partially collapsed areas have decreased sounds. Evaluation establishes areas of exchange and documents baseline to evaluate increasing atelectasis.

Deviation away from affected side may indicate tension hemo/pneumothorax.

Should stabilize if no complications. Advent of crackles may demonstrate developing pulmonary edema, because less lung tissue is carrying the entire circulation.

Cardiac response to hypoxia, stress, pain, altered pH, may indicate impending failure.

Shows rising pulmonary pressures before crackles or other signs of pulmonary edema/failure are present.

Estimate of adequate cerebral perfusion.

Helps maintain patent tubes for drainage. If blockage occurs, tension hemo/pneumothorax may develop. Avoids accidental disconnection or movement. Avoids air leaking back into pleural cavity.

Occurs with increasing/decreasing pressures in pleural cavity with respirations. Will not occur if tubing is obstructed.

Drainage is part of I & O. May demonstrate hemorrhage. Amount should decrease sharply one hour after procedure.

Increases ventilation and reinflation of lung.

Increases ventilation, O_2 usage and cellular perfusion.

Prevent and note possible infection and healing.

MEDICAL MANAGEMENT

Oxygen per nasal cannula/mask.	Increases available oxygen to tissues and decreases dyspnea.
Thoracentesis.	May be done to extract extra fluid/air quickly before chest tubes are inserted.
Chest tubes inserted and connected to closed drainage.	Allow the pleural cavity to be evacuated of air/fluid reestablishing negative pressure allowing for reexpansion of the lung.
Chest x-ray one hour after procedure and daily times 3 postprocedure.	Show placement of chest tube and resolving atelectasis and areas of air/fluid in pleural spaces.
Incentive spirometer.	Assists with reexpansion of lung and removal of secretions.
Antibiotics/bronchodilators.	Prophylactically to prevent infection, depending on cause of pneumothorax; bronchodilators to assist in better gas exchange.
Hematocrit/hemoglobin after 24 hours postinsertion.	Estimate blood loss/hydration.

NURSING DIAGNOSIS:	**Comfort, alteration in, pain.**
SUPPORTING DATA:	**Pain may be caused by initial injury to the chest. Pneumothorax can cause pain due to increased intrapleural pressure and anxiety.**
DESIRED PATIENT OUTCOMES:	**Patient is comfortable.**

INTERVENTIONS	RATIONALE
Document pain, dyspnea, restlessness, and associated symptoms.	May help rule out other causes of chest pain.
Instruct patient not to lie on chest tube site. Pillow may be placed at side to support tubing.	Lying on chest tube elicits pain; pillow decreases tension on site and supports arm on affected side.
Explain to patient reason for necessary procedure prior to movement.	May be better able to relax or cooperate with move and lessen discomfort; sudden movement causes jerky muscle activity that may cause stress on painful areas, increasing pain.
Teach patient to move arm on affected side through ROM exercises several times daily and increase as tolerated.	Patient tends to not move side on which tubing is placed due to discomfort and fear of dislodging tube. Promotes drainage and prevents contractures.
Give information regarding how tubing is secured.	Decrease anxiety about movement.

MEDICAL MANAGEMENT

Analgesics.	Comfort allows patient to rest and decreases metabolic demands; thereby, decreasing dyspnea.

NURSING DIAGNOSIS:	Knowledge deficit, disease and treatment.
SUPPORTING DATA:	Lack of knowledge increases chances for readmission with same process.
DESIRED PATIENT OUTCOMES:	Verbalizes understanding of cause of problem and follows medical routine.

INTERVENTIONS

Instruct patient in what symptoms to be alert for; that is, sudden pain, shortness of breath, dyspnea, signs of infection.

Teach patient to care for wound.

RATIONALE

Early detection of symptoms can reduce chance of severe complications.

Proper care of chest wound will prevent infection at site and intrapleural space.

DIAGNOSIS: Cancer of the Larynx: Radical Neck/Permanent Laryngostomy Procedures

PATIENT DATA BASE

NURSING HISTORY

Most common in men over 50 but other ages and women are also affected.

History of smoking, increased use of vocal cords (singer, auctioneer).

History of hoarseness, voice change, feeling of pressure or "lump" in throat that may be especially noticeable when patient swallows, pain in throat, dysphagia, dyspnea, cough, sore throat of more than six weeks duration.

DIAGNOSTIC STUDIES

Baseline studies: CBC including platelet count, serum electrolytes, BUN, liver function studies, urinalysis.

Immunologic survey and more extensive blood chemistry may be done for patients receiving chemo/immunotherapy.

Chest x-ray: establish baseline and rule out pulmonary disease and metastasis. Other radiographic studies may be used to further evaluate tumor site and involvement; may be plain films, tomograms, or dye studies.

Scan of the bone, liver, brain, and spleen may be indicated for advanced lesions if distant metastasis is suspected.

Computerized axial tomography (CT scan): to locate intracranial lesions that may be extension of head and neck tumors.

Biopsy may be done before or after the diagnostic procedures already noted.

PHYSICAL EXAMINATION

Laryngoscopy: to visualize tumor. If limited to vocal cords, growth may be slow due to relative low vascularity. Carcinoma in situ may be removed without incision.

Enlarged cervical lymph nodes may be present.

Note other systemic symptoms of metastasis: weight loss caused by dysphagia and inadequate nutritional intake or symptoms caused by pressure of enlarging tumor mass.

NURSING PRIORITIES

1. Keep airway patent, patency maintained.
2. Relieve pain/discomfort.
3. Assist patient in developing alternate methods of communication.
4. Provide support for acceptance of altered body image.

NURSING DIAGNOSIS:	Airway clearance, ineffective.
SUPPORTING DATA:	Laryngectomy causes copious secretions, initially, that the patient may not be able to clear without assistance.
DESIRED PATIENT OUTCOMES:	Patent airway is maintained.

INTERVENTIONS

Elevate head of bed 30–40° when stable.

Encourage coughing and deep breathing to dislodge secretions. Suction using sterile technique p.r.n. Suction nasal and oral cavities gently after suctioning laryngectomy.

Cleanse trach/laryngectomy tube inner cannula every four hours and p.r.n.

Maintain proper position of trach/laryngectomy tube.

Provide supplemental humidification.

Observe for signs of respiratory distress; such as increased rate of respirations, restlessness, use of accessory muscles for breathing.

Use narcotics cautiously.

Observe for bleeding, especially in the first 24 hours.

RATIONALE

Facilitates drainage of secretions and respirations.

Prevents secretions build-up that may obstruct airway. Oral/nasal suctioning required as patient is no longer able to blow nose, and mouth secretions may accumulate due to dysphagia.

Prevents build-up of crusts and hardened secretions that may narrow or obstruct airway.

Continual movement of tube promotes irritation and tissue erosion and airway obstruction. Ties should be snug enough to hold tube in place but not constrict major vascular channels. Make sure there is no undue pressure on skin flap, which may impede proper healing.

Normal humidification is bypassed.

May indicate narrowing of the airway.

May depress cough reflex and respiratory rate.

Surgery may weaken tissue support of carotid artery. Small amount of bleeding may indicate small vessel oozing or herald massive carotid bleed.

NURSING DIAGNOSIS:	Comfort, alteration in, pain.
SUPPORTING DATA:	Pain related to incision and placement of nasogastric tube that may irritate throat.
DESIRED PATIENT OUTCOMES:	Patient is comfortable.

INTERVENTIONS

If dysphagia present, allow patient to expectorate saliva or suction secretions; check for presence of pharyngeal suture line trauma.

Avoid swallowing and movement of the NG tube; provide oral irrigations and gargles several times daily.

Avoid hyperextension of neck by supporting back of neck when assisting to sit; teach self-support of neck.

RATIONALE

Swallowing causes muscle activity that may strain suture line and cause trauma. Limitation of swallowing aides healing early in the postop recovery phase.

Tube may cause sore throat or discomfort. Irrigations, anesthetic gargles may ease discomfort.

Prevents strain on suture line. May have some neck weakness and loss of control due to severing of muscles during surgery. Paralysis, numbness, results from muscle and nerve resection/damage and may affect specific areas. Damage to spinal accessory nerve XI results in strength loss of ipsilateral shoulder muscles.

MEDICAL MANAGEMENT

Aspirin, codeine.

For incisional discomfort. Pain is minimal because many nerves are cut by skin flap incisions.

NURSING DIAGNOSIS: **Communication, impaired verbal.**

SUPPORTING DATA: **Vocal cords removed with radical tumor dissection.**

DESIRED PATIENT OUTCOMES: **Able to communicate adequately.**

INTERVENTIONS

Preoperatively, discuss why speech, breathing are altered, using anatomic drawings or models to assist in explanations.

Refer to loss of speech as temporary.

Encourage working with speech therapist preoperatively as well as postop.

Refer to Lost Chord/New Voice Club, International Association of Laryngectomees, postoperatively.

Postop, give call light/bell for summoning nurse. Provide alternate means of communication, that is, magic slate, paper and pencil, letter board. After reading, destroy note in patient's presence. Do not start IV in writing arm if possible.

Anticipate needs. If asking yes or no questions, the patient may not be able to "shake" head in response due to incision. Allow adequate time for communication. Provide nonverbal communication, such as touching and physical presence.

Encourage patient to plan to return to work 4–8 weeks postop.

Encourage wearing of Medic Alert bracelet.

Discuss electronic voice box, esophogeal, speech, recorded tape for reaching fire, police, or help.

RATIONALE

Visualization enhances understanding of normal anatomy and potential alterations.

Alternate means of communication and speech are available.

Allows practice of esophageal speech while able to ask questions.

Give information on esophageal speech and alternate means of communication; offer support to the laryngectomee.

Establishes means of communication and immediate help if it becomes necessary. Destroying notes protects privacy.

Makes communication easier. Adequate time allows patient to fully express needs without abbreviating or eliminating comments because the staff appears rushed or uncaring. Nonverbal communications reassure of worth and acceptance.

Stimulus for mastering esophageal speech. May settle for electronic device if feels too rushed.

Vital information if patient is unconscious.

Allow patient to select appropriate method(s) that will be comfortable.

NURSING DIAGNOSIS: **Injury, potential for, complications.**

SUPPORTING DATA: **Establishment and maintenance of new airway is required. Suture line placement is over an area of high stress and wounds may be easily contaminated or traumatized.**

DESIRED PATIENT OUTCOMES: **Wounds are healed without infection/complications.**

INTERVENTIONS

Note wound drainage; normal or excessive.

Irrigate or "milk" drainage catheters, usually removed in three days.

Note characteristics of drainage and include total amount in total output. Report any milky appearing drainage.

Observe wound for redness, swelling, exudates, temperature elevation; change dressings immediately when they become damp.

Note edema, especially in lower half of face.

Elevate head of bed 30–45° and encourage patient to sleep on unoperated side.

After dressings have been removed, cleanse incisions with sterile saline and peroxide (mixed 1:1).

Take care to prevent direct trauma when irrigating suture lines in oral cavity. Teach patient how to do own irrigations and encourage use of mouth wash when sutures have healed.

Discuss care of intraoral prosthesis, if used.

Thoroughly cleanse around stoma and neck plates with peroxide and rinse with sterile water. Cleanse with cloth, not cotton, tissue, or cut gauze.

Do not use soap or alcohol to cleanse around stoma. Avoid drugs that dry mucosal secretions.

Keep cloth over stoma, one devoid of lint.

RATIONALE

Continuous blood drainage may indicate small vessel oozing that may necessitate ligation. 200–300 ml may collect from wound in first 24 hours but then should steadily decline.

Keeps tubing patent and allows free flow of drainage to collection site. Build-up or drainage retards healing and provides medium for bacterial growth.

Foul, purulent drainage signifies infection. Milky drainage may indicate thoracic lymph duct leakage that may lead to excessive loss of fluids and electrolytes. Leak may heal spontaneously or require closure.

Signs of infections; moisture enhances bacterial growth and may show fistula formation.

Due to excised lymph channels, some edema is to be expected, but should begin to diminish after four days postop.

Prevents or minimizes edema, which slows healing.

Helps remove crusts to minimize scar formation and prevent infection.

Irrigations stimulate blood supply, decrease infection by maintaining clean surgical area and helping control unpleasant mouth odors. Mouth is now underused and secretions may become stagnant. Also makes foods more palatable.

Helps prevent trauma to tissues and infection.

Cleansing aids healing. Materials other than cloth may leave fibers in stoma causing irritation.

Mucosal drying agents, drugs lead to stomal irritation and possible inflammation.

Covering acts as filter preventing inhalation of foreign bodies and aids cosmetic effect.

MEDICAL MANAGEMENT

Antibiotic ointment to external suture lines.

Prevents infection.

NURSING DIAGNOSIS:	**Nutrition, alteration in, less than body requirements.**
SUPPORTING DATA:	**Mode of intake is altered, temporarily or permanently by the surgery. Air flow through the mouth and nose is changed, limiting taste/ smell feedback mechanisms.**
DESIRED PATIENT OUTCOMES:	**Normal body weight is maintained through self-administered feedings.**

INTERVENTIONS

Obtain preoperative nutritional assessment, food likes/dislikes, eating pattern, food intolerances.

Determine caloric needs for body size, healing.

Discuss role of proper nutrition in wound healing and health maintenance.

Weigh twice weekly.

Teach principles of tube feedings as necessary, stressing self-care.

Provide frequent oral hygiene.

When oral feedings begin (usually after 7–10 days to allow for suture line healing), give water and advance as tolerated. Stay with patient during meals for first few days.

Serve food attractively.

When patient is taking oral feedings, inspect tracheal secretions for presence of food particles. If noted, stop oral feedings immediately and notify physician.

RATIONALE

Helps establish baseline for food selection postop.

Assist in return to optimal health status.

Helps patient understand importance of diet in recovery.

Gives rough estimate of fluid/satisfactory nutritional intake.

Prevents complications, speeds feelings of accomplishment and independence.

Freshens mouth and makes food more palatable.

Fluids are easier to swallow than solid foods. Regular diet helps tone esophagus for esophageal speech. Secretions may be raised and require suctioning during meals.

Sight replaces lost sense of acute taste/smell.

Evidence of esophageal fistula, especially common in patients who have received radiation therapy preoperatively.

NURSING DIAGNOSIS:	**Self-concept, disturbance in, altered body image.**
SUPPORTING DATA:	**Procedure alters body function and facial appearance and patient loses ability to blow nose, smell, suck, gargle, whistle, and lift heavy objects.**

DESIRED PATIENT OUTCOMES:	Verbalizes incorporation of body alterations and limitations to formulate and accept new body image.

INTERVENTIONS

Encourage patient/significant others to communicate feelings to each other. Allow patient to discuss concerns re: mutilation, prognosis, rejection, and so forth.

Alert staff that their facial expressions need to convey acceptance and not revulsion of patient's appearance.

Discuss possibilities of masking deformities produced by resection.

Expect expressions of grief (i.e., withdrawal, anger, crying, mood swings) that are usually most intense during 3–4 days postop. Note signs of severe or prolonged depression.

Be aware that female response to physical change may be more intense.

Encourage visits from laryngectomee and significant others.

Caution family members to treat patient normally and not as an invalid.

Answer call bell immediately. Make note at central answering system that patient is not able to speak. Visit patient frequently.

RATIONALE

Helpful in decreasing anxiety, which may then hasten adaptation.

Patient has fears of being unacceptable and repugnant to others; nurse's reaction may confirm or reject this feeling and leave a lasting impression.

Use of cosmetics, prosthetics, clothes may be helpful.

Even though alterations have been discussed, the finality of surgery forces the patient to face permanent losses. Patient may display prolonged depression or make suicidal gestures that require prompt psychiatric referral.

Loss of voice limits expression, which may be viewed as a sexual attribute and, therefore, a loss of femininity.

Support groups provide opportunities for sharing of hopes and fears. Allows former patient to show successful adaptation and can provide encouragement for the patient.

Treating as an invalid encourages depression, view of self as abnormal, dependent; promotes isolation and feelings of rejection.

Helpful in decreasing anxiety related to inability to call for help. Frequent visits increases feelings that someone is always close by and available for assistance.

Refer to Care Plan: Psychosocial Aspects of Care in the Acute Setting.

NURSING DIAGNOSIS:	Knowledge deficit, postoperative care.
SUPPORTING DATA:	Pre/postoperative teaching involves repeated communications to teach details of care involving wounds, laryngectomy, nutrition, mouth care, airway maintenance and protection.

| DESIRED PATIENT OUTCOMES: | Verbalizes steps and rationale of laryngectomy care and demonstrates correct care postoperatively. |

INTERVENTIONS

Consult with other members of the health team including social services, speech therapy, physical/occupational therapy, nutritionist or dietitian, audiology, maxifacial prosthodontist, and respiratory therapy.

Provide information about procedure, equipment to be used, postop appearance and expectations. Allow patient time for asking questions/ventilating feelings.

Give written directions, booklets for patient/ significant others to read.

Teach patient to suction self in front of mirror. Obtain suction machine for home use if necessary. Give positive reinforcement for efforts.

Teach cleansing of laryngectomy tube to be done every 4–5 days; supervise care during entire procedure each day until patient/significant others are comfortable carrying out procedure.

Teach patient to cover stoma before performing activity that may lead to inhalation of foreign particles (e.g., shaving, use of powder).

Discuss importance of reporting stoma narrowing, presence of ''lump'' in throat, dysphagia, or bleeding immediately to caregiver.

Provide information about wearing Medic Alert bracelet, developing a means of communicating at home in case of emergency.

RATIONALE

Evaluation and consultation preoperatively will assist in postoperative adjustments.

Information may need to be reinforced and clarified many times. Correlation of expectations with probable postop realities facilitates adjustment. Ventilation of feelings helps to relieve tensions and may hasten postop adjustment.

Reinforces proper information and may be used as a home reference.

Airway patency is of paramount importance and suctioning must be done frequently at first. Self-care stimulates independence, boosts ego, and assists in adjustment.

Proper care decreases incidence of complications and speeds healing, but may be frightening. Nurse's presence offers immediate assistance if it is required.

Prevents undue obstruction and irritation to trachea, decreases chance of aspiration of foreign material into lungs.

May be sign of recurrent cancer, tracheal stenosis, or carotid erosion.

Provides for care if patient is unconscious. A tape recording of the address to play for the police, fire department can be helpful.

DIAGNOSIS: Adult Respiratory Distress Syndrome (ARDS)

PATIENT DATA BASE

NURSING HISTORY

Respiratory failure of sudden onset may occur in the previously healthy person who has sustained any type of pulmonary or systemic insult; such as anaphylaxis, aspiration, chemical induced lung injury, disseminated intravascular coagulation (DIC), drug ingestion and overdose, fat or air embolus, head injury, interstitial viral pneumonitis, massive blood transfusions, near-drowning, nonthoracic major trauma, oxygen toxicity, pancreatitis, severe pneumonitis (viral and other), prolonged cardiopulmonary bypass, radiation-induced lung injury, sepsis, shock, smoke and gas inhalation, thoracic trauma, and uremia.

An initial insult is usually followed by a latent period when pulmonary function appears normal but ultimately progresses into respiratory failure.

DIAGNOSTIC STUDIES

Chest x-ray: confirmative rather than diagnostic, owing to delay between pathophysiology and diagnostic cues. Shows diffuse alveolar infiltrates in a honeycombed pattern.

Arterial blood gases: serial comparisons show refractory hypoxemia or lowered arterial oxygen tensions that are poorly responsive to increased concentrations of inspired oxygen (decreased PO_2 even with increased forced inspiratory oxygen [FIO_2]). pH elevation is the result of PCO_2 decreases due to the respiratory alkalemia that accompanies the compensatory increase in rate and depth of breathing.

Serum lactate levels, if the initial insult is due to shock or hypoxemia, the pH change may be attributed to lactic acidosis.

Pulmonary function tests: demonstrate decreasing static and dynamic compliance as well as decrease in lung volumes, especially the FRC (functional residual capacity).

Shunt measurement: QP/QS (pulmonary flow versus systemic flow) provides a clinical measurement of intrapulmonary shunting and a basis for prediction of the maintenance of adequate cardiopulmonary state.

Alveolar-arterial gradient (A-a gradient): provides a comparison of the oxygen tension with alveoli and arterial blood. In the clinical setting, this test demonstrates the difficulty with which oxygen crosses the alveolar capillary membrane, which evaluates the amount of shunting present in the cardiopulmonary system. Normal values: room air-less than 15–20 mm Hg; 100 percent oxygen less than 350 mm Hg.

PHYSICAL EXAMINATION

Abnormal findings on physical examination indicate that the disease process has progressed beyond the early stages.

Central and/or peripheral cyanosis if the patient has greater than 5 grams of desaturated hemoglobin, pallor related to compensatory peripheral vasosconstriction.

Tachypnea, dyspnea, increased work of breathing evidenced by use of accessory muscles of neck, shoulders, and the abdominal muscles, intercostal retractions, flaring of nares.

Restlessness progressing to anxiety, irritability, and finally obtundation.

Also phenomenon that relate to the underlying etiology, such as skin, conjunctival and retinal changes with fat embolism, or singed nasal hairs in pulmonary burns.

On palpation: possible decrease in chest wall expansion, fremitus associated with consolidation, diaphoresis and cool skin associated with later stages related to shock symptoms.

Percussion: notes of dullness over consolidated or fluid-filled areas, decreased diaphragmatic excursion possible.

Auscultation: initially is normal, but crackles (rales), wheezes (rhonchi), and bronchial breath sounds may become apparent as the disease state progresses.

NURSING PRIORITIES

1. Promote and maintain adequate ventilation/perfusion state.
2. Promote satisfactory cardiovascular function, tissue perfusion, and stabilization of vital signs.
3. Promote fluid, electrolyte, and nutritional balance.
4. Maintain normal renal function.
5. Prevent and/or minimize complications related to therapies.
6. Promote patient's/significant others' psychologic adaptation.

NURSING DIAGNOSIS: Gas exchange, impaired.

SUPPORTING DATA: The pathologic changes associated with this disease state impede gas diffusion and may include: thickened alveolar walls, interstitial and intra-alveolar hemorrhage, focal atelectasis, congestion of capillaries, surfactant deficiencies, or development of hyaline membrane decreasing lung compliance. Intrapulmonary shunting or ventilation/perfusion mismatch may involve: perfusion of unventilated alveoli (atelectasis, ARDS, hyaline disease), ventilation of unperfused alveoli (pulmonary embolus).

DESIRED PATIENT OUTCOMES: Absence of signs of respiratory distress. Adequate oxygenation and ventilation with arterial blood gases within normal limits.

INTERVENTIONS

Monitor respiratory status through periodic assessment of pulmonary system.

Note changes in respiratory effort and patterns of breathing.

Assess presence of cyanosis.

RATIONALE

Observing for signs of deterioration.

Reflect pulmonary status, i.e., tachypnea is the compensatory mechanism for hypoxemia. Compensatory physical maneuvers, such as use of intercostal muscles and flaring of nares reflects increased respiratory effort and promotes optimum entry of air into the tracheobronchial system.

Result of desaturation of at least 5 gm of hemoglobin and evidence of a ventilation/perfusion imbalance.

Note decrease in chest wall expansion and presence of or increase in fremitus.

Expansion may be limited or unequal due to accumulation of fluid, edema and secretions in sections/lobes. Lung consolidation and fluid filled areas may increase fremitus.

Note characteristics of breath sounds and presence of adventitious breath sounds, such as crackles, wheezes, or pleural rubs.

Provides information about the flow of air through the tracheobronchial tree and indicates the presence of fluid, mucus, or obstruction. Pulmonary congestion (evidenced by crackles and wheezes) can be associated with increased hydrostatic forces in the pulmonary vascular system, which promotes movement of fluid into tissue spaces and increased permeability of the capillary wall caused by the insult predisposing to ARDS.

Monitor effects of fluid regulation: increase in crackles, wheezes, decrease in ventilation/perfusion as evidenced by ABGs, decrease in cardiac output as evidenced by vital signs, patient symptomatology, and invasive monitoring (PAWP), I & O and daily weight.

Excessive fluid accumulation increases total lung water resulting in a decrease in ventilation and perfusion.
Movement of fluid out of the intravascular space leads to a decrease in cardiac output, which can be determined by continuous hemodynamic and vital signs monitoring.

Facilitate patent airways through pulmonary toilet techniques. Assist with most effective techniques for coughing, i.e., sitting position, breathing techniques, and timing of cough.

Often have increased secretions that impair adequate ventilation. Primary, effective means for removing secretions from the airways.

Do nasotracheal suctioning.

Pooling of secretions decreases ventilation effects and increases the chance of infection.

MEDICAL MANAGEMENT

ABGs.

Document suspicions of hyper/hypoventilation and reveal the status of ventilation and perfusion. Pulmonary therapy is based on arterial blood gases.

Humidified oxygen therapy.

Hypoxemia is a primary concern and must be treated early. May assist in thinning of secretions.

Chest physiotherapy, postural drainage, vibration, and percussion (preferably after aerosol therapy).

Uses gravity and percussion to promote secretion drainage from the lung segments into the central bronchi, where they can be coughed or suctioned out. Secretions drain better from dilated airways, thus, aerosol therapy with drugs or saline should precede these techniques.

Bronchodilators.

To improve ventilation and aid in removal of secretions.

Mucolytic agents.

Liquefy secretions.

Diuretics.

Facilitate the reduction of interstitial edema by decreasing the intravascular hydrostatic pressure.

Steroid therapy.

May be of benefit in reversing ARDS due to its ability to decrease the tendency for WBCs to adhere to pulmonary capillary walls, enhance surfactant production and reducing edema formation by decreasing capillary permeability.

Antibiotics.

Inhibit growth of bacteria in the pooled secretions.

IV fluid therapy, crystalloid versus colloid.

Fluid replacement is a controversial topic due to the purpose/function of each IV solution as it relates to the pulmonary vascular status. Colloids prove effective except when the ARDS process involves leaking capillary endothellium, in which case there would be rapid equilibrium of the protein concentrations between vascular and interstitial spaces and the ventilation/perfusion problem would worsen. Crystalloids provide the benefits of being effective, available, and inexpensive.

Mechanical ventilation via endotracheal intubation.

Early intervention is preferred due to the cyclic sequence of events related to deterioration. Promotes more control of respiratory parameters and pulmonary status. (Refer to Care Plan: Ventilatory Assistance.)

Extracorporeal membrane oxygenation.

Has been used experimentally with only limited benefit to date.

NURSING DIAGNOSIS:	**Tissue perfusion, alteration in.**
SUPPORTING DATA:	**Low cardiac output may be associated with the patient with ARDS on a ventilator, especially with the therapeutic use of PEEP due to the increase in intrathoracic pressure and possible decrease in venous return.**
DESIRED PATIENT OUTCOMES:	**Tissue perfusion maintained as evidenced by adequate urinary output, absence of cardiac arrhythmias, and mental status is maintained.**

INTERVENTIONS

Monitor/assess hemodynamic status: blood pressure, mean arterial pressure if available via arterial line. Pulmonary artery pressure (PAP), mean PAP and pulmonary wedge pressure (PWP) and central venous pressure (CVP); cardiac output/index.

RATIONALE

Blood pressure and mean arterial pressure reflect tissue perfusion. Invasive cardiovascular monitoring is helpful in assessing anticipated cardiovascular compromise. Direct measurement of mixed venous and systemic arterial blood gases, CVP and PWP provide data from which a relationship among PEEP, intrapulmonary shunting, and cardiac output can be determined.

Note findings classically related to decreased perfusion: cool, pale, cyanotic, moist skin.

Vasoconstriction allows the available oxygenated blood to be shunted to vital organs, temporarily satisfy oxygenation and perfusion needs, but eventually proves ineffective as evidenced by a decrease in vital signs. Therapeutic intervention may prove more effective when initiated at the first signs of cardiac decompensation.

Monitor blood lactate levels and arterial blood gases noting metabolic acidosis.

Anaerobic metabolism due to decrease tissue perfusion will lead to a rise in lactate levels and progressive metabolic acidosis.

Measure intake and output.

A decrease in urine output is a fairly good indication of decreased renal perfusion. Renal tubular ischemia may result if hypoxemia and vasoconstriction are prolonged. Also, SIADH may occur when decreased venous return and perfusion to vital organs stimulates ADH secretion.

Monitor BUN and creatinine levels as indicated.

Decreased perfusion of the kidneys reduces the filtration and excretion functions causing a rise in BUN and creatinine levels.

Observe for arrhythmias.

Hypoxemia is commonly associated with irritability of myocardial tissue, producing a variety of ectopics/arrhythmias. In addition, sympathetic stimulation may lead to tachyarrhythmias. Acidosis may depress myocardial automaticity and lead to bradyarrhythmias.

Observe for alterations in mental status associated with hypoxemia: restlessness, agitation, irritability, confusion, personality changes, impaired judgment, memory losses, bizarre behavior deteriorating into obtundation and coma.

Hypotension and respiratory failure lead to tissue hypoxia and alterations in level of consciousness.

Assess bowel sounds, abdominal girth, anorexia, nausea/vomiting, constipation, and GI bleeding.

Sympathetic stimulation associated with the stress of altered blood gases and acid-base disturbances produces vasoconstriction and decreased peristalsis of the GI tract. Prolonged vasoconstriction may result in ulceration of the mucosa of the stomach and/or bowel infarction.

MEDICAL MANAGEMENT

Fluid and RBC transfusions.

Appropriate fluids and blood products may facilitate the conversion of a low-flow state to a high-flow state to reverse hypotension.

Cardiotonic/inotropic agents.

May be necessary if the ventilator support (PEEP) needed to achieve adequate pulmonary function decreases the cardiac output status.

Antacids/cimetidine.

Prevent/minimize possibility of GI bleed.

Fluid restriction and/or declomycin.

Control SIADH.

NURSING DIAGNOSIS: **Nutrition, alteration in, less than body requirements.**

SUPPORTING DATA: **An increase in calories/protein is needed to meet the increased energy requirements of stress, healing, and weaning when the patient has been intubated.**

DESIRED PATIENT OUTCOMES:	Positive nitrogen balance is maintained. Weight is maintained within acceptable range.

INTERVENTIONS

Refer to Care Plan: Total Parenteral Nutrition.

RATIONALE

NURSING DIAGNOSIS:	Coping, ineffective, individual/significant others.
SUPPORTING DATA:	Care of the critically ill patient in an ICU involves a variety of mechanisms that may contribute to an inability to cope. Sensory deprivation/overload, sleep deprivation, fear and anxiety about the unknown, and depersonalization because of staff preoccupation with monitors and equipment are examples of what may occur.
DESIRED PATIENT OUTCOMES:	Remains oriented and alert. Depression and psychotic behavior prevented or minimized.

INTERVENTIONS

Give information about progress and activities on an ongoing basis.

Schedule patient activities so periods of rest alternate with nursing care.

Provide for a quiet environment and position equipment out of view as much as possible.

Provide meaningful conversation while performing care.

Use clocks, calendars, bulletin boards, and frequent references to time, place, and so forth.

Refer to Care Plan: Psychosocial Aspects of Care in the Acute Setting.

RATIONALE

When kept abreast of what is happening, anxiety can be minimized and trust established.

Sleep deprivation can easily occur if attention is not given to this factor.

Sensory overload may encourage auditory and visual hallucinations.

Will be helpful to sensory stimulation and personalization.

Facilitates orientation to environment.

CARE PLAN: Ventilatory Assistance (Mechanical)

PATIENT DATA BASE

Mechanical ventilation is initiated whenever the ventilatory function of the patient fails to maintain an adequate pulmonary gas exchange. For data base discussion, refer to care plan appropriate to underlying disease process.

INTERVENTIONS	RATIONALE
Maintain a patent airway by proper endotracheal tube placement/taping.	Due to anatomical structure of the mainstem bronchi, the endotracheal tube may slip into the right mainstem if positioned too low, thereby, obstructing airflow to the left lung.
Inflate tracheal/endotracheal tube cuff using the minimal air leak or occlusive technique.	The cuff must be adequately inflated to provide a closed system between the patient and the respirator. Underinflation of the endotracheal tube cuff may allow aspiration of gastric contents or saliva. Overinflation may cause tracheal tissue necrosis or may herniate the cuff over the tip of the tube causing partial or complete airway obstruction.
Turn patient every 1–2 hours. Alternate side-to-side and semi-Fowler's position.	Both ventilation and perfusion can be preferentially delivered to the segments of the lung through positioning maneuvers that promote drainage of some segments and ventilation of others.
Use nonverbal as well as verbal communication. Provide slate/pencil; maintain IV in nonwriting arm.	Patients experience fear, helplessness, and despair and communication is necessary.
Evaluate respiratory status periodically noting bilateral breath sounds and symmetry of chest movement.	Auscultation provides information regarding the flow of air through the tracheobronchial tree and the presence of fluid, mucus, or obstruction. Evaluation of symmetry with respirations provides information about air flow to lungs and may identify right mainstem intubation.
Suction airway as necessary.	The intubated patient usually has an ineffective cough reflex due to the interference of the tube with glottis closure. Suctioning should not be routine, because unnecessary suctioning may produce excessive tracheal irritation.
Hyperventilation with Ambu bag or ventilator sigh and oxygenation pre/post suctioning, with 100% O_2 for 1–5 minutes.	Hyperventilation minimizes atelectasis related to suctioning. High concentrations of oxygen provided prior to and following suctioning assist in preventing myocardial hypoxia and cardiac arrhythmias.
Monitor ECG during suctioning.	Hypoxia is a common cause of arrhythmias. Ventilated patients have ventilation/perfusion imbalances and often have hypoxia/hypoxemia.

Maintain respiratory parameters within normal limits by frequent checks on ordered ventilatory settings every hour.

Oxygen percentage.

The lowest possible FIO_2 capable of promoting adequate oxygenation should be provided to the patient; lower levels (less than 50%) can be used for long periods of time without evidence of oxygen toxicity.

Tidal volume.

Indicates the amount of air breathed in and out of the airway during a normal respiratory cycle. Changes may indicate leakage through the machine or cuff and will affect oxygenation.

Inspiratory-expiratory ratio.

The relationship of inspiration to expiration is such that expiration is twice the length of the inspiratory phase. Changes in I:E ratio will affect ventilation and perfusion.

Sensitivity.

Determines the amount of negative pressure that the patient must generate in the assist mode to trigger the ventilator. If the sensitivity is not adjusted, the patient can hyperventilate or at the other extreme, fight for air.

Airway pressure.

Once the tidal volume has been established, the airway pressure should remain relatively constant. An increase in the pressure reading on the manometer may reflect an increase in the amount of pressure needed to deliver a set volume of gas as occurs with increases in airway resistance and/or decreases in lung compliance as may occur with pneumothorax, pulmonary edema, misplacement of the ET tube.

Sigh (frequency and volume).

Frequency and volume of sigh affect the ventilation of the alveoli, promote cough, and help prevent atelectasis.

Humidity and temperature.

The usual warming/humidifying function of the nasopharynx has been bypassed with intubation. Humidification is necessary to maintain secretions at normal viscosity. The temperature of inspired gas should be maintained at approximately body temperature.

Rate.

Respirations should be counted for one full minute comparing the patient's respiratory rate with set ventilatory rate. Rapid respiratory rates due to the patient's triggering of the ventilator can produce abnormal blood gas values.

Alarm system.

Mechanical ventilators involve a series of audible and visual alarms to reflect abnormal ventilator changes and increase ventilator efficiency and patient safety, e.g., low/high pressure alarms, I:E ratio alarms, oxygen alarm. These alarms should never be turned off even when suctioning.

Evaluate response to mechanical ventilation:
Level of consciousness and responsiveness and monitor ABGs.

Assessment of orientation is difficult in view of intubation. Changes may be early indicators of hypoxia, as noted by ABGs. Due to nature of illness requiring intubation, frequent status checks, sensory stimuli of respirator and other monitors/equipment, these patients are prone to sensory overload/sleep deprivation, and disorientation.

Patient respirations related to respirator.

If the patient is "fighting the respirator," adjustments can be made to minimize spontaneous respirations. Problem is particularly dangerous because it can lead to pneumothorax, cardiovascular collapse, and airway trauma.

Constant supervision and care are required if Pavulon is used.

Complete paralysis makes the patient totally dependent on respirator for breathing and on nursing staff for general care.

Maintenance of optimal PEEP; avoid routine suctioning.

Each time the ventilator is disconnected, the PEEP is lost and it takes time to reestablish effective alveolar pressures again.

Recognize side effects/complications:
Atelectasis evidenced through auscultation/palpation and tracheal position.

Localized atelectasis may occur as result of retained secretions. Trachea will shift toward the affected side.

Decreased cardiac output evidenced by decrease in blood pressure and pulse.

The positive pressures generated increase the intrathoracic pressure, which can potentially decrease venous return resulting in a decrease in BP and pulses (especially with the use of PEEP).

Monitor signs of pneumothorax (barotrauma):
Asymmetrical chest movements; diminished/absent breath sounds on affected side; tachycardia with weak pulse; cyanosis; hypotension, decreased cardiac output; accumulation of air under skin, crackling of skin with palpation; displacement of trachea. Note tracheal position.

Pressures generated by the PEEP mode of ventilation may promote rupture of the alveoli walls, allowing air leaks into the pleural space, mediastinum and/or subcutaneous spaces, resulting in accumulation of pressures in excess of atmospheric pressure. The lung collapses (pneumothorax), and great vessels in the mediastinum become compressed and occluded, resulting in circulatory collapse. Trachea shifts away from the affected side. Depending on the size of pneumothorax and/or mediastinal or subcutaneous emphysema, chest tubes insertion may be necessary. (Refer to Care Plan: Pneumothorax.)

In preparation for weaning:
Monitor the tests related to respiratory status.

ABGs, electrolytes, measures of lung compliance, and ventilation/perfusion ratio provide information for the weaning decision.

Discuss procedure, length of ventilation; stay with patient during initial periods off ventilator.

Patient has developed a dependence on the ventilator and often feels uncomfortable being alone. This preparation can be helpful psychologically to the patient.

Assess respirations and ventilator breaths per minute; record tidal volume for each during use of IMV for weaning.

Allows the patient's own breathing pattern to be maintained with positive breaths intermittently by the respirator.

Monitor for signs of respiratory distress.	Early detection and treatment of respiratory difficulty will prevent possibility of return to the respirator.

MEDICAL MANAGEMENT

Arterial line and serial ABGs.	To assess effectiveness of ventilator and weaning.
Bronchodilators.	Use may reduce obstruction to gas exchange that may be related to bronchial edema and bronchospasms.
Pavulon.	Sedation or paralysis alleviates the problem of "fighting the respirator." Does make the patient completely dependent on mechanical ventilation.
Sedatives.	The use of Pavulon does not affect the ability to think and sedation is important to reduce the unpleasant feelings that accompany the use of this drug.
Addition of PEEP to ventilator regimen.	Promotes alveolar expansion and helps to prevent shunting of blood through unventilated areas of the lung, thereby increasing FRC and optimizing the oxygen gradient across the alveolar/capillary membrane.
IMV, SIMV, or other appropriate weaning techniques.	Promotes use and gradual strengthening of the respiratory muscles and the central nervous system respiratory centers that are responsible for regulating respiration while providing minimum support by the mechanical ventilator.

BIBLIOGRAPHY

Books and Other Individual Publications

ARMSTRONG, M. (ED.): *Handbook of Clinical Nursing.* McGraw-Hill, New York, 1979.

BAUM, G. (ED.): *Textbook of Pulmonary Diseases,* ed. 2. Little, Brown & Co., Boston, 1974.

BERGERSEN, B. AND KRUG, E.: *Pharmacology in Nursing,* ed. 11. C. V. Mosby, St. Louis, 1969.

BEYERS, M. AND DUDAS, S.: *The Clinical Practice of Medical-Surgical Nursing.* Little, Brown & Company, Boston, 1977.

BLELAND, I.: *Clinical Nursing Pathophysiological and Psychosocial Approaches,* ed. 2. MacMillan, New York, 1970.

BOME, J.: *Management of Thoracic Emergencies,* ed. 3. Appleton-Century-Crofts, New York, 1980.

BURTON, G., GEE, G., AND HUDGKIN, H.: *Respiratory Care, A Guide to Clinical Practice.* J. B. Lippincott, Philadelphia, 1977.

BRUNNER, L. S. AND SUDDARTH, D. S.: *The Lippincott Manual of Nursing Practice,* ed. 2. J. B. Lippincott, Philadelphia, 1980.

BUDASSI, S. H. AND BARBER, J. M.: *Emergency Nursing: Principles and Practice.* C.V. Mosby, St. Louis, 1981.

BURGESS, A. AND LAZARE, A.: *Psychiatric Nursing in the Hospital and in the Community.* Prentice-Hall, Englewood Cliffs, New Jersey, 1976.

COMROE, J.: *Physiology of Respiration,* ed. 2. Year Book Medical Publishers, Chicago, 1975.

CRAYTOR, J. AND FARR, M. L.: *The Nurse and the Cancer Patient, A Programmed Text.* J. B. Lippincott, Philadelphia, 1980.

ELLIS, J. R. AND NOWLIS, E. A.: *Nursing, A Human Needs Approach.* Houghton Mifflin, Boston, 1977.

FISHMAN, A.: *Pulmonary Diseases and Disorders,* McGraw-Hill, New York, 1980.

FRASER, R. AND PARE, J.: *Diagnosis of Diseases of the Chest,* Vol. I, II, III, ed. 2. W. B. Saunders, Philadelphia, 1979.

GUENTER, C. AND WELCH, M.: *Pulmonary Medicine.* J. B. Lippincott, Philadelphia, 1977.

GUYTON, A. C.: *Basic Human Physiology: Normal Function and Mechanisms of Disease.* W. B. Saunders, Philadelphia, 1977.

HART, L. K. ET AL.: *Concepts Common to Acute Illness: Identification and Management.* C. V. Mosby, St. Louis, 1981.

HINSHAW, H. AND MURRY, J.: *Diseases of the Chest,* ed. 4. W. B. Saunders, 1980.

JOHANSON, B. C. ET AL.: *Standards for Critical Care.* C. V. Mosby, St. Louis, 1981.

KIM, M. AND MORITZ, D. (EDS.): *Classification of Nursing Diagnosis.* McGraw-Hill, New York, 1981.

LUCKMAN, J. AND SORENSEN, K. C.: *Medical-Surgical Nursing,* ed. 2. W. B. Saunders, Philadelphia, 1980.

MAYERS, J.: *Human Nutrition, Its Physiological, Medical and Social Aspects.* Charles C Thomas, Springfield, 1979.

RAREY, K. P. AND YOUTSEY, J. W.: *Respiratory Patient Care.* Prentiss-Hall, Englewood Cliffs, New Jersey, 1981.

ROBINSON, C. H. AND LAWLER, M.: *Normal and Therapeutic Nutrition,* ed. 15. Macmillan, New York, 1977.

SECOR, J.: *Patient Care in Respiratory Problems.* W. B. Saunders, Philadelphia, 1969.

SHAPIRO, B., HARRISON, R., AND TROUT, C.: *Clinical Applications of Respiratory Care,* ed. 2. Year Book Medical Publishers, Chicago, 1979.

SLONIM, N. AND HAMILTON, L.: *Respiratory Physiology,* ed. 3. C. V. Mosby, St. Louis, 1976.

SPENCER, H. AND LIEBOW, A.: *Pathology of the Lung (excluding Pulmonary Tuberculosis),* Vol. I, II, ed. 3. Pergamon Press, Oxford, 1977.

SWEETWOOD, H. M.: *Nursing in the Intensive Respiratory Care Unit,* ed. 2. Springer-Verlag, New York, 1979.

TILKIAN, S. M., CONOVER, M. B., AND TILKIAN, A. G.: *Clinical Implications of Laboratory Tests.* C. V. Mosby, St. Louis, 1979.

TUCKER, S. ET AL.: *Patient Care Standards,* ed. 2. C. V. Mosby, St. Louis, 1980.

VREDEVOE, D. L. ET AL.: *Concepts of Oncology Nursing.* Prentiss-Hall, Englewood Cliffs, New Jersey, 1981.

WILKINS, R. W. AND LEVINSKY, N. G. (EDS.): *Medicine, Essentials of Clinical Practice.* Little, Brown & Co., Boston, 1978.

Journal Articles

BROOKS, C. G., JR.: *Artificial mechanical ventilation of the adult. Fine Tuning, Part 2.* CCN, 1:8+, 1981.

CHISHOLM, E.: *Pleural effusion followed by emphysema . . . Community nursing care study.* Nursing Times, Nov. 11/17; 77:1966–68, 1981.

CLINE, C. ET AL.: *ARDS means emergency.* Nursing (Horsham), Feb. 12:62–7, 1982.

DE TOLEDO, L. W.: *Caring for the patient instead of the ventilator.* RN, 43:20–3+, 1980.

FATHERS, B.: *Nursing care study: Mycoplasma pneumonia.* Nursing Times, 1661–64, Vol. 77, No. 39, Sept. 1981.

HARPER, R. W.: *Application of alveolar ventilation physiology.* DCCN, 1:80–6, 1980.

HUNTER, P. M.: *Symposium on respiratory care. Bedside monitoring of respiratory function.* NCNA, 16:211–24, 1981.

JACOBS, M. M. ET AL.: *Proticol; chronic obstructive lung disease.* Nursing Practice, Nov./Dec. 4:11+, 1979.

NETT, L. M.: *Respiratory care today—and tomorrow.* Heart Lung, 11:58–9, 1982.

PETERSON, B.: *Application and assessment of O_2 therapy devices.* Nursing Clinics of North America; Symposium on Respiratory Care, June, 241–258. W. B. Saunders, Philadelphia, 1981.

PULOR, W. H. ET AL.: *Pleural effusions by chromosome analysis.* Chest, Feb.: 81:193–7, 1982.

QUICK, G.: *Penetrating chest wounds* (pictorial). Critical Care Update, 9:14–5+, Jan. 1982.

ROKOSKY, J.: *Assessment of the individual with altered respiratory function.* Nursing Clinics of North America; Symposium on Respiratory Care, June, 195–210. W. B. Saunders, Philadelphia, 1981.

SMITH, M.: *Respiratory emergencies.* Nursing Mirror, 154, Clinical Forum, ii–iv+, Nov. 1980.

STEVENS, G. H.: *The unnecessary stress imposed on ARDS patients.* Respiratory Therapy, Jan./Feb. 12:21–4, 1982.

VAUGHN, P.: *Acute respiratory failure in the patient with chronic obstructive lung disease-home study program.* CCN, 1:44–68, 1981.

CHAPTER 5
NEUROLOGIC

DIAGNOSIS: Headache (Including Migraine)

PATIENT DATA BASE

NURSING HISTORY

Headache may be preceded by aura and/or neurologic disturbances and varies in onset, frequency, duration, characteristics, location, and early symptoms.

Complains of headache, generalized or localized, steady or intermittent, occurring at specific times during the day, aggravated by specific postures, activities.

History of total parenteral nutrition: may cause headache when administered too rapidly.

Recent lumbar puncture.

Use of birth control pills, onset of menses or occurrence of menopause perhaps causing headache due to endocrine change.

Activities that might produce eyestrain, such as close handwork or reading.

History of head trauma, hypertension: family history of headaches.

DIAGNOSTIC STUDIES

Lumbar puncture: to document increased cerebrospinal fluid pressure and presence of abnormal amounts of cells, blood, or infection.

Electroencephalography: record brain activity signifying seizure disorder and/or location of brain lesions.

Brain scan: detect intracranial lesions.

Echoencephalography: for location of normal structures to document displacement because of trauma, cerebrovascular disease, or space-occupying lesion.

CT scan: detect intracranial masses and ventricular shifts.

Cerebral arteriography: substantiate vascular lesions, such as aneurysms, malformation, space-occupying lesion.

CBC: detect leukocytosis signifying systemic infection or anemia, polycythemia.

Skull x-rays: may show one erosion, deviation of structures indicating space-occupying lesion.

PHYSICAL EXAMINATION

Complete ocular exam: to detect abnormalities or muscle control problems.

Ear exam: inspect tympanic membrane for signs of infections, rupture

Exam of nasal structures: increased pain on bending over or pressure over sinuses may indicate infection.

Exam of neck, shoulder, scalp muscles: tenderness/rigidity may indicate tension.

Dental exam: infection, damage that may cause nerve irritation and exposure, to rule out cardiovascular disease as cause of pain referred to teeth, jaw.

Headache can be a symptom of an underlying disorder and may occur with or without the presence of organic disease.

NURSING PRIORITIES

1. Increase patient comfort.
2. Assist in the detection and elimination of underlying disease.
3. Provide patient with information regarding cause/treatment/prevention, and complications.
4. Assist patient/significant others in dealing with lifestyle changes that may be necessary.

NURSING DIAGNOSIS:	**Comfort, alteration in, pain.**
SUPPORTING DATA:	**Irritation/pressure on nerves and increased intracranial pressure produce pain and other associated symptoms.**
DESIRED PATIENT OUTCOMES:	**Pain is minimized/managed and patient is comfortable.**

INTERVENTIONS	RATIONALE
Place in darkened room.	May have photosensitivity, which intensifies attack in migraine/vascular/cluster headaches.
Encourage rest with quiet environment.	Activity increases blood pressure; may worsen headache.
Take vital signs every 30 minutes × 4, then every 3 hours if stable.	Hypertension/hypertensive crisis may cause headache; increased intracranial pressure may cause alteration of vital signs.
Observe for nausea/vomiting.	Frequently occurs in migraines.
Apply cold compresses to forehead.	Soothing and decreases vasodilation fever.
Massage head/neck/shoulder muscles, manually stretching nuchal/occipital muscles.	Relieves tension and promotes relaxation of muscles.

Allow expression of feelings and explore sources of tension by frequent contact, listening.

Enables patient to release tension, recognize nature of feelings and relationship to the pain. May be resentful of the affliction and accompanying disabilities causing anger/depression. Verbal expression of anger can facilitate adjustment.

Give diet as tolerated; for hangover, give high-protein, low-carbohydrate diet.

Stabilizes blood sugar after alcohol ingestion.

Avoid temperature extremes.

Hot/cold may aggravate headache.

Explore the use of therapeutic touch, visualization and imagery, biofeedback, and other alternative methods of healing.

Can be useful tools for relaxation and provide a sense of self-control.

Refer to pain clinic.

May be necessary when problem is chronic and intractable.

MEDICAL MANAGEMENT

Aspirin/Tylenol.

Nonaddicting and may relieve pain.

Ergotamine tartrate.

Give within 30–60 minutes of beginning of migraine attack.

Narcotic analgesics.

May be necessary when pain is severe, or unrelieved by other measures. Should be avoided if possible, as may be habit-forming and great relief and euphoria produced may result in patient unwillingness to accept other forms of therapy. Give only as ordered if intracranial pressure is suspected, as may mask symptoms or depress CNS.

Pressure over unilateral common carotid.

Reduce fluid load to brain.

Sedatives.

May be needed p.r.n. to provide for rest and decreased activity.

Antihypertensives.

When hypertension is the underlying cause.

Prednisone.

Decreases inflammation.

Mannitol, urea.

Causes dehydration of cerebral tissues to decrease pressure.

Antibiotics.

Treats cause of inflammation and swelling.

Refer to appropriate care plans related to the underlying cause, such as hypertension.

NURSING DIAGNOSIS:	**Knowledge deficit, cause/treatment.**
SUPPORTING DATA:	**Headaches have many causes and treatments, and patients need information to make necessary decisions/changes in lifestyle and/or cooperate with medical treatment.**

DESIRED PATIENT OUTCOMES:	Verbalizes causes of headache and regimen necessary for prevention/ treatment.

INTERVENTIONS

RATIONALE

Discuss cause of disease and relationship to headache.

Can relieve anxiety by providing information and clearing up misconceptions.

Discuss medication regimen and side effects.

Important for patient to be aware of all aspects of medication regimen to be able to use appropriately.

Discuss precipitating or aggravating factors.

Avoidance can often prevent development of attacks.

Instruct patient/significant others in massage, exercises and other helpful techniques.

Massage is soothing, helps relax shoulder tension; exercises can relieve shoulder and neck tightness. Refer to Interventions discussed in Nursing Diagnosis: Comfort, alteration in, pain

Discuss importance of raised shoulders, body posture, and tightness.

Lowering shoulders can decrease muscle tension and relaxation of body posture can provide overall relief of tension.

HEADACHES: CHARACTERISTICS AND MANAGEMENT

POST-TRAUMATIC:

Usually caused by local tissue damage.

Characteristics:
Onset is after injury and frequency is variable. They are often associated with vertigo, insomnia, nausea, irritability. Careful evaluation is warranted to identify disorder when legal action is involved.

Management:
Psychologic support, counseling, mild analgesics.

SINUS:

Caused by inflammatory process, injury to sinus because of ostia pressure.

Characteristics:
Onset is gradual with no prodromal symptoms and frequency is variable. Usually begins in AM and subsides in PM. It is dull, aching, worse with change in head position, but no nausea and vomiting. Chronic sinus headache may result in osteomyelitis and adjacent cranial tissue involvement. If persists after drainage of sinuses consider extradural/subdural involvement.

Management:
Analgesics, decongestants, antibiotics after culture of mucus is taken.

EYE:

Characteristics:
Onset is gradual and may be intermittent or continuous. No prodromal symptoms are noted. Nausea and vomiting may accompany it; location is behind the eyes or may be generalized; iritis may cause it.

Management:
Correction of conditions producing strain; aspirin/Tylenol. Treatment of trauma, eye patch, immobilization of iris, prednisone to decrease inflammation. Decrease lighting and cool cloth on forehead and eyes may provide symptomatic relief.

MUSCLE TENSION:

Caused by sustained contraction of face, scalp, neck muscles.

Characteristics:
Onset is gradual with no prodromal symptoms. Pain may last for hours, days, or years. It is nonpulsatile, unilateral/bilateral, head-band location, tightness, muscles may become tender and patient limits use. May be aggravated by cold; pressure on tender muscles increases intensity of pain, tinnitus, dizziness, lacrimation, or these may occur spontaneously.

Management:
Psychologic support, massage, manual stretching of nuchal and occipital muscles. Aspirin/Tylenol, phenobarbital (30mg TID), muscle relaxants, heat, and time.

TEETH:

Due to irritation of branches of fifth cranial nerve from extractions, inflammation.

Characteristics:
Onset is variable after trauma or onset of disease. It is continuous with no prodromal symptoms. Usually pain is distributed along trigeminal branches causing surface hypersensitivity, eye pain, redness, and may cause aching of other head areas.

Management:
Aspirin/Tylenol, warm compress, if possible, to inflamed area. Antibiotics if indicated. Dental care.

EAR:

Pain from pressure, irritation of nerves and surrounding areas, contraction of surrounding muscles (e.g., acute otitis media, ruptured tympanic membrane, fractured bone).

Characteristics:
Variable occurrence after onset of disease/trauma. No prodromal symptoms; continuous or intermittent depending on cause. May be accompanied by vertigo, fever. Pain is usually well localized but may be generalized and deceptive.

Management:
Aspirin/Tylenol, warm compresses to area, antibiotics as indicated, immobilization.

INCREASED INTRACRANIAL PRESSURE:

Caused by irritation of pain-sensitive structures. Usually caused by space-occupying lesion or inflammation.

Characteristics:
Insidious onset; steady and continuous and may be accompanied by abnormal neurologic signs. Most commonly frontal or occipital but may be anywhere, generalized or localized. Deep, aching, usually more intense in AM, aggravated by stooping, straining, or other activities that increase intracranial pressure. Does not interfere with sleep. May intermittently block cerebral ventricular system causing marked, sudden increase in intracranial pressure that may be fatal; lasts approximately 30 minutes and ends abruptly. Inflammation causes pain that may be pulsatile.

Management:
ASA, cold packs, removal of mass. Transient decompression; increased doses of corticosteroids, IV mannitol, urea, irradiation; ventricular drainage/shunting. Antibiotics as needed.

VASCULAR (MIGRAINE OR CLUSTER):

May be caused by sepsis, carbon monoxide, epilepsy, hangover, rectal/urinary bladder distention, hypertension, inflamed cerebral tissues.

Characteristics:
Migraines more common in women; cluster headaches more common in men, aged 20–40. Rapid onset, may occur frequently or infrequently, lasts hours to days. Variable symptoms one hour prior to occurrence. Temporal, frontal, supraorbital most common, but may be any location. May be associated with neck/face pain. May have atypical neuralgia, unusually forceful throbbing in neck area. May be accompanied by vomiting, photophobia, vertigo, redness of eyes, lacrimation, epistaxis, nasal congestion. Cluster headaches may wake patient. May be aggravated by some foods, such as wine, cheese, chocolate.

Management:
ASA, antiemetics, narcotics. Pressure on common carotid and affected artery. Ergotrate, Cafergot, sedatives. Methysergide as serotonin antagonist to prevent occurrence. Antihypertensives, prednisone, Inderal, lithium, Bellergal.

HANGOVER

Give high-protein, low-carbohydrate diet.

DIAGNOSIS: Seizure Disorders

PATIENT DATA BASE

NURSING HISTORY

History of seizures observed by others.

Complains of blackout spells, periods of amnesia, mental disturbances, muscle tremors, uncontrolled muscle movements, loss of muscle tone, abnormal sensations or hallucinations, other bodily disturbances.

SEIZURE ACTIVITY

May be secondary to hyperpyrexia, CNS disease or trauma, hypoxia, toxic agents, metabolic disturbances, anaphylaxis, degenerative brain disorders and may be transient or recurring.

IDIOPATHIC SEIZURES

Usually begin before age 20 and rarely after age 30 and may be due to congenital defects, birth injuries. May be elicited by sudden loud noise, music, flickering lights, exhaustion, drugs, sleep, and perhaps emotional stimuli.

LABORATORY EVALUATION

EEG: may help locate specific cerebral area of malfunction, type of episode, characteristics.

Telemetry computer equipment monitors brain electrical activity to help identify prodromal period of seizure so that occurrences may be predicted and/or controlled.

Skull x-rays to note changes, space-occupying lesions.

CT scan to detect congenital abnormalities, masses.

Lumbar puncture may detect abnormal pressure or show signs of bleeding or infection.

Cerebral angiography shows area of mass, atherosclerosis.

PHYSICAL EXAMINATION

Neurologic exam noting signs of increased intracranial pressure, cranial nerve dysfunction, altered deep tendon reflexes.

Disturbance of perception, mentation, special senses, involuntary movements, recurrent loss of or altered consciousness.

Areas of paralysis, paresthesia, hypersensitivity, abnormal deep tendon reflexes.

SEIZURES: CHARACTERISTICS

Grand mal: with petit mal, make up only 10 percent of all seizure activity. Grand mal lasts 2–5 minutes; tonic phase lasts 30–60 seconds, pupils dilate, respirations jerky and stertorous, excessive saliva blown from mouth creating froth. Postictally, sleep 30 minutes to several hours followed by confusion and amnesia for the episode, nausea, stiff and sore muscles, injuries may be present from unprotected fall.

Petit mal: periods of altered consciousness lasting 5–30 seconds. Minor motor seizures may be akinetic (loss of movement), myoclonic (repetitive motor contractions), or atonic (loss of muscle tone).

Psychomotor: arise from the temporal lobe. Patient generally remains conscious while involuntary motor symptoms occur. May display psychologic reactions, such as irritability, hostility, or fear, and behaviors that appear purposeful but are inappropriate. Postictally the patient has no memory for these events.

Focal-Motor: arise from the posterior frontal lobe (motor cortex); sensory arise from the parietal (numbness, tingling), occipital (bright, flashing lights); posterior temporal (difficulty speaking). Often preceded by aura and last 2–15 minutes and may produce drowsiness postictally. If restrained during seizure, may exhibit combative and uncooperative behavior.

Status epilepticus: continuous seizure activity usually because of abrupt withdrawal of anticonvulsants and other metabolic phenomena.

NURSING PRIORITIES

1. Protect from injury.
2. Provide information to assist patient/significant others to deal with necessary lifestyle alterations.

NURSING DIAGNOSIS: **Injury, potential for.**

SUPPORTING DATA: **Seizures usually involve loss of muscle control/consciousness, patients are prone to injuries.**

DESIRED PATIENT OUTCOMES: **Seizure activity is controlled/eliminated and injuries are prevented.**

INTERVENTIONS	RATIONALE
Assess for signs/symptoms of hypoglycemia.	May precipitate seizure activity.
Keep accurate intake and output and electrolyte levels.	Imbalances may affect/predispose to seizure activity.
Observe for side effects and effectiveness of drug therapy. Monitor drug blood levels.	Therapeutic level may be close to toxic level.
Observe for respiratory depression, arrhythmias.	May result from drug therapy.
Do neurologic check after seizure and p.r.n.	Documents postictal state and helps differentiate site of seizure stimulus.
Identify and avoid precipitating factors.	Prevents seizure activity.
Seizure precautions:	
Keep on strict bed rest; do not allow up to bathroom.	Often patients will become restless or feel need to defecate prior to seizuring.
Keep side rails up and fully padded.	Minimizes injury.

Keep bite stick/airway at bed with suction equipment.	If inserted prior to seizure, bite stick may help prevent biting of tongue during seizure; some sources believe bite stick creates more harm because of injuries sustained when inserted after seizure begins. Wooden tongue blades should not be used as they may splinter and break in the patient's mouth causing further injuries.
Do not allow any unsupervised smoking.	May cause minor or serious burns if accidentally dropped.
During seizure, protect patient:	
Loosen clothing, turn to side, move away from dangerous areas/objects.	Prevent airway obstruction and injuries.
Do not attempt to restrain.	May injure restraining person or increase erratic movement.
Surround with padding if possible, especially under head.	Prevents head and body injuries.
Suction p.r.n.	Maintain airway and prevent aspiration when salivation is excessive.
During seizure note:	
If aura was present, how seizure began and progressed, how long seizure lasted, if cyanosis and incontinence occurred, deviation of eyes, postictal symptoms.	Helps locate area of brain involvement that stimulated seizure.
After seizure:	
Take vital signs every 5 and then every 15 minutes, reorient, place on bed rest until fully recovered.	

MEDICAL MANAGEMENT

High doses of oral anticonvulsants.	Raise the seizure threshold. Large doses of a single drug seem to be more effective than smaller doses of several drugs.
Ancillary drugs, i.e., Diamox, Dexedrine.	May enhance effects of major anticonvulsants.
IV anticonvulsant (Dilantin), Valium, phenobarbital.	For status epilepticus: may lead to brain damage because during this time brain glucose and oxygenation are inadequate due to increased metabolic demands.
Oxygen, Ambu bag.	Increase available oxygen during seizure activity and limit hypoxia.
Surgery.	May be useful in limited cases with well-defined ectopic foci and inadequate control with drug therapy.

NURSING DIAGNOSIS:	**Knowledge deficit, disease management.**

SUPPORTING DATA:	Lack of information, societal attitudes, and amnesia of events create an anxiety-producing situation.
DESIRED PATIENT OUTCOMES:	Verbalizes reason for seizure disorder, and treatment regimen.

INTERVENTIONS

Avoid overprotecting patient; allow to partake in as many activities as possible with adequate supervision.

Teach significant others care of patient during and after seizure.

Wear ID (MedicAlert) tag stating they have epilepsy and name of physician.

Discuss importance of maintaining good general health with adequate diet, rest, avoidance of alcohol, caffeine and stimulant drugs; and activity short of fatigue.

Discuss feelings regarding diagnosis of epilepsy.

Discuss and stress importance of taking drugs as ordered.

Discuss side effects of prescribed drug therapy: gingival hypertrophy, visual disturbances nausea/vomiting, rashes, syncope/ataxia, confusion.

CBC every 6 months, or if sore throat and fever occur.

Discuss need for good oral hygiene/regular dental care.

Take medications with meals.

Do not take/discontinue drugs without permission of physician.

Refer to National Epilepsy League or National Association to Control Epilepsy, Inc.

RATIONALE

Participating in as many experiences as possible can lessen depression about limitations.

Decreases feelings of helplessness and dependence. May prevent complications and brings incurred injuries to attention of medical personnel for treatment.

Expedites treatment in emergencies.

Deficiencies, exhaustion, alcohol, emotional upsets tend to precipitate seizures.

Important to allow patient to verbalize fears, anger, and concerns about future implications.

Need to know risk of status epilepticus resulting from abrupt withdrawal of anticonvulsants.

Important for patient/significant others to verbalize knowledge of potential problems from long-term drug use and take appropriate action to minimize/control.

Testing necessary to monitor for serious side effect of agranulocytosis.

Prevent oral infections

If nausea/vomiting is present.

Prescribed drugs may have many interactions with other drugs.

Opportunity to gain further information, support, and ideas for dealing with problems from others with same diagnosis.

DIAGNOSIS: Increased Intracranial Pressure

PATIENT DATA BASE

NURSING HISTORY

History of drug overdose, poisoning, head trauma, loss of consciousness, neurologic disease and treatment, infection.

History of sudden short episodes of dizziness, frequent headache (especially early morning), loss of ability to speak, blackout spells, syncope.

History of hypertension, obesity, diabetes mellitus, heart disease, vascular disease, embolic disease, transient ischemic attacks (TIAs), elevated serum cholesterol, cigarette smoking.

Progressive changes in mental status, confusion, lethargy, agitation, drowsiness, changes in motor function, weakness, unsteady gait, temporary paresthesia/paralysis.

Changes in visual acuity, loss of part of visual field, deviation of eyes to one side.

Presence of nausea, projectile vomiting, vomiting with or without nausea.

Symptoms may have progressed rapidly or insidiously.

Changes may be noted by family rather than patient.

DIAGNOSTIC STUDIES

ABGs may be needed to assess adequacy of ventilation.

Skull films done to note changes in bony structure, shift of midline structures, changes consistent with chronic increased intracranial pressure.

Chest x-ray for baseline data, presence of pulmonary disease that may influence ABGs.

ECG: checks for arrhythmias, ST segment abnormalities may be generated by intracranial process.

Toxin screen for possible cause of unconsciousness.

Hematocrit and hemoglobin, platelet, WBC and differential may suggest chronic disease (infection, neoplasm).

Serum anticonvulsant level may predispose epileptic patient to seizures/unconsciousness.

Urine, specific gravity and Na$^+$, K$^+$ for estimate of hydration.

Serum electrolyte levels: sodium may be especially altered.

Echoencephalograms demonstrate lateral shift of midline structures (limited use in adults).

Cerebral angiograms to pinpoint hemorrhage sites and abnormal vascular patterns (tumors, aneurysms).

Brain scan to demonstrate damaged brain tissue or tumors.

EEG helps in localizing tumors.

CT scan identifies space-occupying lesions: hemorrhage, neoplasms, abcesses.

Intracranial pressure monitoring catheter may be inserted into ventricle and pressure recordings made (normal = 1–10 mm Hg).

Pneumoencephalograms: displacement/deformity of ventricles.

Lumbar puncture is not normally done because of risk of brain herniation.

PHYSICAL EXAMINATION

The extent of physical assessment must be adjusted to the condition of the patient. With rapidly deteriorating condition, a medical emergency exists, and respiratory status, vital signs, pupil check, and spinal reflexes may be the only areas assessed.

Interview family of unconscious patient for gradual versus rapid onset of symptoms, past medical history, lifestyle, use of alcohol or drugs, which may contribute to present condition.

Skin: note needle marks/venipunctures, which may indicate addiction or diabetes.
   Edema may indicate kidney disease, result from toxic drug reaction, trauma.
   Pallor may indicate bleeding/shock.
   Rubor may indicate carbon monoxide poisoning, hypertension, alcoholism.
   Jaundice may indicate hepatic encephalopathy.
   Cyanosis indicates hypoxia.
   Petechiae may indicate blood dyscrasias.

Level of consciousness: note response to questions, commands. Note ability to speak clearly and appropriately, occurrence of repetitive speech, or memory defict.

Respiratory status: assess for obstruction; monitor respiratory rate, depth, and pattern. Be alert for periods of apnea and note length of occurrence.

Vital signs: hypertension, elevated temperature, slow pulse, rapid pulse.

Eyes: look for pupillary changes; measure pupil size, response to light, brisk or sluggish, symmetry in size and response. Check for deviation of eye or eyes to one side. Use ophthalmoscope to check for papilledema. Note occurrence of "doll's eyes" response.

Injuries: check head and face for bruising, lacerations, abrasions, healing or new.

Motor function: in the ambulatory patient, look for unsteady gait, assess for hemiplegia; check handgrasps for strength, symmetry, ability to move all extremities and strength of movements, nuchal rigidity, involuntary movement.

NURSING PRIORITIES

1. Monitor and support vital functions.
2. Provide for maximizing potential for self-care.
3. Provide information to assist with rehabilitation/psychosocial needs resulting from brain injury.

NURSING DIAGNOSIS:	Sensory perception, alterations in.
SUPPORTING DATA:	Actual loss/destruction of tissue because of interruption/lack of circulation resulting in altered levels of consciousness.
DESIRED PATIENT OUTCOMES:	Present level of consciousness maintained or improved. Further increased intracranial pressure does not occur.

INTERVENTIONS

Assess ability to speak, response to simple commands; response to painful stimuli and whether response is appropriate, immediate, or delayed.

RATIONALE

Changes may indicate deteriorating condition or improvement.

Provide sensory stimulation including familiar smells, sounds, tactile stimulation with a variety of objects, changing of light intensity, and so forth. Encourage significant others to bring in familiar objects and to talk to and touch the patient frequently.

Helps maintain neurologic pathways even though the patient may not respond.

Explain procedures and provide means of communication, if indicated.

Fear and anxiety may lead to increased blood and intracranial pressure.

Speak to the unresponsive patient during care.

Provides auditory stimulation and may help keep patient oriented.

NURSING DIAGNOSIS:	**Breathing patterns, ineffective.**
SUPPORTING DATA:	**Compression of the brain may impair action of autonomic nervous system.**
DESIRED PATIENT OUTCOMES:	**Respiratory functioning is supported while patient is unable to breathe effectively. Symptoms of respiratory dysfunction are absent.**

INTERVENTIONS

Monitor for breathing irregularities.

Position on side or prone and elevate head, as indicated.

Assess respiratory rate, rhythm, regularity, blood cell count, ABGs, gag/swallow reflex, skin color, breath sounds, chest expansion and x-ray.

Encourage deep breathing if patient is conscious or hyperventilate with Ambu bag p.r.n.

Use extreme caution if suctioning of respiratory secretions is necessary.

Monitor every shift for calf tenderness, redness, increased PCO_2, decreased PO_2, and chest pain.

Avoid administration of tranquilizers, sedatives, narcotics.

RATIONALE

Slow respiratory rate, Cheyne-Stokes respirations or apnea may indicate need for mechanical ventilation.

Facilitates maximum ventilation and avoids pressure on neck veins that may obstruct venous outflow and cause rebound increase in blood and intracranial pressure. Side position also prevents obstruction of airway by tongue or other oral contents and devices.

If respiratory effort is not adequate may lead to hypoxia, which increases intracranial pressure caused by increasing cerebral blood flow.

Prevents atelectasis.

May cause stress and initiate cough reflex, both of which increase intracranial pressure.

Thrombophlebitis leading to pulmonary embolism may occur due to prolonged bed rest and other risk factors.

Decrease respiratory effort predisposing to pneumonia, atelectasis. May also alter mental status making neurologic assessment difficult.

MEDICAL MANAGEMENT

Oxygen therapy.	Maximizes arterial PO$_2$ and prevents hypoxia.
Respiratory support or maintenance.	Respiratory centers may be depressed and support is required to maintain life.

Refer to Care Plan: Ventilatory Assistance (Mechanical).

NURSING DIAGNOSIS:	**Injury, potential for.**
SUPPORTING DATA:	**Edema associated with: tissue injury/inflammation, hypoxia and/ or hemorrhage, can cause excessive pressure on the brain due to the space-limiting effect of the cranium. This pressure can compromise CNS function/regulation and even lead to death.**
DESIRED PATIENT OUTCOMES:	**Pressure is decreased and brain functioning is maintained.**

INTERVENTIONS

RATIONALE

Monitor vital signs at regular intervals; every 15 minutes until stable. If on hypo/hypertensive drug therapy, monitor continuously.	Reflect changes in condition. Declining blood pressure may compromise cerebral blood flow. May necessitate adjustment according to response. A rise in blood pressure and fall in pulse and respiratory rate indicates increasing intracranial pressure.
Check pupils for equality, reactivity, accommodation.	Unequal pupils, changes in reactivity imply pressure on brain tissue/nerves.
Assess ability to move all extremities, hand grips, move eyes and focus in any direction.	Focal signs may suggest etiology or indicate deterioration. Third nerve palsies may accompany increased pressure.
Note occurrence of restlessness, irritability.	May indicate advent of seizuring or further CNS deterioration. (Refer to Care Plan: Seizure Disorders.)
Elevate head of bed, 30–45°; keep head aligned with neck at midline.	Assist venous drainage from head decreasing intracranial pressure. Minimizes headache.
Check presence of deep tendon reflexes, gag/ cough reflexes.	Decrease in activity signals further deterioration.

MEDICAL MANAGEMENT

Mannitol.	Reduces pressure by osmotic diuresis.
Decadron.	Reduces pressure by relieving inflammation and cerebral edema.

Oxygen if indicated.

Minimizes hypoxia, which can increase intracranial pressure.

Antipyretics (avoid aspirin-containing drugs).

Temperature increase will increase cerebral metabolism and potentiate edema formation.

Barbiturates.

Sedative effect can decrease brain metabolism as well as blood pressure and general intracranial pressure.

Hyperventilation.

If on mechanical ventilation, creates respiratory alkalosis and cerebral vasoconstriction, thereby reducing cerebral blood flow and intracranial pressure.

Intracranial monitoring.

Can provide more accurate assessment of pressure fluctuations and allows for removal of cerebrospinal fluid to decrease pressure.

Surgery.

Craniotomy may be necessary to relieve pressure.

NURSING DIAGNOSIS: **Fluid volume, alteration in, imbalance, potential.**

SUPPORTING DATA: **Fluid excess increases intracranial pressure. Diuretics distend the vascular tree.**

DESIRED PATIENT OUTCOMES: **Fluid balance is maintained and intracranial pressure is not increased.**

INTERVENTIONS

RATIONALE

Note occurrence of nausea and vomiting.

May be due to direct stimulation of emetic center in medulla caused by pressure, or reflex action to dehydrate body in presence of increased intracranial pressure.

Monitor I & O, electrolyte balance.

Overhydration can cause increased intracranial pressure. The use of mannitol will cause diuresis and possible altered electrolyte balance.

Check urine/serum electrolytes.

Decreased sodium, increased fluid retention may occur from interference with ADH secretion due to cerebral swelling. Dehydration predisposes to increased levels of serum sodium.

If osmotic diuretics are given, monitor for congestive heart failure, hypovolemia.

Encourage flow of fluids from tissues into vascular space for filtering and excretion by kidneys: expanded intravascular load may overtax myocardial function.

Monitor cardiac enzymes and ECG.

Establishes baseline and documents myocardial damage that may decrease cardiac output and compromise cerebral flow.

MEDICAL MANAGEMENT

Antiemetics.	May be helpful when nausea is present.
Indwelling catheter.	May need to monitor urine output and prevent distention of bladder.
Diuretics, steroids.	Promote diuresis and decrease edema.

NURSING DIAGNOSIS:	**Nutrition, alteration in, less than body requirements (potential).**
SUPPORTING DATA:	**Altered level of consciousness disturbs normal intake of nutrients.**
DESIRED PATIENT OUTCOMES:	**Nutritional levels maintained.**

INTERVENTIONS

RATIONALE

Assess ability to swallow, respond, and restrict oral intake, if necessary.

Inability to swallow, chew may result in aspiration.

Provide soft, semiliquid diet.

Requires limited mastication and more easily managed orally.

Provide for care of feeding tube:

Check placement of tube prior to feeding by aspiration of gastric contents or injection of air into NG tube and listening for gurgling with stethoscope over epigastric area.

May change with movement. Assures proper placement and prevents accidental flow of formula into bronchi.

Divide feedings into small amounts and give every 2–3 hours.

Allows for normal gastric functioning.

Add food coloring.

Helpful in assessing regurgitation/aspiration.

Place head of bed at 30° or more during and for one hour after feedings.

Prevents regurgitation and aspiration.

Clear tube with 25–50 ml of water after each feeding.

Prevents precipitates from obstructing tube.

If continuous feedings are used: check gastric residual periodically and flush tube with cranberry juice.

Prevents gastric distention/regurgitation if decreased motility or ileus occurs. Acidity limits/clears particles of curdled formula from tube.

Give nostril care where tube is inserted.

Prevent breakdown and soreness.

Swab lips, tongue, mouth at least twice per shift or as needed with lemon and glycerine.

Many unconscious patients are mouth breathers due to lack of muscle tone/nerve innervation to jaw.

MEDICAL MANAGEMENT

Nutritional support team and appropriate diet.

Determine optimal diet for individual.

NURSING DIAGNOSIS:	Skin integrity, alteration in.
SUPPORTING DATA:	Prolonged immobility is associated with development of pressure areas.
DESIRED PATIENT OUTCOMES:	Tissue breakdown does not occur.

INTERVENTIONS	RATIONALE

Refer to Care Plan: Long-Term Care, Nursing Diagnosis: Skin integrity, impairment of, actual, potential.

NURSING DIAGNOSIS:	Fear (specify).
SUPPORTING DATA:	Placed in unfamiliar surroundings, patient may not be able to perceive environment and may or may not be aware of deficiencies. Patient may perceive significant others' concern about the seriousness of the patient's condition, fear of outcome, death, or incapacity and react with anxiety.
DESIRED PATIENT OUTCOMES:	Anxiety is reduced to manageable level.

INTERVENTIONS	RATIONALE
Assess level of anxiety: restlessness, asking of questions, not following directions, verbalization of anxiety, and overt anxiety.	Increasing/decreasing levels need to be verified by talking to the patient/significant others.
Encourage expression of concerns about seriousness of disease, possibility of death, or incapacity.	Verbalization of fears can decrease anxiety.
Explain procedures and reinforce explanations given by others.	Knowledge can be helpful in decreasing fear.
Provide information about disease process in relationship to symptoms.	Helpful for understanding what is happening.

NURSING DIAGNOSIS:	Knowledge deficit, disease process/ treatment and prognosis.

SUPPORTING DATA:	Varying degrees of brain damage and disability may result from different conditions that cause increased intracranial pressure. Patient/significant others need information to deal effectively with long-term needs.
DESIRED PATIENT OUTCOMES:	Verbalizes rationale for treatment, expected outcomes. Follows regimen for rehabilitation.

INTERVENTIONS

Discuss prescribed activity and limitations; dietary regimen; medications, including dosage, frequency, expected results, and potential side effects.

Provide written instructions.

Encourage and discuss plans for self-care with patient and significant others.

Refer to community agencies as indicated.

If patient remains comatose, discuss plans for future with significant others.

RATIONALE

Prognosis largely depends on discharge planning and followup.

Helpful to refer to at home when questions arise.

Allows for increase of strength, becoming more independent and increasing self-esteem.

May benefit from consultation with VNA, professional counseling, or other resources according to individual needs.

May need to be moved to a long-term care facility. If death is anticipated, significant others will need support and help with planning for funeral arrangements.

DIAGNOSIS: Cerebrovascular Accident/Hemorrhage

PATIENT DATA BASE

Cerebrovascular disease refers to any functional abnormality of the central nervous system caused by a pathologic condition of the cerebral vessels or of the entire cerebral vascular system. It either causes hemorrhage from a tear in the vessel wall or impairs the cerebral circulation by a partial or complete occlusion of the vessel lumen.

Hemorrhage: intracerebral, subarachnoid, aneurysm.

Occlusion: embolus, arterial spasm, transient ischemic attack (TIA), thrombosis.

NURSING HISTORY

Hemorrhage: usually has sudden onset, while the patient is active may have headache, nausea/vomiting, decreased level of consciousness that may lead to coma and death.

Subarachnoid hemorrhage: excruciating headache, nausea/vomiting with a decrease in consciousness or seizure. May complain of a stiff neck.

Embolism, TIAs: may complain of transient episodes of memory impairment, visual disturbances, and numbness or paralysis.

Thrombosis: symptoms result from area of infarction; slow development of symptoms. May experience dizziness, mental disturbances or convulsions, transient loss of speech, right/left-sided paralysis, or paresthesias.

History of arteriosclerosis, hypertension, diabetes, recent emboli in other areas of the body, headaches, recent head injury, or epilepsy.

Determine whether patient is a cigarette smoker, obese, or has any chronic lung problems.

History of oral contraceptive use.

Family history of cerebrovascular disease.

DIAGNOSTIC STUDIES

CBC: may show anemia or polycythemia.

Mild leukocytosis may be present in thrombosis or embolism and hemorrhage.

Blood sugar: may show transient hyperglycemia.

Blood lipids: may be elevated.

Urine studies: may show albumin and casts. Associated renal disease may cause an elevation in blood urea nitrogen. Glycosuria may be present.

Lumbar puncture: the pressure is normal in cerebral thrombosis, embolism and TIA and is usually clear. In subarachnoid and intracerebral hemorrhage, the pressure is usually elevated and the fluid is grossly bloody. Total protein level may be elevated in cases of thrombosis due to the inflammatory process.

Electroencephalogram: may be helpful in locating an area of damage (of limited value in distinguishing hemorrhage from infarction).

ECG: rule out presence of silent myocardial infarction and determine presence of arrhythmias.

X-rays: *chest:* presence of cardiomegaly or pulmonary congestion; *skull:* may show shift of pineal gland to the opposite side from an expanding mass; calcifications of the internal carotid may be visible in cerebral thrombosis; partial calcification of walls of an aneurysm may be noted in subarachnoid hemorrhage.

Cerebral angiography: may demonstrate arterial obstruction or narrowing of arterial Circle of Willis or branches. A typical aneurysm pattern may be noted or cerebral arteriovenous malformations. In cerebral hemorrhage, the hemorrhagic area is seen as an avascular zone surrounded by displaced arteries and veins.

CT scan: can show density changes of the brain and differentiate blood clot formation.

PHYSICAL EXAMINATION

Examination of head for evidence of injury.

Note pupil size and reaction; pupillary deviations: in general is toward the lesion in hemispheric abnormalities and away from the lesion in brain stem abnormalities; examine optic disc for papilledema; sclerotic changes in retinal vessels.

Nuchal rigidity may be present.

Assess character of respiration, pulse rate, and blood pressure. Cheyne-Stokes respirations may be present.

Temperature elevation may indicate impairment of thermoregulator centers. (Vital signs may be normal if hemorrhage is small.)

Presence of jugular bruits indicate atherosclerosis.

Neurologic exam: presence of hemiplegia; changes in reflexes.

NURSING PRIORITIES

1. Promote oxygenation to minimize cerebral damage.
2. Provide for physical care until able to care for self.
3. Prevent deformities and complications and retain function present.
4. Assist patient to gain independence in daily living activities.
5. Assist patient/significant others to deal with psychologic needs of rehabilitation.

NURSING DIAGNOSIS:	Tissue perfusion, alterations in.
SUPPORTING DATA:	Changes of atherosclerosis predispose to ischemia; thrombi may cause infarction and/or hemorrhage; aneurysms may rupture resulting in hemorrhage, all of which may impair circulation to the brain.
DESIRED PATIENT OUTCOMES:	Perfusion and cerebral blood flow are maintained.

INTERVENTIONS

Monitor blood pressure, pulse, and level of consciousness.

Assess neurologic status; response to stimuli, movement, speech.

Monitor I & O, ABGs.

RATIONALE

Indicators of increasing intracranial/circulatory collapse.

Identify changes and take appropriate action to prevent serious complications if functioning is compromised.

Dehydration causes hemoconcentration and may decrease cerebral blood flow. Assess PO_2.

MEDICAL MANAGEMENT

Fluids IV.	Maintain level of hydration.
Oxygen.	Maintains arterial PO$_2$ at desired level.
Hyperbaric chamber.	Has been used with some success to increase amount of oxygen available to the tissues.

Refer to Care Plan: Increased Intracranial Pressure.

NURSING DIAGNOSIS:	**Mobility, impaired, physical.**
SUPPORTING DATA:	**Hemiparesis, hemiplegia may occur as a result of damage to motor areas of the brain. Immobility and bed rest can create problems of contractures and loss of muscle tone.**
DESIRED PATIENT OUTCOMES:	**Mobility is maintained at an optimal level and deformities are minimized.**

INTERVENTIONS

RATIONALE

INTERVENTIONS	RATIONALE
Begin range of motion of all extremities on admission.	Minimizes loss of muscle tone, promotes circulation, and prevents contractures.
Assess extent of paralysis initially and on a regular basis.	Identify extension of damage.
Maintain patient in functional position, and body in alignment with extremities supported.	Prevents contractures.
Support affected arm in a functional position with hand and arm slightly higher than level of the heart.	Promotes drainage and prevents edema and fibrosis.
Use trochanter roll along the outer aspect of the thigh.	Prevents external rotation.
Change position every two hours, turning on unaffected side.	Minimizes edema.
Place in prone position twice a day.	Maintain hyperextension of hip joints necessary to normal gait.
Keep flat or slightly elevate head of bed when on back.	Prevents hip flexion contractures.
Use footboard.	Prevents footdrop.
Explain all procedures as they are done.	Minimizes anxiety about what is happening to patient.
Involve family and patient in exercise program.	Enhances feeling of control and sense of involvement in situation where many factors are not in their control.

Sit in chair and begin ambulation as soon as vital signs are stable.

Resumption of activity as quickly as possible promotes maximum return of functioning.

NURSING DIAGNOSIS:	Communication, impaired, verbal and/or written.
SUPPORTING DATA:	Depending on area of the brain involved, impairment of speech and/or understanding may occur.
DESIRED PATIENT OUTCOMES:	Communication is maintained.

INTERVENTIONS

Assess degree of dysfunction.

Make note at nurses' station about speech impairment. Provide special call bell if necessary.

Talk directly to the patient, speaking slowly and distinctly.

Anticipate and provide for the patient's needs.

Provide alternative methods of communication.

RATIONALE

Does the patient hear words, process, and respond? Determine the degree of difficulty patient has with any or all steps of the process.

Will be helpful to allay anxiety related to inability to communicate. Call bell that is activated by minimal pressure is useful when patient is unable to use a regular bell.

Regardless of the level of response, it is important to continue to treat the patient in a normal manner. The stimulation and sense of being included are important to recovery.

Helpful in decreasing frustration when dependent on others and unable to communicate desires.

Depending on impairment, writing or felt board, pictures, and so forth can be helpful.

MEDICAL MANAGEMENT

Consult with speech therapist.

Assesses patient's verbal capabilities, sensory, motor, and cognitive functioning and develops therapy plan for nurse, patient, and significant others.

NURSING DIAGNOSIS:	Sensory perception, alterations in.
SUPPORTING DATA:	Because of neurologic deficits, may not perceive external stimuli, sounds, sights, sensations, such as pain, pressure, temperature, and visual loss.
DESIRED PATIENT OUTCOMES:	Sensory impairments are recognized and managed.

INTERVENTIONS

Assess for sensory awareness.

Talk to patient while giving care, telling them what has occured.

Reorient to time, place, and events when conscious.

Assess type of sensory deficits present.

Arrange bed, personal articles, and food trays and approach patient on unaffected side.

Describe where affected areas of body are when moving patient.

Provide tactile stimulation as care is given.

RATIONALE

Stimulus of hot/cold; dull/sharp; awareness of motion and location of body parts.

Hearing seems to be the last sense lost and patient may receive information when still unconscious or unresponsive. Provides auditory stimulation and a sense of being included in what is going on.

Will diminish sense of alienation and fear.

Restriction of field of vision, symmetry of dilation, eye movements may be present.

Plan to take advantage of functional vision.

May have loss of ability to know the location of parts of body in space.

Touching is an important part of caring and is a deep psychologic need.

NURSING DIAGNOSIS:	**Nutrition, alteration in, less than body requirements.**
SUPPORTING DATA:	**Extent of paralysis, level of consciousness affect ability to maintain adequate nutritional intake.**
DESIRED PATIENT OUTCOMES:	**Nutritional balance is maintained.**

INTERVENTIONS

Assess ability to swallow, level of consciousness, extent of paralysis.

Maintain accurate I & O.

Increase diet from soft to select as tolerated, providing easily managed foods, such as finger foods, and assisting as necessary with eating.

RATIONALE

Individualize intake to ability to eat and drink.

Be aware of fluid intake and potential deficiencies.

As ability to chew, swallow, and manage food increases, self-feeding, as much as possible, will increase feelings of independence and allow for increased intake.

MEDICAL MANAGEMENT

IV fluids.

Tube feedings.

Refer to Care Plan: Total Parenteral Nutrition.

May be necessary for fluid replacement the first 24–48 hours when unable to take anything orally.

May be necessary if prolonged coma exists or if dysphagia persists.

173

NURSING DIAGNOSIS:	Self-care deficit (specify feeding, bathing, hygiene, dressing, grooming, or toilet).
SUPPORTING DATA:	Depending on extent of involvement, patient will have varying degrees of disability, such as hemiplegia, dysphagia, urinary and/or bowel incontinence.
DESIRED PATIENT OUTCOMES:	Functioning at maximum level of ability.

INTERVENTIONS

RATIONALE

Avoid doing things for the patient that the patient can do; assisting as necessary.

Hemiplegics may become fearful and dependent and while assistance is helpful in preventing frustration, it is important for the patient to do as much as possible.

Maintain a supportive, firm attitude.

Patients will need empathy but need to know caregivers will be consistent in their assistance.

Provide self-help devices as needed.

Depending on the need, many things are available to help, such as knife-fork combinations, long-handled brushes, extensions for picking things up from floor

Take to the bathroom every two hours for voiding.

May have physical, emotional interferences; may be inattentive or unable to communicate needs.

Identify normal bowel habits, and establish regimen based on previous habits.

Will assist in development of retraining program.

Provide for bulk in diet, encourage fluid intake and increased activity.

To aid in preventing constipation and impaction.

MEDICAL MANAGEMENT

Suppositories and stool softeners.

May be necessary at first to aid in establishing regular bowel function.

Consult with physical/occupational therapist.

To assess and develop a therapy plan and identify special equipment required.

NURSING DIAGNOSIS:	Coping ineffective, individual, family.
SUPPORTING DATA:	Patients with hemiplegia are often emotionally labile, confused, forgetful, and frustrated. Finding themselves in a strange environ-

ment, unable to communicate, or move one side of their body, they can become depressed, hostile, and believe life is not worth living.

DESIRED PATIENT OUTCOMES: Patient expresses interest in and is participating in rehabilitation activities.

INTERVENTIONS

Assess ability to understand.

Identify previous activities: occupation and leisure.

Give explanations of all activities that are happening.

Have same personnel take care of patient as often as possible.

Treat patient with courtesy and respect. Converse as with anyone.

RATIONALE

It is very difficult to grasp full extent of patient's abilities. Lack of concern may indicate brain damage; may have impaired intellectual ability, judgment, reasoning, and comprehension.

Depending upon degree of physical and language impairment, may be unable to resume previous employment and interests.

Information can be useful in allaying fear and concern.

Establishes trusting environment in which patient can express fears and begin to learn ways of dealing with situation.

Although body image has been altered, will allow patient to see self as a worthwhile person again.

DIAGNOSIS: Intracranial Infections: Meningitis, Encephalitis, Brain Abscess

PATIENT DATA BASE

NURSING HISTORY

History of upper respiratory infection or other site of infection, recent lumbar puncture, surgery, skull fracture, middle ear infection, mastoiditis, head injury or trauma, sinus infection, ingestion of toxins or poisons.

Recent immunization, exposure to meningitis, mumps, virus, herpes simplex, animal bites, recent travel, epidemic outbreaks, mononucleosis.

History of drug use: brain abscess may occur from injected bacteria; nonbacterial meningitis due to drug hypersensitivity reaction.

History of sickle cell anemia: functional splenectomy predisposes to bacteremia.

Concurent medical problems and treatment: debility, alcoholism, diabetes mellitus, radiation therapy increase risk of the development of sepsis, which may result in intracranial infection.

Living conditions: meningococcal meningitis more common in areas of close, crowded, living/working conditions.

Certain types of meningitis and encephalitis have seasonal patterns.

Complains of fever, severe headache, stiff neck, photophobia, pain with ocular movements, malaise, aches, sore throat, nausea, vomiting, backache, diplopia.

Change in behavior noted by significant others, altered communication abilities.

Seizure activity (noted by others), nystagmus (continuous movement of the eyeball), ptosis (drooping of the upper eyelid), tachycardia, respiratory distress, arrhythmias.

DIAGNOSTIC STUDIES

Cerebrospinal fluid exam per lumbar puncture: pleocytosis, increased pressure and protein, decreased glucose in bacterial meningitis.

Smear and culture of fluid helps identify organism, e.g., Haemophilus influenzae and pneumococcus. Meningococcal meningitis often follows viral diseases. Alcoholics may develop unusual types of meningitis, such as Klebsiella. Sensitivity establishes effective drug treatment.

BUN, creatinine, urinalysis help assess state of hydration.

Brain scan may assist in identifying area of involvement.

Brain biopsy may help identify difficult organisms.

Serum electrolytes (often show hyponatremia/chloremia), hemoglobin, hematocrit, platelets, WBC level, sedimentation rate, clotting profile, toxin screens, anticonvulsant drug levels help assess present levels of health, concurrent disease, or cause of illness.

Arterial blood gases: respiratory baseline function.

Culture and sensitivity of blood, urine, sputum, oropharyngeal area, wounds, cerebrospinal fluid in an effort to help establish causative organism.

ECG and EEG to establish baseline and note abnormalities.

PHYSICAL EXAMINATION

Nuchal rigidity, opisthotonos may be present in severe cases. Altered level of consciousness varying from mild confusion to delirium to unconsciousness.

Positive meningeal signs, i.e., Brudzinski, Kernig, weakness, aphasia, ataxia, involuntary movement, olfactory/gustatory hallucinations, temporal lobe seizures, anosmia (loss of smell), rash, palsies, burning/itching/tingling along distribution of nerve showing irritation.

Check for reticuloendothelial system malignancies.

Tachycardia, altered respiratory patterns, slightly elevated blood pressure, temperature elevation.

NURSING PRIORITIES

1. Maintain and prevent deterioration of CNS functions.
2. Prevent complications caused by disease and treatments.
3. Return to previous level of ADL, within limitations of condition.

NURSING DIAGNOSIS:	**Breathing pattern, ineffective.**
SUPPORTING DATA:	**Increasing intracranial pressure may depress respiratory effort, alter ability to handle secretions and result in airway obstruction. Pneumonia is a frequent complication.**
DESIRED PATIENT OUTCOMES:	**Normal respiratory pattern and blood gases maintained. Symptoms of hypoxia are absent and aspiration of secretions is avoided.**

INTERVENTIONS

Monitor respiratory rate, pattern, quality, airway patency, ABGs, chest x-ray, breath sounds.

Encourage deep breathing, position change, increase activity as tolerated. Discourage coughing.

Monitor for restlessness not attributable to other causes (e.g., full bladder).

Monitor skin/nailbed color, vital signs.

Observe for nausea/vomiting and keep NPO, if occurs.

RATIONALE

May indicate ability/inability to handle secretions. Hypoxia increases intracranial pressure. May be altered with developing obstruction of airway. Breath sounds estimate quality of aeration and note developing pulmonary infiltrate or obstruction.

Stimulates mobilization of secretions to prevent stasis and infection; coughing increases intracranial pressure.

Hypoxia causes restlessness.

Cyanosis, increased respiratory rate, decreasing blood pressure may occur with hypoxia.

May be indicative of increasing pressure; decreases risk of aspiration if vomiting occurs or are unable to handle oral secretions.

Test for gag/swallow relex every two hours.

Deterioration may be sign of increasing neurologic deterioration.

Suction p.r.n.

Need to prevent possibility of aspiration if vomiting occurs or are unable to handle oral secretions.

Maintain strict isolation, if indicated, until 24 hours after start of antibiotic therapy.

Meningococcal meningitis can occur in epidemic form and secretions from nose and throat may be infectious.

MEDICAL MANAGEMENT

Oral airway.

Maintains position of tongue and minimizes upper airway obstruction.

Supplemental O_2.

Increases available oxygen.

Endotracheal tube/tracheostomy.

May be necessary if unable to clear airway.

Ventilatory assistance.

May be necessary to support respiratory functioning.

Surgery.

May be needed to drain and relieve pressure when abscess formation occurs.

Refer to Care Plan: Ventilatory Assistance (Mechanical).

NURSING DIAGNOSIS:	**Injury, potential, seizure.**
SUPPORTING DATA:	**Inflammation of cerebral tissue or abscess formation occupies space in closed cranium causing an increase in intracranial pressure that may result in seizure.**
DESIRED PATIENT OUTCOMES:	**Seizures prevented; brain damage is minimized/prevented.**

INTERVENTIONS

RATIONALE

Assess motor-sensory-perceptual function including level of consciousness, neurologic responses, pupillary responses, Kernig and Brudzinski signs, posturing (normal versus decerebrate/decorticate).

Establishes baseline data against which to measure changes.

Keep side rails up at all times; take seizure precautions. Note occurrence of associated symptoms and so forth. (Refer to Care Plan: Seizure Disorders.)

Seizures may occur that can result in self-injury.

Maintain quiet environment, avoid sudden movement, loud noises.

Excessive stimuli may trigger seizures.

Provide explanation to patient/significiant others when restraints are necessary. Reaffirm temporary nature and remove frequently when supervised. Remove one at a time and reapply as indicated.

Can decrease anxiety that patient is uncontrollable; removal allows for exercise of extremities.

MEDICAL MANAGEMENT

Antibiotics IV and/or intrathecally.

Penicillin, ampicillin, or chloramphenicol are usually drugs of choice for meningococcal meningitis and must be administered IV/intrathecally because most antibiotics do not diffuse well into the CSF. Culture and sensitivity will influence drug of choice.

Steroids.

Reduce cerebral inflammation.

Anticonvulsants or Valium.

Prevent seizure activity.

Restraints.

May be necessary if it is the only way to protect the patient. Patient safety must be weighed against fighting restraints, which can cause Valsalva maneuver and act to increase intracranial pressure.

NURSING DIAGNOSIS:	**Thought processes, alterations in.**
SUPPORTING DATA:	**Increased intracranial pressure resulting from infection, decreases level of consciousness and ability to function.**
DESIRED PATIENT OUTCOMES:	**Able to think as prior to illness. Neurologic deficits and symptoms of increased intracranial pressure are not present.**

INTERVENTIONS

Monitor and document vital signs every two hours and p.r.n.

Do neurologic checks every two hours; note changes and decrease in level of consciousness.

Test ability to receive and send communications; if unable to communicate verbally, establish alternate means.

Reorient to time/place/person as needed and note results.

Keep familiar objects, pictures around patient.

Refer to Care Plan: Increased Intracranial Pressure.

RATIONALE

Bradycardia and hypertension suggest rising intracranial pressure.

May indicate development of brain abcess, hydrocephalus.

Being unable to make wishes known is very anxiety-provoking.

Inability to maintain orientation is a sign of deterioration.

Aids in keeping patient oriented.

179

NURSING DIAGNOSIS:	Tissue perfusion, alteration in.
SUPPORTING DATA:	Development of shock, hypovolemia limits circulation to tissues. Rising intracranial pressure due to inflammation may result in decreased pulse and increased blood pressure.
DESIRED PATIENT OUTCOMES:	Shock/hypovolemia are prevented/treated and perfusion to tissues is maintained.

INTERVENTIONS

Monitor vital signs, neuro status every 1–2 hours as indicated; monitor CVP if available.

Observe for increasing temperature, decreasing blood pressure, and development of petechia, especially on trunk/legs, which may progress to large ecchymotic areas or purpuric lesions.

Observe skin, mucous membranes for pallor, cyanosis, mottling or coolness of extremities.

Do ROM at least four times/day and reposition often.

MEDICAL MANAGEMENT

Steroids.

Fluid replacement.

RATIONALE

Increased pulse and blood pressure, decreased respiration and pulse rate, reflex bradycardia indicate increasing intracranial pressure. Increasing blood pressure, CVP may indicate overhydration. Decreasing blood pressure, CVP may indicate dehydration or developing shock, especially from sepsis.

Petechial rash is especially seen in meningococcal disease. May be indicative of impending shock.

May be caused by decreased blood pressure, cardiac output.

Stimulates circulation to tissues and prevents prolonged pressure on susceptible areas, which may impede circulation.

Anti-inflammatory action may decrease cerebral edema.

May be necessary if dehydration occurs. (Refer to next nursing diagnosis.)

NURSING DIAGNOSIS:	Fluid volume, alteration in, excess, potential.
SUPPORTING DATA:	Increasing intracranial pressure alters hormonal influence on fluid and electrolytes.
DESIRED PATIENT OUTCOMES:	Fluid and electrolyte balance is maintained.

INTERVENTIONS

Maintain accurate I & O. Evaluate for decreased output.

Monitor serum electrolytes, weight, temperature, presence of nausea/vomiting.

Test urine specific gravity every two hours.

Provide diet as tolerated.

RATIONALE

Fluid overload, sodium retention may occur due to inappropriate ADH secretion stimulated by cerebral edema.

Note impending imbalance.

Concentrated urine may signal developing inappropriate secretion of ADH.

Maintain fluid/nutrient levels.

MEDICAL MANAGEMENT

Mannitol, fluid restrictions.

IV fluids.

NG feedings.

Decreases fluid load, acts to dehydrate, and pulls fluid from the brain tissues.

Maintain fluid level/renal functioning if unable to use other routes of intake.

If unable to take food in adequate amounts orally.

NURSING DIAGNOSIS:	**Fluid volume deficit, potential, hemorrhage.**
SUPPORTING DATA:	**Increased intracranial pressure may alter hormone balance and predispose to development of stress ulcers, GI bleeding and DIC.**
DESIRED PATIENT OUTCOMES:	**Complications of bleeding are minimized/prevented.**

INTERVENTIONS

Monitor vital signs.

Note abdominal tenderness, distention.

Guaic test emesis, feces, urine as indicated.

Evaluate hydration; encourage increased intake unless contraindicated.

RATIONALE

Decreasing blood pressure, increasing pulse may indicate bleeding.

May be sign of GI irritation due to bleeding.

Identifies occult bleeding.

Prevents hypovolemia, which may worsen developing shock.

MEDICAL MANAGEMENT

Cimetidine, antacids.

Blood/plasma expanders.

Decrease gastric irritation, stress ulcers.

Replace and maintain circulating volume.

NURSING DIAGNOSIS:	Comfort, alteration in.
SUPPORTING DATA:	Bed confinement in neurologic disease may promote muscle soreness, decubitus ulcer development. Temperature variations, symptomatology (frequently, headache that is worse in the morning), required treatments may be uncomfortable.
DESIRED PATIENT OUTCOMES:	Comfort level is attained/maintained.

INTERVENTIONS

Log roll patient to turn.

Reposition at least every two hours, prop with pillows, massage bony prominences, tense or rigid areas frequently.

Check bed linens and change when damp.

Give sponge baths as needed.

Monitor bowel sounds/distention and bladder distention and take appropriate measures to relieve pressure.

Darken room and use ice bag for head. Dark glasses may be helpful.

Apply patch to one eye; alternate every few hours.

Avoid reaching, stretching, blowing nose, holding breath.

MEDICAL MANAGEMENT

Analgesics.

Hyper/hypothermia.

Antipyretics.

Lumbar puncture, ventricular tap.

Stool softeners.

RATIONALE

Avoids movement of neck that may be very painful in meningeal irritation.

Decreases risk of skin and pulmonary complications.

Temperature variations often result in diaphoresis and a wet bed can be uncomfortable.

Reduce temperature and provide comfort.

Restlessness and discomfort may be due to development of other complications, such as paralytic ileus.

Headache and photophobia may be present with increased pressure and meningeal irritation.

If diplopia is present, can cause headaches and decrease visual acuity.

Activities that can cause pressure against closed glottis will increase intracranial pressure.

Relieve headache and discomfort.

Temperature extremes may occur due to pressure on hypothalamus.

Decrease temperature.

May be necessary to decrease pressure, obtain specimen for identification of invading organism.

Prevent constipation and straining.

NURSING DIAGNOSIS:	Fear of dying.
SUPPORTING DATA:	May be aware of neurologic deficits and if unable to interpret the meaning of procedures and disease, may make assumption about outcome.
DESIRED PATIENT OUTCOMES:	Trusting relationship is developed in which support and information is provided for patient/significant others.

INTERVENTIONS

Allow time to verbalize thoughts and fears.

Answer questions honestly and give information about favorable prognosis.

Provide explanation of relationship between disease process and symptoms.

Explain and prepare for procedures beforehand.

Involve patient/significant others in care, daily planning, decision-making as much as possible. Encourage independence, diversional activity.

Support planning for realistic lifestyle after illness within limitations but fully using capabilities.

Explore sources of support; significant others, clergy, professional counseling.

RATIONALE

Will bring fears into the open where they can be addressed.

Important to the establishing of trust as the diagnosis of meningitis may be frightening and honesty and accurate information can provide reassurance.

Lessens mystery and unpredictability of disease that may increase anxiety.

Alleviate apprehension when testing involves the brain.

Increases feeling of control.

May have residual limitations or deficits.

May have need for further assistance. (Refer to Care Plan: Psychosocial Aspects of Care in the Acute Setting.)

NURSING DIAGNOSIS:	Knowledge deficit, disease/treatment.
SUPPORTING DATA:	May have misunderstandings/ misinformation about what is happening. May have residual disabilities that may require physical therapy and/or educational programs.

DESIRED PATIENT OUTCOMES:	Verbalizes relationship of appropriate pathophysiology and occurrence of symptoms; rationale of treatment and symptoms of drug toxicity, relapse.

INTERVENTIONS

Assess level of knowledge and reinforce relationship of symptoms to pathophysiology (e.g., muscle weakness, level of consciousness related to intracranial pressure).

Discuss importance of avoiding factors that may promote recurrence of disease and communicability of disease to others.

Teach proper control of airborne droplets, disposal of secretions and tissues and importance of good handwashing.

Discuss dosage, time, rationale, and side effects for each drug.

Discuss followup care, signs and symptoms to be reported.

Discuss chemoprophylaxis for those having close contact with patient prior to start of antibiotic therapy.

RATIONALE

Can be helpful in decreasing anxiety of the unknown and seeing the predictability of symptoms.

Close contacts of patients with meningococcal meningitis may need chemoprophylaxis.

Prevents spread of infection.

May be discharged on antibiotics or other medications to control symptoms.

Seizures, hearing loss, focal signs, late obtundation, behavioral defects should be reported immediately. Relapse due to brain abscess is common.

Meningococcal meningitis is communicable and vaccine or rifampin may be given.

DIAGNOSIS: Herniated Nucleus Pulposus
(Herniated Intervertebral Disk)

PATIENT DATA BASE

NURSING HISTORY

Symptoms depend on site, severity, whether acute or chronic, and the effects on the surrounding structures.

History of acute episode of low back pain with or without pain radiating down one or both legs.

May have periodic episodes of back pain that are becoming more severe.

Pain may be associated with numbness or weakness in one or both lower extremities; with cervical disk, the upper extremities and head may be affected.

Note patient's description of pain and precipitating cause. Is this new or ongoing symptom?

Occupation may give insight into physical/psychologic stress.

Hobbies can give insight into lifestyle, physical stress activities.

Evaluate patient for back injury history: accident, on-job injury, psychologic stress, weight compared to ideal body weight.

Current medications give insight into drug tolerance/dependence.

Note allergies. (May have significance in relation to diagnostic procedures.)

DIAGNOSTIC STUDIES

Myelogram may show evidence of herniated disks.

X-ray of area; cervical, lumbar, rule out other lesions.

Electromyography may be done to determine muscle strength.

Spinal fluid to rule out other conditions; presence of blood, and so forth.

PHYSICAL EXAMINATION

Pain aggravated by coughing, sneezing, or defecation.

Muscle spasm is prominent.

Note changes in posture. May have dropped shoulder or a tilt to one side.

Motion may be restricted by pain.

Straight-leg raising aggravates sciatic pain (Lasègue sign).

Neurologic exam may reveal muscle weakness, alterations in reflexes and sensory changes.

NURSING PRIORITIES

1. Reduce stress, muscle spasm and promote optimal functioning.
2. Provide information about proper care of back and necessary lifestyle modifications.
3. Prepare patient/significant others for surgery, if indicated.

NURSING DIAGNOSIS:	Comfort, alterations in, pain.
SUPPORTING DATA:	Protrusion of the nucleus of the disk causes compression of the nerve. Severe muscle spasm is painful; pain increases muscle spasm that further increases pain.
DESIRED PATIENT OUTCOMES:	Pain is relieved/controlled.

INTERVENTIONS

RATIONALE

Assess complaints of pain; site, duration, activity, visitors, or stress associated with onset.

Determination of related factors allows for more effective interventions.

Promote bed rest and change position from flat to mild jackknife to high-Fowler's.

Relieve muscle spasm, reduce edema, and reduce stress of above structures on involved disk.

Place board under mattress or provide orthopedic bed.

Holds body firmly and reduces spinal flexion.

Provide opportunities to talk and listen to concerns.

Helpful to determine stress factors in illness as well as those created by hospitalization.

Instruct in relaxation/visualization techniques.

Assists in healing by reducing muscle tension.

MEDICAL MANAGEMENT

Heating pad.

Relaxes muscles. Use caution when sensory nerve involvement is present.

Traction, cervical or pelvic.

Increases vertebral space and relieves pressure. Begin with short periods and extend time as tolerated. Provides relief of muscle spasm.

Cervical collar.

May be used in addition to or instead of traction.

Analgesics and muscle relaxants.

Decrease pain and muscle spasm, which promotes general relaxation.

Brace.

Immobilizes area when ambulating to prevent spinal flexion and pain.

Physical therapy.

Heat, massage, whirlpool may relieve muscle spasm.

NURSING DIAGNOSIS:	Bowel elimination, alteration in, constipation.
SUPPORTING DATA:	Immobilization, pain on defecation, and possible neurologic involvement can interfere with elimination.
DESIRED PATIENT OUTCOMES:	Normal bowel function maintained.

INTERVENTIONS

Identify patient's normal routine.

Increase intake of fruit juices and liquids.

Promote increased bulk and fiber in the diet.

MEDICAL MANAGEMENT

Bulk extenders, such as Metamucil and/or stool softeners.

Laxatives and enemas.

RATIONALE

Maintenance of normal routine is more effective and less stressful.

Maintain soft consistency of stool.

May be used for brief periods of time to avoid constipation/straining.

May be necessary when inactivity and pain interfere with normal bowel activity.

NURSING DIAGNOSIS:	**Urinary elimination, alteration in pattern.**
SUPPORTING DATA:	**Herniated disk may produce neurologic involvement to the lower extremities, which interferes with bladder functioning.**
DESIRED PATIENT OUTCOMES:	**Bladder is emptied at each voiding.**

INTERVENTIONS

Keep intake/output, recording amount and frequency.

Check for bladder distention.

MEDICAL MANAGEMENT

Check urinary residual, if indicated.

RATIONALE

Difficulty in voiding may indicate neurologic involvement.

May be retaining urine even though voiding.

To assess retention.

NURSING DIAGNOSIS:	**Knowledge deficit, disease process and treatment.**
SUPPORTING DATA:	**Misinformation or lack of knowledge of disease and/or therapies may lead to anxiety or failure to follow prescribed regimen. Patients often believe that problems and/or surgery on the spine will lead to paralysis.**
DESIRED PATIENT OUTCOMES:	**Able to describe what is causing pain and what changes in occupation, lifestyle, and/or other activities will be necessary.**

INTERVENTIONS	RATIONALE
Assess knowledge of disorder. Is this the initial episode or recurrence?	Can build on information and understanding the patient already possesses.
Allow opportunities for discussing understanding, giving information, and reinforcing previous explanations.	Helpful in clarifying and developing understanding and acceptance of necessary lifestlye changes. When the problem is in the cervical area, convalescence can be expected to extend to 6 weeks, although lifetime changes will probably be necessary.
Discuss sleep patterns.	Cervical: use soft pillow, i.e., feathers. Lumbar: avoid prone position, sleep on side with knees flexed.
Avoid riding in a car for long periods.	Can aggravate pressure on disk.
Discuss medications, their actions and side effects.	When patient has information, can make decisions and participate in therapy more fully.
Give information about and discuss importance of proper body mechanics and exercise routine. Include proper posture for standing, sitting, as well as lifting.	Changing old habits is more easily accomplished when patient has sufficient information and understands how change will be helpful. With cervical problems it is important to avoid extreme flexion; lumbar, lift with straight back, bent knees, and no lifting above the elbows.
Provide information about what symptoms need to be reported to the physician for further evaluation.	Progression of the process may necessitate further treatment and/or surgery. Chemonucleolysis is an alternative to surgery. An enzyme, chymopapain, is injected into the disk causing depolymerization of the mucoprotein without effect on the surrounding collagenous structures.

NURSING DIAGNOSIS:	**Mobility, impaired physical.**
SUPPORTING DATA:	**Pain, muscle spasms, and diagnostic procedures can interfere with mobility.**
DESIRED PATIENT OUTCOMES:	**Mobility is maintained at a satisfactory level.**

INTERVENTIONS	RATIONALE
Prepare for and give explanation of any diagnostic procedures being done.	Knowledge of expectations can decrease anxiety and enhance cooperation.
Instruct in postmyelography procedures.	Explanation of procedure will help patient understand need to force fluids and lie flat or at 30° elevation as indicated for specified number of hours.

NURSING DIAGNOSIS:	Coping, ineffective, individual.
SUPPORTING DATA:	Recurrent disorder and continuing pain can create situation in which the individual feels helpless and hopeless.
DESIRED PATIENT OUTCOMES:	Patient is coping with disorder by verbalization of reasons for pain, treatments, and necessary lifestyle changes.

INTERVENTIONS

Assess level of anxiety and how patient is coping.

Provide accurate information and honest answers to questions.

Provide opportunity for expression of concerns about possible paralysis and sexual dysfunction.

If surgery has been recommended, discuss procedure and concerns, as well as postoperative expectations.

RATIONALE

Important to know how the individual patient is dealing with the situation to be able to provide appropriate assistance.

Enables patient to make decisions based on knowledge.

Most patients have these concerns and they need to be expressed and responded to with accurate information.

Provide for opportunity to deal with feared situation more productively.

CARE PLAN: Laminectomy

PATIENT DATA BASE

NURSING HISTORY

Laminectomy may be done as an emergency procedure following trauma; when there is progressive nerve involvement with muscle weakness and impairment; and for recurring episodes of herniation. Spinal fusion may be done when the spine is unstable due to anatomic or degenerative changes.

History of conservative treatment that has not been successful.

Continuing complaints of pain.

See Care Plan: Herniated Nucleus Pulposus for additional data base.

NURSING PRIORITIES

1. Promote comfort and healing.
2. Prevent bowel and urinary complications.
3. Help patient/significant others deal with necessary lifestyle changes.

Refer to Care Plans: Surgical Intervention; Herniated Nucleus Pulposus.

NURSING DIAGNOSIS: **Comfort, alteration in, pain. Note additional edema.**

SUPPORTING DATA: **Although pain from pressure of the disk has been removed, edema will be present postoperatively, which causes continuing pain.**

DESIRED PATIENT OUTCOMES: **Pain will be controlled/managed.**

INTERVENTIONS

Assess amount, description, and site of pain. Note additional edema.

May be allowed to assume position of comfort. Use logroll for position change.

Provide explanation of the possibility of various manifestations of pain and other sensations.

MEDICAL MANAGEMENT

Narcotics and sedatives.

RATIONALE

May vary from mild to severe. When graft has been taken from the iliac crest, pain may be more severe at the donor site than the surgical area. When cervical area is involved, may complain of sore throat; pain may occur in legs/arms due to swelling in the operative area.

Surgeons may have differing opinions about positioning. Avoids tension on operative area.

Edema, swelling of compressed nerve, and inflammatory changes may cause pressure on various nerves with differing results.

Given as pain indicates. Often, narcotics are necessary in the immediate postop period, while lesser medication suffices as recuperation progresses.

NURSING DIAGNOSIS:	Mobility, impaired physical.
SUPPORTING DATA:	Usually the patient is kept supine for a period of time immediately postop. With a laminectomy, ambulation is usually permitted the second postop day. With a fusion, the patient will be ambulated with a brace.
DESIRED PATIENT OUTCOMES:	Mobility will be regained without incident.

INTERVENTIONS

CERVICAL:

Check neurologic and vital signs frequently.

May be allowed to sit up the evening of surgery.

LUMBAR:

Check movement and sensation of lower extremities and feet as well as vital signs.

Logroll the patient from side to side, keeping the back straight. Use a turning sheet and sufficient personnel when turning.

Use pillows between knees during position change and when on side.

With a laminectomy, movement is allowed more freely than when a fusion is done.

MEDICAL MANAGEMENT

Give pain medication ½ hour before turning.

Brace may be worn when patient is ambulated.

Physical therapy consultation.

RATIONALE

Nerve damage may occur with resulting paralysis and respiratory difficulty.

If a brace is in place. A Philadelphia collar may have been applied in the operating room. Tongs also may be used with a brace to maintain stability.

Edema and swelling of the tissues may press on the nerves.

Maintain body alignment as twisting motion may interfere with the graft and healing process.

Maintain alignment.

Fusion graft may be dislodged with activity.

Patients anticipate pain with turning and may become tense. Medication will be helpful for relieving pain and allowing for better relaxation and cooperation with movement.

When a fusion is done, the brace is applied with the patient lying in bed before being assisted to an upright position.

Strengthening exercises and ambulatory devices may be necessary.

NURSING DIAGNOSIS:	Fluid volume deficit, potential, hemorrhage.

SUPPORTING DATA:	Hematoma is likely to develop in the surgical area, more so with a fusion.
DESIRED PATIENT OUTCOMES:	Bleeding is minimized/controlled.

INTERVENTIONS	RATIONALE
Patient may be kept flat on back for several hours postop.	Provides more pressure on area.
Observe for bleeding as well as change in contour of the operative site when turning the patient. When the patient remains flat, it is important to feel underneath.	Allow for early intervention. Wetness may indicate excess drainage or bleeding.
Check vital signs.	Hypotension may indicate blood loss.
Observe for the presence of a large amount of light pinkish tinged, clear drainage.	May indicate a "dura leak," which is usually treated by keeping the patient in mild Trendelenburg position for a number of days.

NURSING DIAGNOSIS:	Bowel elimination, alteration in, constipation.
SUPPORTING DATA:	Pain and swelling in surgical area, and immobilization interfere with functioning of the bowel. Ileus is a common complication.
DESIRED PATIENT OUTCOMES:	Elimination returns to normal.

INTERVENTIONS	RATIONALE
Note abdominal distention and listen for return of bowel sounds.	Distention and lack of bowel sounds indicate bowel is not functioning.
Limit oral intake.	Until danger of ileus is past.

MEDICAL MANAGEMENT

Rectal tube, suppositories, enemas.	Used as necessary to relieve abdominal distention.
NG tube.	May be necessary to decompress GI tract if ileus occurs.

NURSING DIAGNOSIS:	Urinary elimination, alteration in pattern.

SUPPORTING DATA:	Bladder dysfunction is common for several days. Pain and swelling in operative area and necessity for remaining flat in bed makes voiding difficult.
DESIRED PATIENT OUTCOMES:	Bladder is emptied adequately.

INTERVENTIONS

Observe and record amount and time of voiding.

Palpate for bladder distention.

MEDICAL MANAGEMENT

An indwelling catheter may be used.

RATIONALE

Determine whether bladder is being emptied.

May indicate retention.

May be necessary for several postop days until swelling decreases allowing for normal voiding.

NURSING DIAGNOSIS:	Knowledge deficit, disease, postoperative treatment and possible alterations in lifestyle.
SUPPORTING DATA:	Length of recuperation time and necessary changes in lifestyle vary with the extent of the surgical procedure. In general, at least 6 weeks are required for initial healing and as long as a year may be necessary for return to normal activities. Changes in occupation and other activities may be necessary to avoid further problems.
DESIRED PATIENT OUTCOMES:	Verbalizes nature of the surgery performed, expectations for return to ADL and any restrictions that may be necessary on an individual basis.

INTERVENTIONS

Discuss return to activities, increasing as tolerated.

RATIONALE

Individual needs dictate tolerance levels.

Avoid activities that increase the flexion of the spinal column.

Make time for regular rest periods.

Use heat in the form of warm packs, showers, or heating pad. Tub baths are permitted after healing is sufficient.

Do not resume heavy work until 2–4 months after surgery.

Develop regular exercise program.

Instruct in use of brace.

Refer to Care Plan: Surgical Intervention.

Climbing stairs, automobile riding, bending at the waist with knees straight, and twisting of the spine.

Important to allow for healing and recuperation.

Aid in resolution of exudates.

Allows sufficient time for healing.

Strengthens abdominal muscles and erector muscles of spine.

Important to have correct application to gain most benefit.

DIAGNOSIS: Paraplegia/Quadriplegia: Acute Phase

PATIENT DATA BASE

NURSING HISTORY

History of a recent accident: e.g., car accidents (number 1 cause of para/quadriplegics in this country) or falls.

History of multiple sclerosis, neoplastic disease, vascular deficiency to the spinal column, or tuberculosis.

Determine current level of the spinal cord damage and control of bladder, bowels, sexual ability, respiratory difficulties, spasms.

Note use of a brace/corset because of previous injury/surgery.

Previous surgical intervention since injury, if applicable.

Note signs of depression.

Previous occupation, family dynamics, home environment, and financial situation.

Current/past medication use.

DIAGNOSTIC STUDIES

X-ray of spinal column: note level and type of injury.

X-ray of chest: rule out pneumonias, which are common in cervical and thoracic injuries because of inability to cough well.

Hct, Hb: note blood loss.

ABGs: note oxygenation of tissues.

Electrolytes: baseline and to note shifts.

Type/crossmatch if new injury, hemorrhage may occur.

Tidal volumes may be done on patients with high cord level injury to note respiratory capacity.

PHYSICAL EXAMINATION

Neurologic examination: level of function, sensation, reflex activity, hyper/hyporeflexia.

Blood pressure, pulse: bradycardia may be due to sympathetic impairment.

Lung sounds to determine respiratory status: may indicate progressing spinal shock.

Note skin integrity.

Abdominal exam: injuries present; bladder full, uncontrolled urination. Bowel sounds: often cease for 3–4 days post injury.

NURSING PRIORITIES

1. Prevent further injury and support respiratory/cardiovascular function.
2. Reduce/control pain.

3. Promote bladder/bowel control.
4. Provide information to assist patient/significant others in dealing with rehabilitation/psychosocial aspects and necessary lifestyle changes.

NURSING DIAGNOSIS:	Mobility, impaired physical.
SUPPORTING DATA:	Injury/illness may result in paraplegia, quadriplegia depending on the level of impairment to the spinal column; cervical, high-thoracic, thoracic, lumbar, low-sacral. Twisting or turning of the body can result in further injury to the spinal cord.
DESIRED PATIENT OUTCOMES:	Maintains optimal function/activity.

INTERVENTIONS

When turning patient, use several staff making turn in one motion. Using clear commands can coordinate movement.

Turn carefully following instructions for specialized beds and/or traction.

Document all positions and times of turning.

Turn at least every two hours.

Position to maintain proper alignment.

Do passive ROM, progressing to active exercises as condition allows.

Maintain ankles at 90°, with padded footboard.

Observe for pressure on heels; use trochanter rolls along thighs.

RATIONALE

Logrolling or moving with one motion and supporting the patient will prevent further injury. Depending on the type of traction, and/or bed, the turn needs to be made so the field is clear for treating the patient and support is available, as indicated.

Halo-pelvic traction, Crutchfield or Vinke tongs, Stryker or Foster frames, and CircOlectric bed are used to prevent twisting/extension movement of spinal column.

Ensure continuity in rotation schedule.

Prevent statsis, and pressure sores.

Prevents further cord damage, contractures, and joint freezing.

Strengthen muscles and prevent joint freezing and contractures.

Prevents footdrop.

The patient may not be aware of pressure because of loss of sensation. Prevent external rotation of the hips.

NURSING DIAGNOSIS:	Injury, potential for, spinal shock.

SUPPORTING DATA:	During spinal shock (which may last several days to many weeks but usually averages approximately three months), complete motor paralysis occurs with flaccidity, areflexia below the site of the lesion, loss of deep tendon and superficial reflexes, bladder and bowel paralysis, lack of vasomotor control, blood pressure drop, and lack of perspiration. May progress to hyperreflexia with spastic and involuntary movements.
DESIRED PATIENT OUTCOMES:	Spinal shock is treated and further injury is prevented.

INTERVENTIONS

Assess frequently for motor and sensory changes.

CERVICAL:

Assess breathing depth and pattern. Note decreasing tidal volumes.

Assess bowel sounds.

Assess edema of feet/ankles and elevate lower extremities periodically.

Keep room cool and use minimal covers but avoid exposure to drafts.

Give cool sponge baths.

Provide meticulous skin care according to level of immobility.

Patient may be placed in a head down position.

Consult with physician before encouraging coughing.

MEDICAL MANAGEMENT

IPPB, percussion, deep breathing, coughing.

RATIONALE

May indicate transection or increasing edema.

Nerve innervation to respiratory muscles may be interrupted.

Will return when peristalsis is regained. In spinal shock, may return in 48–72 hours or longer.

Loss of vascular tone and "muscle action" on vessels results in pooling of blood in lower extremities.

Inadequate thermal regulation caused by loss of vasomotor control.

Frequent febrile episodes.

Loss of sensation and paralysis result in easy pressure sore formation. (Refer to Care Plan: Long-Term Care, Skin integrity, impairment of, actual, decubitus ulcer.)

To allow bronchial secretions to drain by gravity.

Increases spinal pressure and may be contraindicated.

Decrease chances for secretions to accumulate in the bronchial tree. In thoracic injuries, may splint chest and have shallow respirations.

197

NG tube, on low suction.	May be necessary if paralytic ileus occurs.
Antiemboli stockings/abdominal binders.	Decrease pooling of blood in abdomen and legs and assist in venous return.
Corticosteroids.	May be useful to prevent/alleviate spinal cord edema.
Ventilatory assistance.	Necessary if unable to expand lungs owing to paralysis. Refer to Care Plan: Ventilatory Assistance (Mechanical).
Laminectomy.	May be necessary to reduce fracture/evacuate fragments and relieve compression of cord, which could cause further injury to the cord.
Experimentally:	
Alpha-methyltyrosine.	Blocks synthesis of norepinephrine, which causes vascular constriction decreasing blood supply to the cord in the immediate postinjury period.
Hyperbaric chamber.	Increases amount of oxygen dissolved in blood, thereby increases oxygen to the spinal cord.

NURSING DIAGNOSIS:	**Comfort, alteration in, pain/ discomfort.**
SUPPORTING DATA:	**After spinal shock, spasticity and muscle spasms may occur indefinitely and may be triggered by emotional factors, cutaneous stimuli and visceral stimulation.**
DESIRED PATIENT OUTCOMES:	**Comfort is maintained.**

INTERVENTIONS

RATIONALE

Maintain proper positioning: hips extended, shoulders abducted, feet at a 90° angle.	Decreased chance for spasticity.
Assess for pain.	Root pain may be present due to damage or irritation of the affected nerve roots.
Assist patient in recognizing predisposing factors of pain.	Burning pain and muscle spasms are aggravated by multiple factors (e.g., anxiety, tension, sitting for long periods of time, bladder stones).
Provide for position changes, massage, touch, and other measures, such as diversional activities.	Often medications for pain may produce undesirable side effects due to compromised respiratory ability; therefore, alternate measures for pain control should be used.

MEDICAL MANAGEMENT

Muscle relaxants.	Reduce spasms.
Analgesics; aspirin.	Relieve pain.

Narcotics.	Used for brief periods in acute stage. Use cautiously with cervical injuries, as they may increase respiratory depression. Addiction can be a problem with long-term use.
Sedatives/tranquilizers.	To control anxiety/fear and assist in decrease of pain.
Selective nerve block or surgical sectioning.	For severe pain unrelieved by other measures.

NURSING DIAGNOSIS:	**Bowel elimination, alteration in, constipation.**
SUPPORTING DATA:	**In spinal shock, reflex activity of the bowel is absent and paralytic ileus may occur.**
DESIRED PATIENT OUTCOMES:	**Functioning is restored/maintained.**

INTERVENTIONS

RATIONALE

Measure abdominal girth and ascultate bowel sounds.	With loss of sensation patient may not be aware of feelings that may be signs of ileus/impaction.
Promote adequate fluid intake, including prune juice.	Aid in maintaining stool consistency.
Document bowel movement and frequency.	Daily bowel movement can avoid impactions and distention.
Observe for incontinence and provide for cleansing and care of the skin.	Loss of sphincter control may occur.
Begin bowel-training program, as indicated by loss of function.	Will be important to social acceptance and independent functioning.
Control type of diet, avoid irritating foods.	Affects fecal consistency.

MEDICAL MANAGEMENT

NG tube to low suction.	Prevent vomiting, aspiration and relieve distention.
Rectal tube.	Pass flatus and relieve distention.
Glycerine suppository.	Stimulate peristalsis.
Stool softeners, laxatives, enemas.	Used with discretion as needed. May be necessary during spinal shock period.

NURSING DIAGNOSIS:	**Urinary elimination, alteration in pattern.**

199

SUPPORTING DATA:	In spinal shock, reflex activity of the bladder is absent. The neck of the bladder is constricted, dilation is increased and there is a lack of muscle tone. Incontinence occurs as an over-flow phenomenon and output is decreased.
DESIRED PATIENT OUTCOMES:	Urinary elimination is re-established/maintained.

INTERVENTIONS

Monitor intake and output. Encourage intake up to 3–4000 ml/day including cranberry juice.

Check for bladder distention on a regular basis and observe for overflow.

Clean perineal area t.i.d. and keep dry.

Institute appropriate bladder training program when catheter is removed.

MEDICAL MANAGEMENT

Indwelling catheter to closed drainage and/or intermittent catheterization schedule.

Vitamin C, Mandelamine.

RATIONALE

Helpful in maintaining renal function and prevention of infection and urinary stones.

Urinary retention may result in multiple complications, such as infection and autonomic hyperreflexia.

Decrease chance of infection and/or skin breakdown.

Depending on level of injury and amount of control remaining.

Keep bladder deflated.

Maintain acidic environment to discourage bacterial growth.

NURSING DIAGNOSIS:	Injury, potential for, autonomic hyperreflexia.
SUPPORTING DATA:	Exaggerated autonomic response can occur in patients with injury above T7 creating a medical emergency that can lead to cerebral hemorrhage and/or death.
DESIRED PATIENT OUTCOMES:	Complication is avoided/minimized.

INTERVENTIONS

Be aware of precipitating factors:
  Stimulation of pain receptors, bladder/bowel distention or manipulation, pressure on penis/testes.

RATIONALE

Visceral distention is most common cause of hyperreflexia.

Observe for symptoms; i.e., sudden severe rise in blood pressure, pounding headache, blurred vision, flushed face, restlessness, severe diaphoresis above level of injury, bradycardia, nasal congestion.

Early detection of impending emergency to initiate therapy.

Elevate head of bed immediately or place in sitting position.

Lower blood pressure and prevent CVA.

Check for bladder distention/obstruction of indwelling catheter.

Frequent precipitating factor.

Assess for fecal impaction, apply local anesthetic ointment in rectum and remove impaction after symptoms are alleviated.

Use of anesthetic agent will block autonomic stimulation allowing removal of impaction without further symptoms.

Assess room for other possible sources of sympathetic stimulation, i.e., cold air drafts.

Also precipitating factors.

MEDICAL MANAGEMENT

Ganglion blockers IV.

Blocks nerve transmission.

Atropine sulfate, Hyperstat.

Increase heart rate and decrease blood pressure.

Adrenergic blockers.

May be used prophylactically if problem is chronic.

Pelvic/pudendal nerve block or posterior rhizotomy.

If chronic problem, and/or does not respond to other therapies.

NURSING DIAGNOSIS:	**Knowledge deficit, diagnosis/prognosis.**
SUPPORTING DATA:	**Immobility, paralysis, and treatment result in anxiety and depression because of the unknown environment and fear of long-term consequences.**
DESIRED PATIENT OUTCOMES:	**Knowledge base will be expanded to allow for effective decision-making and anxiety and depression will be relieved.**

INTERVENTIONS

RATIONALE

Be available for listening, answering questions, and providing information, factually and honestly.

Will provide emotional support and establish rapport in which the patient can begin to deal with the traumatic changes that have occurred.

Be alert to depression and suicidal signals/gestures and provide close monitoring.

Often feel helpless and powerless.

Explain and involve patient in plan of care.

Provides information about what is happening, encourages autonomy, and promotes involvement in the rehabilitation process.

Have patient assist with care when physically and medically feasible.

Provides feeling of self-control.

Provide for sexual counseling.

Need to adapt to new expressions of sexuality. Paraplegic women can conceive, usually 3–8 months postinjury. Men may have penile implant if they are appropriate candidates. May be able to elicit reflex erection. Alternate methods of sexual satisfaction can be explored on an individual basis.

Teach signs/symptoms of autonomic hyperreflexia and appropriate interventions.

Immediate treatment reduces possibility of complications.

MEDICAL MANAGEMENT

Arrange for psychiatric/social services consult.

Need for long-term changes in life makes early intervention important.

Refer to Care Plan: Psychosocial Aspects of Care in the Acute Setting.

Note: Although strides are being made in the use of computerized electrical stimulus of muscles, the focus of learning must be based on handling the extent of the existing handicap until these advances are more widely available.

202

DIAGNOSIS: Guillain-Barré Syndrome, Polyradiculitis

PATIENT DATA BASE

NURSING HISTORY

History of mild respiratory or gastrointestinal infection 1–3 weeks prior to onset of symptoms in 50 percent of patients.

Complains of numbness, pain, tingling, and other sensations usually beginning in the lower extremities. Weakness, paralysis of muscles, usually involvement is bilateral progressing to the trunk, arms, and cranial nerves. Disease progressively continues for 10–14 days (paralysis of phrenic and intercostal nerves may result in respiratory failure).

History of recent vaccination or immunization. May be allergic or immunologic reaction.

History of past surgeries/injuries: in 10 percent of cases, this disease follows a surgical procedure.

Occurs equally in both sexes, in all seasons of the year, favors the young adult.

DIAGNOSTIC STUDIES

Baseline CBC, electrolytes.

Chest x-ray: prone to respiratory infections, especially if coughing is compromised.

ABGs: may reveal hypoventilation if respiratory function is compromised.

Urinalysis, specific gravity, osmolarity: baseline and estimation of hydration.

ECG: baseline and to rule out cardiac involvement.

Respiratory function tests.

Nerve conduction velocities may be decreased and show evidence of demyelination.

Cerebral spinal fluid tests: normal pressure and normal WBC count with increased protein. Protein continues to rise and reaches peak in 4–6 weeks and is thought to be due to release of plasma proteins from the inflammation, degeneration, and damage of nerve roots.

PHYSICAL EXAMINATION

Muscle weakness, flaccid paralysis, symmetrical, particularly in the lower extremities, sometimes in upper extremities and face.

Check for presence of paresthesias, other sensory disturbances.

Assess occurrence of hyper/hypotension, diaphoresis, and flushing which may indicate involvement of vagus (X) and hypoglossal (XII) cranial nerves.

Mental status exam.

NURSING PRIORITIES

1. Maintain/support respiratory function.
2. Maintain fluid and electrolyte balance.
3. Maintain body functioning, nutrition and elimination.
4. Assist patient/significant others with dealing with psychologic aspects of situation.

NURSING DIAGNOSIS:	Breathing pattern, ineffective.
SUPPORTING DATA:	Involvement of intercostal and abdominal muscles decreases respiratory effort. Involvement of cranial nerves produces loss of gag/swallow reflex.
DESIRED PATIENT OUTCOMES:	Normal ABGs, respiratory pattern and effort maintained.

INTERVENTIONS

RATIONALE

Assess respiratory rate, rhythm, tidal volume, and breath sounds every hour.

Respiratory insufficiency/paralysis may lead to pneumonia. Paralysis may occur insidiously and is shown by decreasing pulmonary volumes. Acute respiratory distress may be the first evidence of distress.

Note decrease in gag/swallow reflex and keep NPO.

Aspiration pneumonia may develop.

Monitor ABGs.

Prone to hypoxemia and hypercapnia.

Monitor for signs/symptoms of thrombophlebitis, pulmonary embolism.

Immobility predisposes to clot formation.

Keep on side if decreased gag/swallow reflex is present.

Maintain airway.

MEDICAL MANAGEMENT

Oxygen.

For hypoxemia and hypercapnia.

Antiembolic stockings.

Assist venous return.

Intubation/ventilation.

May be required when respiratory paralysis is severe (Refer to Care Plan: Ventilatory Assistance [Mechanical].)

NURSING DIAGNOSIS:	Fluid volume deficit, potential.
SUPPORTING DATA:	Decreased mobility may predispose to decreased function of bowel, sensitivity to bladder fullness. Loss of muscle tone, ventilators may lead to prerenal azotemia.
DESIRED PATIENT OUTCOMES:	Fluid/electrolyte balance is maintained.

INTERVENTIONS

Observe for dry mucous membranes, dry cracked lips, poor skin turgor, decreasing level of consciousness, thirst, and weight loss. Monitor for increasing hematocrit, BUN, creatinine and sodium.

Measure output and note amount of emesis and diarrhea as well.

Calculate insensible loss and output.

Monitor for abdominal tenderness, distention.

Guaiac all emesis and stools.

Oral medications may need to be crushed and given through feeding tube.

MEDICAL MANAGEMENT

IV fluids.

Antacids/cimetidine.

Serial chest x-rays.

RATIONALE

Signs of dehydration; extrarenal azotemia occurs with volume depletion; hypernatremia occurs with loss of free water.

Estimate of adequate hydration, bowel elimination.

Output should be at least 30 ml/hour. Insensible losses may be increased when the patient is on mechanical ventilation.

May indicate GI bleeding, fecal impaction.

May be prone to stress ulcers, when on mechanical ventilation.

If unable to swallow.

Prevent/control dehydration.

If gastric irritation/ulcers are present.

Observe fluid overload/pulmonary edema.

NURSING DIAGNOSIS:	**Elimination, alterations in, urinary/bowel, potential.**
SUPPORTING DATA:	**Immobility, decreased sensation may disturb normal signals for elimination.**
DESIRED PATIENT OUTCOMES:	**Elimination patterns are maintained adequately.**

INTERVENTIONS

Determine patient's previous patterns and aids used.

Evaluate intake and output. Unless contraindicated, intake should be 2–3000 ml/fluid/day; total intake should equal output, considering insensible losses.

Check for bladder distention.

Evaluate bowel sounds.

RATIONALE

Establishes goal for return to normal function.

Adequate hydration encourages normal bowel function; decreases risk of urinary tract infection and is a check for adequate hydration.

Sphincters are rarely involved but urinary retention may occur.

Hypoactive/absent sounds may signify ileus due to potassium imbalance, immobility.

Evaluate bowel movements for adequacy considering intake; place on bowel regimen, involving patient in planning if possible.

Avoids uncomfortable impaction. Patient's help will allow for some feelings of control in this situation where there is considerable loss of control.

MEDICAL MANAGEMENT

Stool softeners, laxatives as indicated.

May be needed to assist in bowel program.

Foley catheter.

If urinary retention occurs.

NURSING DIAGNOSIS:	**Nutrition, alteration in, less than body requirements.**
SUPPORTING DATA:	**Varying degrees of involvement and immobility can interfere with ability to chew and/or swallow.**
DESIRED PATIENT OUTCOMES:	**Weight is maintained at a desirable level.**

INTERVENTIONS

RATIONALE

Assess ability to chew and swallow.

Individual degree of impairment will dictate diet.

Assist with eating as indicated.

May need help with placement of food or may need to be fed.

MEDICAL MANAGEMENT

Nasogastric tube feedings.

May be used if dysphagia is present.

Refer to Care Plan: Total Parenteral Nutrition.

In severe cases, may need added intake.

NURSING DIAGNOSIS:	**Injury, potential for, skin integrity and infection.**
SUPPORTING DATA:	**Decreased muscle tone, absent reflexes, and immobility can lead to tissue breakdown. These patients are subject to infections that can result in death.**
DESIRED PATIENT OUTCOMES:	**Infection/problems of immobility do not occur.**

INTERVENTIONS

RATIONALE

Turn every two hours. Do range of motion on all extremities.

Prevent decubiti and/or flexion contractures and maintain muscle tone. Prevent complications of pneumonia/thrombophlebitis.

Be careful not to overexercise with passive range of motion in the early stages.	May overstretch muscle tissue or joints.
Provide for frequent rest periods.	May be exhausting due to required effort of weakened muscles.
Monitor vital signs; take blood cultures and CBC if temperature spikes.	Sepsis must be recognized early and treated aggressively.
Check IV sites every shift.	With loss of sensation, patient may not be aware of infiltration, phlebitis, and so forth.
Patch/tape eyes as indicated.	Prevents corneal ulcerations and abrasions when paralysis prevents eyelid closure.

MEDICAL MANAGEMENT

Alternating pressure mattress.	Decreases pressure on bony promininences to reduce risk of decubitus.
Antibiotics.	If infection occurs.
Analgesics.	Neuropathy/immobility may cause muscle aching and pain.
Artificial tears.	Protect eyes when blink reflex is absent.

NURSING DIAGNOSIS: **Coping, ineffective, individual/family.**

SUPPORTING DATA: **Paralysis is very frightening, and although it is usually temporary, it may be difficult to deal with slow and unknown outcome.**

DESIRED PATIENT OUTCOMES: **Coping skills are adequate to handle the situation, and anxiety is decreased to a manageable level.**

INTERVENTIONS

RATIONALE

Assess level of anxiety.	Provides a baseline for interventions and referrals.
Allow patient to react in own way without judgment by the staff, providing support as indicated.	Helpful in establishing trust and allowing for acceptance of individual reactions to the situation.
Provide information about the disease progression and therapy.	Helpful to know the recovery will be slow, and while there is no cure, supportive treatment will prevent/minimize complications. Information will help the patient/significant others recognize progress that is being made.
Assess functional capacity and place needed/familiar objects within sight.	Generalized weakness may limit patient independence and increase anxiety.
Establish communication and ways of contacting staff.	Critical for a patient whose communicating ability may become impaired as the disease progresses.

NURSING DIAGNOSIS:	Knowledge deficit, disease and prognosis.
SUPPORTING DATA:	Frightening onset of disease/paralysis creates concern re outcome of situation.
DESIRED PATIENT OUTCOMES:	Verbalizes expected outcomes of individual situation.

INTERVENTIONS

Inform patient/significant others about procedures and reasons for actions.

Review symptoms and discuss importance of contacting physician when problems arise.

Discuss probability of complete recovery with no residual deficits, with recovery phase usually lasting 3–6 months but some cases may last several years.

Discuss activity requirements and restrictions.

MEDICAL MANAGEMENT

Physical therapy consultation.

RATIONALE

Provide information for understanding.

Although disease is usually transient, symptoms may recur.

Information will be helpful to·planning for convalescence and may be helpful in lessening anxiety. (Refer to Care Plan: Psychosocial Aspects of Care in the Acute Setting.)

Exercises are increased slowly as tolerance increases. Overexertion and lack of precautions may lead to injuries.

May need additional assistance during long, slow convalescence.

DIAGNOSIS: Alzheimer's Disease

PATIENT DATA BASE

NURSING HISTORY

Patient may deny symptoms and/or describe vague complaints of fatigue, dizziness, or occasional headaches.

History of recent viral illness, recent head trauma may be associated with disorientation. Rule out reversible causes of confusion. Seizures may occur.

May present a total healthy picture except for memory/behavioral changes.

History from significant others who report an insidious decline in capabilities, behavior, and thought processes.

May report impaired recent memory with impaired motor skills.

May be suspicious or fearful of imaginary people and situations, misperceives environment, misidentifies objects and people, clings to significant others, claims misplaced objects are stolen.

May have impaired communication: unable to find correct words, substitutes meaningless words, conversation repetitive or drifts into nonsense, gradually loses ability to write or read.

Emotional lability: cries easily, laughs inappropriately, variable mood changes (apathy, lethargy, restlessness, irritability), sudden angry outbursts (catastrophic reactions), sleep disturbances.

Multiple losses, changes in body image, self-concept, self-esteem, may show depression overlay.

Current medications: may aggravate or precipitate reversible confusional states. Rule out drug toxicity or drug induced confusion.

Diet history: who provides and prepares meals? May forget mealtime, depends on others to cook, reports changes in taste, inability to: chew, feed self, use utensils or may refuse to eat.

Elimination: urgency may indicate loss of muscle tone, may be incontinent as disease progresses, or may be prone to constipation, forgets to go to bathroom or unable to find it.

Smoking habits: potential safety hazard if smokes.

Occupation: may have been forced to retire. Psychosocial factors, individuality and prior personality influence present altered behavioral patterns.

Hobbies: waning interest in usual activities.

May conceal inabilities, may thumb through a book without reading it. Content watching others, main activity may be hoarding inanimate objects, hiding articles, or wandering.

Sex, race, or familial tendencies not proven; disease process may begin in middle years and up.

DIAGNOSTIC STUDIES

CBC, VDRL, electrolytes, thyroid studies may determine and/or eliminate treatable, reversible dysfunctions.

B_{12}: if low, may disclose a nutritional deficit.

ECG: may show cardiac insufficiency.

EEG: may be normal or show some slowing, aids in establishing treatable brain dysfunctions.

Skull x-rays may be normal.

Vision and hearing deficits may be the cause of disorientation, mood swings, or altered sensory perceptions rather than an intellectual dysfunction.
CT scan may show widening of ventricles, cortical atrophy.

PHYSICAL EXAMINATION

Neurologic status: cognitive function, memory, orientation, confusion, disorientation to time and place. (May laugh at or feel threatened by these exams.) Orientation to person usually remains until late in the disease, being the last sense lost. Impaired recent memory, intact remote memory is typical of Alzheimer's. May change answers during the interview. Unable to do simple calculations, or repeat the names of three objects.
Evaluate gait, tremors, rigidity, and speech, which may be fragmented: aphasia and dysphasia may be present.
Evaluate reflexes: primitive reflexes (positive snout, suck, palmar) may be present.

Rule out treatable depressed state.

NURSING PRIORITIES

1. Limit aggressive behavior, promote socially acceptable responses.
2. Maintain reality orientation, prevent sensory deprivation/overload.
3. Protect patient from injury, complications.
4. Encourage participation in self-care within individual limitations.
5. Facilitate communication with patient/significant others.
6. Promote coping mechanisms of patient/significant others.
7. Assist patient/significant others in grieving process.

NURSING DIAGNOSIS:	**Thought processes, alteration in.**
SUPPORTING DATA:	**Neuronal degeneration produces varied neurobehavioral dysfunctions.**
DESIRED PATIENT OUTCOMES:	**Undesired behaviors, threats, and confusion are decreased by simplified communication.**

INTERVENTIONS	RATIONALE
Approach in a slow, calm manner.	Soothes and lessens the momentum of the short-lived anger and inner agitation that surges in the individual who misperceives or feels threatened by imaginary people and/or situations.
Maintain a pleasant, quiet environment.	Reduces distorted input; whereas, crowds, clutter, noise generate overload that irritates the impaired neurons.
Give simple directions, one at a time using short words and simple sentences.	As the disease progresses, the communication centers in the brain become impaired, hindering the individual's ability to decipher complex messages.
Decrease tone and rate when speaking.	Increases the chance for comprehension.

Pause between phrases or questions and open-ended phrases when possible.	Invites a response and may increase comprehension.
Face the individual.	Maintains reality, expresses interest, and arouses attention.
Listen with regard.	Conveys interest and worth to the individual with the inability to process messages or to formulate meaningful ideas into a sentence.
Decipher meaningful statements: offer positive feedback.	Helpful to state concrete ideas leaving out extraneous material so frustration is decreased. May not always comprehend but patient is aware of own confusion.
Reduce provacative stimuli: negative criticism, arguments, confrontations.	Any provocation is interpreted as a threat that may trigger a fight or flight response.
Assist with finding misplaced items or label drawers.	Decreases defensiveness when being accused of stealing a misplaced, hoarded, or hidden item. To refute the accusation won't change the belief and may create a catastrophic reaction.
Refrain from forcing activities and communications.	Force intimidates, accentuates suspiciousness, and intensifies confusion.
Focus on appropriate behavior, give positive responses.	Reinforces and soothes dulled senses.
Respect individuality and evaluate individual needs.	This person deserves respect in the same way an unimpaired individual does.
Respect personal space.	Intrusion threatens and potentiates a catastrophic reaction.
Use touch judiciously.	Frequently transcends verbal interchange, conveying warmth and reality.
Use humor with interactions.	Laughter can assist in dealing with the emotional lability of this individual.
Call by name.	Names form the self-identity, establish reality and individual recognition. These patients tend to misidentify and/or fail to recognize others before losing self-recognition.
Encourage the use of the telephone. (Post significant telephone numbers in a prominent place; secure long-distance numbers).	Can be used as a reality orientation but impaired judgment does not allow for distinguishing long-distance numbers.
Allow personal belongings.	Enhances sense of self and avoids feelings of deprivation.
Permit hoarding.	An activity that preserves security and counterbalances irrevocable losses.

NURSING DIAGNOSIS: **Memory deficit.**

SUPPORTING DATA: **Irreversible neuronal degeneration causes memory loss.**

| DESIRED PATIENT OUTCOMES: | Promote reality to aid memory gaps. |

INTERVENTIONS

Maintain a reality-oriented relationship and environment.

Provide clues for orientation (calendars, clocks, notecards).

Indulge in reminiscence (e.g., old time music, war stories).

Supply with mementos (e.g., pictures).

RATIONALE

Reduces confusion and deters painful, frustrating struggles while easing adaptation to the altered environment.

Clues are tangible reminders that aid recognition and permeate memory gaps.

Awakens memories and aids in the preservation of individuality while easing adaptation to a changed environment.

Stimulate recollections and increase feelings of security.

NURSING DIAGNOSIS:	Diversional activity, deficit.
SUPPORTING DATA:	Disease process causes a decreased attention span, restlessness, confined feelings. Premature retirement can cause boredom.
DESIRED PATIENT OUTCOMES:	Participates in activities compatible with ability.

INTERVENTIONS

Provide simple outings, short walks.

Create simple activities paced to the individual's speed.

Refer to interventions of previous nursing diagnosis.

RATIONALE

Nerve degeneration results in weakness and decreases motor functioning. Promote balanced physiologic functions, preserve mobility and reduce the potential for bone and muscle atrophy. Outings refresh reality, provide sensory stimuli that can deter suspiciousness, hallucinations, or feelings of imprisonment.

May be threatened by activities that may lead to failure. Motivate patient and reinforce usefulness and self-worth.

| NURSING DIAGNOSIS: | Rest-activity pattern, ineffective. |
| SUPPORTING DATA: | Neurologic impairment potentiates irritability, disorientation, poor judgment, which increase aimless wandering. |

DESIRED PATIENT OUTCOMES:	Rest-activity pattern is established and wandering is reduced.

INTERVENTIONS

Provide for rest/naps; reduce mental activity late in the day.

Avoid use of restraints.

Provide with an identification bracelet showing disease, name, and telephone number.

RATIONALE

Physical and mental activity result in fatigue; confusion increases with fatigue.

Invite humiliation, increase agitation, which restricts rest in addition to endangering the individual who succeeds in partial removal of restraints.

Facilitates safe return if lost. These individuals may be detained in jail as a consequence of confused wandering, irritable/violent outburtsts, and poor judgment.

NURSING DIAGNOSIS:	Injury, potential for, impaired judgment.
SUPPORTING DATA:	Wandering, forgetful, misidentifies objects.
DESIRED PATIENT OUTCOMES:	Injury is prevented.

INTERVENTIONS

Dress according to physical environment.

Be attentive to nonverbal physiologic symptoms.

Be alert to underlying meaning of verbal statements.

Minimize potential hazards in the environment.

Use child proof locks; lock medications, poisons, and so forth.

Teach significant others to be alert for potential hazards and how to avoid them.

RATIONALE

The general slowing of the metatolic processes results in less body heat. A leading cause of death is pneumonia.

Due to sensory loss and language dysfunction may express thirst by panting, pain by sweating, doubling over, and so forth.

May direct a question to another, such as "Are you cold/tired?" meaning they are cold/tired.

A confused individual is prone to accidental injury, because of the inability to take responsibility for basic safety needs or to evaluate the unforseen consequences (e.g., may light a stove/cigarette and forget it, mistake plastic fruit and eat it, misjudge stairs).

As the disease progressively worsens the individual is less able to take responsibility for basic safety needs. May fiddle with objects, locks or put small items in mouth, which potentiates opportunity for accidental injury/death.

Of utmost importance to prevent injury.

NURSING DIAGNOSIS:	Self-care deficit.
SUPPORTING DATA:	Increasing inability to cope with daily activities, frustration, misuse/ misidentification of objects, forgetfulness creates a situation in which the person needs additional care.
DESIRED PATIENT OUTCOMES:	Care provided sustaining as much independence as possible.

INTERVENTIONS	RATIONALE
Supervise but allow as much autonomy as possible.	Eases the frustration over lost independence.
Anticipate hygenic needs and assist with as needed. May include: care of nails, clean glasses, skin care, dental checks.	As the brain deterioration worsens, the individual neglects basic hygiene that may lead to harm or infection. Patient/caregivers may be irritated or intimidated by these problems.
Allot plenty of time to perform tasks.	Tasks once easy (e.g., dressing, bathing) are now complicated by decreased motor skills, mental and physical fatigue. Time and patience reduce chaos.
Assist with neat dressing, provide colorful clothes.	Enhance esteem, may diminish sense of sensory loss and convey aliveness.
Offer one item of clothing at a time, step by step.	Simplicity is the key to the prevention of rage and despair.
Allow to sleep in shoes/clothing.	Providing no harm is done, altering the ''normal'' lessens the rebellion and allows sleep.
When a problem arises, wait and/or change the time to approach dressing/hygiene.	Like the short-term memory, anger is quickly forgotten and another time or approach may be acceptable.

NURSING DIAGNOSIS:	Nutrition, alteration in, potential.
SUPPORTING DATA:	Impaired judgment and coordination, forgetfulness, regressed habits, and concealment can affect daily food intake and result in under/overeating with loss/gain of weight.
DESIRED PATIENT OUTCOMES:	Nutritional balance/weight is maintained.

INTERVENTIONS

Determine who prepares meals and that person's knowledge of dietary needs.

Offer/provide assistance in menu selection.

Provide privacy.

Offer small feedings and/or snacks.

Allow ample time for eating.

Allow automony in feeding.

Anticipate needs: cut foods, provide soft/finger foods. Offer a spoon. Avoid baby and hot foods.

RATIONALE

Will need assistance, as the individual may forget it is mealtime or be unable to cook/shop for self.

Is indecisive, overwhelmed by choices, or unaware of the need to maintain elemental nutrition. Metabolic rate decreases with age requiring calorie adjustment.

Aids esteem. Socially unacceptable and embarrassing eating habits develop as the disease progresses.

Large feedings may overload the patient resulting either in complete abstinence or bulimia.

A leisurely approach facilitates digestion and enables an individual with a decrease in motor functioning time to chew.

Decreases potential catastrophic reactions at mealtime. (Finger foods, sandwiches ease inabilities.)

Coordination decreases with the progression of the disease process. The ability to chew and handle utensils becomes impaired. Baby foods lack fiber, taste, and add to humiliation. Hot foods may burn or result in refusal to eat.

NURSING DIAGNOSIS: **Elimination, alteration in patterns.**

SUPPORTING DATA: **A potential for incontinence/constipation exists because of urgency, disorientation, lost neurologic functioning, or inability to locate the bathroom.**

DESIRED PATIENT OUTCOMES: **Problems of elimination are minimized/managed.**

INTERVENTIONS

Locate near a bathroom; make signs for or color-code door.

Provide adequate lighting particularly at night.

Take to the toilet at regular intervals.

Encourage adequate fluid intake during the day; limit intake during the late evening and at bedtime.

Be alert to nonverbal cues.

RATIONALE

Location, adequate lighting, signs, and/or color coding enhance orientation.

Incontinence may be attributed to inability to find a toilet.

Adherence to a daily and regular schedule may prevent accidents.

Essential for bodily functions and prevents potential constipation. Restricting intake in evening reduces frequency during the night.

Such as restlessness, holding self, or picking at clothes may signal urgency.

MEDICAL MANAGEMENT

Stool softeners or Metamucil.

May be necessary to facilitate regular bowel movement.

NURSING DIAGNOSIS:	**Sexual dysfunction.**
SUPPORTING DATA:	**Confusion, forgetfulness, and disorientation to place or person can lead to unacceptable/undesirable behaviors.**
DESIRED PATIENT OUTCOMES:	**Able to meet own sexual needs in an acceptable manner.**

INTERVENTIONS

Show affection.

Assure privacy.

RATIONALE

The intellectually confused retain the basic needs of affection, love, acceptance, and sexual expression.

Sexual expression or behavior may differ. The individual may masturbate, expose self. Privacy allows sexual expression without embarrassment and the objections of others.

NURSING DIAGNOSIS:	**Coping, ineffective family (compromised or disabling).**
SUPPORTING DATA:	**The patient's behavior is disruptive to the family, socially immobilizing and embarrassing. The family grieves over their helplessness while watching their loved one deteriorate. Home maintenance is extremely difficult leading to difficult decisions with legal/financial problems.**
DESIRED PATIENT OUTCOMES:	**Family better able to cope with long-term incapacitation of the family member.**

INTERVENTIONS

Include all significant others in teaching and planning for home care.

RATIONALE

Can ease the burden of home management and adaptation. Comfortable and familiar lifestyle at home is helpful in preserving the need for belonging for the affected individual.

Allow for unlimited visitation.

Provides a reassuring freedom from loneliness and contact with familiarity, which can maintain a base of reality for the individual.

Provide comfort for significant others.

The self-sacrificing, painful nature of the care in this disease requires support and comfort to let them know they are doing their best and to ease the process of adaptation and grievance.

Refer to local resources:
Adult day care, respite care, Homemaker Services, or a local chapter of ADRDA (Alzheimer's Disease and Related Disorders Association).

Coping with this individual is a fulltime, frustrating task. Respite care may lighten the burden, reduce potential social isolation, and prevent family burnout. ADRDA is a national organization with many local chapters that provide group support, family teaching and promote research. Local groups provide a social outlet for sharing grief and promote problem-solving with such matters as financial and legal advice, home care, and so forth.

Nursing Home placement may need to be considered; support significant others' needs around such a decision.

Constant care needs may be more than can be managed. Support aids this difficult guilt-producing decision that may become a financial burden also.

BIBLIOGRAPHY

Books and Other Individual Publications

ADAMS, J. C.: *Outline of Orthopaedics,* ed. 9, Churchill Livingston, Edinburgh, 1981.

BEYERS, M. AND DUDAS, S.: *The Clinical Practice of Medical Surgical Nursing.* Little, Brown & Co., Boston, 1977.

BRUNNER, L. S. AND SUDDARTH, D. S.: *The Lippincott Manual,* ed. 2. J. B. Lippincott, Philadelphia, 1980.

BUDASSI, S. H. AND BARBER, J. M.: *Emergency Nursing: Principles and Practice.* C. V. Mosby, St. Louis, 1981.

BURNSIDE, I. M.: *Nursing and the Aged.* McGraw-Hill, New York, 1981.

CAMPBELL, C.: *Nursing Diagnosis and Intervention in Nursing Practice.* John Wiley & Sons, New York, 1978.

DAVIS, J. E. AND MASON, C. B.: *Neurologic Critical Care.* C. V. Mosby, St. Louis, 1981.

HART, L. K. ET AL.: *Concepts Common to Acute Illness: Identification and Management.* C. V. Mosby, St. Louis, 1981.

JOHANSON, B. C. ET AL.: *Standards for Critical Care.* C. V. Mosby, St. Louis, 1981.

KIM, M. AND MORITZ D. (EDS.): *Classifications of Nursing Diagnosis.* McGraw-Hill, New York, 1981.

LUCKMANN, J. AND SORENSEN, K. C.: *Medical-Surgical Nursing,* ed. 2. W. B. Saunders, Philadelphia, 1980.

MACE, N. AND RABINS, P. V.: *The 36-Hour Day: A Family Guide to Caring for Persons with Alzheimer's Disease, Related Dementing Illnesses, and Memory Loss in Later Life.* The Johns Hopkins University Press, Baltimore, 1981.

PHIPPS, W. J., LONG, B. C. AND WOODS, N. F.: *Medical-Surgical Nursing.* C. V. Mosby, St. Louis, 1979.

ROAF, R. AND HODKINSON, L.: *Textbook of Orthopaedic Nursing,* ed. 3, Blackwell Scientific Publishers, Oxford, London, 1980.

STRUB, R. L. AND BLACK, F. W.: *Organic Brain Syndromes: An Introduction to Neurobehavioral Disorders.* F. A. Davis, Philadelphia, 1981.

TILKIAN, S. M., CONOVER, M. B., AND TILKIAN, A. G.: *Clinical Implications of Lab Tests.* C. V. Mosby, St. Louis, 1979.

TUCKER, S. ET AL.: *Patient Care Standards,* ed. 2. C. V. Mosby, St. Louis, 1980.

WILKINS, R. W. AND LEVINSKY, N. G. (EDS.): *Medicine, Essentials of Clinical Practice.* Little, Brown & Co., Boston, 1978.

WOLANIN, M. AND PHILLIPS, L.: *Confusion.* C. V. Mosby, St. Louis, 1981.

Journal Articles

ALVAREZ, S. E. ET AL.: *Respiratory treatment of the adult patient with spinal cord injury.* Physical Therapy, J. of the Amer. Physical Therapy Assoc., Dec.:61:1737–45, 1981.

ALZHEIMER'S DISEASE. Special Issue: The J. of Gerontological Nursing, 8(2):1–120, Feb. 1982.

BARTOL, M. A.: *A therapeutic approach to patients with Alzheimer's disease.* Presentation at the Fourth National Symposium on Psychiatric/Mental Health Nursing co-sponsored by the J. of Psychosoc. Nurs. Mental Health Services and the Shc. of Nurs., Univ. of CA, San Francisco, April 26, 1982.

BARTOL, M.A.: *Non-verbal communication in patients with Alzheimer's disease.* J. of Gerontological Nursing, 5(4):21–31, July/August 1979.

BUTLER, R.: *Aging: Research leads and needs.* Forum on medicine, 716–725, Nov. 1979.

BUTLER, R.: *White House conference on Alzheimer's disease-senile dementia and related disorders.* National Institute on Aging, 1978.

BYRNE, C.: *Coping with brain disease: It's like a funeral that never ends.* The Minneapolis Star, (ADRDA Reprint), Nov. 13, 1978.

CAMERON, I. ET AL.: *Assessing and managing dementia.* Patient Care, 2(20):90–116, November 30, 1977.

DONOVAN, W. AND BEDBROOK, B.: *Comprehensive management of spinal cord injury.* Clinical Symposia, Ciba Vol. 34, No. 2, 1982.

Katzman, R.: *Early detection of senile dementia.* Hospital Practice, 16(6):61–76, June 1981.

LEZAK, M. D.: *Living with the characteriologically altered brain injured patient.* The Journal of Clinical Psychiatry, 39(1):99–15, July 1978.

Living with paraplegia: day by day (Peter S.) (case study). Nurs. Mirror, Mar. 17:154–44–5, 1982

MASTRIAN, K. G.: *Of course you can manage head and trauma patients.* RN, 44:44–51, 1981.

MILLER, M.: *Symposium on emergency nursing. Emergency management of the unconscious patient.* NCNA, 16:59–73, 1981.

MORTIMER, J.: *Research on Alzheimer's disease.* ADRDA, Chicago, 1980.

NORMAN, S. E. ET AL.: *Seizure disorders.* AJN, 81:983–1000, 1981.

People with spinal injuries: Treatment and care. (pictorial) Nurs. Times, Feb. 24/Mar. 2:78:(spinal injuries suppl) 1–4, 1982.

The Alzheimer's disease and related disorders association, (a series of quarterly newsletters), 1(1–3), March 1981–Winter 1982.

Alzheimer's disease: A scientific guide for health practioners. U.S. Dept. of Health and Human Services, (NIH Pub. No. 81-2251), U.S. Govt. Printing Off., Washington, D. C., 1980.

Progress report on senile dementia of the Alzheimer's type. U.S. Dept. for Health and Human Services, (NIH Pub. No. 81-2343), Prepared for the White House Conference on Aging, U.S. Govt. Printing Off., Washington, D. C., Sept. 1981.

The dementias. U.S. Dept. of Health and Human Services, (NIH Pub. No. 81-2252), U.S. Govt. Printing Off., Washington, D. C., March 1981.

CHAPTER **6**
OPHTHALMOLOGY

DIAGNOSIS: Ocular Disorders and Surgery (Detached Retina, Cataracts, Glaucoma)

PATIENT DATA BASE

NURSING HISTORY

Detached Retina:
  May have history of trauma.
  May complain of blurred vision, flashes of light, particles floating in the visual field, veil-like curtain that reduces visual field. Generally is free of pain.

Cataracts:
  Most frequently seen in adults after age 40.
  Complains of visual distortion (blurred/hazy), bright light causing a glare, and gradual loss of vision.
  History of exposure to hair/eyelash dyes.
  Does not complain of pain.
  Pupil may appear gray or milky white.

Glaucoma:
  Most frequently seen in adults after age 35.
  Primary: cause unknown but associated with history of stress, allergy, vasomotor disturbances, endocrine imbalance, heredity.
  Secondary: history of hemorrhage, trauma, ocular disease, tumor.
  Chronic: complains of mild discomfort (e.g., eyes feeling tired), halos around lights, and loss of peripheral vision.
  Acute: complains of cloudy/blurred vision, sudden/severe pain in and around eyes, appearance of rainbows in artificial light, nausea/vomiting, dilation of pupils.

DIAGNOSTIC STUDIES

CBC, sedimentation rate: rule out systemic infection or anemia.

EEG: rule out neurologic disease.

ECG, serum cholestrol and lipid studies: rule out atherosclerosis, coronary artery disease.

Tonography measurement assesses intraocular pressure (normal: 12-25 mm Hg).

Gonioscopy measurement helps differentiate open-angle from angle-closure glaucoma.

PHYSICAL EXAMINATION

Snellen eye chart: assess visual acuity and central vision (may be impaired by defects in cornea, lens, aqueous or vitreous humor, refractive error, or disease of the nervous system supplying the retina or optic pathway).

Assess peripheral visual field (reduction may be caused by CVA, pituitary, brain tumor mass, carotid or cerebral artery pathology).

Assess coordination of extraocular optic muscles with corneal light reflex.

Examine eye for presence of exudate, excessive lacrimation/dryness, redness of sclera or lids, position of eyelids when eyes are fully open/closed, abnormal nodules in or around eye structures.

Note position of eyeballs in socket: normal versus deep or protruding.

Assess pupil size and accommodation.

Examine internal ocular structures with ophthalmoscope to assess presence of glaucoma, optic disk atrophy, papilledema, retinal hemorrhage, and microaneurysms.

Eye may appear inflamed, cornea steamy, anterior chamber shallow, aqueous turbid, pupil may be moderately dilated and may not respond to light.

NURSING PRIORITIES

1. Prevent further visual deterioration.
2. Assist patient in coping with reduced visual acuity, lifestyle changes (if necessary), and treatments.
3. Assist in learning principles of eye care and disease prevention.

NURSING DIAGNOSIS:	**Injury, potential for, infection/ wound dehiscence/increased intra-ocular pressure.**
SUPPORTING DATA:	**Many normal patient activities may cause intraocular pressure to rise, which may rupture ocular wound. The eye is often touched and can easily be contaminated.**
DESIRED PATIENT OUTCOMES:	**Exhibits no symptoms of eye infection or incisional dehiscence.**

INTERVENTIONS

Discuss postoperative expectations; pain, restrictions, appearance, eye bandaging, availability of staff, and anticipated routine. Allow verbalization of fears and concerns.

RATIONALE

Can be helpful to allay fears and enhance cooperation with necessary restrictions.

If advisable, assist with shaving, washing hair; secure or braid long hair. Eyebrows are never shaved; eyelashes may be trimmed during surgery.

These activities may be temporarily curtailed postop. Eyebrows may not regrow into same pattern if shaved.

When returning from surgery, transfer from stretcher to bed in horizontal position. Patient may assist while nurse supports head.

Patient is not to strain. Neutral position avoids pressure on new suture line.

Generally may lie on back or unoperated side. In the case of detached retina, position is prescribed according to location of injury.

Avoids pressure on newly operated eye. Area of retinal detachment should be kept dependent.

Avoid bumping bed.

May startle patient who is attempting to lie quietly and may also cause detachment of retina.

Keep lighting subdued.

Preferable to bright light that may cause patient to close eyes tightly, exerting pressure on new suture line.

Observe for hyphema (bleeding in the eye) postop, especially in cateract removal.

May occur due to strain or for no apparent reason, healing tissue is highly vascular and capillaries are fragile.

Observe for bulging of wound, flat anterior chamber, pear-shaped pupil.

Denotes prolapse of iris or wound rupture caused by loosened sutures or pressure on eye.

Encourage frequent deep breathing, but not coughing.

Coughing increases intraocular pressure.

Encourage activity, ambulation, active/passive ROM exercises several times daily as allowed by individual situation.

Some surgical interventions require avoiding movement postop, while others have minimal restrictions.

Postop, may be allowed up to bathroom with assistance.

Requires less strain than use of bedpan, which could increase intraocular pressure.

Place needed items, call bell within easy reach on unoperated side.

Allows patient to see objects more easily and avoids straining.

Limit activities that may increase intraocular pressure: avoid sudden movement of the head, rubbing eyes, bending/stooping.

May stress operative area or worsen glaucoma.

Discuss importance of not touching operated eye.

Prevent contamination.

Observe for nausea/vomiting. Roll toward unoperated side if vomiting.

Prevent contamination of dressing.

Use sterile technique when performing eye care.

Helps prevent intraocular infection, which may have severe results.

If dressing becomes loose, secure and replace eye shield over dressing.

Many physicians prefer to change dressings to observe the wound. If dressing is not dislodged or otherwise contaminated, reinforce position with silk or paper tape.

Observe for complaints of sharp eye pain that is unrelieved, restlessness, disorientation, signs of upper respiratory infection, disturbance of dressing, and contraindicated activities.

May indicate hemorrhage, infection, occurrence or risk of complications.

Avoid use of talcums, spices.

May cause sneezing or coughing.

Limit use of opiates.

Caution not to use soiled tissue to wipe eyes.

May cause vomiting.

May introduce bacteria into eye.

MEDICAL MANAGEMENT

Antiemetics.

Prevent vomiting with resulting rise in intraocular pressure.

Eye drops: parasympathomimetics, (miotics).

Contracts pupil, drawing iris from cornea and allowing drainage of aqueous humor.

Sympathomimetics.

Decreases production of aqueous humor.

Beta-blockers.

Decreases intraocular pressure.

IV/po:

Carbonic anhydrase inhibitors.

Restricts enzymatic action in production of aqueous humor.

Hyperosmotic agents.

Increased blood osmolality; thereby, pulling fluid from tissues and decreasing intraocular pressure.

Antibiotic ointments.

Prophylactic or if infection does occur.

Stool softeners.

Avoid straining at stool, which may increase intraocular pressure.

Light restraints.

May be needed if uncooperative and touching bandage.

Warm, sterile compresses.

Facilitate resolution of infection and increase patient comfort. Infection may result in adhesions that may impede aqueous outflow, produce traction on retina. Metabolism of lens may be altered by outflow, producing cataract formation.

Trabeculectomy/trephining.

Filtering operations that create an opening between the anterior chamber and the subjunctival spaces so that aqueous humor can bypass the trabecular mesh block.

Cataract extraction.

May be elected prior to glaucoma surgery. Most treatments for glaucoma speed up cataract formation and extraction may favorably affect the glaucoma course.

Iridectomy in upper segment of iris.

Treatment of choice in narrow-angle glaucoma. Upper iris usually is covered with upper eyelid and flow of tears washes bacteria downward. Prophylactic iridectomy is performed because glaucoma is bilateral and will usually develop in the other eye.

Alternate dilatation and constriction by the use of eye drops.

Mobilize pupil and prevent posterior synechia.

Steroids.

May be used to decrease inflammation.

Massage eye.

May be ordered to encourage continued flow of fluids through surgical opening.

NURSING DIAGNOSIS:	Comfort, alteration in, pain.
SUPPORTING DATA:	Some surgical techniques may produce moderate pain postop. Pain causes restlessness and increases activity that may increase intraocular pressures causing rupture of suture line or iris prolapse.
DESIRED PATIENT OUTCOMES:	Comfort is maintained and no undesired complications occur.

INTERVENTIONS

Assess pain.

Provide for comfort measures, such as position changes, and back rub.

Observe for vomiting.

RATIONALE

May indicate hemorrhage and/or increased intraocular pressure.

Minimize restlessness and maintain restricted activity level.

May indicate or cause increased intraocular pressure and pain.

MEDICAL MANAGEMENT

Analgesics.

Cold compresses.

For mild to severe discomfort.

May soothe red, swollen tissues and reduce edema.

NURSING DIAGNOSIS:	Sensory perception, alteration in.
SUPPORTING DATA:	Disease condition, surgical procedures and bandages may limit sight.
DESIRED PATIENT OUTCOMES:	Experiences minimum of untoward reactions because of sight limitation.

INTERVENTIONS

Orient to room, staff, other patients in the room preoperatively.

Observe for signs of disorientation, especially toward evening.

Speak and touch often; encourage significant others to stay with patient as much as possible.

RATIONALE

Provides for increased comfort level and familiarity and reduces postop disorientation.

May become more pronounced during evening hours.

Provides increased sensory stimulation that offsets isolation and occurrence of confusion.

Caution about dim or blurred vision, irritation of eye, which may occur when using eye drops.

May last for 1–2 hours after use but gradually decreases with use. Local irritation should be reported to the physician but do not stop use of the drug in the interim.

Provide diversional activities as able; such as radio, conversation, talking books.

Provide other sensory input and passes time more easily.

Keep side rails up at all times.

Decreases risk of falling, as patient may be unfamiliar with size of bed.

Position call bell within reach and orient patient to its location.

Facilitates patient calling for assistance as needed.

Position doors so they are completely opened or closed and position furniture out of the travel pathways.

Decreased peripheral vision or altered depth perception may cause patient to walk into partially opened door, trip over footstools, and so forth.

Describe food when patient cannot see; feed slowly with small bites.

Increases differences in taste perceptions; decreases chance of choking/vomiting.

May remove patch from unaffected eye during meals or at prescribed intervals.

Decreases disorientation and anxiety; promotes relaxation.

MEDICAL MANAGEMENT

Pinhole glasses.

Decrease eye movement and facilitate rest and healing.

Neo-Synephrine, Cyclogyl, mydriatics.

May be used in retinal detachment to dilate pupil to facilitate retinal visualization.

NURSING DIAGNOSIS:	**Knowledge deficit, disease and complications.**
SUPPORTING DATA:	**Complications/disease progression may cause few symptoms but may result in permanent blindness. Lack of knowledge can lead to improper care.**
DESIRED PATIENT OUTCOMES:	**Avoids activities that may aggravate condition or increase risk of eye damage.**

INTERVENTIONS

Encourage periodic checkups.

RATIONALE

Prior disease/injury of the eye may predispose to the development of further eye disease. There is a hereditary tendency associated with the most common forms of glaucoma.

Review symptoms that are important to report to the physician: progressive dimming of vision, "floaters" or sparks, partial/complete loss of vision.

May signal acute attack of glaucoma, retinal detachment, or side effect of drugs or other disease. Occurrence of retinal detachment may release blood cells and pieces of retinal pigment into vitreous that are seen as sparks and floaters.

Discuss the importance of avoiding or limiting emotionally stressful situations, tight-fitting clothing, lifting or straining, bending, upper respiratory infections, excessive fluid intake, rubbing eyes, sexual activities, smoking, reading, shower/tub baths, shampooing, and mydriatic drugs (atropine).

Activities that increase eye strain or intraocular pressure may compromise surgical results and cause severe complications.

Discuss modifications of or alternative sexual activities.

Unless alternatives are found, patient may not adhere to restrictions.

Advise to cough with mouth wide open.

Minimizes increased pressure build-up.

Discuss reduced accommodation that occurs with use of miotic drugs and may cause compromised vision, especially in poorly lit areas.

With miotics, less light may enter pupil to reflect image on retina.

Aphakic (without lens) patients require retraining for depth perception.

Glasses enlarge objects by 1/3 and alter perception. (Less distortion with use of contact lenses.) If only one eye has no crystalline base, binocular vision is impossible without corrective lenses. Requires patience and practice for use.

Ocular conditions may require lifelong treatment. Review drug dosage and side effects. Avoid use of medications/eye washes not specifically prescribed by the physician.

Conditions may be controlled rather than cured; awareness of this can enhance cooperation with necessary treatment/lifestyle changes.

Encourage wearing eye shield at night.

Protects eye from inadvertent injury.

Teach general principles for prevention of eye injuries:

Use eye protective devices or shelter.

Protect eyes from flying objects and harmful agents that have a potential for damaging the internal or external structures.

If foreign matter enters eye, irrigate with copious amounts of tap water or allow eye to wash itself with tears by displacing top eyelid manually over lower eyelid.

Irrigation neutralizes and washes irritating or harmful substances out of eye. Allows tears to wash over orbit and flow foreign matter into lower lid pocket or out of eye.

Seek immediate medical care if damage is suspected or symptoms unrelieved.

Prevent serious complications, including loss of vision.

Glaucoma patients should be encouraged to carry medical identification.

In case of accident, information will be helpful as some medical treatments may be contraindicated.

BIBLIOGRAPHY

Books and Other Individual Publications

BEYERS, M. AND DUDAS, S.: *The Clinical Practice of Medical-Surgical Nursing.* Little, Brown & Co., Boston, 1977.

BRUNNER, L. S. AND SUDDARTH, D. S.: *Textbook of Medical-Surgical Nursing,* ed. 3. J. B. Lippincott, Philadelphia, 1975.

BRUNNER, L. S. AND SUDDARTH, D. S.: *Lippincott Manual of Nursing Practice.* J. B. Lippincott, Philadelphia, 1978.

KIM, M. AND MORITZ, D. (EDS.): *Classification of Nursing Diagnosis.* McGraw-Hill, New York, 1981.

PHIPPS, W. J., LONG, B. C., AND WOODS, N. F.: *Medical-Surgical Nursing.* C. V. Mosby, St. Louis, 1979.

TILKIAN, S. M., CONOVER, M. B., AND TILKIAN, A. G.: *Clinical Implications of Laboratory Tests.* C. V. Mosby, 1979.

WILKINS, R. W. AND LEVINSKY, N. G. (EDS.): *Medicine, Essentials of Clinical Practice.* Little, Brown & Co., Boston, 1978.

CHAPTER 7

GASTROENTEROLOGY

DIAGNOSIS: Eating Disorders: Anorexia Nervosa; Anorexia Nervosa-Bulimia

PATIENT DATA BASE

NURSING HISTORY

Asterisks indicate DSM III (*Diagnostic and Statistical Manual of Mental Disorders*) diagnostic criteria.

*Onset before age 25 to early 30s.

*Disturbed (unrealistic) body image. Reports self as fat regardless of weight; sees thin body as fat.

*Expresses intense fear of gaining weight.

*No medical illness evident to account for weight loss.

Exhibits a distorted attitude toward eating, food, and weight.

Denies hunger; appetite rarely vanishes, may be normal or exaggerated.

Displays an unrealistic pleasure in weight loss, while denying self-pleasure in other areas.

Refuses to maintain normal weight for age and height.

Exhibits sense of helplessness.

Often no other psychiatric illness is present and no evidence of the presence of a thought disorder.

May have a hysterical or obsessive personality style.

Displays appropriate affect, except in regard to body and eating.

Usually intelligent and a good student. Often middle-class family.

History of being a quiet, cooperative child.

May be evidence of an emotional crisis of some sort; such as the onset of puberty or a family move.

May be an avid exerciser.

May complain of feeling cold even when room is warm.

Disturbed sleep patterns, commonly early morning insomnia.

Loss of sexual interest.

In bulimia, weight remains near normal, with ingestion of huge amounts of food, often in binges, followed by self-induced vomiting, use of laxatives and/or fasting.

May have epileptic seizures.

May binge secretively and in private, and usually does not present early for treatment.

DIAGNOSTIC STUDIES

Endocrine studies:
Usually has normal thyroxine levels, however, circulating triiodothyronine (T_3) levels are low.

Pituitary Function:
TSH (Thyroid Stimulating Hormone) response to TRF (thyrotropin releasing factor) is abnormal in anorexia nervosa.
Propranolol-glucagon stimulation test studies the response of human growth hormone. In anorexia nervosa there is a depressed level of growth hormone.
Gonadotropic hypofunction.

Hypothalamic function tests: abnormality may be a cause of anorexia (rare).

Cortisol metabolism abnormalities are present (elevated).

Leukopenia, elevated BUN, elevated SGOT, hypercarotenemia, anemia.

Abnormal ECG, low voltage, T-wave inversion.

Electrolyte derangements: decreased K^+ and Cl^-, increased CO_2.

Urinalysis and renal function tests as indicated.

PHYSICAL EXAMINATION

(Asterisks indicate DSM III diagnostic criteria).

*Presence of weight loss of 25% or more of total body weight.

Cachectic appearing.

*Amenorrhea. May be the presenting symptom.

*May exhibit periods of hyperactivity.

*Increased hair growth on body.

*May have low BP and bradycardia (less than 60/min).

*Vomiting may occur: may have binge-purge syndrome (bulimia) with subsequent stomach problems.

Dehydration may be evident.

Tooth decay may be present, due to acidity from vomiting.

Mental status exam may reveal mental changes brought on by malnutrition (starvation).

Constipation may be present; determine use of laxatives and/or diuretics.

Polyuria.

May have swollen salivary glands, benign, not painful; and constant sore throat.

NURSING PRIORITIES:

1. Reestablish adequate nutrition to remedy/prevent malnutrition.
2. Remedy fluid and electrolyte imbalance to prevent death.

3. Establish a therapeutic nurse/patient relationship in which the patient can begin to assume responsibility for self.
4. Cooperate with other disciplines in a total treatment program to provide consistent effective care.

NURSING DIAGNOSIS:	Nutrition, alteration in, less than body requirements.
SUPPORTING DATA:	Inadequate food intake leads to malnutrition. Distorted attitude toward food, unusual hoarding or handling of food. Cure of the underlying problem cannot happen without improved nutritional status. Internal control mechanisms of hunger and/or satiation may be lost.
DESIRED PATIENT OUTCOMES:	Adequate nutritional intake with weight gain to within normal limits.

INTERVENTIONS

May need to be hospitalized for nutrition therapy. Make selective menu available.

Provide regular diet and snacks with substitutes and preferred foods available.

Allow patient to control choices.

Use a consistent approach. Present and remove food without persuasion and/or comment.

Sit with patient while the patient is eating. Make no comment on food.

Be alert to choices of low-calorie foods; hoarding food; disposing of food in various places, such as pockets or wastebaskets.

Behavior modification program may be instituted. Involve patient in setting up program. Provide reward for weight gain, ignore loss.

Provide one to one supervision. Have the patient remain in the room with no bathroom privileges for a specified period (½ hour) following eating.

RATIONALE

Controlled environment; food intake and output, medication, and activities can be monitored. Separates from family who may be causative factor; although family therapy may be the treatment of choice.

Having a variety of foods available will enable the patient to have a choice of potentially enjoyable foods.

Patient needs to gain confidence in self and feel in control of environment.

Patient detects urgency and reacts to pressure. When staff responds in a consistent manner, patient can begin to trust their responses. Avoids manipulative games.

Coercion provides focus on food. May experience guilt if forced to eat.

Patient will try to avoid taking in what the patient views as too many calories.

Provides structured eating situation while allowing patient some control in choices. Behavior modification may be effective only in mild cases or for short-term weight gain.

Prevent vomiting during/after eating. Sometimes patient desires food and uses a binge-purge syndrome to maintain weight.

Monitor exercise program and set limits on physical activities. Chart activity level of work (e.g., pacing).	Patient will exercise excessively to burn calories.
Establish a minimum weight goal.	When this is agreed upon, psychologic work can begin.
Maintain a regular weighing schedule, such as M–W–F before breakfast in same attire and graph results.	Provides accurate ongoing record of weight loss and/or gain. Also may prevent obsessing about gains and/or losses.
Do not give laxatives.	Often used by patient to rid body of food/calories.
Limit room checks and control devices.	Usually not helpful, as may reinforce feelings of powerlessness.
Be alert to possibility of patient disconnecting tube and emptying hyperalimentation. Check measurements and tape tubing snugly.	Sabotage behavior is common in attempt to prevent weight gain.

MEDICAL MANAGEMENT

Total liquid diet and/or tube feedings.	When calorie intake is insufficient to sustain metabolic needs, tube feedings can be used to prevent malnutrition and death while therapy is continuing.
May blend and tube feed anything left on the tray after a given period of time.	As part of behavior modification program.
High-calorie liquid feedings.	May be given as medication.
Electroshock therapy.	In difficult cases when malnutrition is severe and may be life-threatening, a short-term EST series may enable the patient to begin eating and become accessible to psychotherapy.

NURSING DIAGNOSIS: **Fluid volume, deficit, potential.**

SUPPORTING DATA: **Malnutrition, dehydration, toxicity and electrolyte imbalances occur with inadequate intake of food and liquids and/or consistent self-induced vomiting.**

DESIRED PATIENT OUTCOMES: **Adequate hydration and electrolyte balance are maintained.**

INTERVENTIONS

RATIONALE

Refer to Nursing Diagnosis: Nutrition, alteration in, less than body requirements.

Measure urine output accurately. Be aware of diet soft drink intake.	Reduced urinary output is a direct result of reduced food intake. Not true when there is an increased intake of diet soft drinks.
Monitor vital signs.	May be prone to hypotension, tachycardia may reflect dehydration.

MEDICAL MANAGEMENT

I.V., hyperalimentation.

Used as an emergency measure to correct malnutrition. Refer to Care Plan: Total Parentenal Nutrition.

Potassium supplements, oral or I.V.

Restore electrolyte balance.

Refer to Care Plan: Fluid and Electrolyte Imbalances.

NURSING DIAGNOSIS:	Self-concepts, disturbance in: Body image, self-esteem.
SUPPORTING DATA:	Has distorted body image as fat, even in the presence of severe emaciation. Expresses little concern, uses denial. Perceptual disturbances with failure to recognize hunger; fatigue, anxiety, and depression also occur.
DESIRED PATIENT OUTCOMES:	More realistic body image is established. Patient acknowledges self as an individual who has responsibility for self.

INTERVENTIONS

Establish a therapeutic nurse-patient relationship.

Work with self-concept without moral judgment.

State rules re:weighing schedule; remaining in sight during medication and eating times. Be consistent in carrying out rules without undue comment.

Respond with reality when patient makes unrealistic statements, such as "I'm gaining weight, so there's nothing really wrong with me."

Avoid arguing. Be aware of own reaction to the patient's behavior.

Assist the patient to assume control in areas other than dieting/weight loss.

RATIONALE

Within a helping relationship, the individual can begin to trust and try out new thinking and behaviors.

Individual sees self as weak-willed, even though a part of the person may feel a sense of power and control.

Tend to be obsessive about weight fluctuations. Can be an important indicator of nutritional state. Consistency is important in establishing trust.

These patients need to be confronted because they deny the psychologic aspects of their situation, and are often expressing their sense of inadequacy and depression.

Feelings of disgust, hostility, and infuriation are not uncommon when caring for these patients. The nurse needs to deal with these feelings so that they do not interfere with the care of the patient.

Feelings of helplessness, personal ineffectiveness, low self-esteem, and perfectionism are often part of the problem.

Assist patient in dealing with unacknowledged sexual fears.

Major physical/psychologic changes in adolescence can contribute to development of this problem. Lack of control of feelings, in particular sexual, sensations, and physical development lead to an unconscious desire to desexualize themselves. Often believe they can control this by dieting.

Assist the patient in making own decisions and accepting self as is, encouraging patient to accept inadequacies as well as strengths.

Often these patients don't know what they want for themselves. Parents (mother) usually make decisions for them. They believe they have to be the best in everything and hold themselves responsible for being perfect.

Encourage patient to take charge of own life in a more healthful way.

Can develop a sense of identity as separate from family and maintain sense of control in other areas, besides dieting and weight loss,

Acknowledge anger when it is verbalized.

Important to know that anger is part of self and as such is acceptable.

Teach strategies other than eating for dealing with feelings.

Feelings are the underlying issue and patients often use food instead of dealing with them appropriately.

Involve in group therapy.

Provides an opportunity to talk about feelings and try out new behaviors.

Refer to National Association of Anorexia Nervosa and Associated Disorders.

Source for support and information for patient and significant others.

Refer to Care Plan: Psychosocial Aspects of Care in the Acute Setting.

NURSING DIAGNOSIS: Family dynamics, alteration in.

SUPPORTING DATA: The patient's not eating is often controlled by the way the patient and the patient's parents transact issues of control. This is a pattern of behavior rather than the individual's actions. Patient feels internally helpless and controlled by environment.

DESIRED PATIENT OUTCOMES: The individual's coping behaviors are more autonomous; family boundaries are more clearly defined. Conflict is recognized and appropriately resolved by the individuals involved.

INTERVENTIONS

Identify patterns of interaction. Encourage each family member to speak for oneself. Don't allow two members to discuss a third without that member's participation.

RATIONALE

Helpful information for planning interventions. The enmeshed, overinvolved family members often speak for each other and need to learn to be responsible for their own words and actions.

Discourage members from asking for approval from each other. Be alert to verbal or nonverbal checking with others for approval. Acknowledge competent actions of patient.

Each individual needs to develop an internal sense of self-esteem. Individual often is living up to others' (family's) expectations rather than making own choices. Provides recognition of self in positive ways.

Pay attention to the patient when the patient speaks.

Gives a sense of competence in that the patient has been heard and attended to.

Encourage individuals not to answer to everything.

Reinforces individualization and return to privacy.

Communicate message of separation.

Needs reinforcement. Confronts rigidity and opens options for different behaviors.

Encourage and allow expression of feelings (e.g., crying, anger) by individuals.

Often these families have not allowed free expression of feelings and will need help and permission to learn and accept this.

Prevent intrusion in dyads by other members of the family.

Inappropriate interventions in family subsystems prevent individuals from working out problems successfully.

Reinforce importance of parents as a couple who have rights of their own.

Child is caught in adolescent dependent/independent conflict.

Prevent patient from intervening in conflicts between parents. Assist parents in identifying and solving their marital differences.

Triangulation occurs in which a parent-child coalition occurs. Sometimes the child is openly pressed to ally with one parent against the other. The symptom (anorexia) is the regulator in the family system and the parents deny their own conflicts to protect the child.

Be aware and confront sabotage behavior on the part of family members.

Feelings of blame, shame, and helplessness may lead to unconscious behavior designed to maintain the status quo.

NURSING DIAGNOSIS:	**Thought processes, impaired.**
SUPPORTING DATA:	**Severe malnutrition impairs thinking ability.**
DESIRED PATIENT OUTCOMES:	**Nutritional status is improved so thinking is not impaired and the patient is available for psychiatric intervention.**

INTERVENTIONS

Be aware of patient's distorted thinking ability.

Listen to and do not challenge irrational, illogical thinking. Present reality concisely and briefly.

Adhere strictly to nutrition regimen.

RATIONALE

Knowing thinking ability is impaired allows the caregiver to lower expectations and provide information and help.

It is not possible to respond logically when thinking ability is physiologically impaired. The patient needs to hear reality, but challenging will lead to distrust and frustration.

Refer to Nursing Diagnosis: Nutrition, alteration in, less than body requirements.

NURSING DIAGNOSIS:	Skin integrity, impairment, potential.
SUPPORTING DATA:	Dehydrated, cachectic, and malnourished. Skin is dry, hair is brittle and dry.
DESIRED PATIENT OUTCOMES:	Skin remains intact, soft, and supple. Hydration is adequate.

INTERVENTIONS

Discourage frequent bathing.

Use skin cream twice a day and after bathing.

Massage skin, especially over bony prominences.

RATIONALE

Frequent baths contribute to dryness of the skin.

Will contribute to lubrication of the skin.

Improves circulation to the skin and skin tone.

DIAGNOSIS: Eating Disorders: Obesity

PATIENT DATA BASE

NURSING HISTORY

Identify presence of associated diseases, cardiovascular, hypertension, diabetes and endocrine disturbance.

Determine when problem began; lifetime or related to life event.

Note family history of obesity.

Identify whether weight is a problem to the patient.

How does the patient perceive own body image?

What are the patterns of gaining and losing weight?

Identify the kinds of diets tried in the past. How successful were these measures?

What is the daily calorie intake? Type of foods and eating habits.

Identify the emotions and events associated with eating.

Determine the level of nutritional knowledge.

Note type and amount of exercise done on a routine basis.

Identify motivation for change.

Determine the presence of pertinent psychologic factors.

Note the presence of significant others. Are they helpful or nonhelpful?

Note the influence of cultural factors, such as a value for thinness.

DIAGNOSTIC STUDIES

Complete workup essential to determine effect of obesity on body systems.

Complete blood count and urinalysis.

Chest x-ray.

Endocrine studies as indicated, i.e., thyroid series and pituitary function.

PHYSICAL EXAMINATION

Do complete physical.

Measure height and weight and record.

Do body measurements, including skinfold estimate of fat.

Evaluate gross body size, proportions of body fat, lean body mass and distribution of weight.

NURSING PRIORITIES

1. Provide a pattern of weight control that contains needed nutrients.
2. Assist patient to improve self-concept and body image.
3. Change health practices to provide for weight control throughout life.

NURSING DIAGNOSIS: **Nutrition, alteration in, more than body requirements.**

SUPPORTING DATA:	Food intake exceeds body needs, may be due to psychosocial factors. May deny excessive food intake. Weight of 20% or more over optimum body weight.
DESIRED PATIENT OUTCOMES:	Desirable body size and composition is attained, with optimal maintenance of health and reduction of existing illness factors, such as decreased BP and controlled diabetes.

INTERVENTIONS

In consultation with the patient, determine the diet to be used, avoiding fad diets. Use knowledge of height, body build, age, gender, and individual patterns of eating. Stress the importance of a balanced diet.

Discuss realistic goals for weekly weight loss. May be increment goals.

Reassess calorie requirements q 2–4 weeks to determine need for adjustment. Be aware of plateaus where weight remains stable for periods of time. May need emotional support at this time.

Determine current activity levels and plan increasing exercise program tailored to the individual goals and choice.

Develop an appetite reeducation plan with the patient.

Stress the importance of avoiding tension at mealtimes as well as not eating too fast.

RATIONALE

The patient will be more apt to adhere to a diet that the patient has developed and agreed to. Diet needs to provide nutrients with fewer calories than energy expenditure. There is no basis for recommending one diet over another. Standard tables are subject to error when applied to individual situations. Circadian rhythms and lifestyle patterns need to be considered. Elimination of carbohydrates from the diet can lead to metabolic acidosis (ketosis) and fatigue, headache, instability, and weakness.

One–two pounds per week is reasonable and achieves a more lasting loss. Too rapid loss may result in fatigue and irritability, which may lead to failure in meeting goals and losing weight. Motivation may be more easily maintained by meeting stair-step goals instead of one large goal of total amount.

Changes in weight and exercise will necessitate changes in diet. As weight is lost, changes in metabolism occur. Distrust and accusations of "cheating" on the calorie intake are not helpful.

Added activity increases energy output and tones the muscles. Commitment on the part of the patient will enable setting more realistic goals and adhering to the plan. No evidence exists that spot reducing or mechanical devices aid in weight loss in specific areas. Loss occurs on a generalized overall basis. Exercise further aids in weight loss by reducing appetite and enhancing sense of well-being and accomplishment.

Signals of hunger and fullness often have become distorted, ignored, and are not recognized without reeducation.

Reducing stress provides an opportunity for a more relaxed eating atmosphere and more leisurely eating patterns. A period of time is required for the appestat mechanism to know the stomach is full.

Eat only at a table or designated eating place and avoid eating standing. Behavior modification techniques may be helpful.

MEDICAL MANAGEMENT

May be hospitalized for fasting regimen.

Determine calorie requirements and goal for individual weight loss. (Actual weight minus 15 lbs. should be used for very obese patients.)

Appetite-suppresant drugs.

Salt restriction and diuretic drugs.

Hormonal therapy, such as thyroid.

Vitamin, mineral supplementation.

Refer to Care Plan: Obesity, Surgical Interventions.

A designated place is helpful in avoiding snacking.

May be tolerated for limited periods. Program can be monitored more effectively in a controlled setting. Initial rapid weight loss may encourage adherence to long-term program. Complications of postural hypotension, anemia, cardiac irregularities, decreased uric acid excretion with hyperuricemia may occur.

Several formulas are used to determine daily needs for each individual. Usually based on the basal calorie requirement for 24 hours. For the very obese person, may be the patient's own rather than an ideal goal. Use nutritional team, if available.

Used with caution at the beginning of a weight loss program. They are only effective for a few weeks and cause problems of addiction in some people.

Water retention may be a problem because of increased fluid intake, as well as the result of fat metabolism.

May be necessary when hypothyroidism is present. Replacement when no deficiency is present is not helpful and may be harmful. Other hormonal treatments, such as human chorionic gonadotropin (HCG), although widely publicized, have no documented evidence of value.

While obese individuals have large fuel reserves, this does not hold true for vitamins and minerals.

NURSING DIAGNOSIS:	Self-concept, disturbance in.
SUPPORTING DATA:	Self and body image is how one views oneself. A person's mental image often does not match that person's physical reality. Slimness is valued in this society. Mixed messages are received when advertising stresses thinness; families and subcultures encourage overeating; sedentary lifestyles; affluence and availability of high-calorie "fast" foods; and socialization around food all promote intake of more calories than are necessary to maintain optimal weight.

DESIRED PATIENT OUTCOMES:	**Patient verbalizes a more realistic self-concept, regarding mental and physical body image. Demonstrates acceptance of self as is rather than an idealized image.**

INTERVENTIONS

RATIONALE

Discuss the patient's view of being fat and what being fat does for the patient.

Mental image includes our ideal and is usually not up to date. Fat and compulsive eating behaviors may have deep-rooted psychologic implications, i.e., compensating for love and nurturing, as well as a defense against intimacy. People often eat because of depression, anger, and guilt.

Determine the patient's motivation for weight loss and set goals.

If patient is losing weight for someone else, patient is not likely to be successful on a long-term basis.

Be alert to myths the patient and significant others may have about weight and weight loss.

Beliefs about what an ideal body looks like and unconscious motivations, such as the feminine thought, "If I become thin, men will follow me, throw me on the ground, and rape me;" the masculine counterpart, "I don't trust myself to stay in control of my feelings," as well as issues of strength, power, and "good cook," can lead to frustration, fear, and sabotage behavior.

Assist patient to identify emotions that lead to compulsive eating. Keeping a diary can be helpful. Develop strategies for doing something besides eating for dealing with these emotions.

Awareness of emotions that lead to overeating can be the first step in behavior change.

Graph weight on a weekly basis.

Provides ongoing visual evidence of weight changes and is reality oriented.

Be alert to binge-eating and develop strategies for dealing with it.

The patient has a considerable amount of guilt related to this behavior and this is counterproductive to success.

May join a support and/or therapy group.

Group therapy can be helpful in dealing with underlying psychologic concerns. Support groups can provide companionship, increase motivation, decrease loneliness and social ostracism, and give practical solutions to common problems.

Be sure responsibilities of patient and nurse are clear.

It is helpful to the individual to understand areas of responsibility. Misunderstandings do not arise as often.

Provide for privacy as care is given.

May experience sense of shame due to stigma of being fat.

Staff needs to be aware of and deal with own feelings when taking care of these patients.

Judgmental attitudes, feelings of disgust, anger, weariness, and despair can interfere with care.

Refer to Care Plan: Psychosocial Aspects of Care in the Acute Setting.

NURSING DIAGNOSIS:	**Breathing pattern, alteration in, pickwickian syndrome.**

SUPPORTING DATA:	Central and obstructive apnea result in restlessness/sleep deprivation, and decreased respiratory drive.
DESIRED PATIENT OUTCOMES:	Breathing patterns remain stable and effective.

INTERVENTIONS

Note respiratory patterns and air exchange.

Document periods of restlessness at night and somnolence during the day.

Position patient prone with head elevated for sleep.

Encourage weight reduction.

MEDICAL MANAGEMENT

Progesterone.

Tricyclic antidepressants.

Tracheotomy.

RATIONALE

In central apnea, respiratory effort is irregular with periods of apnea lasting 15–90 seconds. Obstructive apnea results in chest movement without air exchange.

Central apnea periods may occur hundreds of times during sleep causing patient to awaken breathless. Daytime somnolence is a result of recurrent interrupted sleep pattern.

Helps to minimize effects of anatomical problems, such as short neck, receding jaw, large tongue, and hypertrophied tonsils/adenoids that can cause obstructive apnea.

Excessive weight on chest wall combined with abdominal fat, can impede thoracic/diaphragmatic movement.

Stimulates respirations.

Mechanism of positive effect has not yet been identified.

May be necessary when episodes of obstructive apnea are life-threatening.

CARE PLAN: Obesity, Surgical Interventions (Jejunoilea Bypass, Gastric Partitioning)

Jejunoileal Bypass: shunt between the jejunum and terminal ileum leaving 14 to 18 inches of small intestine.

Gastric Partitioning: a small pouch is created by two rows of staples across the stomach 1½ cm distal to the gastroesophageal junction leaving a small opening through which food passes. This operation is simpler, requiring less anesthesia, and having fewer complications. Patients are satisfied after taking in small amounts of food and do not experience the nutritional problems of the bypass.

PATIENT DATA BASE

NURSING HISTORY/CRITERIA

Morbid obesity, weight exceeding twice ideal body weight, or more than 100 lbs.

Presence of chronic conditions, such as hypertension, diabetes, and arthritis, pickwickian syndrome, infertility, which may benefit from weight loss.

No previous liver or renal dysfunction, myocardial or bowel disease.

Age range: late teens to 50s, average mid-thirties.

Motivated to lose weight for oneself, not for gratification of others. Rule out those hostile to family and physicians.

Adequate trials and failure of other treatment approaches.

Agreement to extensive medical followup.

Refer to Care Plan: Eating Disorders: Obesity.

DIAGNOSTIC STUDIES

Most done to r/o underlying diseases.

Serum iron and iron binding capacity.

Protein level for indication of nutritional status.

CBC, check for signs of existing infection and/or anemia.

Liver function tests; including enzymes, clotting profile, and platelet count and alkaline phosphatase.

Renal testing: urinalysis, BUN, creatinine.

AGBs to determine O_2 perfusion.

FBS, cholesterol and triglycerides.

Chest x-ray and pulmonary function test.

GI Series, gallbladder series, barium enema, and IVP.

ECG and stress testing, urinalysis.

PHYSICAL EXAMINATION

Psychiatric evaluation (major psychiatric disorders are a countraindication).

Refer to Care Plan: Eating Disorders: Obesity.

NURSING PRIORITIES: (Jejunoileal Bypass)

1. Provide preoperative teaching about anticipated problems specific to obesity.
2. Identification and minimizing of postoperative complications.
3. Managing altered bowel function, nutrition, and diarrhea.

(Care of these patients in general falls under Care Plan: Intestinal Surgery, ostomy not anticipated. Because of increased risk factors and severity of complications seen in this patient group, special problems and interventions are highlighted here.)

NURSING DIAGNOSIS: Breathing patterns, ineffective.

SUPPORTING DATA: Large body mass compromises lung capacity, diaphragmatic breathing inhibited by incision. Drugs and positioning further reduce depth and rate of breathing.

DESIRED PATIENT OUTCOMES: Adequate oxygenation is maintained and no infection is present.

INTERVENTIONS	RATIONALE
Elevate head of bed 30°.	Encourages optimal lung expansion and minimizes pressure of abdominal contents on the respiratory cavity.
Deep breathing exercise and cough q2h first two days postop. Use incentive breathing device q4h × 2 days.	Promotes maximal lung expansion and aids in clearing the airways.
Turn q2h and ambulate within first 24h.	Position changes encourage aeration of different segments of the lung, mobilizing and aiding in removal of secretions.
Pad the siderails and teach the patient to use them as arm rests.	Using the siderail as an armrest, allows for greater chest expansion.
Use small pillow for head, when indicated.	Many obese patients have large, thick necks and use of large, fluffy pillows may obstruct the airway.
Avoid use of abdominal binders.	Usually don't fit and tend to restrict lung expansion.

MEDICAL MANAGEMENT

Supplemental O₂.	Increases available oxygen.
IPPB and/or incentive spirometer, and so forth.	Enhance lung expansion, reduce atelectasis.

NURSING DIAGNOSIS: Injury, potential for, thrombophlebitis.

SUPPORTING DATA:	**Immobility leads to venous stasis resulting in thrombus formation. Activity is especially difficult for these patients when they are confined to bed.**
DESIRED PATIENT OUTCOMES:	**Thrombophlebitis does not occur.**

INTERVENTIONS

Provide adequate/appropriate equipment and sufficient staff for handling patient.

Range of motion exercises legs and ankles q2–3h × 24 hours.

Early ambulation, discourage sitting and/or dangling at the bedside.

Assess for Homans sign, redness, and edema.

RATIONALE

Will be helpful in dealing with the bulk of the patient for moving, bowel care, and ambulating.

Circulation is stimulated in the lower extremities.

Sitting constricts venous flow, whereas walking encourages venous return.

Early and may be only indicator of clot formation.

MEDICAL MANAGEMENT

Minidose heparin therapy preop and up to five days postop.

Inhibits the clotting process.

NURSING DIAGNOSIS:	**Skin integrity, impairment of, actual.**
SUPPORTING DATA:	**Reduced vascularity and difficulty in approximation of suture line of fatty tissue results in poor wound healing with potential of infection and hernia formation.**
DESIRED PATIENT OUTCOMES:	**Wound heals without complications.**

INTERVENTIONS

Routine incisional care, being careful to keep dressings dry and sterile.

Pay particular attention to cleanliness of skin folds.

Support incision when turning, coughing, deep breathing, and ambulating. Avoid bending and lifting.

RATIONALE

Reduces chances of nosocomial infections. The presence of drains in the subcutaneous layers results in accumulation of serosanguinous drainage, which serves as a media for bacterial growth.

Excoriation enhances growth of bacteria that can lead to postop infection.

Reduces possibility of dehiscence and later incisional hernia.

NURSING DIAGNOSIS:	Bowel elimination, alteration in, diarrhea.
SUPPORTING DATA:	Six to eight stools per day normally occur due to induced malabsorption. Stools may be more frequent.
DESIRED PATIENT OUTCOMES:	Patient manages new bowel pattern and complications are kept to a minimum.

INTERVENTIONS

As diet resumes, encourage diet high in bulk, with moderate fluid intake.

Observe for signs of "dumping syndrome," sweating and weakness after eating.

Assist with frequent peri-care using ointments as indicated.

RATIONALE

Increases consistency of the effluent. While sufficient fluid is necessary for optimal renal function, excessive amounts contribute to diarrhea.

Rapid emptying of food from the stomach may result in these symptoms. Refer to Care Plan: Gastric Resection.

Anal irritation, excoriation, and pruritus occur because of diarrhea. The patient often cannot reach the area for proper cleansing and may be embarrassed to ask for help.

NURSING DIAGNOSIS:	Fluid volume, deficit, potential.
SUPPORTING DATA:	Excessive stools, nasogastric suction result in loss of electrolytes in particular, potassium, but also magnesium and calcium.
DESIRED PATIENT OUTCOMES:	Fluid and electrolyte balance is maintained.

INTERVENTIONS

Assess neuromuscular weakness; irregular, weak pulse; muscle cramps in legs; postural hypotension.

Monitor diarrhea and NG suction.

Instruct patient to watch for signs of hypokalemia.

Instruct in importance of eating foods/fluids high in potassium.

RATIONALE

Potassium is most frequent electrolyte lost. If below 2.5 mEq/L, respiratory/cardiac arrest may occur.

Large amounts may result in decreased Mg^{++} and calcium. Neuromuscular weakness/tetany may occur.

Diarrhea, muscle weakness of lower extremities and flaccid paralysis, and cardiac arrhythmias may be symptoms.

Milk, coffee, cola, potatoes, carrots, bananas, and oranges.

NURSING DIAGNOSIS:	**Nutrition, alteration in, less than body requirements.**
SUPPORTING DATA:	**Frequent stools, malabsorption of nutrients, impaired absorption of vitamins can result in malnutrition.**
DESIRED PATIENT OUTCOMES:	**Nutrition is maintained at an optimum level.**

INTERVENTIONS

Provide diet, liquid advancing to soft, high in protein and bulk, and low in fat.

Determine foods that are gas-forming.

Discuss food preferences with patient and include in diet.

MEDICAL MANAGEMENT

Refer to the dietitian if indicated.

Vitamin supplements as well as B_{12} injections.

RATIONALE

Provides nutrients without additional calories.

Avoiding foods that are a problem for the individual and may interfere with appetite/digestion, assists with optimal nutritional intake.

May be helpful in eliminating foods that are inappropriate.

May need assistance in planning a diet that meets nutritional needs.

Absorption may be impaired.

NURSING DIAGNOSIS:	**Injury, potential for, infection.**
SUPPORTING DATA:	**Immediately postop; and later developing wound infections and/or dehiscence may occur due to poor healing of fatty tissues. Urinary tract infections are common.**
DESIRED PATIENT OUTCOMES:	**Infections are minimized or do not occur.**

INTERVENTIONS

Use strict aseptic technique in dressing changes and catheter care.

Instruct women in proper cleansing of perineum.

Maintain accurate I & O.

Encourage patient to drink acid-ash juices, such as cranberry.

RATIONALE

Minimize source of infections.

Prevent ascending bladder infections to which women are prone.

Early assessment of possible kidney problems.

Maintain urine acidity to retard bacterial growth.

NURSING DIAGNOSIS:	Knowledge deficit, postoperative care.
SUPPORTING DATA:	The possibility of complications necessitates ongoing medical supervision as well as assistance with the lifestyle changes necessary related to the weight loss.
DESIRED PATIENT OUTCOMES:	Verbalizes/cooperates with regimen for followup care.

INTERVENTIONS

Discuss with patient/significant others, responsibility for self-care.

Stress importance of regular medical checkup; including CBC and electrolytes; and possible health problems that may occur.

Discuss medication regimen; dosage and side effects.

Discuss necessity for avoiding the use of alcohol.

Discuss problems of learning to live with decreased body size and altered body image. May need referral to support/therapy group.

RATIONALE

Full cooperation is important for successful outcome after bypass.

Every three months is the recommended period for most patients. Liver dysfunction, malnutrition, electrolyte imbalances, and kidney stones are some problems that may develop.

Knowledge can be helpful in maintaining the schedule.

May contribute to liver/pancreatic dysfunction.

Anticipation of problems can be helpful in dealing with situations that arise.

CARE PLAN: Reconstructive Facial Surgery

PATIENT DATA BASE

NURSING HISTORY

Presence of physical attributes that the patient believes are disfiguring or unacceptable.

Determine patient expectations. May need psychiatric evaluation.

Recent injury to bony framework, cartilagenous structures or soft tissues. Trauma deformities should be repaired as soon as possible to achieve best results.

Family or personal history of diabetes, keloid formation (or other major disease), which may predispose to infection, affect healing, and lead to disappointing results.

DIAGNOSTIC STUDIES

Blood glucose levels: check for diabetes mellitus or high glucose levels.

Clotting studies give information about coagulation defects which may lead to hemorrhage.

PHYSICAL EXAMINATION

Absence of skin infections (if surgery is elective).

Check nutritional status, deficiencies, especially protein, may interfere with healing.

Determine airway patency: examine oropharynx for foreign materials, e.g., broken dentures, vomitus, external debris that could obstruct airway.

NURSING PRIORITIES

1. Assure patent airway.
2. Prevent/control hemorrhage.
3. Help patient set realistic expectations and adjust to new appearance.

NURSING DIAGNOSIS:	**Gas exchange, impaired.**
SUPPORTING DATA:	**Trauma to soft tissues and airway because of surgery and/or injuries.**
DESIRED PATIENT OUTCOMES:	**Airway patency and normal respiratory pattern maintained.**

INTERVENTIONS	RATIONALE
Observe for change in respiratory rate, rhythm. Note use of accessory muscles, hoarseness, high-pitched cough, wheezing, surrounding tissue edema.	May indicate impending respiratory distress. Trauma to soft tissue and bone usually produces marked edema, which may develop to its maximum 24 hours after the trauma/surgery.
Keep tracheotomy tray at bedside.	Readily available for emergency use.

Do neuro checks if facial injury due to trauma. Check for rhinorrhea, otorrhea.

Head injuries may have occurred concurrently with facial injuries. May indicate leaking cerebrospinal fluid with communication between brain and outside, predisposing to meningitis.

Examine floor of mouth for swelling, discoloration.

Bleeding in this area is masked because of tissue looseness; careful examination is required.

Note patient's complaint of increasing dysphagia.

May indicate soft tissue swelling in the posterior pharnyx.

Keep wirecutters at bedside.

When the fractured jaw is wired, there are usually 2–6 major wires that require cutting to release entire wired area and open airway.

Check in mouth for accumulation of oral secretions, blood. Suction as necessary.

Keeps airway clear.

MEDICAL MANAGEMENT

Penrose drain.

Bleeding in area may need evacuation.

Tracheotomy.

If airway patency is threatened by swelling.

Antiemetics.

Prevent vomiting, which may obstruct airway.

NURSING DIAGNOSIS:	Comfort, alteration in, pain.
SUPPORTING DATA:	Tissue and bone trauma. Nasal congestion.
DESIRED PATIENT OUTCOMES:	Pain is controlled/minimized.

INTERVENTIONS

RATIONALE

Give information about donor site pain.

Loss of epidermis exposes nerve endings. Knowing what to expect can prevent surprises and resultant anxiety.

Examine mouth for loose or protruding wires.

May irritate or damage surrounding tissues.

Support immobilized areas with sand bags, rolled pads.

Helps maintain proper positioning and prevents undue stress on supporting musculature.

Massage, do passive/active ROM to unaffected areas.

Helps reduce stiffness, encourages circulation that may be sluggish due to bed rest and areas of edema.

Allow time for ventilation of feelings.

Anxiety may increase pain and can be decreased by having time to talk about concerns and fears.

MEDICAL MANAGEMENT

Analgesics.

Usually a great deal of discomfort is present.

Warm/cold compresses.

Relieve congestion and provide relief of pain.

Nasal decongestants.

Helps shrink upper airway mucous membranes to relieve congestion, which gives a feeling of suffocation and may be frightening to a patient whose teeth may be wired and whose eyes may be swollen shut.

NURSING DIAGNOSIS:	Communication, impaired verbal.
SUPPORTING DATA:	Edema of mouth and surrounding structures. Pain on jaw movement. Jaws may be wired shut.
DESIRED PATIENT OUTCOMES:	Patient able to communicate satisfactorily.

INTERVENTIONS

Explore alternate means of communication, such as pencil and pad, magic slate, or bell.

Place call light where patient can reach it, and answer promptly.

Make note at nurses' station.

RATIONALE

May not be able to verbally communicate.

Helps alleviate anxiety that patient may not be able to call for help if needed.

May not be able to enunciate clearly. If vomiting occurs, airway may be compromised.

NURSING DIAGNOSIS:	Nutrition, alteration in, potential for less than body requirements.
SUPPORTING DATA:	Reduced pharyngeal lumen; limited accessibility to pharnyx. Inability to masticate.
DESIRED PATIENT OUTCOMES:	Loss of weight is minimized/prevented.

INTERVENTIONS

Give diet high in calories, vitamins, and proteins.

Weigh patient 2 x /week.

Give fluids ad lib; ice chips or water may be given as soon as nausea subsides.

Provide foods of acceptable consistency, such as pureed or liquid. Serve each food in individual container.

Proceed to diet as tolerated; may gradually return to normal diet in 5–6 weeks postop.

RATIONALE

Adequate nutrition is important to the healing process.

Ascertain weight loss.

Prevents dehydration.

Patient may be unable to masticate or feeding must be given by NG tube. Being able to identify various flavors adds to the pleasure of eating.

Muscle stiffness, dental malocclusion may delay capability for normal foods.

MEDICAL MANAGEMENT

Dietary supplements.

Addition of calories/protein to liquified diet may be beneficial.

NURSING DIAGNOSIS:	Skin integrity, impairment of, potential.
SUPPORTING DATA:	Graft failure causes degradation of epidermis.
DESIRED PATIENT OUTCOMES:	Healed incisional areas.

INTERVENTIONS

Apply mittens or restraints as necessary.

Immobilize grafted area. If rhytidoplasty, have patient avoid excessive talking for several days postop.

Elevate grafted area. Check for increase in edema.

Cleanse mouth frequently and especially after each feeding with lukewarm water and peroxide, noting location of sutures. Avoid disturbing sutures. Waterpik may be used.

Check hematocrit and hemoglobin, clotting tendencies.

Note continuance or increase in pain.

RATIONALE

Keeps patient from disturbing graft/donor sites. Prevents contamination/damage to operative areas.

Movement encourages bleeding and leads to hematoma formation, which causes pulling and distortion of suture lines.

Reduces edema formation, which may stress graft and increase the probability of graft failure. Edema recedes in 4–7 days.

Promotes healing by discouraging infection, keeping suture line intact.

Influences healing; abnormalities encourage bleeding and hematoma formation.

May indicate infection, which accentuates pain. Any jaw fracture involving a tooth-bearing portion is considered a compound fracture, even if there is no break in the soft tissue because a tooth acts to allow communication between the mouth and the fracture that may lead to infection; this may lead to the development of gangrene (even gas gangrene), or abcess formation that may involve the oropharynx and endanger airway patency.

MEDICAL MANAGEMENT

Change graft dressings carefully.

Examine graft for indications of "take," necrosis, or infections.

Note fluid accumulation under graft and aspirate with sterile needle or "roll" out with sterile swab.

Dressing may stick to graft, pulling it away from dermis or causing avulsion of graft margins.

Vascularization begins in 3–5 days after grafting. Infections are the major cause of graft failure.

Delays graft healing.

Wet dressings, ointments to graft sites and suture lines maintaining sterile technique.	Reduces topical bacteria and keeps graft pliable; prevents eschar accumulation, which interferes with fine line suture healing.
Systemic antibiotics.	Combats infection.
Tranquilizers.	Promote rest and relaxation.

NURSING DIAGNOSIS: Tissue perfusion, alteration in.

SUPPORTING DATA: Concurrent injuries may decrease cardiac output or restrict proper circulation to extremities.

DESIRED PATIENT OUTCOMES: Extremities demonstrate normal color and pulses.

INTERVENTIONS

Observe color of extremities.

RATIONALE

Should be normal, even if face is purplish, because of venous congestion from tissue trauma and edema. Mottled extremities indicate inadequate circulation, the cause of which necessitates immediate investigation.

NURSING DIAGNOSIS: Injury, potential for, hemorrhage.

SUPPORTING DATA: With surgical incisions and trauma, there is risk of hemorrhage. Loss of skin surface allows oozing of body fluids.

DESIRED PATIENT OUTCOMES: Hemorrhage is managed and/or does not occur.

INTERVENTIONS

Apply pressure dressings to donor sites for 24 hours. Dressings may be removed down to a single layer of nonadherent gauze material.

RATIONALE

Hemorrhage, large fluid losses may occur from denuded areas; pressure closes surface vessels and encourages clotting. Nonadherent dressings (opsite, biobrane), act to protect donor/graft sites as a biological dressing that keeps site moist and pliable, and will separate from site as healing takes place.

Dressings may be reinforced and kept in place an additional 12–24 hours.

If excessive oozing or bleeding occurs.

NURSING DIAGNOSIS: Coping, ineffective, potential.

SUPPORTING DATA: Altered physical appearance may lead to disturbance in self-image.

DESIRED PATIENT OUTCOMES:	Verbalizes knowledge about what to expect in regard to surgical procedure, realistic expectations of surgical outcome(s), and demonstrates acceptable behavior patterns.

INTERVENTIONS

Explore reasons for seeking surgery, attitude toward physical imperfections, how patient feels physical appearance affects life.

Help patient formulate realistic expectations in regard to surgical results.

Prepare patient and significant others for postoperative appearance; encourage significant others to support patient. If appearance is temporary, assure that it will change in time. Explain size of bandage.

Take suicide precautions if patient has been disfigured; elicit psychologic support if necessary. Investigate possibility of plastic surgery repair at a later date.

Be alert for signs of depression. Acquaint with others who have had similar procedures. Be available for support and help.

Refer to Care Plan: Psychosocial Aspects of Care in the Acute Setting.

RATIONALE

When surgery is elective, this helps define expectations, gives opportunity to give information about surgical limitations.

Increase satisfaction with surgical results.

Significant bone splintering affects physical contours. Exact replication of features may not be possible. Preparation of significant others prevents visual shock being communicated to patient.

An emotional reaction occurs when the face is disfigured; need to adjust to new appearance. Coping depends on pretrauma abilities.

Many operations may be necessary. Healing and waiting periods between repairs may be long and it is easy to become discouraged.

DIAGNOSIS: Achalasia

PATIENT DATA BASE

NURSING HISTORY

More common in men in their 40s–50s.

Onset is unusually insidious.

Most prominent symptom is dysphagia for both liquid and solid foods.

Meals may be interrupted by the necessity to regurgitate the swallowed food.

Nocturnal regurgitation may result in aspiration, resulting in chronic pulmonary infections or sudden death.

Aggravated by emotional upset, sudden shock, or deviations from dietary restrictions.

May lose weight and may be malnourished, secondary to fear of eating and beginning the discomfort and dysphagia again.

May complain of substernal pressure, fullness, and often heartburn or pain in the midthoracic area secondary to dysphagia.

DIAGNOSTIC STUDIES

Barium swallow: peristaltic wave is weak and the collection of barium in the lower esophagus gives it a funnel-like appearance.

Administration of small doses of a cholinergic or parasympathomimetic drug causes marked contraction and emptying of the esophagus and confirms the diagnosis.

Esophageal mobility studies may be helpful in the early diagnosis. Manometric measurements in these studies reveal that the lower esphogeal sphincter fails to relax with swallowing. The resting pressure of the lower esophageal sphincter may be normal or slightly elevated.

Esophagoscopy with biopsy and cytology to determine evidence of esophagitis or rule out carcinoma.

SMA studies: anemia and electrolyte imbalances secondary to malnutrition may be present.

PHYSICAL EXAMINATION

May have emaciated and/or dehydrated appearance with decreased skin turgor.

Chest ascultation may determine if pulmonary complications secondary to aspiration have occurred.

NURSING PRIORITIES

1. Improve nutritional status.
2. Prevent aspiration.
3. Provide information and assistance to enable patient/significant others to develop coping skills to deal with chronic condition.

NURSING DIAGNOSIS:	**Nutrition, alteration in, less than body requirements.**
SUPPORTING DATA:	**The patient often experiences pain when swallowing (dysphagia) and may often regurgitate resulting in reluctance to eat.**

DESIRED PATIENT OUTCOMES:	Nutritional intake is adequate for metabolic needs.

INTERVENTIONS

Encourage patient to chew food thoroughly.

Swallow liquids with food.

Encourage patient to eat slowly. Provide a quiet nonstressed environment.

Avoid alcohol, hot, cold, or spicy foods.

Provide explanation of the need for increased nutritional intake.

MEDICAL MANAGEMENT

Vitamin and iron supplements.

Dilatation of the lower esophagus with a mercury filled tube (bougie) or a pneumatic bag.

Heller procedure.

RATIONALE

Breaks down the food well and adds saliva to the food, which will aid its passage.

Facilitates passage of food by slightly dilating the esophagus.

Rapid eating is stressful and may further aggravate swallowing difficulties.

May promote esophageal spasm.

Patient cooperation is necessary to maintain proper diet.

May be deficient in the presence of anemia and malnutrition.

May allow passage of fluid/foods more easily and increase intake. (There is no known way to restore esophageal muscle function.)

May be done if dilatation is unsuccessful, or too temporary, to enlarge the mucosa and allow food to pass more easily.

NURSING DIAGNOSIS:	Airway clearance, ineffective.
SUPPORTING DATA:	Secondary respiratory problems, such as pneumonitis, lung abscess, or bronchiectasis, are common in achalasia due to nocturnal regurgitation and aspiration during dysphagia. This continues as a concern even after dilatation is done.
DESIRED PATIENT OUTCOMES:	Normal lung function without aspiration complications.

INTERVENTIONS

Elevate head of the bed 10–12 inches.

Instruct patient not to eat/drink 2–3 hrs before lying down.

Avoid drugs such as Butazolidin.

Encourage bland diet.

RATIONALE

Regurgitation and aspiration of stomach and esophageal contents is prevented.

This allows the passage of most food into the bowels and minimizes possible reflux/aspiration when lying down.

May lead to ulceration if aspirated.

Minimize irritation.

MEDICAL MANAGEMENT

Frequent pulmonary evaluations, e.g., auscultation, chest x-ray, and/or bronchoscopy and treatment as necessary.

Will identify/prevent serious infections or chronic problems.

Antispasmodic drugs are not recommended.

They have been found to give little or no decrease in symptoms.

Pulmonary care and antibiotics.

May be given a few days before and following dilatation and/or surgery. May decrease the chance of pulmonary infections directly related to the structure change during surgery.

NURSING DIAGNOSIS:	Knowledge deficit, disease process and management.
SUPPORTING DATA:	Treatment of achalasia is at the best palliative because, as yet, there is no way to restore normal esophogeal muscle function.
DESIRED PATIENT OUTCOMES:	Patient/significant others can verbalize disease pathology and symptoms of complications that should be reported to the physician. Are able to maintain the necessary lifestyle and dietary changes.

INTERVENTIONS

Assist patient in identifying support person(s).

Assist patient/significant others to understand how and why to avoid stress and stressful situations.

Reinforce instruction about this disease process, and the reasons only palliative treatment can be given.

Instruct patient and significant others in recognition of signs and symptoms of possible complications, such as increased respiratory problems, fever, or hematemesis and predisposition to cancer of the esophagus.

Instruct and reemphasize the importance of good nutrition and necessary precautions while eating. Provide written diet instructions.

RATIONALE

This is a chronic disease and may be very frustrating to a patient so support systems are very important in maintaining the necessary lifestyle changes.

Stress may exacerbate symptoms of dysphagia and, therefore, the patient must be aware and know how to manage stress successfully. Refer to Care Plan: Psychosocial Aspects of Care in the Acute Setting.

An informed and knowledgeable patient has more control of own care as well as understanding and patience with the therapy, especially as it is essentially palliative.

Prompt physician notification of symptoms may prevent long and serious complications.

Proper dietary intake will promote well-being and increased strength to maintain the necessary self-management. Written instructions may be referred to periodically at home.

DIAGNOSIS: Hiatal Hernia With Reflux

PATIENT DATA BASE

NURSING HISTORY

Seen more frequently in men in their 30s–50s. Up to 50% of the general population may have hiatal hernias, only approximately 5% have reflux symptoms.

Of little consequence unless associated with reflux.

May have noticed a slow increase in difficulty in swallowing liquids or solids.

May notice ease in swallowing when drinking fluids after swallowing food.

History may include previous intake of a corrosive chemical causing damage.

Symptoms may have a sudden onset with varying severity.

May complain of substernal pressure (heartburn), or hot, burning pain behind the xiphoid or sternum; epigastric pain or some abdominal fullness with or without regurgitation.

Recumbency may increase symptoms.

Pain may increase with ingestion of citrus liquids, alcohol, extremes of hot or cold fluids, spicy foods, chocolate, cola drinks, or coffee: cigarette smoking may increase reflux.

Pain associated with feelings of fullness, belching, nausea/vomiting, usually gone 1 hour after meal.

Pain may mimic peptic ulcer, and at times, angina pectoris.

Symptoms may be worsened by increases in intra-abdominal pressure when bending over, lifting heavy objects, or straining to pass stool.

Relief may be obtained by taking water, milk, antacids, gaviscon or by standing rather than lying down.

May have history of bleeding, melena, or hematemesis.

May have nocturnal "cigarette cough," possibly secondary to aspirated gastric reflux.

Patient may notice weight loss secondary to decreased intake and its association with pain.

DIAGNOSTIC STUDIES

CBC, electrolytes, urinalysis; assess nutritional status or anemia secondary to a mild GI bleed from irritated esophagus.

Thyroid function tests: r/o thyroid abnormality (enlargement).

ECG: r/o cardiac origin of pain.

Upper GI series: may show the hernia, may or may not demonstrate reflux.

Barium swallow: may show dilatation and elongation of the esophagus and demonstrates the procedure of swallowing and emptying of the esophagus. May also r/o cancer of the lower esophagus.

Esophagoscopy or endoscopy may exclude neoplasms, demonstrate the presence of reflux, or observe the esophageal/cardia stricture. Mucosal changes may be noted and biopsy obtained.

Structure of lower esophagus noted secondary to recurrent reflux.

Chest x-ray: r/o aspiration pneumonia, abscess, or other pulmonary complications secondary to aspiration.

Stool guaiac: GI bleeding may be present.

Esophageal pH measuring, to document reflux of gastric contents, infrequently performed.

PHYSICAL EXAMINATION

Physical findings are often not specific.

Head and neck exam for enlarged thyroid or a mass that blocks swallowing.

Auscultate lungs; possible pulmonary complications secondary to aspiration of reflux contents.

Cardiac exam to r/o cardiac involvement when patient presents with complaints of chest pain.

Abdominal exam to include palpitation for tenderness or bloating.

May be obese, especially when c/o reflux symptoms.

Observe for signs of decreased nutritional intake, decreased skin turgor, weight loss or emaciation, as patient attempts to avoid precipitating pain.

NURSING PRIORITIES

1. Promote comfort.
2. Improve nutritional status if necessary.
3. Minimize complications.
4. Provide information about the disease process; necessary lifestyle changes; and medical therapy.

NURSING DIAGNOSIS:	**Comfort, alteration in, pain.**
SUPPORTING DATA:	**Hiatal hernia is of little concern unless it is accompanied by gastric reflux, which is usually the reason patients enter the health care system.**
DESIRED PATIENT OUTCOMES:	**Patient will experience little or no discomfort or pain.**

INTERVENTIONS

Avoid bending forward, coughing, straining at stool, tight fitting clothing, and heavy lifting.

Decrease fat, alcohol, chocolate intake, discontinue smoking.

Encourage frequent small feedings.

Avoid extremely hot or cold beverages and foods that increase pain; e.g., coffee, spicy foods.

Learn to decrease or effectively handle stress.

Instruct the patient not to recline for 3–4 h after meals and to elevate the head of the bed 8–10 inches for sleeping.

Reduce weight, if obese.

RATIONALE

Increases gastric reflux and possible pain.

These have been found to decrease the lower esophageal tone and can promote reflux.

Large meals overload stomach and promote reflux.

May cause esophageal spasm and increase acid secretory response in the stomach.

Stress increases gastric acid production, which may be easily refluxed.

Prevents reflux and aspiration by using gravity to decrease the gastro-esophageal pressure gradient. Decreases nocturnal reflux.

Intensifies herniation reflux.

MEDICAL MANAGEMENT

Antacids.

Routine use can neutralize gastric acidity and gastric contents when refluxed and prevent esophageal irritation.

Stool softeners.

Prevent straining at stool.

Cimetidine, bethanechol chloride, or Reglan.

Systematically decreases gastric acid production and gastric spasm.

Surgical procedure: Nissen or Belsy operation.

Performed on large hiatus hernias, those of the para-esophageal type, to relieve pain and discomfort of reflux not relieved by conventional therapy. Refer to Care Plan: Surgical Intervention.

NURSING DIAGNOSIS:	**Knowledge deficit, disease process, complications, and medical management.**
SUPPORTING DATA:	**Chronic nature of the disease process requires complete patient participation in care to prevent worsening of symptoms and complications.**
DESIRED PATIENT OUTCOMES:	**Patient/significant others able to verbalize the basics of the pathology of the disease and necessary lifestyle alterations.**

INTERVENTIONS

Instruct and stress dietary and dietary pattern changes necessary.

Instruct the patient on the importance of effective stress management.

Provide nutritional counseling, reduction diet and referral to group as indicated. Refer to Care Plans: Eating Disorders: Obesity; Obesity, Surgical Interventions.

Stress the importance of daily precautions to prevent reflux; e.g., no bending or heavy lifting.

Reinforce instruction about the disease process of hiatal hernia, its chronicity and the reasons for the medical therapy regimen.

Instruct patient/significant others: re: signs and symptoms of possible worsening of condition and/or complications: i.e., greatly increasing pain, hematemesis, or swallowing difficulties.

RATIONALE

Proper adherence to diet regimen will minimize reflux and accompanying discomfort.

Stress may exacerbate reflux and its pain.

When obesity is a factor, weight reduction can provide symptomatic relief.

Patient must have a thorough awareness in order to avoid activities that increase reflux.

An informed and knowledgeable patient has more control of own care and the medical therapy will be more effective.

Prompt physician notification of such symptoms may prevent long and serious complications.

DIAGNOSIS: Mallory-Weiss Syndrome

PATIENT DATA BASE

NURSING HISTORY

Mallory-Weiss syndrome accounts for 5–15% of all acute Upper GI bleeds needing hospital admission, but is rarely a cause of continuous bleeding.

May have history of severe vomiting, consisting of fluids in the stomach, followed by sudden hematemesis. May rarely follow an epileptic seizure or status asthmaticus, severe coughing, straining at stool, hyperemesis gravidarum, poisoning, heavy lifting, or external cardiac massage.

Determine any history of alcohol abuse, frequently is a causative factor in development of this syndrome.

May have a history of hiatal hernia.

DIAGNOSTIC STUDIES

If bleeding has been prolonged, anemia may be present, but rarely is severe enough to require transfusion.

GI x-ray may be inconclusive.

Endoscopy provides the best and most accurate evaluation.

PT, PTT for clotting times.

Chest x-ray, to rule out aspiration.

Blood alcohol level may reveal recent abuse as a contributing factor.

PHYSICAL EXAMINATION

Note amount and character of bleeding; may be mild to severe; up to 80% of the cases stop spontaneously.

May not have significant abdominal complaints.

Vital signs may be within normal limits as this is usually a self-limited bleed.

Stools may be positive for blood, depending on length of bleed.

NURSING PRIORITIES

1. Monitor/prevent complications secondary to hemorrhage.
2. Promote comfort and ensure rest.
3. Provide psychologic support and prevent future problems.

NURSING DIAGNOSIS:	Fluid volume, deficit, potential, hemorrhage.

258

SUPPORTING DATA:	Mallory-Weiss syndrome is a linear muscular tear at the esophagogastric junction. The bleeding is usually self-limiting, but the potential for severe hemorrhage is present.
DESIRED PATIENT OUTCOMES:	Bleeding is controlled/limited.

INTERVENTIONS

Monitor vital signs.

Obtain Hct & Hb and type and cross-match as indicated.

Keep the patient calm and quiet.

Keep patient NPO, and maintain accurate I & O.

RATIONALE

Indicate severe blood loss.

Indications of actual total blood loss and prepare to replace if necessary.

Because the bleed is usually self-limited, decreased movement promotes circulatory rest and hopefully will result in cessation of bleeding.

Permit GI rest and provide information about fluid balance.

MEDICAL MANAGEMENT

Replace losses/maintain adequate fluid volume.

NG tube.

Ice water lavage.

Endoscopy.

Intra-arterial infusion of drugs, such as vasopressin may be indicated.

Direct suture repair of the lacerated mucosa.

Refer to Care Plan: Esophageal Varices.

Prevent dehydration.

May be indicated if severe bleeding occurs.

Causes vasoconstriction and promotes decrease or resolution of the bleeding.

May be necessary to determine the exact diagnosis or site of bleeding. Needs to be selectively used because it may aggravate a bleeding site.

Acts as a vasoconstrictor, may decrease the frequency of the need for surgical repair.

Only performed if bleeding is not self-limited (less than 5% of all cases).

If bleeding problems are severe.

NURSING DIAGNOSIS:	Knowledge deficit; of the acute process and medical management.
SUPPORTING DATA:	An acute process without previous illness, as in the Mallory-Weiss syndrome, results in need for information about what is occurring as this is usually sudden and unexpected with no previous history of GI problems.

INTERVENTIONS

Give explanations as care is given.

Give information about the possible etiology of the bleeding.

Review signs of recurrence, such as melena.

RATIONALE

Can decrease patient's/significant others' fear and promote cooperation.

Can begin briefly during the bleed and continued/reinforced after it is controlled to help alleviate anxiety of the unknown.

Need to be alert to hidden bleeding.

DIAGNOSIS: Esophageal Varices

PATIENT DATA BASE

NURSING HISTORY

Sudden loss of blood in large quantities through the mouth or rectum.

Hematemesis (usually bright red blood but may be darker), or melena (passing of blood clots rectally).

May have history of hepatitis, or known cirrhosis, especially postnecrotic cirrhosis.

Usually does not complain of pain.

History of alcohol and tobacco use.

History of recent extreme physical exertion, mechanical trauma, e.g., ingestion of coarse food, coughing, sneezing, straining at stool, nausea, or vomiting.

May have allergies.

Occupation: stressful either physically or emotionally.

Note effect of symptoms on client, fear and anxiety.

Check history of ulcers (rule out gastric bleed).

DIAGNOSTIC STUDIES

Anemia (may be severe) depending on extent/duration of bleed.

Hct, Hb, direct platelet count, WBC, PT, PTT.

Guaiac stools for presence of blood.

Arterial blood gases may indicate need for supplemental O_2.

High blood alcohol may be present.

SGOT, SGPT, LDH, alkphosphatase, indicators of liver involvement. Liver function tests to reconfirm cause as cirrhosis.

Esophagoscopy to note exact location of the bleed (gastric versus esophageal), must be done with great caution. If massive bleed of unknown etiology occurring, arteriography may be necessary.

PHYSICAL EXAMINATION

Note amount and character of bleeding.

Stools with melena or bright red blood may be very loose.

Abdominal exam shows enlarged, possibly tender liver with abdominal distention; may be shriveled and shrunken in later stages; ascites may be present.

Decreased BP, increased thready pulse (possibly quite shocky, depending on length of the hemorrhage).

Increased respiratory rate.

Ascultate chest to r/o aspiration.

May be anxious and/or disoriented.

Neurologic check may give indications of hepatic encephalopathy.

Skin pale in color, poor turgor.

After acute stage is stabilized, complete physical.

NURSING PRIORITIES

1. Promote comfort.
2. Maintain a patent airway and adequate respiratory function.
3. Observe for complications of hemorrhage, and so forth.
4. Provide information to assist patient in dealing with disease management.
5. Assist in dealing with psychologic aspects of illness.

Refer to Care Plan: Cirrhosis of the Liver for nursing diagnoses and care as the majority of esophageal varices are related to cirrhosis.

NURSING DIAGNOSIS:	**Knowledge deficit, disease process, complications, and medical management.**
SUPPORTING DATA:	**Esophageal varices bleed quite suddenly and severely and management requires patient cooperation.**
DESIRED PATIENT OUTCOMES:	**Patient/significant others verbalize understanding of the cause and management of the bleeding and cooperate with care to their level of ability.**

INTERVENTIONS

Explain each intervention before and as it is occurring.

Give information about the etiology of the varices, especially focusing on the role of alcoholism in its development, when appropriate.

Reinforce the above information after the bleed has been controlled and the patient is rested.

RATIONALE

Helpful in decreasing fear and promoting cooperation.

While this is a very traumatic occurrence, the information is essential and may be helpful in making the decision to quit, when alcohol is the causative factor.

An acute bleed of great quantity affects the ability of the patient to comprehend all that is occurring, especially if the patient is in near shock secondary to the bleed.

DIAGNOSIS: Gastritis, Acute/Chronic

PATIENT DATA BASE

NURSING HISTORY

Complains of indigestion, anorexia, nausea, vomiting, hematemesis, hiccups, heartburn, burping with sour taste, headache, fatigue. Symptoms appear after ingestion of certain foods or irritants or may be unpredictable; may appear on empty stomach or a specific time interval following ingestion of contaminated food.

Patient may have a habit of eating food rapidly or in excessive quantity.

Patient confirms ingestion of spicy or irritating foods.

History of ingestion of drugs, such as aspirin, digitalis, iodides, alcohol, or corrosive chemicals.

May have bacterial/viral infection accompanied by cramps/diarrhea.

History of irradiation of gastric area; gastric ulcer disease; gastric surgery: removal of pylorus may allow bile reflux causing symptoms of gastritis/esophagitis, unrelieved by vomiting or eating, but which will respond to binding agents, such as cholestyramine, aluminum hydroxide gel.

History of allergic reactions, especially aspirin.

Assess stress level.

May have no specific symptoms with chronic gastritis.

DIAGNOSTIC STUDIES

Fiberoptic endoscopy:

Acute gastritis: shows hyperemic and edematous gastric mucosa; it may also show erosion.

Chronic gastritis: the mucosal membranes are at first thickened and the rugae prominent, but eventually they become thinned and secretions decrease. Chronic gastritis may lead to gastric cancer, therefore, ulcerations should be biopsied to rule out benign or malignant ulcerations as the cause of symptoms.

Serum BUN and creatinine: elevated levels may indicate uremia, which may be associated with chronic gastritis.

Upper GI series: no abnormality demonstrated in gastritis; ulcerative disease, however, will be visualized.

In acute hemorrhagic gastritis, hemoglobin and hematocrit levels may be low.

PHYSICAL EXAMINATION

General appearance may show signs of systemic disease as a cause of the symptomatology.

Spider angiomas, palmer erythema, palpable liver or signs of portal hypertension may indicate hepatic disease as a cause of gastritis due to chronic congestion of the stomach wall.

Vital signs within normal limits or slightly elevated.

Examine skin turgor, moistness of mucous membranes for signs of dehydration.

In corrosive gastritis, such as that caused by ingestion of lye and so forth, bloody vomitus, stools, and collapse may lead to death due to blood loss or perforation.

NURSING PRIORITIES

1. Maintenance/restoration of fluid and electrolyte balance.
2. Support/maintain adequate nutritional intake.
3. Minimize/prevent recurrence.

NURSING DIAGNOSIS: **Fluid volume, deficit, potential.**

SUPPORTING DATA: **Symptoms lead to decreased intake with excessive output and potential of subsequent imbalance.**

DESIRED PATIENT OUTCOMES: **Regain and maintain adequate fluid/electrolyte balance.**

INTERVENTIONS

Assess electrolyte balance per lab data and observation daily and p.r.n.

Assess hydration and record I & O accurately; note sources of insensible loss.

Encourage oral intake when vomiting ceases, starting with clear liquids and advancing as tolerated, avoiding acid/irritating fluids. Offer small amounts (30–60 ml)/hour initially.

MEDICAL MANAGEMENT

Intravenous therapy with electrolyte replacement.

Antiemetics.

RATIONALE

Vomiting, poor intake may cause loss of essential electrolytes, especially H^-, Cl^-, and K^-, and may produce alkalosis.

Output may exceed intake, which may already be inadequate to meet insensible losses. Dehydration may increase glomerular filtration rate (GFR) making output inadequate to properly clear wastes and lead to increased BUN and altered electrolyte assay.

Maintain hydration and minimize side effects of anticholinergics.

May be necessary to maintain hydration and electrolyte balance.

Helpful when vomiting is present.

NURSING DIAGNOSIS: **Nutrition, alteration in, less than body requirements.**

SUPPORTING DATA: **Patient experiencing anorexia, nausea, and vomiting depending upon cause and varying degrees of severity of disease process.**

DESIRED PATIENT OUTCOMES: **Minimize weight loss and establish adequate nutritional intake.**

INTERVENTIONS

Keep NPO until acute symptoms subside, usually within hours or days.

Observe for increased salivation, sweating, trembling, blood pressure, pulse, irregular respirations.

Observe characteristics of vomitus.

Clean area immediately, keep environment pleasant, well-ventilated; avoid unpleasant odors and sights; promote restful atmosphere.

Encourage and provide frequent oral care, including brushing teeth.

Offer ice chips, tea, 7-Up before other foods.

Give regular milk, not skim.

Give small, frequent meals of bland foods.

Avoid caffeinated beverages.

Ascertain patient's preferred foods.

Observe for symptoms of other diseases that may cause gastritis symptoms.

RATIONALE

Allows gastric mucosa rest and time for healing so oral intake can be resumed as tolerated.

Exaggerated vasomotor activity often preceeds vomiting.

May be helpful in differentiating cause of gastric distress. Yellow-green may indicate bile content and implies that the pylorus is open. Fecal content indicates bowel obstruction. Bloody: Bright red signals recent or arterial bleeding, perhaps due to gastric ulceration; dark red may be old blood or venous bleeding from varices. Coffee-grounds are suggestive of partially digested blood from slowly oozing area. Undigested food indicates obstruction or gastric tumor.

Symptoms may be stimulated by upsetting emotional experiences and noxious odors. Quiet surroundings decrease response to stimuli and promote relaxation.

Halitosis from stagnant oral secretions are unappetizing and may aggravate symptoms. Gingivitis and dental problems may arise.

Small amounts of clear liquids are more easily tolerated by irritated gastric mucosa.

Fat in regular milk decreases HCl secretion; calcium of skim milk acts to increase secretion of HCl.

Small feedings do not distend gastric area, act to neutralize gastric acids and dilute stomach contents.

Stimulates HCl production.

May respond more favorably and digest accustomed foods more easily if altered cultural changes are consistent with dietary restrictions.

Uremia, pernicious anemia, gastric ulcer disease, hiatal hernia, portal hypertension, pregnancy, poisoning, psychosomatic disease, hypoxia, visual or middle ear abnormalities, pancreatitis, cholecystitis, intestinal obstruction, hepatic disease, migraines, and CNS disease may cause symptoms.

MEDICAL MANAGEMENT

Antacids.

Sedatives.

Anticholinergics and cimetidine.

Antacids neutralize acids, which then relieve gastric discomfort.

Promote relaxation.

Suppress gastric secretions of HCl and delay emptying.

Supplementary vitamin B_{12}.	In diffuse atrophic gastritis, the intrinsic factor necessary for B_{12} absorption from the GI tract is not secreted and may develop pernicious anemia.
Antibiotics.	When infection is the cause.

NURSING DIAGNOSIS:	**Knowledge deficit, disease process.**
SUPPORTING DATA:	**Wide range of causative factors in susceptible individuals can result in recurrent episodes of gastritis.**
DESIRED PATIENT OUTCOMES:	**Minimize or prevent recurrent episodes.**

INTERVENTIONS

Provide information about underlying disease process.

Emphasize that patient needs to avoid certain foods and emotional situations that are suspect or known to produce symptoms.

Suggest small, frequent meals. Provide explanation of the value of such a regimen.

Discuss avoidance of drugs that cause gastric irritation.

If patient smokes, may need to discuss advisability of quitting and methods to help accomplish this (Stop Smoking Clinic and so forth).

Help patient identify and learn stress reduction and relaxation techniques.

Stress importance of followup care.

Refer to Care Plan: Psychosocial Aspects of Care in the Acute Setting.

RATIONALE

Varied causes of gastritis may require broader knowledge base to enable patient to deal adequately with the total problem. (Refer to specific care as indicated, e.g., ulcers, cancer.)

Decreases extrinsic stimulation of HCl and avoid recurrence of gastritis symptoms.

Frequent eating keeps HCl neutralized, dilutes stomach contents to minimize action of acid on gastric mucosa, which produces symptoms of gastritis.

Identification of drugs that are irritating to the individual patient will allow for choice in avoiding them. Emphasize importance of reading content labels of over-the-counter medications.

Smoking increases intestinal motility.

Promotes reduction of physiologic/psychologic stress that may be a precipitating factor.

Chronic gastritis predisposes to gastric cancer.

DIAGNOSIS: Ulcers

PATIENT DATA BASE

NURSING HISTORY

Complains of epigastric pain; nausea and vomiting; weight loss; dyspepsia; eructation.

History of epigastric pain that is absent or diminished in the morning, present two or three hours after meals and most severe at night.

Episodes of pain may last a period of days or weeks interspersed by pain-free intervals of weeks or months. Pain is unrelated to body motion. Pain may be alleviated after vomiting.

Dietary history to specifically include relationship of: a) symptomatic relief of pain in response to food; b) nausea and vomiting in response to food; c) calorie count in response to weight loss.

Note amount and frequency of ingestion of caffeine-containing beverages and alcohol.

Note changes in bowel pattern; diarrhea, tarry stools, or the presence of frothy, foul-smelling stools (steatorrhea: may be indicative of Zollinger-Ellison syndrome).

If smoker, determine pattern and amount of daily consumption.

Past and current medications: to determine if ulcers are a side effect of ingestion of medications.

Recent/concurrent serious illness/trauma, hospitalization that may result in Curling's ulcer, occurring in burns and stress ulcers seen in ICU.

Psychologic history to specifically include anxiety and irritability.

Relationships of type of work, socioeconomic class, blood type.

DIAGNOSTIC STUDIES

Gastrointestinal series: determine presence of ulcerations.

Gastric analysis: determines amount of hydrochloric acid (increased amount indicative of duodenal ulcer; decreased or normal amount indicative of gastric ulcer; enormous hypersecretion and acidity may be diagnostic of Zollinger-Ellison syndrome.

Stools for occult blood: determines occurrence of GI bleeding.

Endoscopy: determines location of ulcers; allows visual evaluation; biopsy may be taken.

CBC: determines baseline blood count; anemia; assists in determining dehydration.

PHYSICAL EXAMINATION

Observe abdomen for distention.

Auscultate for bowel sounds, note increase in number of bowel sounds.

Palpate abdomen for tenderness and rebound pain.

Observe for signs of dehydration.

Observe nonverbal behavior indicative of anxiety and irritability.

NURSING PRIORITIES

1. Control of pain and bleeding.
2. Promote physical and mental rest to enhance healing process.
3. Prevention of recurrence and complications.

NURSING DIAGNOSIS:	Comfort, alteration in, pain.
SUPPORTING DATA:	Characteristic pain depends on sites of erosion.
DESIRED PATIENT OUTCOMES:	Pain, as a result of ulcer, is alleviated.

INTERVENTIONS

Diet may range from NPO to as tolerated.

Provide small frequent meals when indicated for individual patient.

Avoid gastric irritants, such as caffeine, alcohol, smoking, individual food intolerances. Identify relationship of food intake and precipitation of or relief from epigastric pain.

Use regular rather than skim milk.

MEDICAL MANAGEMENT

Analgesics.

Antacids.

Anticholinergics, such as belladonna, atropine.

Histamine antagonists, cimetidine. Avoid the use of antacids within 1 hr after oral administration.

RATIONALE

Depending on severity of bleeding present.

Has an acid neutralizing effect, as well as diluting the gastric contents. Small meals prevent distention and the release of gastrin.

Caffeine and smoking stimulate gastric acidity. Alcohol contributes to erosion of gastric mucosa. Individuals may find that certain foods increase pain. Food should not be used as an antacid; stimulates acid secretions.

Fat in regular milk decreases gastric secretions while the calcium in skim milk increases them.

Promote physical and mental rest.

Decrease gastric acidity by physical absorption or by chemical neutralization. Evaluate type of antacid in regard to total health picture; e.g., sodium restriction.

Decrease gastric motility and are effective in relieving nocturnal pain.

Decrease secretion of gastric acid by inhibiting the action of histamine H_2 receptors of the parietal cells. Antacids block the absorption of cimetidine.

NURSING DIAGNOSIS:	Fluid volume deficit, potential.
SUPPORTING DATA:	Bleeding often occurs with ulceration, may be insidious or in the form of sudden hemorrhage.
DESIRED PATIENT OUTCOMES:	Circulating blood volume is maintained.

INTERVENTIONS

Monitor lab studies. Hb/Hct, occult blood.

Note amount and color of any emesis.

RATIONALE

Indicative of developing blood loss.

Determine current or old bleed.

Check vital signs on a regular schedule, noting signs of hypovolemia.

Tachycardia, sweating, coldness of extremities, fainting and/or orthostatic hypotension, and dyspnea with activity.

Bed rest.

Conserve energy.

Monitor I & O.

Document adequate hydration and renal function. Decreasing urinary output can be an early warning of impending hypovolemia.

MEDICAL MANAGEMENT

Mild sedation.

Promotes rest, may reduce intensity of bleed, and alleviates pain but does not mask signs of impending hypovolemia.

NG suction.

Monitors rate of bleeding and empty clots.

Ice saline lavage (levophed may be added to solution).

Aids in localized vasoconstriction.

Antacid per NG tube.

Neutralizes gastric secretions.

Cimetidine, IV.

Decreases acid production in the gastric lining.

IV fluid and/or blood replacement.

Maintain adequate circulating volume and prevent hypovolemic shock.

Gastroscopy.

Visualization aids in accurately locating sites of erosion and bleeding status.

Surgery. (Repair/resection.)

If hemorrhage persists or perforation occurs.

NURSING DIAGNOSIS: **Coping, ineffective, individual.**

SUPPORTING DATA: **Emotional factors influence the function of the stomach. People who develop ulcers often are unhappy, tense, perfectionistic individuals who require changes in lifestyle, which in themselves are stressful.**

DESIRED PATIENT OUTCOMES: **Demonstrates acceptance of unavoidable stressful situations without reactivation of ulcer.**

INTERVENTIONS

Allow time for and encourage verbalization.

RATIONALE

Trusting and understanding relationship promotes credibility between patient and health caregiver, reducing anxiety about current condition.

Encourage communication with significant others.

Development of a significant support system assists in maintaining healthful behaviors.

Encourage and support patient in evaluating lifestyle.

Evaluation of lifestyle with potential changes may be necessary to avoid recurrence of ulcer condition.

MEDICAL MANAGEMENT

Refer to professional therapy.

Necessary if evaluation and control of lifestyle is not within current capability of patient.

Refer to Care Plan: Psychosocial Aspects of Care in the Acute Setting.

NURSING DIAGNOSIS:	**Knowledge deficit, disease process and management.**
SUPPORTING DATA:	**Lack of knowledge re varied causative factors may result in recurrence of GI bleed.**
DESIRED PATIENT OUTCOMES:	**Verbalizes knowledge of causative factors and demonstrates modification of behavior as needed.**

INTERVENTIONS

Stress importance that patient be aware of cause/effect relationships of lifestyle behaviors and epigastric pain/bleeding.

Instruct and emphasize the importance of rest and the use of effective coping mechanisms (see previous nursing diagnosis).

Instruct and assist patient and significant others in understanding the effects of smoking, alcohol, and caffeine on the ulcerative process.

Inform patient regarding the need to avoid taking over-the-counter medication without checking with the physician; especially medications containing acetylsalicylic acid.

Assist patient in identifying and developing significant others for support.

RATIONALE

Precipitating factors of epigastric pain is individual; therefore, the patient needs to be aware of what foods, fluids, and lifestyle factors precipitate these episodes.

Rest and avoidance of stress will promote recovery.

Cooperation with the minimal use of alcohol, smoking, and caffeine will assist in the recovery process and aid in preventing further recurrence.

Acetylsalicylic acid ingestion is firmly associated with ulcer development.

Due to probable alterations in lifestyle, support persons are important in maintaining changes of behavior.

NURSING DIAGNOSIS:	**Knowledge deficit, recognizing signs of complications.**
SUPPORTING DATA:	**Complications may develop after discharge. Early detection may prevent or limit life-threatening situations.**
DESIRED PATIENT OUTCOMES:	**Patient and significant others verbalize recognition of signs of complications of ulcers.**

INTERVENTIONS

Instruct patient and significant others of signs of hemorrhage, such as vomiting blood, tarry stools, faintness, dizziness, thirst, apprehensiveness, restlessness, dyspnea.

Instruct re signs of pyloric obstruction, such as epigastric fullness, pain, sitophobia (morbid fear of food), projectile vomiting, dehydration, and weight loss.

Instruct re signs of perforation, such as sudden, sharp abdominal pain; tender board-like abdomen; rapid, shallow respirations; profuse perspiration; and referred pain to shoulder region (phrenic nerve irritation).

Instruct about reporting amount and/or duration of bleeding.

RATIONALE

Bleeding may indicate reactivation of and/or development of new ulcer. It is the most common complication. May need to r/o Zollinger-Ellison syndrome.

Approximately 10% of patients develop pyloric obstruction. Usually seen in patients with long-standing disease.

Approximately 4% experience perforation. Findings on physical examination are: no bowel sounds, abdominal guarding, direct and rebound tenderness. It is usually considered a surgical emergency.

May be indication of Zollinger-Ellison syndrome.

Zollinger-Ellison Syndrome:
Usually presents with symptoms of peptic ulcer disease caused by malignant/benign tumor of gastrin-producing cells (gastrinoma) or tumors of nonbeta islet cells of the pancreas. These tumors cause excessive production of gastrin resulting in hypersecretion of acid by the parietal cells.
The syndrome is an inactivation of lipase by the lowered pH in the duodenum and jejunum, thus resulting in pancreatic insufficiency and inability to digest fats.

Less than 20% of the islet cell tumors are resectable and treatment is therefore directed at the "target" organ. The intervention of choice has been total gastrectomy (see Care Plan: Gastric Resection). Recent studies using cimetidine to reduce hypersecretion have had promising results in the controlled setting but require further study before the surgical intervention is abandoned.

CARE PLAN: Gastric Resection (Surgical Removal of Part of the Stomach)

PATIENT DATA BASE

Refer to Care Plans: Gastritis; Ulcers.

NURSING PRIORITIES

1. Promote healing and adequate nutritional intake.
2. Prevent complications.
3. Assist patient/significant others with potential changes in lifestyle.
Refer to Care Plans: Surgical Intervention; Intestinal Surgery.

NURSING DIAGNOSIS: Nutrition, alteration in, less than body requirements.

SUPPORTING DATA: Conditions requiring sub/total gastrectomy as well as pre/postoperative restriction of fluids and food to decrease motor and secretory activity interfere with nutritional intake for significant periods of time resulting in some degree of malnutrition.

DESIRED PATIENT OUTCOMES: Nutritional needs will be met.

INTERVENTIONS	RATIONALE
Maintain patency of NG tube. *Do not* reposition tube if it becomes dislodged.	Prevents gastric distention with accumulated secretions that may cause stress on the sutures and possible rupture of the stump. The tube is placed during surgery and needs to be repositioned by the physician to prevent injury to the operative area.
Note character and amount of NG drainage.	Will be bloody for first 12 hours, and then be clearing.
Provide oral hygiene on a regular, frequent basis using glycerine and lemon juice swabs.	Prevent discomfort of dry mouth and cracked lips caused by fluid restriction and the NG tube.
Caution the patient to limit the intake of ice chips.	Sodium and potassium will be removed by the NG tube along with liquid.
Maintain accurate I & O.	Necessary guide for fluid replacement.
Monitor Hb, Hct, and electrolytes.	Detect complications.
Auscultate for bowel sounds and note passage of flatus.	Peristalsis can be expected to return about the third postop day.
Monitor tolerance to fluid and food intake.	Complications of paralytic ileus, obstruction, and gastric dilatation may occur.
Avoid the use of milk in the diet.	May trigger "dumping syndrome."

MEDICAL MANAGEMENT

IV fluids and electrolytes.

Replacement therapy.

Progressive diet; clear liquid to bland diet with several small feedings.

Usually NG tube is clamped for periods of time when peristalsis returns, to determine tolerance. After NG tube is removed, intake is advanced gradually.

Vitamin supplements, including B_{12}.

Removal of the stomach prevents absorption due to loss of intrinsic factor and can result in pernicious anemia.

Protein supplements.

Helpful for tissue repair and healing.

NURSING DIAGNOSIS:	**Knowledge deficit, postoperative care.**
SUPPORTING DATA:	**With removal of part or all of the stomach, changes in eating habits will be necessary to avoid complications, such as "dumping syndrome."**
DESIRED PATIENT OUTCOMES:	**Verbalizes successful adjustment to new eating regimen.**

INTERVENTIONS

Discuss symptoms that may indicate "dumping syndrome."

Discuss the importance of eating small frequent meals; avoid high intake of sugars and salt; take fluids between meals rather than with food; eat slowly and in a relaxed atmosphere resting after meals.

Instruct in avoiding fibrous foods and chewing food well.

Discuss and identify stress situations and how to avoid them.

Review diet regimen and importance of maintaining vitamin supplementation.

Discuss importance of regular checkup with physician.

RATIONALE

Weakness, profuse perspiration, nausea, vomiting, faintness, flushing, epigastric discomfort, and palpitation occurring within 15 minutes after eating.

Measures that can be helpful in avoiding occurrence of "dumping syndrome" and hypoglycemic reactions.

Remaining gastric tissue may not be able to digest such foods as citrus skins and seeds and these may collect and form a mass (phytobezoar formation), which is not excreted.

Can interfere with optimal digestion. Refer to Care Plan: Psychosocial Apsects of Care in the Acute Setting.

Will be helpful to patient in understanding changes. Provides opportunity for questions and clarifications.

Detect complications, such as anemia, problems with nutrition, and/or recurrence of disease.

DIAGNOSIS: Regional Enteritis, Ileocolitis, Transmural Colitis, Colitis, Granulomatous Colitis, Crohn's Disease

PATIENT DATA BASE

NURSING HISTORY

Disturbance in elimination, frequent diarrhea (three to five stools daily), increased peristalsis, anorexia aggravated by illness and emotional upset, nausea and abdominal cramping, particularly after meals and especially in the right lower abdominal quadrant.

Higher incidence in English, Jewish, high stress-oriented young adults between ages 20–30, peaks again between ages 40–50.

Familial occurrence.

Episodes precipitated by dietary indiscretions, especially dairy products and fatty foods.

Family history of inflammatory bowel disease.

Weight loss may be insidious, progressing to severe loss.

History of chronicity helps differentiate from acute appendicitis.

DIAGNOSTIC STUDIES

X-rays: barium swallow to demonstrate luminal narrowing in the terminal ileum, stiffening of the bowel wall, mucosal irritability or ulceration.

Barium enema: to differentiate from other gastrointestinal diseases, such as diverticulosis or cancer. In regional enteritis, the small bowel is nearly always involved but the rectal area is affected only 50% of the time. Fistulas are frequent, and are usually found in the terminal ileum but may be present in segments throughout the gastrointestinal tract as well.

Urine culture: if E. Coli are present, suspect fistula formation to bladder.

Altered albumin-globulin ratio caused by blood loss.

Sigmoidoscopic examination: edematous hyperemic mucosa or a discrete ulcer when the colon is involved.

Complete blood count: shows increased white blood cells, increased sedimentation rate, and with temperature elevation may reflect inflammation.

Decreased serum iron-binding capacity caused by chronic infection or secondary to blood loss.

Anemia: hypochromic (occasionally macrocytic) anemia. Does not occur often with ileitis except with iron, folic acid, or vitamin B_{12} deficiency due to nutrition or malabsorption. Depressed bone marrow function due to chronic inflammatory process.

Stool examination: occult blood may be positive due to mucosal erosion; stools are negative for dysentery; steatorrhea may be found.

Clotting studies: alterations may occur due to poor vitamin B_{12} absorption.

Electrolytes: decreased potassium, calcium, and magnesium with increased sodium; dehydration may be present. Acute episodes may deplete electrolytes rapidly.

PHYSICAL EXAMINATION

In acute regional enteritis, abdominal pain is usually severe and may be localized in right lower quadrant, necessitating surgical intervention to establish a differential diagnosis.

Fistula formation or right quadrant mass; tenderness in periumbilical region.

Hyperactive bowel sounds, especially in right lower quadrant.

Evacuation urgency of soft or semi-liquid stool even at night; flatus or blood may indicate ulcerations; presence of steatorrhea indicates loss of absorption and derangement of bile salts from impaired enterohepatic recirculation.

Colicky, abdominal pain, often relieved by bowel movement.

Anorexia, flatulence, malaise, weight loss.

Inspection of perineum for fistula formulations; inflamed areas are suspect of occult fistula formation.

NURSING PRIORITIES

1. Maintenance of fluid and electrolyte balance, and adequate nutrition.
2. Promote patient comfort.
3. Provide knowledge of disease process and treatment regimen.
4. Assist patient in developing appropriate interventions to deal with long-term aspects of recurrent disease process.

NURSING DIAGNOSIS:	**Fluid volume deficit, potential.**
SUPPORTING DATA:	**Patient exhibits anorexia and food avoidance because of cramping. Fluids and electrolytes are lost in excess with prolonged diarrhea.**
DESIRED PATIENT OUTCOMES:	**Maintaining normal hydration and electrolyte levels, particularly potassium.**

INTERVENTIONS

Accurate intake and output, daily weights. Note weight decrease of more than four pounds per week.

Give fluids in amounts necessary to maintain hydration.

Monitor electrolytes, especially potassium, and possible acid-base disorders. Note muscle weakness or cardiac arrhythmias.

RATIONALE

Dehydration occurs easily with diarrhea.

1000 ml/24 hours is minimum fluid intake that will meet basic body fluid requirements; more is required if insensible loss is increased or diarrhea is present.

Potassium is necessary for proper skeletal and cardiac muscle function. Minor alterations in serum levels may result in profound and/or life-threatening symptoms. Diarrhea can lead to metabolic acidosis (loss of HCO_2).

MEDICAL MANAGEMENT

Potassium supplementation with at least 4 oz. of water or juice.

Maintains potassium levels and minimizes gastric irritation.

NURSING DIAGNOSIS:	Comfort, alterations in, pain.
SUPPORTING DATA:	Frequent abdominal cramping, evacuation urgency, excoriation of the anus.
DESIRED PATIENT OUTCOMES:	Patient verbalizes lessening or absence of pain. Symptoms of fistula formation or obstruction are absent.

INTERVENTIONS

Observe and record changes in description of pain, location, frequency, duration, characteristics, and precipitating events.

Observe and record distention, increased temperature, decreased blood pressure, rectal bleeding, or ischiorectal and perianal fistulas.

Cleanse rectal area with mild soap and water; apply ointments as indicated.

MEDICAL MANAGEMENT

Analgesics.

Anticholinergics.

Sitz baths.

RATIONALE

Pinpoints causative factors, such as stressful events, food intolerance, and developing complications.

An increase in pain and tenderness may indicate developing obstruction from inflammation, edema, and scarring. Fistulas may develop from erosion and weakening of bowel wall.

Constant irritation with undigested bowel contents leads to skin breakdown and ulceration.

Pain varies from mild to severe and necessitates management to facilitate adequate rest and recovery, and to avoid problems of dependency.

Relieve spasm of the GI tract.

For local soothing and comfort.

NURSING DIAGNOSIS:	Nutrition, alteration in, less than body requirements, potential.
SUPPORTING DATA:	Cramping and diarrhea may prevent/inhibit patient from eating. Hyperactivity of the bowel reduces transit time and decreases absorption of nutrients.
DESIRED PATIENT OUTCOMES:	Weight stabilized and/or weight gain attained as individually indicated.

INTERVENTIONS

Encourage bed rest and/or limited activity during acute phase of illness.

RATIONALE

Decreases calorie depletion and conserves energy.

Provide necessary comfort measures, including oral hygiene and opportunity for rest before serving meals.

A clean mouth can enhance the taste of food. Rest before meals quiets peristalsis, increases available energy for eating.

Give small, frequent feedings.

Large meals act to distend gastric pouch, stimulating peristalsis.

Have patient participate in dietary planning.

Gives patient active participation in disease regimen.

Note clotting studies; observe for overt or occult bleeding.

Inadequate diet and decreased absorption may lead to vitamin K deficiency and defects in coagulation.

Assess individual need for limitation of fats, spicy foods, and milk products.

Some foods may be poorly tolerated or result in allergic reactions, manifested by increased diarrhea.

Serve allowed foods in well-ventilated, pleasant surroundings with unhurried atmosphere, congenial company; may give appetite stimulants, such as wine.

Avoids unpleasant distractions and encourages intake. Wine may be given to some patients to stimulate appetite.

MEDICAL MANAGEMENT

Iron supplementation, by injection.

Oral route for iron supplementation is ineffective due to intestinal alterations that severely reduce absorption.

Keep NPO until vomiting subsides; IV therapy, TPN (Total Parenteral Nutrition) may be indicated.

This regimen rests the gastrointestinal tract while providing essential nutrients; gradual resumption of normal diet minimizes return of symptoms, TPN may be necessary if patient is unable to tolerate any oral feedings. (Refer to Care Plan: Total Parenteral Nutrition.)

Clear liquids, progressing to bland, low-residue diet.

Given in small amounts as tolerated to allow intestinal tract to readjust to digestive process.

Provide high-protein, high-calorie, and low-fiber diet. May need to supplement diet with vitamin B_{12}, folic acid.

Protein is necessary for tissue integrity and repair; low bulk decreases peristaltic response to meal. Marked loss of ileum results in reduced absorption of B_{12}. Vitamin B_{12} supplementation aids in reversing bone depression caused by prolonged inflammatory process.

Antiemetics p.r.n.

Prevents vomiting and further nutritional losses.

NURSING DIAGNOSIS:	**Bowel elimination, alteration in, diarrhea.**
SUPPORTING DATA:	**Toxic elements produced by inflammation, segmental narrowing of the lumen and increased peristalsis, act to decrease transit time of bowel contents, thereby producing diarrhea.**

| DESIRED PATIENT OUTCOMES: | **Reduction of frequency of stools and return to more normal stool consistency.** |

INTERVENTIONS

INTERVENTIONS	RATIONALE
Make bathroom/bedpan facilities readily available.	Defecation urges may occur without warning and be uncontrollable.
Remove stool promptly. Use room deodorizers.	Reduce room odors to avoid undue patient embarrassment.
Observe and record frequency, characteristics, amount, and precipitation factors of occurrence of diarrhea.	Helps differentiate from other diseases and assesses severity of episode.
Restrict foods and fluids that precipitate diarrhea, such as raw vegetables and fruits, whole grain cereals, condiments, and carbonated drinks.	Promotes intestinal rest.
Provide opportunity to vent frustrations related to disease process.	Unknown cause/cure/surgical alternatives lead to stress that may aggravate condition.

MEDICAL MANAGEMENT

MEDICAL MANAGEMENT	
Antidiarrheals, such as Lomotil.	Decrease peristalsis, relieves cramping and diarrhea.
Anticholinergics. (Do not give in presence of symptoms of obstruction.) Watch for urinary retention.	Given before meals to decrease peristalsis. Side effects of drugs containing atropine.
Steroids.	Steroids are given to decrease inflammatory process, thereby decreasing occurrence of diarrhea.
Antibiotics.	To treat local suppurative infection.
Antacids.	Decrease gastric irritation.
Hydrophyllic mucilloids, such as Metamucil.	Provides bulk in a low-residue diet; decrease fluidity and number of stools, thus decreasing perianal irritation.
Cholestyramine.	Absorption of bile salts may be impaired. Salts pass into the colon and increase absorption of water and electrolytes, which then leads to diarrhea. Cholestyramine binds bile salts to block this cycle.

| **NURSING DIAGNOSIS:** | **Knowledge deficit, disease process.** |
| **SUPPORTING DATA:** | **Chronic disease has no cure and requires patient knowledge for cooperation to help avoid and minimize symptoms.** |

| DESIRED PATIENT OUTCOMES: | Patient is able to verbalize and initiate appropriate interventions to deal with prescribed regimen in chronic illness. |

INTERVENTIONS

Provide patient/significant others information about disease process, medications and symptoms of complications.

Help patient identify foods/fluids and situations that may precipitate attacks.

Avoid laxatives and drugs that may irritate tne gastrointestinal tract.

Make referrals to outside resources as indicated; such as Public Health Nurse, Ostomy Association, and patient groups.

Refer to Care Plan: Psychosocial Aspects of Care in the Acute Setting.

RATIONALE

Factual information increases patient understanding of disease process and affords opportunities for some control over exacerbations through modification of lifestyle.

Avoidance allows resting of the gastrointestinal tract, minimizing symptoms.

Decreases further irritation of the intestinal mucosa and exacerbation of the disease process.

Resources can be helpful in disease management.

To assist in dealing with long-term aspects of this disease.

DIAGNOSIS: Ulcerative Colitis

PATIENT DATA BASE

NURSING HISTORY

Bloody diarrhea with urgency, cramping, tenesmus coupled with malaise, occasional nausea, vomiting, anorexia, and weight loss.

History of disease may help distinguish type of ulcerative colitis:
  a) relapsing or remitting type, which is milder, involving rectal area only; remission occurs in weeks to months.
  b) chronic or continuous type, which is an ongoing disease involving areas above the rectal area.
  c) acute or fulminating type, which is uncommon; there is a rapid progression and deterioration of the disease.

Exacerbations are usually due to dietary indiscretions, emotional upsets, gastrointestinal irritants (such as medications), overexertions and fatigue, upper respiratory or other infections, and pregnancy.

Special attention to gastrointestinal complaints and recent emotional stresses including patient and family reaction to the illness may help to rule out gastroenteritis.

Arthritis, skin lesions, finger clubbing, anemia, fatty liver infiltration, herpes zoster, biliary cirrhosis, and nephrolithiasis may accompany ulcerative colitis.

Note patient's behavior during the assessment, as well as patient's ability to communicate and understand. During exacerbation patient can become discouraged and withdraw.

Note expressions of food habits, fatigue or overwork that may have produced anxiety or tension.

Typical patient is young adult (ages 20–40), slightly more common in women, higher incidence found in Jewish population; question of familial predisposition.

DIAGNOSTIC STUDIES

Stool specimens will be positive for blood. Also examine for intestinal organisms, especially Entamoeba histolytica. In the active stage, the stool is mainly composed of mucus, blood, and pus. Stool examinations can be used in initial diagnosis and to follow disease progression.

CBC: patients with active disease usually have hyperchromic anemia. Anemia is generally present due to blood loss and iron deficiency; bone marrow depression may be present after long inflammatory process.

WBC: leukocytosis may occur, especially in fulminating or complicated cases and in those on steroid therapy.

Bone marrow: a generalized bone marrow depression is common in fulminating types.

Serum iron level is lowered due to blood loss.

Prothrombin time is prolonged in severe cases from altered factors VII and X caused by vitamin K deficiency. This usually correlates with severe disease.

The sedimentation rate is increased according to the severity of the illness.

Thrombocytosis may occur due to the inflammatory disease process.

Electrolyte disturbances, especially a decrease in potassium, is common in severe disease.

Albumin level is decreased and negative nitrogen balance is evident due to loss of plasma proteins.

Alkaline phosphotase is increased, along with serum cholesterol and hypoproteinemia indicating disturbed liver function.

Proctosigmoidoscopy shows the texture of the mucous membranes: ulcerations, friability and hemorrhagic areas occur in 85% of these patients and is caused by necrosis and ulceration. The degree of edema and hyperemia can be visualized. Inflammation is the result of a secondary infection of the mucosa and submucosa.

Neoplastic changes can be detected on biopsy, as well as characteristic inflammatory infiltrate called crypt abscess.

When inner muscle destruction occurs, it is replaced with granulation tissue; diffuse vs segmental process as seen in Crohn's disease. Initial involvement is of the rectum and affects the colon with upward progression.

Barium enema should be done after visual examination has been done. (Do not prepare the patient by purging because enemas produce hyperemia and edema that can be confused with colitis.)

PHYSICAL EXAMINATION

Endocrine factors, such as menses, menopause, and hyperthyroidism, may be related to periods of crisis.

The patient frequently appears apprehensive, tense, and is pale and weak with an obvious weight loss; edema may be present.

Abdominal examination may reveal rebound tenderness and guarding in the right lower quadrant.

Bowel sounds may be present but are most often quiet with peristalsis absent.

The liver may be palpated.

Distention over the transverse colon is usually a poor prognostic sign indicating the presence of toxic megacolon.

The rectal examination may be painful so should be done as carefully as possible. The anal sphincter may be spastic or relaxed. Pseudopolyps may be palpated. Blood, mucus, or pus may present as exudate on examination glove. The examination may show perianal irritation, fissures, hemorrhoids, fistulas, and abcesses. The rectal lumen is often narrowed and tubular with stenosis when the disease is active. If the disease is inactive, the findings are similar except that congestion and edema are not found. The patient may present with minimal exudate or none at all.

Symptoms of nutritional deficiencies may be evident.

Anemia may be evidenced by pallor of the skin, mucous membranes, and nail beds.

The psychologic status needs careful evaluation. Individuals with ulcerative colitis are usually passive and anxious to please. Periods of stress may aggravate symptoms. Although depression is common, hostile behavior may be observed.

NURSING PRIORITIES

1. Maintain fluid balance and nutrition.
2. Control inflammation and prevent infections.
3. Provide physical rest and minimize emotional upsets.
4. Provide knowledge of disease process and treatment regimen.

NURSING DIAGNOSIS:	**Bowel elimination, alteration in, diarrhea.**
SUPPORTING DATA:	**Frequent watery stools are typical in the acute phase of illness. The need to defecate may be sudden and painful.**

DESIRED PATIENT OUTCOMES:	Stools are of normal consistency and frequency is minimized.

INTERVENTIONS

See Care Plan: Regional Enteritis for initial nursing intervention.

Observe for fever, tachycardia, lethargy, leukocytosis, decreased serum protein, anxiety, and prostration.

Observe for side effects if steroids are given on a long-term basis.

RATIONALE

May signify that perforation and peritonitis are imminent and bowel must be put to rest immediately.

Used to control inflammation to effect a remission of the disease. Side effects may include GI upset, masking of infections, and lowered resistance and fluid retention.

MEDICAL MANAGEMENT

Tincture of belladonna, atropine, Lomotil, anodyne suppositories.

Discontinue above drugs if decreased bowel sounds, distention, gas, hypermotility or hypokalemia occur.

Azulfidine, steroids, Imuran.

Sedatives and tranquilizers.

Surgery (Refer to Care Plans: Intestinal Surgery; Fecal Diversion.

Relieve rectal spasms. Decrease number and increase consistency of stools.

Antispasmotics may cause toxic megacolon.

Act upon sub-epithelial connective tissue, which is affected in ulcerative colitis. Decrease infection and inflammation. Autoimmune reaction is thought to be a possible cause of this disease.

Promote general rest as well as decreasing peristalsis, allowing inflamed bowel to rest. Use opiates with caution as they may precipitate toxic megacolon.

May be indicated due to complications of hemorrhage, fistula formation and perforation, and/or long-standing problem of anemia, malnutrition or excessive diarrhea.

NURSING DIAGNOSIS:	Fluid volume deficit, potential.
SUPPORTING DATA:	Stools are watery and frequent. Excessive diarrhea and denuded bowel loses plasma and electrolytes profusely.
DESIRED PATIENT OUTCOMES:	Diarrhea is controlled. Fluid and electrolyte balance is maintained. Protein loss is replaced.

INTERVENTIONS

Maintain accurate intake and output (include number, character, and amount of liquid stools).

RATIONALE

Dehydration occurs easily with diarrhea.

Weigh daily.

Overall indication of fluid and nutritional status.

Monitor serum electrolytes (Na^+, K^+, Cl^-, HCO_3^-, pH).

Fluids and electrolytes are lost in large amounts by denuded, ulcerated bowel. Patients with severe diarrhea may lose 500–1700ml of H_2O and 2–8 gms Na^+ in 24 hrs.

Observe for excessively dry skin and mucous membranes, decreased skin turgor, oliguria, decreased temperature, weakness, increased Hct and Hb, elevated BUN, and urine specific gravity.

Indicators of excessive fluid loss with resultant dehydration, hemoconcentration and decreased glomerular filtration rate.

MEDICAL MANAGEMENT

Blood, plasma, or serum albumin transfusions.

Correct anemia.

Refer to Care Plan: Regional Enteritis.

NURSING DIAGNOSIS:	Nutrition, alteration in, less than body requirements, potential.
SUPPORTING DATA:	With decreased transit time, absorption of fluids and nutrients is decreased. Scarred and denuded bowel is unable to absorb nutrients properly. Nausea, odor, resultant cramping, and diarrhea decrease patient's inclination for food.
DESIRED PATIENT OUTCOMES:	Weight stabilized and/or gain as individually indicated.

Refer to Care Plan: Regional Enteritis.

NURSING DIAGNOSIS:	Knowledge deficit, disease process.

Refer to Care Plan: Regional Enteritis.

NURSING DIAGNOSIS:	Coping, ineffective, individual.
SUPPORTING DATA:	Recurrent episodes often lead to discouragement, anxiety, and preoccupation with the physical self.
DESIRED PATIENT OUTCOMES:	Recurrent episodes are limited/prevented.

INTERVENTIONS

Assess patient's and significant others' understanding and previous methods of dealing with disease process.

Assess outside stresses, such as family, social, or work environment. Avoid extreme changes in environment or nursing management. Provide for necessary changes gradually.

Refer to outside resources, as appropriate.

Refer to Care Plan: Psychosocial Aspects in the Acute Setting.

RATIONALE

Enables the nurse to deal more realistically with current problems. Anxiety and other factors may have interfered with previous health teaching/patient learning.

These areas may be presenting difficulties that contribute to problems of coping. Continuity of care can lessen the stress of constantly adjusting to changing personnel.

May need additional support and counseling.

NURSING DIAGNOSIS:	**Comfort, alteration in, pain.**
SUPPORTING DATA:	**Presence of diarrhea, cramping, skin irritation.**
DESIRED PATIENT OUTCOMES:	**Diarrhea is controlled. Excoriation of perineal area is minimized or prevented. Patient is comfortable.**

INTERVENTIONS

Refer to Care Plan: Regional Enteritis.

RATIONALE

CARE PLAN: Fecal Diversion

Ileostomy: diversion of the effluent of the small intestines, usually permanent.
Colostomy: diversion of the effluent of the colon, which may be temporary or permanent.

PATIENT DATA BASE

NURSING HISTORY

Causative factors may include:
1. Obstruction: mechanical, vascular, or neurogenic.
2. Perforation: trauma, ruptured diverticulum, or inflammation.
3. Inflammation: ulcerative colitis, Crohn's disease.

PHYSICAL EXAMINATION

Evaluate general condition.

Note type of ostomy: end, loop (with or without rod), or double barrel.

Determine presence or absence of mucous fistula.

Examine stoma for: position, size, color, texture, shape, proximity to suture lines or drains, and character of effluent.

Examine peristoma skin for irregularities and integrity.

NURSING PRIORITIES

Refer to Care Plans: Surgical Intervention; Intestinal Surgery.

1. Assist patient and family in acceptance of the ostomy.
2. Return to homeostasis.
3. Provide adequate collecting device for the ostomy, and maintain skin integrity.
4. Instruct patient and significant others in self-care.
5. Provide support and information of community resources, e.g., Ostomy Club, supply outlets, and counseling if indicated.

NURSING DIAGNOSIS:	**Self-concept, disturbance in.**
SUPPORTING DATA:	**Stoma presents distorted body image. Loss of control of bowel elimination. Dealing with disease process that necessitated ostomy, such as cancer, and may require further surgery and/or treatment.**
DESIRED PATIENT OUTCOMES:	**Within 2–3 days, patient has viewed stoma, begun to talk about and constructively deal with feelings.**

INTERVENTIONS

Begin counseling when the first discussion arises about the possibility and/or necessity of an ostomy.

Encourage the patient and significant others to verbalize feelings regarding the ostomy. Acknowledge feelings of anger and depression as normal.

Provide means for patient to deal with ostomy through self-care.

Discuss possibility of contacting ostomy visitor and make arrangements for visit, if desired.

RATIONALE

It is important to begin counseling at this time to provide the most help available, keeping in mind that the patient will have limited capability for absorbing information depending on emotional state and whether it is a planned or emergency procedure.

These patients can be helped to realize they need not feel guilty for feelings they experience. They need to recognize feelings before they can deal with them effectively.

Independence in self-care helps to improve self-esteem.

Can provide a good support system. Helps to reinforce teachings by sharing experiences.

NURSING DIAGNOSIS:	**Fluid volume deficit, potential.**
SUPPORTING DATA:	**Preoperatively, patient may have been dehydrated from emesis, diarrhea, diaphoresis, and NPO.**
DESIRED PATIENT OUTCOMES:	**Adequate hydration maintained.**

INTERVENTIONS

Monitor I & O carefully, including liquid stool.

Monitor BP, pulse, and weight.

Monitor Hct & electrolytes.

Instruct patient re need for increased fluid intake during warm weather months.

May need to decrease salt intake.

IV fluid and electrolyte replacement.

RATIONALE

Patient can become hypovolemic very rapidly.

Lab tests are a resource for detecting homeostasis or imbalance.

Loss of normal colon function of conserving water and electrolytes can lead to dehydration.

Increases ileal output.

Fluid loss must be replaced to maintain homeostasis.

NURSING DIAGNOSIS:	**Comfort, alteration in, pain.**
SUPPORTING DATA:	**Intensity of pain will be influenced by activity of disease process and psychologic factors. Fear of injuring stoma may cause patient to restrict movements that intensify pain.**

DESIRED PATIENT OUTCOMES: Verbalizes or displays relief of pain and demonstrates ability to assist in care through use of general comfort measures.

INTERVENTIONS

Report and document nature and site of pain.

Reposition and use proper support measures as needed. Assure patient that position change will not injure stoma.

Encourage patient to verbalize.

Actively listen and provide support.

Document relief of pain.

RATIONALE

Aids in identification of cause of pain.

Proper positioning can reduce or eliminate the need for pain medication.

Fear can enhance pain.

Can sometimes reduce or eliminate need for pain medication.

Helps to determine the effectiveness of comfort measures and medication.

MEDICAL MANAGEMENT

Analgesics.

Relieve pain and enhance comfort.

NURSING DIAGNOSIS: Sleep pattern, disturbance in.

SUPPORTING DATA: Patient is disturbed frequently for routine postoperative care. Patient may feel insecure and afraid to sleep because of leakage of pouch and/or injury to stoma. Excessive flatus or ostomy effluent may necessitate emptying during the night.

DESIRED PATIENT OUTCOMES: Able to sleep/rest between disturbances and cooperates with routine postoperative care.

INTERVENTIONS

Explain necessity for disturbances to monitor vital signs and functions.

Provide adequate collecting device. Tell patient that stoma will not be injured when sleeping.

Determine cause of excessive flatus and effluent. If diet related, confer with dietitian regarding restriction of foods. If disease or medication related, confer with physician regarding corrective measures.

RATIONALE

Patient is more apt to be tolerant of disturbances if patient understands the reasons for and importance of the care.

Patient will be able to rest better if feeling secure about stoma and ostomy.

Excessive flatus or effluent can cause enough pressure to cause leakage. Identification of cause enables institution of corrective measures that may interfere with sleep/rest.

Empty pouch before retiring and, if necessary, on a preagreed schedule.

May have excessive flatus and effluent despite interventions. Emptying on a schedule will minimize threat of leakage.

NURSING DIAGNOSIS:	**Skin integrity, impairment of, potential.**
SUPPORTING DATA:	**No sphincter control of stoma, stool and flatus flow from ostomy. Peristomal skin is susceptible to breakdown from bacteria and/or enzymes in the effluent. Consistency of effluent will be affected by the disease process, location of the ostomy, and medications.**
DESIRED PATIENT OUTCOMES:	**Skin integrity maintained.**

INTERVENTIONS

Measure stoma and order correct size and make of an odorproof drainable pouch.

Use effective skin barriers, such as Stomahesive (Squibb), karaya gum, Reliaseal (Davol), and similar products.

Opening on adhesive backing of pouch should only be ⅛ inch larger than the base of the stoma with adequate adhesiveness left to apply pouch.

Provide proper equipment to empty and cleanse ostomy pouch when necessary.

RATIONALE

Proper fitting appliance will be worn by patient so effluent is collected as it flows from the ostomy, thus preventing contact with the skin.

Protects skin from pouch adhesive, enhances adhesiveness of pouch, and facilitates removal of pouch when necessary.

Proper size opening will prevent trauma to the stoma tissue and protect the peristomal skin. Adequate adhesive area is important to maintain a seal.

Frequent pouch changes should be avoided as they will irritate the skin. Emptying and rinsing the pouch with the proper solution not only allows for cleaning of odor-causing stool and flatus but also deodorizes the pouch.

NURSING DIAGNOSIS:	**Skin integrity, impairment of, actual.**
SUPPORTING DATA:	**Some patients develop reactions to products used. Depending on the level of the ostomy, the effluent contains varied amounts of digestive enzymes that cause excoriation if protective barrier or appliance application is inadequate.**
DESIRED PATIENT OUTCOMES:	**Skin integrity is restored and maintained.**

INTERVENTIONS

Evaluate adhesive product and appliance fit.

Experiment with alternate adhesive protective barriers.

Antacids may be applied to the skin.

Refer to ostomy nurse or other available resources.

RATIONALE

To determine the basis of the problem and formulate solutions.

Product allergy must be considered in the absence of appliance/barrier problems.

Helps to neutralize the enzymes and lessen irritation.

In the presence of persistent or recurring problems, which do not respond to simple measures, the ostomy resource may have a wider range of knowledge.

MEDICAL MANAGEMENT

Corticosteroid aerosol spray and nystatin powders.

Assist in healing. Have potential detrimental side effects and should be used sparingly.

NURSING DIAGNOSIS: **Nutrition, alteration in, less than body requirements, potential.**

SUPPORTING DATA: **May be undernourished from disease process or illness. Some foods are gas and odor forming in the digestive process and individual sensitivities to some foods may result in diarrhea/constipation. Bulk and residue may need to be restricted depending upon bowel activity.**

DESIRED PATIENT OUTCOMES: **Patient is able to plan a diet that meets nutritional needs and limits gastrointestinal disturbances.**

INTERVENTIONS

Do thorough nutritional assessment. Confer with physician and dietitian to correct deficiencies.

Identify offensive foods and temporarily restrict from diet. Gradually reintroduce one food at a time.

Document those foods that continue to be a source of flatus (i.e., carbonated drinks, beer, beans, cabbage family, onions, fish, and highly seasoned foods) or odor (i.e., onions, cabbage family, eggs, fish, and beans).

Increase use of yogurt, buttermilk, and cranberry juice.

RATIONALE

Deficiencies need to be corrected before recovery can occur.

Sensitivity to certain foods is not uncommon following intestinal surgery. Patient can experiment with food several times before determining if it is offensive.

Those foods that do cause excessive flatus or odor can be restricted or eliminated. It may be necessary to empty the pouch more frequently if they are ingested.

May help decrease odor.

Discuss the mechanics of swallowed air as a factor in the formation of flatus and some ways the patient can exercise control.

Factors that affect the amount of flatus from swallowed air include drinking through a straw, snoring, anxiety, smoking, ill-fitting dentures, and gulping down food. Too much flatus not only necessitates frequent emptying, but can be a causative factor in leakage from too much pressure within the pouch.

Avoid cellulose products, e.g., peanuts.

Digestion requires colon bacteria.

Exercise caution in the use of prunes, dates, stewed apricots, strawberries, grapes, bananas, cabbage family, beans, and nuts.

These products increase ileal effluent.

Discuss with the physician the patient's nutritional needs and have the dietitian discuss meal planning with the patient and significant others before discharge.

Proper nutrition is important for recovery and maintenance. Improper diet will interfere with the function of the ostomy.

MEDICAL MANAGEMENT

Total parenteral nutrition.

In the presence of severe debilitation and/or patients who do not tolerate oral intake, TPN (hyperalimentation) can be used to supply needed components for healing and prevention of catabolic state. (Refer to Care Plan: Total Parenteral Nutrition.)

NURSING DIAGNOSIS:	**Bowel elimination, alteration in, constipation.**
SUPPORTING DATA:	**Ostomies in the descending or sigmoid colon allow more time for reabsorption of fluid from the effluent.**
DESIRED PATIENT OUTCOMES:	**Patient establishes an elimination pattern suitable to physical needs and lifestyle.**

INTERVENTIONS

Assess the fluid intake to determine adequacy.

Review dietary pattern.

Review physiology of the colon and discuss the use of irrigation in management.

Review patient's normal bowel pattern and lifestyle.

May use a 120 ml asepto syringe and inject 400 ml normal saline every 10 minutes until relief is obtained.

RATIONALE

The amount of fluid is an important factor in determining the consistency of the stool.

Adequate intake of fiber and roughage is important in the control of constipation.

Will enable the patient to understand the use of these procedures.

Will assist in formulation of an effective schedule.

May be used to relieve constipation when immediate relief is desired.

Irrigations may be used on a daily basis, or for special occasions.

There are differing views on the use of daily irrigations. Some believe they are helpful in cleaning the bowel on a regular basis. Others believe that this interferes with normal functioning. Most authorities agree that occasional irrigating is useful for emptying the bowel to avoid leakage.

Inform the patient who has an ileostomy that the discharge will be liquid. If constipation occurs, check with physician before attempting irrigation.

Later, the small intestines will begin to take on water-absorbing function to permit a more semi-solid, pasty discharge. Constipation may indicate an obstruction.

As the effluent becomes more manageable, use a closed end pouch or a patch.

Less expensive than regular colostomy pouches. Patient may feel more comfortable socially.

Allow the patient to be involved in the care of the ostomy on an increasing basis.

Rehabilitation can be facilitated by allowing the patient to gain as much control over the ostomy care as possible.

NURSING DIAGNOSIS: **Sexual dysfunction.**

SUPPORTING DATA: **More common in cancer-related causes because of tumor spread and radical resection that may be required. More common in men due to narrow pelvis and because of active sex organ (penis must become erect prior to penetration), women have a passive sex organ that is receptive despite dysfunction. May have psychologic origin, due to body image and self-esteem issues, or may be physiologic due to nerve damage. Acceptance or rejection by significant others will influence.**

DESIRED PATIENT OUTCOMES: **Patient and significant other are willing to resume sexual relationship and explore alternate methods of sexual satisfaction as indicated.**

INTERVENTIONS

Encourage patient and significant other to verbalize feelings about stoma.

Review with the patient and significant other basic anatomy and physiology of the sex organs.

Reinforce information given by the physician.

RATIONALE

Identify feelings and fears so they may be dealt with constructively.

Understanding normal physiology helps the patient and significant other to understand the mechanisms of nerve damage, and the need for exploring alternate methods of satisfaction.

It may take up to two years to regain potency.

Discuss how proper stimulation by alternate methods may help to achieve sexual fulfillment.

Include information that impotency does not mean the patient is sterile.

Discuss possibility of having ostomy visitor come who can be helpful with this discussion.

Assess the patient's sexual relationships prior to the disease and/or surgery and consider the following:
1. Counseling, individual or couple.
2. Investigation of the possibility of penile prosthesis.
3. Be aware of factors that might be distracting, such as unpleasant odors and pouch leakage.
4. May use an attractive pouch cover.
5. Sense of humor.

If they are willing to try new ideas, can be helpful in adjustment.

The review of anatomy will be helpful to this understanding.

May be able to share resolutions to some of these problems.

Sexual needs are very basic. Patient will be rehabilitated more successfully if a satisfying sexual relationship is developed.

DIAGNOSIS: Appendicitis

PATIENT DATA BASE

NURSING HISTORY

More common among men. Occurs most frequently between the ages of 10–30, although it may occur at any age. Elderly people may experience only dull pain and often delay seeking medical help, possibly until rupture occurs.

History of sudden onset, although may have experienced previous episodes of abdominal pain or distress that were not identified as symptoms of illness.

Early pain is often experienced as discomfort that might be relieved by a laxative or bowel movement (check whether or not patient has taken laxative); patient may complain of constipation.

DIAGNOSTIC STUDIES

Leukocytosis above 10,000/cu mm.

Neutrophil count elevated to 75%.

Urinalysis normal.

PHYSICAL EXAMINATION

Classic symptoms begin with abdominal pain around the epigastrium and umbilicus, which becomes increasingly severe and localizes at McBurney's point (halfway between umbilicus and crest of right ileum). Symptoms may be less clearly defined due to location of appendix retrocecally or next to ureter.

Light palpation of the abdomen may reveal tenderness/rigidity indicative of rupture and peritonitis.

Often patient is observed lying on side or back with knees flexed to decrease pain; extension of right leg will increase RLQ pain. If standing, note posture. It is difficult to stand up straight.

Anorexia, nausea, and vomiting may be present; low grade temperature, tachycardia may be present.

Have patient cough. If inflammation is present, pain will often localize in inflamed area.

Careful evaluation is necessary to rule out other diseases as appendicitis is called "The Great Impersonator" and often mimics other diseases, such as acute pyelitis, ureteral stone, acute salpingitis, and regional ileitis.

NURSING PRIORITIES

1. Prepare for surgery.
2. Promote comfort.
3. Prevent complications.

Surgery is the treatment of choice for appendicitis. It will usually progress to rupture with resultant peritonitis, abscess, and the possibility of death due to sepsis. Refer to Care Plan: Surgical Intervention.

NURSING DIAGNOSIS:	**Comfort, alteration in, pain.**
SUPPORTING DATA:	**Inflammation distends intestinal tissues and causes pain.**

DESIRED PATIENT OUTCOMES: *Pain is minimized; comfort level is maintained.*

INTERVENTIONS	RATIONALE
Keep at rest in Fowler's position.	Gravity localizes inflammatory exudate into lower abdomen or pelvis relieving abdominal tension, which is accentuated by prostrate position.
Ice bag may be placed on abdomen (never heat).	Soothes and relieves pain through desensitization of nerve endings. Heat may cause tissue congestion with subsequent rupture of appendix.
Keep NPO; inquire what time food/fluids by mouth were last taken.	Decreases intestinal peristalsis. An empty stomach decreases the risk of aspiration during and after surgery and also decreases intestinal peristalsis.
Give frequent mouth care with special attention to protection of the lips.	Dehydration results in drying and painful cracking of the lips and mouth.

MEDICAL MANAGEMENT

Analgesics after diagnosis is made.	Use of adequate medication allows for optimum cooperation with necessary procedures; e.g., preoperative teaching and surgical preparation.

NURSING DIAGNOSIS: **Injury, potential for, interruption in gastrointestinal tract integrity.**

SUPPORTING DATA: **When the appendix perforates or ruptures, peritonitis or abscess formation occurs.**

DESIRED PATIENT OUTCOMES: **Absence of symptoms of infection; temperature normal.**

INTERVENTIONS	RATIONALE
Monitor vital signs.	Provides data regarding possible spread of infection and impending septic shock.
Do not give laxatives.	Increase peristalsis and risk of rupture.
Give no narcotics until diagnosis is made.	Relieving the pain might mask the symptoms and make diagnosis more difficult.

MEDICAL MANAGEMENT

Antibiotics.	Reduce number of multiplying organisms to decrease spread and seeding of the abdominal cavity.

Refer to Care Plans: Surgical Intervention; Peritonitis.

```
┌─────────────────────────────────────────────────────────────────┐
│                                                                   │
│  NURSING DIAGNOSIS:        Fluid volume deficit, potential.       │
│                                                                   │
│  SUPPORTING DATA:          The infectious process results in in-  │
│                            creased blood flow to the perito-      │
│                            neum with resultant accumulation       │
│                            of large amounts of fluid in the ab-   │
│                            domen. Vomiting and inability to       │
│                            take fluids by mouth increase fluid    │
│                            loss.                                   │
│                                                                   │
│  DESIRED PATIENT OUTCOMES: Fluid and electrolyte balance main-    │
│                            tained.                                 │
│                                                                   │
└─────────────────────────────────────────────────────────────────┘
```

INTERVENTIONS

Keep NPO.

Monitor CVP (central venous pressure), BP, and pulse.

Monitor intake and output; report output of less than 30ml/hour.

MEDICAL MANAGEMENT

Gastric/intestinal suction.

IV fluids and electrolytes.

RATIONALE

Decrease vomiting and subsequent fluid/electrolyte losses.

CVP decrease may be an early indication of hypovolemia; variations in vital signs help identify fluctuating intravascular volumes.

Adequate output helps assess circulating volume, cardiac output, and GFR.

An NG tube is usually inserted to reduce vomiting, prevent fluid loss, reduce pressure in the bowel, and promote intestinal rest.

The peritoneum reacts to irritation/infection by producing large amounts of fluid that may reduce the circulating blood volume resulting in hypovolemia. Dehydration and relative electrolyte imbalances and hypoproteinemia may occur intravascularly and extracellularly.

295

DIAGNOSIS: Peritonitis

PATIENT DATA BASE

NURSING HISTORY

History of recent trauma with abdominal penetration, e.g., abdominal gunshot or stab wound, and/or blunt trauma where external evidence of internal injury may not be visible.

History of illness of the gastrointestinal tract, such as appendicitis, ulcer, gallbladder disease, cancer, diverticulitis.

In young women, note history of salpingitis.

May have had recent surgery, inadequate surgical prep or intraoperative technical problems; or poor wound healing secondary to malnutrition, diabetes, obesity, or other illness.

Assess medications patient is taking; especially laxatives and steroids.

Assess patient knowledge of disease process and treatment course.

DIAGNOSTIC STUDIES

Leukocytosis.

Urinalysis to rule out urinary tract involvement.

Peritoneal aspiration if necessary to obtain responsible organism; culture and sensitivity to identify offending organism.

X-ray of abdomen to demonstrate abnormal fluid and gas levels found in perforation.

Hematocrit, arterial blood gases, electrolyte levels for baseline measurement, as these may need support with the onset of septicemia.

PHYSICAL EXAMINATION

Abdominal pain may be localized or generalized, and is intensified by movement.

Abdominal rigidity and distention, rebound tenderness, and paralytic ileus may be present.

Bowel sounds are decreased or absent.

Nausea and vomiting may occur; anorexia is present.

Temperature elevation; may be low-grade at first; tachycardia, weakness, diaphoresis, pallor, shallow respirations due to attempt to immobilize muscles to avoid pain.

Assess for signs of shock: decreased blood pressure and so forth.

NURSING PRIORITIES

1. Assist in establishing a diagnosis.
2. Prevent complications and spread of infection.
3. Promote patient comfort.

NURSING DIAGNOSIS: **Injury, potential for, infection, actual/potential.**

SUPPORTING DATA:	An inflammation of the peritoneum usually occurs because of a break in the gastrointestinal tract continuity that allows organisms to enter the peritoneal cavity. May range from minimal irritation to a full blown infectious process.
DESIRED PATIENT OUTCOMES:	Infection is resolved and complications are minimized/prevented. Blood studies, vital signs are within acceptable limits.

INTERVENTIONS

Assess possible sources of contamination, such as appendicitis or ruptured diverticula.

In the presence of an open wound, maintain strict aseptic technique, changing dressings as indicated.

MEDICAL MANAGEMENT

Antimicrobials.

Surgery, if indicated. (For further information, refer to Care Plans: Surgical Intervention; Intestinal Surgery.)

RATIONALE

With early identification and treatment of possible sources of contamination, organisms have less of an opportunity to extend the infection.

Decrease spread and seeding of infection throughout the abdomen.

Reduce number of multiplying microorganisms.

If patient's condition permits, surgery to prevent or correct the perforation is essential; also, an abscess may form that can be surgically drained.

NURSING DIAGNOSIS:	Nutrition, alteration in, less than body requirements.
SUPPORTING DATA:	Nausea/vomiting, infection with resultant interruption of function necessitates putting the GI tract at rest limiting nutritional intake.
DESIRED PATIENT OUTCOMES:	Nutritional intake is reestablished.

INTERVENTIONS

Assess abdomen for size.

Maintain gastric or intestinal suction. Keep patient NPO until normal bowel function returns.

Assess for return of normal bowel function as indicated by soft abdomen, presence of bowel sounds and the passing of flatus.

Resume clear liquid to soft diet as tolerated.

RATIONALE

Note increasing distention.

Usually an NG tube is inserted to reduce pressure in the bowel and decrease peristalsis.

In some cases, conservative measures result in resolution of the inflammation.

Maintain fluid/nutritional intake.

MEDICAL MANAGEMENT

TPN. (Refer to Care Plan: Total Parenteral Nutrition.)

If nausea/vomiting, infectious process persists beyond five days, parenteral nutrition may be instituted to maintain level and promote healing.

NURSING DIAGNOSIS:	**Fluid volume, deficit (actual and potential).**
SUPPORTING DATA:	**The infectious process results in increased blood flow to the peritoneum with resultant accumulation of large amounts of fluid.**
DESIRED PATIENT OUTCOMES:	**Fluid and electrolyte balance maintained.**

INTERVENTIONS

Monitor CVP (central venous pressure), blood pressure, and pulse.

Monitor intake and output; and report output of less than 30ml/hour.

Monitor hematocrit and electrolytes.

MEDICAL MANAGEMENT

Intravenous fluids and electrolytes.

RATIONALE

CVP decrease may be an early indication of hypovolemia; variations in vital signs help identify fluctuating intravascular volumes.

Adequate output helps assess hydration and alerts nurse to decreasing and/or impending hypovolemia with resultant kidney failure.

Provides information re hydration.

The peritoneum reacts to infection by producing large amounts (up to 5L/da) of fluid that may reduce the circulating blood volume resulting in hypovolemia. Dehydration and relative electrolyte imbalances and hypoproteinemia may occur intravascularly and extracellularly.

NURSING DIAGNOSIS:	**Comfort, alteration in, pain.**
SUPPORTING DATA:	**The infectious process, dehydration, abdominal pressure, and surgical incisions result in pain and discomfort.**
DESIRED PATIENT OUTCOMES:	**Pain is minimized; comfort level is maintained.**

INTERVENTIONS

Observe and describe complaints of pain.

Give frequent mouth care with special attention to protection of the lips.

Maintain semi-Fowler's position.

Do not give analgesics until diagnosis is made.

Do not give laxatives or apply heat to abdomen.

Insert rectal tube.

RATIONALE

Pain and tenderness may change in character and site and thorough documentation may assist in accurate diagnosis.

Dehydration results in drying and painful cracking of the lips and mouth. NG tube is irritating to the mucous membranes.

Gravity localizes inflammatory exudate into the lower abdomen or pelvis allowing deeper inspiratory effort with less discomfort.

Medications may mask symptoms and interfere with diagnosis. Use of adequate medication allows for optimum cooperation with necessary procedures, e.g., TCDB, postop activity and enhances healing.

May precipitate rupture and/or further damage.

To help with expelling flatus when peristalsis is reduced or halted by inflammation.

MEDICAL MANAGEMENT

Analgesics, narcotics.

Medicate for pain as necessary after diagnosis has been made.

NURSING DIAGNOSIS:	**Fear, severe illness.**
SUPPORTING DATA:	**Patient may be extremely apprehensive when numerous tests are performed and diagnosis is delayed; patient may be acutely aware of or suspect the seriousness of situation.**
DESIRED PATIENT OUTCOMES:	**Patient copes effectively with situation by cooperating with treatment regimen. Patient demonstrates appropriate range of feelings.**

INTERVENTIONS

Assess anxiety level by monitoring patient's verbal and nonverbal responses; allow free expression of emotions.

Provide information regarding seriousness/treatability of condition.

RATIONALE

The patient's apprehension may be escalated by severe pain, increasingly ill feelings, urgency of diagnostic procedures, and the possibility of surgery.

Patient/significant others may lack information regarding seriousness of disease progression, which may affect their response to treatment regimen.

For further information, refer to Care Plan: Psychosocial Aspects of Care in the Acute Setting.

DIAGNOSIS: Diverticulitis

PATIENT DATA BASE

NURSING HISTORY:

Usually occurs in individuals over age 40.

May complain of long-standing constipation from spastic colon syndrome.

Alterations in bowel habits may include constipation, diarrhea, or a combination of both.

DIAGNOSTIC STUDIES

White blood count and sedimentation rate are elevated with exacerbations of the disease.

Occult blood may be positive in the stool in about 20% of the cases. Pus and mucus may appear in the stools also.

Anemia may be evident if bleeding has persisted.

Sigmoidoscopy should be done to inspect the lumen. In diverticulitis is usually normal.

Colonoscopy may show the diverticulum.

Barium enema is the main diagnostic test: postevacuation films show distortions, pouches, or narrowing of the bowel.

While air contrast studies are useful in visualizing diverticulum, they are usually contraindicated when diverticulitis is suspected as perforation can occur.

PHYSICAL EXAMINATION

Areas of emphasis are similar to those in Care Plan: Ulcerative Colitis.

Tenderness is present over the affected bowel upon palpation and may occur across the entire hypogastric area.

The sigmoid colon may be felt as a firm distinct tender mass.

A tender induration may be felt on digital rectal examination.

Abdominal rigidity, rebound tenderness, and fever are present.

Crampy pain in the lower left quadrant is usually present.

Narrow stools may be noted due to fibrotic strictures of the colon.

Rectal bleeding may be present.

NURSING PRIORITIES

1. Promote and maintain normal bowel elimination.
2. Promote patient comfort.
3. Minimize development of complications, infection, and hemorrhage.

NURSING DIAGNOSIS:	**Bowel elimination, alteration in, constipation.**
SUPPORTING DATA:	**Inflammation with fibrotic stricture, narrowing of the colon.**

DESIRED PATIENT OUTCOMES:	Stool passes easily through the colon. No straining during defecation.

INTERVENTIONS

Observe color, consistency, and frequency.

Promote adequate fluid intake.

Provide soft, high-residue, low-roughage, low-sugar diet.

Bran products may be used to add bulk.

Assist patient in assessing individual response to diet. May need to reduce residue.

Assist patient in establishing regular bowel habits.

MEDICAL MANAGEMENT

Bulk laxatives, such as Metamucil, and stool softeners, such as Colace.

Warm oil retention enemas.

Vitamin B_{12} supplements.

RATIONALE

Change in bowel habits and character of the stool can indicate improvement or development of complications.

Increased fluid content minimizes constipation.

Increased fiber provides bulk that gives the stool more consistency.

Avoids the collection of feces in diverticulum, minimizing inflammation.

Increased bulk may result in increased symptoms for some patients.

Promotes complete evacuation of stool.

Softening the stool minimizes straining for defecation, which increases pressure in the intestine and may lead to further formation of diverticula and/or perforation.

To treat local inflammation and soften the stool.

Small bowel involvement may result in stasis and bacterial overgrowth, causing malabsorption of fat and Vitamin B_{12}.

NURSING DIAGNOSIS:	Comfort, alteration in, pain.
SUPPORTING DATA:	Pain and discomfort because of inflammation and/or infection.
DESIRED PATIENT OUTCOMES:	Comfort level is maintained, complications are minimized.

INTERVENTIONS

Observe for signs and location of pain; determine type and severity.

Palpate abdomen to determine tenderness or rigidity.

MEDICAL MANAGEMENT

Nonopiate analgesics, anticholinergics or antispasmotics.

RATIONALE

Indicative of site of diverticulum and extent of inflammation.

Indication of possible perforation and developing peritonitis.

Opiates may mask signs of perforation. Morphine increases tension in the lumen of the colon and can aggravate the condition. Anticholinergics decrease spasms of the colon.

NURSING DIAGNOSIS:	Injury, potential for, infection/hemorrhage.
SUPPORTING DATA:	Abscess or perforation with resultant peritonitis.
DESIRED PATIENT OUTCOMES:	No infection or hemorrhage occurs.

INTERVENTIONS

Monitor vital signs.

Note onset or change in patient description of character and site of pain.

Note laboratory data:
  WBC, Sedimentation rate, Hb/Hct.

Check stools for occult blood and note signs of shock or fresh rectal bleeding

Keep NPO.

Promote hydration/diet as tolerated.

Bed rest while inflammation is present.

Avoid straining at stool, excess bending, lifting, and coughing.

MEDICAL MANAGEMENT

IVs and electrolytes.

Antibiotics.

Parenteral vitamin K.

Refer to Care Plan: Ulcerative Colitis.

RATIONALE

Increased temperature may be indicative of infection.

Early changes may indicate development of obstruction, fistula and/or sepsis, which may spread through portal vein to liver, causing abscess formation.

Increase/elevation are indicators of infection and volume shifts.

Development of granulation tissue may lead to bleeding and resultant anemia. Massive bleeding caused by erosion into branches of arterial circulation is more common and occurs in 10–20% of patients.

During inflammatory phase to rest the bowel and prevent perforation.

Normal stool consistency minimizes straining for defecation, which can place high pressure on the intestinal wall and may lead to further diverticulum formation or perforation.

Allows body energy to be used in combating infection.

Increases intraabdominal pressure, which can trigger attacks.

To maintain hydration when NPO if perforation and peritonitis is possible.

To combat infection.

May be lost due to interference with synthesis in the bowel. Necessary ingredient for clotting to prevent hemorrhage.

DIAGNOSIS: Herniorrhaphy

PATIENT DATA BASE

NURSING HISTORY

Hernias are classified according to location and severity.

Occurs more frequently in men than women.

Although hernias may occur in many areas of the body, they are most commonly seen in the anterior pelvic area.

Lump or swelling that was reducible, may have been previously noted.

Occurrence or increase in size is directly related to an increase in intraabdominal pressure, such as obesity, pregnancy and lifting heavy objects.

Assess activities of daily living; areas to be considered are occupation, usual activity, lifting or straining activities, and body mechanics.

Assessment of the patient's preoperative respiratory status should be emphasized. If an upper respiratory infection, chronic cough from smoking, or sneezing due to allergies is present, surgery may be delayed, because these might produce sneezing or coughing postoperatively and thus weaken the wound.

May c/o constipation.

DIAGNOSTIC STUDIES

Elevated WBC.

Chest x-ray: r/o respiratory infections.

PHYSICAL EXAMINATION

Symptoms of intestinal obstruction, such as nausea, vomiting, and distention may or may not be present with an incarcerated (irreducible) hernia.

Complaints of localized pain, which may be colicky in nature.

Bowel sounds may be high pitched/hyperactive in mechanical obstruction progressing to decreased/absent.

Fever.

Palpation of the herniated area will reveal the contents of the sac. An attempt to replace or reduce the sac is contraindicated because rupture may occur.

NURSING PRIORITIES

1. Prepare patient for surgery. Refer to Care Plans: Surgical Intervention; Intestinal Surgery.
2. Maximize incision healing.
3. Minimize complications.

NURSING DIAGNOSIS:	Injury, potential for, interruption of incision.

SUPPORTING DATA:	Weakened area has been repaired by surgery (may include synthetic graft) and is susceptible to recurrent injury during the healing period.
DESIRED PATIENT OUTCOMES:	Healing is completed without recurrence of hernia.

INTERVENTIONS

Encourage deep breathing and turning instead of coughing. Splint incision if patient does cough.

Encourage early ambulation.

Use appropriate nursing measures to encourage voiding. Stand at side of bed as tolerated.

Provide adequate hydration and return to full diet as soon as possible. Assist to use toilet to defecate.

Examine scrotum at regular intervals to note any occurrence of swelling.

RATIONALE

Coughing increases intraabdominal pressure, stressing the incision.

Depending on type of anesthesia; encourages return to normal body functioning.

Urinary retention is a frequent complication. Bladder distention can result in stress on the incision.

Promoting normal bowel function minimizes straining during defecation, which could cause incisional stress.

Following inguinal herniorrhaphy, swelling may occur because of inflammation, edema, or hemorrhage.

MEDICAL MANAGEMENT

Use a scrotal support.

Apply ice bags to scrotum as indicated.

Catheterize if unable to void.

Laxatives and/or stool softeners.

Analgesics.

Antibiotics.

Prevents tension of spermatic cord and minimizes edema and swelling.

Relieves swelling and pain.

Prevent bladder distention.

Prevent and/or relieve constipation.

Relieve pain.

Prevent the development of epididymitis.

NURSING DIAGNOSIS:	Knowledge deficit, restriction of activities.
SUPPORTING DATA:	Lack of knowledge about post-surgical physical condition. Concern about sexual functioning because of area of the body involved.
DESIRED PATIENT OUTCOMES:	Verbalizes knowledge of activities that will be allowed upon discharge.

INTERVENTIONS

Instruct patient on necessity of restricting strenuous activities, including a review of occupational dutues.

Discuss importance and methods of avoiding constipation.

Assess body mechanics and provide information needed to improve.

Give information about ability to return to normal sexual activity as soon as healing and pain allow.

RATIONALE

May range from minimal to major restrictions depending upon the extent of the surgery. Occupational duties may need to be curtailed for a period of time.

Prevent stress on the healing incision.

Prevent recurrence.

Sexual functioning is not affected.

CARE PLANS: Intestinal Surgery (for diagnosis and treatment of bleeding, bowel perforation, peritonitis, cancer staging). For specific procedures refer to Care Plans: Fecal Diversion, Obesity, Surgical Interventions (Jejunoileal Bypass)

PATIENT DATA BASE

NURSING HISTORY; DIAGNOSTIC STUDIES; PHYSICAL EXAMINATION see Care Plan: Surgical Intervention.

NURSING PRIORITIES

1. Promote optimal physical condition preoperatively.
2. Alleviate psychosocial concerns.
3. Meet nutritional needs and promote proper GI functioning postoperatively.
4. Prevent complications.

Refer to Care Plan: Surgical Intervention for additional nursing diagnoses as indicated.

NURSING DIAGNOSIS:	**Nutrition, alteration in, less than body requirements, potential.**
SUPPORTING DATA:	**In an elective procedure, it is helpful to diminish the amount of bowel contents preoperatively, while providing adequate calorie intake. May be malnourished due to long-standing illness, such as cancer of the bowel.**
DESIRED PATIENT OUTCOMES:	**Nutritional balance is maintained and/or improved as measured by weight stabilization.**

INTERVENTIONS	RATIONALE
Diet low in residue, high in protein, carbohydrates, and calories.	Given up to five days preoperatively to increase nutrition and decrease peristaltic response that would cause abdominal cramping and/or partial obstruction of the lumen.
Adjust to clear or full liquid diet five days before surgery.	Decreases fecal bulk prior to surgery. May want to avoid milk to decrease gas in the bowel.
Consider likes/dislikes of patient for dietary choices.	Increases patient cooperation with dietary regimen.
Weigh and record as indicated.	Indication of meeting current metabolic needs.
Record intake & output.	Indicator of weight fluctuations related to extracellular fluid status.

MEDICAL MANAGEMENT

Vitamin supplements, with particular attention to vitamin K, parenterally.

Cathartics used may deplete vitamin supply and intestinal problems may block absorption of vitamins. Sterilized bowel cannot synthesize vitamin K resulting in decreased coagulation potential.

IV therapy, including blood replacement and albumin as indicated.

Correct fluid and electrolyte imbalances. Restricted diet and the use of laxatives may result in imbalance, especially sodium and potassium. Inflammation, mucosal erosion, infection, or neoplasm may lead to anemia or malnutrition. Reduces delivery of nutrients at the cellular level. Decreased serum albumin will decrease colloidal osmotic pressure resulting in edema, ascites formation or effusion. Immunodeficiency can predispose patient to wound infection or prolong wound healing.

MEDICAL MANAGEMENT

Consult with the nutritional support team re individual needs, such as TPN.

Many of these patients present with marked weight loss and are generally debilitated, thus being at greater risk for postoperative complications. Refer to Care Plan: Total Parenteral Nutrition.

NURSING DIAGNOSIS:	Injury, potential for, infection.
SUPPORTING DATA:	Opening of the bowel results in contamination of the abdominal cavity.
DESIRED PATIENT OUTCOMES:	No infection is present.

INTERVENTIONS

Postoperatively take vital signs q4h, note temperature elevation.

RATIONALE

Evening temperature spike that returns to normal level in the morning is characteristic of infection. Fever soon after surgery is usually either aspiration pneumonia or urinary tract infection. Temperature elevation 4–7 days postop is often wound abscess or fluid leak formed at anastomosis site.

MEDICAL MANAGEMENT

Bowel prep several days preop:
   Nonabsorbable antibiotic agents, such as Sulfasuxidine and neomycin; observe for possible adverse reaction, such as skin rash, urticaria, hearing loss, difficulty swallowing, or partial loss of taste.

To suppress colon microflora. If renal function is impaired, toxic drug levels may occur, resulting in eighth cranial nerve damage.

Dietary restrictions (as mentioned) and use of laxatives or saline cathartics and enemas.

To reduce colonic contents.

NG tube.

Decompress GI tract to control distention and vomiting.

Culture suspected infection site; if wound, culture both center and outer edges of wound and obtain anaerobic cultures as well.

Frequent multiple organisms involved and anaerobic bacteria, such as Bacteroides fragilis (more common after bowel surgery), can only be detected by anaerobic cultures. Identifying all organisms involved allows more specific choice of effective antibiotic therapy.

Aseptic wound care and frequent dressing changes with use of Montgomery straps to secure dressings.

To protect patient from secondary infections from staff members. Wet dressings act as retrograde wick, drawing in external contaminants. Frequent removal of tape may cause skin abrasion, which can also become a site of infection.

MEDICAL MANAGEMENT

Antibiotic therapy.

Combat infection.

Wound irrigations.

Done to combat infection when present.

NURSING DIAGNOSIS:	**Nutrition, alteration in, actual.**
SUPPORTING DATA:	**Alimental route for nutrition is restricted due to cessation of peristalsis from intraoperative handling of intestines and/or potassium loss with resultant decreased smooth muscle contractility.**
DESIRED PATIENT OUTCOMES:	**As soon as intestinal functioning returns, alimental feeding is resumed.**

INTERVENTIONS

RATIONALE

Maintain patency of NG tube.

Vomiting increases intraabdominal pressure, patient discomfort, and is stressful to the incision. Resumption of fluid and nutritional intake depends on return of bowel activity.

Observe/record quantity, amount, and character of NG drainage. Test pH as indicated. Monitor lab values.

Excessive fluid output may cause electrolyte imbalance and metabolic alkalosis with further loss of potassium by the kidneys attempting to compensate. Hyperacidity, as indicated by pH of less than 5, may identify patients at risk, such as those with previous history of ulcers and/or those with potential for stress ulcer formation.

Do guaiac test on stool.

Microscopic bleeding may not be evident.

Encourage and assist with frequent changes of position.

Prevents formation of magenstrasse in the stomach, which can channel gastric fluid and air past tip of NG tube into duodenum.

Give frequent oral care, use water soluble lubricant to the nares. Tape tube so there is no pressure on the nares.

Palpate abdomen and auscultate for bowel sounds. Record passage of flatus.

MEDICAL MANAGEMENT

Antiemetics, antacids and/or medications, e.g., cimetidine.

IV fluids, electrolyte and nutritional support.

Liquids, progressing to clear liquid, full diet as tolerated after NG tube is removed.

Irritation of mucous membranes causes patient to swallow more frequently and results in increased ingestion of air.

To determine return of peristalsis (usually within 2–4 days).

Prevent vomiting, neutralize or decrease acid formation to prevent mucosal erosion and possible ulceration.

Replacement, see Nursing Diagnosis: Nutrition, alteration in, less than body requirements, potential.

Resumption of fluids and diet is essential to return of normal intestinal functioning and promotes adequate nutritional intake.

NURSING DIAGNOSIS: **Skin integrity, impairment of, actual, surgical incision.**

SUPPORTING DATA: **Factors that may interfere with wound healing include radiation, medication, altered nutritional state, e.g., obesity and malnutrition, altered circulation, immunologic deficit, and may result in infection and/or dehiscence.**

DESIRED PATIENT OUTCOMES: **Wound heals without complications.**

INTERVENTIONS

Monitor vital signs frequently noting increased pulse, tachypnea, and apprehension. Check dressings and wound frequently during first 24 hours for signs of bright blood or excessive incisional swelling.

Splint incision during coughing and breathing exercises. Use scultetus binder for obese and elderly patients.

Review lab values for evidence of anemia and decreased serum albumin. Note leukocyte count.

RATIONALE

Early signs of hemorrhage and/or hematoma formation, which may contribute to delayed wound healing and may progress to hypovolemic shock.

Minimizes stress/tension on healing wound edges. Fatty tissue is difficult to approximate and suture line is more easily disrupted. The aging process and atherosclerosis contribute to diminished circulation to the wound.

Anemia results in decreased oxygen. Altered colloidal osmotic pressures result in edema formation, which may interfere with healing. Steroid therapy or anticancer drugs reduce leukocyte count and suppress capillary formation and fibrogenesis.

Encourage adequate nutrition with emphasis on protein intake and vitamin C.

Prime contributors to tissue maintenance and repair. Malnutrition is a factor in lowered resistance to infection.

Note signs of infection. (Refer to Nursing Diagnosis: Injury, potential for, infection.)

Be aware of further risk factors, i.e., malignancies, such as lymphosarcoma and multiple myeloma; radiation therapy of operative site.

Reduces immunocompetence thus interfering with wound healing and resistance to infection. Promotes vasculitis and fibrosis in connective tissue interfering with delivery of oxygen and nutrients for healing.

If dehiscence does occur:
Maintain calm attitude. Notify physician. Keep patient on complete bed rest. Position with knees bent. Take baseline vital signs. Stabilize wound edges with butterfly strips.

Stressful situation in which it is extremely important to prevent panic in both the patient and the nurse. Reduces intraabdominal tension. May prevent evisceration from occurring.

If evisceration occurs:
Cover exposed intestines with sterile moist dressings. Prepare for surgical repair of wound.

To prevent drying of mucosal tissue.

NURSING DIAGNOSIS:	Urinary elimination, alteration in pattern.
SUPPORTING DATA:	Retention may occur due to anesthesia effects, pain, fear, tension, and anxiety.
DESIRED PATIENT OUTCOMES:	Urinary output is maintained at no less than obligatory levels.

INTERVENTIONS

Observe and record I & O for 24–48h postoperative period.

Promote privacy and use nursing measures to promote relaxation of the sphincter muscle. Place in semi-Fowler's or standing position.

When voiding has not occurred within 8–10 hours, depending on intake, palpate bladder for distention.

MEDICAL MANAGEMENT

Catheterize.

RATIONALE

Adequate intake is essential for urine formation.

Psychologic factors and pain may increase muscle tension. Increases intraabdominal pressure, which may aid in micturition.

Bladder distention may not be apparent to patient if it has occurred slowly or been masked by pain medication.

Single/multiple straight catheterization as well as Foley insertion is used.

DIAGNOSIS: Cholecystitis With Cholelithiasis

PATIENT DATA BASE

NURSING HISTORY

In acute attack, patient may be very ill, usually with an abrupt onset. May have history of intolerance of fatty foods and recurrent indigestion.

More common in women than in men. While "fair, fat, and forty" is often accurate, there is an increasing incidence among younger women following pregnancy and delivery.

More common in obese patients.

Change in stools; clay-colored.

DIAGNOSTIC STUDIES

In chronic cholecystitis:
 CBC, urinalysis, and liver and pancreatic function tests may be normal. Bilirubin may be increased.

In acute cholecystitis:
 Moderate leukocytosis is seen on the CBC.

 Serum bilirubin is elevated.

 Serum electrolytes may be altered.

 Reduced prothrombin levels and failure of the normal clotting process occurs when an obstruction to the flow of bile into the intestine decreases absorption of vitamin K.

Ultrasound reveals calculi, with gallbladder and/or bile duct distention.

Liver scan with radioactive dye may show obstruction of the biliary tree.

Chest x-ray to rule out pneumonitis.

Multi-position abdominal films may reveal radiopaque (calcified) gallstones, calcification of the wall or enlargement of the gallbladder.

In chronic disease, oral cholecystograms usually reveal stones in the biliary system. (Oral cholecystograms are contraindicated in acute cholecystitis because the patient is too ill to take the dye by mouth, also the gallbladder will not visualize because the absorption and excretion of the contrast agent during an attack is unpredictable.)

PHYSICAL EXAMINATION

Elevated temperature, tachycardia, and increased respiratory rate. Splinted respiration marked by short, shallow breathing may be noted.

Anorexia, nausea, and vomiting may be present, especially in acute episodes. Flatulence may be a complaint in both acute and chronic. Fatty and "gas-former" foods (brussel sprouts, cabbage, cauliflower) intolerance.

Abdominal distention with a palpable mass in the upper right quadrant is occasionally found.

Severe pain, with rebound tenderness and muscle guarding or rigidity noted upon palpation of the RUQ.

Jaundice may be noted, with dry, itching skin.

NURSING PRIORITIES

1. Relieve pain and promote rest.
2. Maintain fluid and electrolyte balance.

3. Provide information to enable patient to avoid further problems.
4. Prevent complications.

NURSING DIAGNOSIS:	Comfort, alterations in, pain.
SUPPORTING DATA:	Obstruction, inflammatory process, and resultant distention of tissues contribute to pain and discomfort. Biliary colic is an intense incapacitating pain.
DESIRED PATIENT OUTCOMES:	Pain is minimized and/or controlled.

INTERVENTIONS

Observe and document location, severity, and character of pain.

Bed rest, allowing patient to assume position of comfort.

Be available to patient by listening to complaints and by frequent contact.

Note response to medication and report to physician if pain is not relieved.

MEDICAL MANAGEMENT

Demerol, anticholinergics and sedatives.

Avoid the use of morphine.

RATIONALE

Will assist in pain management.

Will naturally assume least painful position. Reduces intraabdominal pressures.

Helpful in alleviating anxiety.

Severe pain may not be relieved by routine measures and may need increased medication.

Assist in pain management.

Thought to increase spasms of the biliary sphincter.

NURSING DIAGNOSIS:	Fluid volume, deficit, potential.
SUPPORTING DATA:	Vomiting, distention, and gastric hypermotility can lead to excessive losses of fluid and electrolytes.
DESIRED PATIENT OUTCOMES:	Vomiting is controlled and fluid and electrolyte balance is maintained.

INTERVENTIONS

Maintain accurate I & O.

Observe for dry skin and mouth, muscle cramps, and so forth. Review lab work.

RATIONALE

Provides information about balance and whether replacement is needed.

Signs of dehydration and electrolyte imbalances.

Keep NPO as ordered. If not NPO, limit oral intake.

Do frequent oral hygiene.

Maintain patency of NG tube when present.

Decrease gastrointestinal motility and stimulation of the gallbladder.

Decrease dryness of mouth.

Vomiting may occur if tube becomes plugged.

MEDICAL MANAGEMENT

NG tube, connect to suction.

Antiemetics.

IV fluids and electrolytes.

Rest gastrointestinal tract.

Reduce vomiting.

Replacement therapy.

NURSING DIAGNOSIS: **Knowledge deficit, diagnostic tests and possibility of surgery.**

SUPPORTING DATA: **Lack of knowledge about process of and necessity for testing can be anxiety-producing. Impending surgery can create a stressful situation.**

DESIRED PATIENT OUTCOMES: **Information will be given appropriate to the individual situation and the patient will verbalize understanding and demonstrate lessened anxiety.**

INTERVENTIONS

Give careful explanations of reasons for, preparation needed, and test procedures.

Discuss hospitalization and prospective surgery with patient.

Be available and provide time for listening to the patient.

Provide proper physical preparation of the patient.

RATIONALE

Information can decrease anxiety thereby reducing sympathetic stimulation.

Effective communication and support at this time can diminish anxiety and promote healing.

Enables nurse to more accurately assess the needs of the individual.

Prevent problems of testing that may interfere with the results.

NURSING DIAGNOSIS: **Nutrition, alteration in, less than body requirements.**

SUPPORTING DATA: **In acute attack, continued vomiting and inability to retain food and fluids may result in loss of weight and nutritional deficiencies.**

| **DESIRED PATIENT OUTCOMES:** | **Nausea and vomiting are relieved. Weight is regained and/or maintained at an optimal level.** |

INTERVENTIONS

Begin low-fat liquid diet after NG tube is removed.

Increase diet as tolerated, usually low-fat, high-carbohydrate and protein.

Consult with patient about likes and dislikes, foods that cause distress, and preferred meal schedule.

Keep comments about appetite to a minimum.

Provide a pleasant atmosphere at mealtime.

Have patient do oral hygiene before meals.

Offer effervescent drinks with meals.

Ambulate and increase activity as tolerated.

RATIONALE

Limiting fat content helpful in preventing recurrence.

Increased intake of foods, which do not aggravate condition, assist in recuperation and regaining weight.

Involving patient in planning enables patient to have a sense of control and encourages patient to eat.

Focusing on problem creates a negative atmosphere.

Useful in promoting appetite.

Clean mouth helpful in enhancing appetite.

May lessen nausea and relieve gas.

Helpful to overall recovery and sense of well-being contributing to increasing appetite. Decrease possibility of secondary problems related to decreased mobility.

CARE PLAN: CHOLECYSTECTOMY

PATIENT DATA BASE

Refer to Care Plan: Cholecystitis With Cholelithiasis

The treatment of choice for cholecystitis is surgery. In acute episodes it may be an emergency procedure. Surgery is the only way to remove stones that may be present. (Chenodeoxycholic acid, a natural bile acid, is currently being used experimentally to dissolve cholesterol stones.)

NURSING DIAGNOSIS:	**Injury, potential for, infection and hemorrhage.**
SUPPORTING DATA:	**The patient with severe hepatic or biliary disease is a ready candidate for infection because protein metabolism and use of vitamins are decreased. Resistance is low so that infections are easily acquired. Peritonitis may occur as a result of acute cholecystitis, perforation, or rupture of the gallbladder, as well as postoperatively, if bile escapes into the peritoneal cavity because of seepage at the sutures or slippage of the T-tube. When the bile flow is obstructed, blood prothrombin is lowered and the coagulation time is prolonged resulting in increased bleeding tendencies.**
DESIRED PATIENT OUTCOMES:	**Infection and/or hemorrhage does not occur or is effectively treated.**

INTERVENTIONS

Protect from exposure to infection of any kind.

If seriously ill, provide a private room and screen visitors for colds or other infections. (Includes medical and nursing staff.)

Monitor vital signs.

Observe for signs of bleeding.

Plan for doing several blood samples for testing with one venipuncture.

RATIONALE

Prevention.

Additional protection.

Early detection of developing infection/ hemorrhage.

When bile flow is obstructed, the blood prothrombin will be lowered, and coagulation time prolonged.

These measures reduce number of punctures and possible hematoma formation.

Use sharp, small gauge needles for injections and apply firm pressure for longer than usual after venipuncture.	Reduces bleeding/trauma.
Have the patient use cotton swabs and mouthwash instead of a toothbrush.	Avoid trauma and bleeding of the gums.

MEDICAL MANAGEMENT

Antibiotics.	Prevent/treat infection.
Vitamin K.	Replacement.
Transfusions of whole blood.	Maintain clotting mechanisms and in circulating volume.

NURSING DIAGNOSIS:	**Skin integrity, impairment of, potential.**
SUPPORTING DATA:	**In choledocholithiasis with biliary obstruction, bile does not drain normally into the duodenum and jaundice occurs. Postoperatively it is important to maintain bile flow either through the drainage tubes or into the intestines so it is not forced into the liver and/or bloodstream. Drainage is potentially irritating to the skin around the incision.**
DESIRED PATIENT OUTCOMES:	**Pruritus and skin integrity are effectively managed and controlled. Bile drainage is managed until normal flow of bile is reestablished and jaundice does not occur.**

INTERVENTIONS

RATIONALE

Check the T-tube upon return from the recovery room. If clamped, unclamp and make sure it is free flowing.	Prevent backup of the bile in the operative area.
Observe the color and character of the drainage.	Initially, may contain blood and blood-stained fluid, changing to greenish brown after the first several hours.
Place patient in low Fowler's position, later semi-Fowler's.	Facilitate drainage.
Anchor tube, allowing sufficient tubing to permit free turning, and avoid kinks and twists.	Avoid dislodging and/or occlusion of the lumen of the tube.

Record amount of drainage on I & O.	200–500 ml of drainage is normal initially, decreasing as more bile enters the intestine. Continuing large amounts may be an indication of obstruction. Occasionally, a biliary fistula may develop.
Observe for signs of dislodgment of T-tube.	Include hiccups (diaphragmatic irritation), abdominal distention, and signs of peritonitis.
Change dressings as often as necessary. Clean the skin with soap and water. Use sterile Vaseline gauze, zinc oxide, or karaya powder around the incision.	To keep the skin around the incision clean and free from excoriation because of bile drainage.
Use Montgomery straps.	Facilitates frequent dressing changes and minimizes skin trauma.
A disposable colostomy bag may be used over a stab wound drain.	Collect heavy drainage for more accurate output and to protect skin.
Observe skin, sclerae, urine. Refer to Care Plan: Cirrhosis of the Liver.	Jaundice indicates obstruction of bile flow.
Note color and consistency of stools.	Clay-colored stools result when bile is not present in the intestines.

MEDICAL MANAGEMENT

Clamp T-tube.	Tests the patency of the common bile duct.
Zanchol or dicholin sodium.	Oral replacement of bile salts to facilitate fat absorption.
Feed the patients their own bile, either orally or through NG tube. The bile is chilled, strained, and given with salt or diluted in chilled fruit juice. Do not tell the patient what the liquid is.	On rare occasion is used when excessive or chronic bile losses occur. Prevents the patient from losing the benefit of the constituents necessary for digestion.

NURSING DIAGNOSIS:	**Breathing patterns, ineffective.**
SUPPORTING DATA:	**The incision is fairly high on the abdomen and full chest expansion is painful. Often the patient holds the breath and/or takes shallow breaths and avoids coughing in order to splint the incision. These factors, along with age and obesity, predispose the patient to respiratory complications, usually within the first 48 hours.**
DESIRED PATIENT OUTCOMES:	**Effective breathing patterns are established and no complications occur.**

INTERVENTIONS

Observe for shallow breathing, splinting with respirations, holding breath, decreased breath sounds, and/or respiratory distress.

Auscultate lungs q2h.

Turn, cough, and deep breath every 1–2 hours, splinting incision. Instruct in effective breathing techniques.

Maintain low Fowler's position.

Use abdominal binder when ambulating.

MEDICAL MANAGEMENT

Incentive spirometer.

Analgesics.

RATIONALE

May result in atelectasis/pneumonia.

Monitor development of congestion.

Mobilize secretions and prevent atelectasis.

Facilitates lung expansion.

Splinting incision may allow patient better incisional support and promote ambulation.

Maximize expansion of lungs.

Facilitate more effective coughing, deep breathing and activity.

NURSING DIAGNOSIS:	**Bowel elimination, alteration in, diarrhea.**
SUPPORTING DATA:	**Bile release is continuous when the gallbladder has been removed and this can stimulate motility.**
DESIRED PATIENT OUTCOMES:	**Return of normal bowel habit within a year.**

INTERVENTIONS

Tell patient that loose stools, up to 3/day, may occur for several months.

Dietary changes are not usually necessary, although the patient may be advised to note and avoid foods that seem to aggravate the diarrhea.

Refer to Care Plan: Surgical Intervention for additional

RATIONALE

Body will adjust to the continuous output of bile.

Fats in small amounts usually are tolerated. After a period of adjustment, patients usually do not have problems with most foods.

information and nursing diagnoses.

DIAGNOSIS: Hepatitis

PATIENT DATA BASE

NURSING HISTORY

Loss of appetite with subsequent loss of weight, abdominal cramping and diarrhea or constipation, clay-colored stools, dark urine, anorexia, nausea and vomiting, itching, myalgias, fatigue, headache, and general malaise are common symptoms.

History of known or possible exposure to virus, bacteria or toxins (through contaminated food, water, needles, surgical equipment or blood transfusions), or carriers (symptomatic or asymptomatic).

History of recent surgical procedure with use of halothane anesthesia.

Length of incubation period may help differentiate between types of hepatitis. Type A may be 3–7 weeks with a mean of 4; type B, 6 weeks to 6 months with mean of between 2½–3 months. Type A is more prevalent in fall and winter.

Socioeconomic status/lifestyle and health habits may give clue to definitive cause of illness.

Age susceptibility is highest between 6 and 25, but may occur at any age.

May have recently developed an aversion to cigarette smoking.

DIAGNOSTIC STUDIES

Elevated SGOT/PT. SGPT levels may rise one to two weeks before jaundice is apparent.

Anemia due to decreased life of RBC with liver enzyme alterations, or may be result of hemorrhage; leukopenia, thrombocytopenia may be due to splenomegaly.

Clay-colored stools, steatorrhea due to decreased hepatic function.

Abnormal liver function tests (4–10 times normal values).

Hypoalbuminemia.

Transient hyper/hypoglycemia due to altered liver function.

HBsAG may be positive (type B) or negative (type A); may be diagnostic before clinical symptoms occur.

Prothrombin time may be prolonged due to liver dysfunction.

Liver biopsy defines diagnosis and extent of necrosis.

Urinalysis to rule out renal disease and show elevated bilirubin levels; proteinemia/hematuria may be present.

Serum bilirubin above 2.5 mg/100ml. If above 200 mg/100ml, poor prognosis is probable due to increased cellular necrosis.

PHYSICAL EXAMINATION

Some patients exhibit minimal or no symptoms at all.

May c/o headache, anorexia, N & V, fatigue and weakness, myalgias, fever.

Assess overall physical status. Note presence of other diseases, such as diabetes, congestive heart failure, malignancy or renal disease. Check for injection sites.

Right upper quadrant tenderness.

Preicteric phase; lasts approximately one week.

Icteric phase: reaches intensity in 2 weeks and may last from 1–2 weeks. (Initially, may be observed in sclera.)

Pruitus. Dark urine due to excretion of bilirubin. (Urine may produce foamy head when shaken).

Palpable enlarged liver.

Spider angiomas, palmer erythema, gynecomastia in men.

Splenomegaly, posterior cervical nodes enlargement may occur.

Irritability and drowsiness, asterixis may indicate impending hepatic coma.

NURSING PRIORITIES

1. Reduce demands on liver while promoting physical well-being.
2. Minimize disturbance in self-concept due to communicability of disease.
3. Relieve symptoms and increase patient comfort.
4. Promote patient understanding of disease process and rationale of treatment.
5. Be aware of potential complications, such as hemorrhage, hepatic coma, and permanent liver damage (see Care Plan: Cirrhosis of the Liver).

NURSING DIAGNOSIS:	**Mobility, impaired physical.**
SUPPORTING DATA:	**Intolerance to activity with decreased strength and endurance because of decreased energy metabolism by the liver. Imposed activity restrictions, pain, and depression also lessen mobility.**
DESIRED PATIENT OUTCOMES:	**Normal activities are resumed.**

INTERVENTIONS

Promote bed rest with bathroom privileges only. Help patient learn relaxation techniques.

Change position frequently.

Provide good skin care and daily hygiene.

Provide a quiet environment; visitors may need to be limited.

Do necessary tasks quickly and at one time.

Increase activity as tolerated.

Monitor serum enzyme levels to help determine levels of activity.

Observe for recurrence of anorexia and liver tenderness and/or enlargement.

RATIONALE

Available energy is used for healing. Activity and an upright position are believed to decrease hepatic blood flow, which prevents optimal circulation to the liver cells.

Promotes optimal respiratory function and minimizes pressure areas.

Maintains skin integrity.

Promotes rest and relaxation.

Allows extended periods of uninterrupted rest.

Prolonged bed rest can be debilitating. This can be offset by limited activity with rest periods after eating.

Premature increase in activity can lead to relapse.

Also indicates lack of resolution and/or exacerbation of the disease.

MEDICAL MANAGEMENT

Sedatives and tranquilizers.

To assist in managing required rest. Avoid barbiturates and tranquilizers, such as Compazine and Thorazine, which are known to have hepatotoxic effects.

NURSING DIAGNOSIS:	**Nutrition, alteration in, less than body requirements.**
SUPPORTING DATA:	**Anorexia, nausea, and vomiting may be due to visceral reflexes that may reduce peristalsis. Bile stasis, altered absorption, and metabolism of ingested foods may also produce these symptoms. Calorie needs for tissue healing are increased.**
DESIRED PATIENT OUTCOMES:	**Adequate calorie intake and satisfactory nutritional status is maintained. Weight is stable at or progressing toward a satisfactory goal.**

INTERVENTIONS

Diet is ordered according to patient's need.

May need to give several small feedings vs three large meals.

Offer largest meal at breakfast.

Give fruit juices, carbonated beverages, and hard candy, throughout the day.

Counsel patient on avoidance of alcoholic beverages.

MEDICAL MANAGEMENT

Fat and protein intake, as tolerated.

Protein restriction.

Antiemetics ½ hour before meals.

Antacids.

Vitamin K supplements.

RATIONALE

Allow recovery of injured liver cells.

Large amounts are difficult to manage when patient is anorexic.

Anorexia may worsen during the day.

Easily digested and may be tolerated when other foods are not. Also supplies extra calories.

Increases hepatic irritation and may interfere with recovery.

Fat metabolism varies according to bile production and excretion. If tolerated, a normal or increased protein intake will help with tissue repair.

May be indicated in severe disease and/or impending coma.

Will reduce nausea and may increase food tolerance. (Be sure the drug is not hepatotoxic.)

Counteract gastric acidity.

Coagulation problems may occur if prothrombin time is depressed.

Vitamin B complex, vitamin C, and other dietary supplements.

Correct deficiencies and aid in the healing process.

IV and TPN.

When nausea and vomiting are severe, fluid and electrolyte replacement is needed. TPN may be necessary to meet calorie requirements if symptoms are prolonged. Refer to Care Plan: Total Parenteral Nutrition.

Steroid therapy.

Antiinflammatory effect may be useful in severe cases to reduce nausea/vomiting and enable patient to retain food and fluids. May decrease serum aminotransferases and bilirubin levels; but has no effect on liver necrosis or regeneration.

NURSING DIAGNOSIS:	**Fluid volume deficit, potential.**
SUPPORTING DATA:	**Severe continuing vomiting and diarrhea may occur. May have third-space shift if ascites present.**
DESIRED PATIENT OUTCOMES:	**Adequate hydration is maintained.**

INTERVENTIONS

RATIONALE

Monitor intake and output. Check for ascites or edema formation. Note enteric losses, such as vomiting and diarrhea.

Some patients with severe viral hepatitis may excrete more or less than normal amounts of fluid.

Do daily weights.

Assist in monitoring fluid retention.

Monitor lab values, Hb, Hct, Na$^+$, albumin.

Identifies Na$^+$ retention, which may lead to edema formation.

MEDICAL MANAGEMENT

IV therapy, usually glucose, electrolytes, and protein hydrolysates.

Provide fluid and electrolyte replacement and nutritional support.

NURSING DIAGNOSIS:	**Self-concept, disturbance in.**
SUPPORTING DATA:	**Necessity for isolation measures to prevent cross-contamination. Severity of the disease varies according to individual. Annoying symptoms, confinement, isolation, and length of illness may lead to feelings of depression.**
DESIRED PATIENT OUTCOMES:	**Depression is relieved and patient cooperates with necessary restrictions with minimal loss of self-esteem.**

INTERVENTIONS	RATIONALE
Establish isolation techniques for enteric and respiratory infections according to hospital procedure manual, include effective handwashing.	Prevents transmission of disease to others. Thorough handwashing is effective in preventing virus transmission. Type A (infectious) is transmitted by oral-fecal route, contaminated water, milk, and food, especially inadequately cooked shellfish. Type B (serum) is transmitted by contaminated blood, blood products, needle punctures, open wounds, ingestion, saliva, urine, stool, and semen. Incidence of both has increased among hospital personnel and high-risk patients. Toxic and alcoholic hepatitis are not communicable.
Explain isolation procedures to patient/SOs.	Understanding of reasons for safeguarding themselves and others can lessen feelings of isolation and stigmatization.
Give information regarding availability of gamma globulin through health department or family physician.	May be effective in preventing type A hepatitis in those who have been exposed.
Contract with patient regarding time for listening.	Opportunity to express feelings will allow patient to feel more in control of the situation. Verbalization decreases anxiety and depression and facilitates positive coping behaviors. Patient may need to express feelings about being ill, length and cost of illness, possibility of infecting others, and in severe illness, the possibility of death. May have concerns regarding the stigma of the disease. Establishing time will enhance trusting relationship.
Assess effect of illness on economic factors. Make appropriate referrals for help, as needed.	Financial problems may exist because of loss of patient's role functioning in the family. Use of discharge planners, social services, and/or other community agencies can facilitate problem-solving.
Offer diversional activities based on energy levels.	Enables patient to use time and energy in constructive ways that enhance self-esteem and minimize anxiety and depression.

Refer to Care Plan: Psychosocial Aspects of Care in the Acute Setting.

NURSING DIAGNOSIS:	**Skin integrity, impairment of, actual.**
SUPPORTING DATA:	**Bile salt accumulation in skin results in pruritus.**
DESIRED PATIENT OUTCOMES:	**Itching is relieved and skin integrity is maintained.**

INTERVENTIONS

Use cool showers and baking soda or starch baths.

Calamine lotion may be used.

Assist patient with reducing tendency to scratch by providing diversional activities, keeping fingernails cut short, and providing gloves to wear at night.

Soothing massage at bedtime.

Avoid comments re patient's appearance.

MEDICAL MANAGEMENT

Antihistamines.

Questran. (Note side effects of nausea and constipation.)

RATIONALE

Provides relief from itching.

Minimize trauma to skin.

May be helpful in getting to sleep.

Minimize psychologic stress.

Relieve itching.

May be used to bind bile acids in the intestine and prevent their absorption.

NURSING DIAGNOSIS:	**Bowel elimination, alteration in, diarrhea/constipation.**
SUPPORTING DATA:	**Alterations in digestive processes.**
DESIRED PATIENT OUTCOMES:	**Normal bowel function.**

INTERVENTIONS

Provide adequate dietary and fluid intake.

Observe color, consistency, frequency, and amount of stools.

RATIONALE

Promotes normal stool consistency.

With resolution of the hepatitis, normal bowel function and color will return.

NURSING DIAGNOSIS:	**Knowledge deficit, disease process and necessary lifestyle changes.**
SUPPORTING DATA:	**Lack of exposure to information and unfamiliarity with community resources.**
DESIRED PATIENT OUTCOMES:	**Knowledgeable about the disease and is using appropriate self-care measures and community resources. No relapse or recurrence.**

INTERVENTIONS

Assess level of understanding of disease process.

Provide specific information re prevention/transmission of disease:

Contacts may receive gamma globulin; personal items should not be shared; strict handwashing and sanitizing of clothes, dishes, and toilet facilities is necessary; while liver enzymes are elevated, avoid mucous membrane contact, such as kissing and sexual contact.

Plan resumption of activity as tolerated with adequate periods of rest.

Monitor lab values.

Help patient identify diversional activities.

Discuss the side-effects of and dangers of taking OTC and prescribed medications.

Be aware of restrictions for blood donating.

Emphasize importance of follow-up physical examination and lab evaluation.

RATIONALE

Additional information can be given as necessary.

Teaching needs will vary with the causative agent.

Physical activity needs to be limited until the liver returns to normal size. Patients begin to feel better and need to understand the importance of adequate rest in preventing relapse or recurrence. (Relapse occurs in 5–25% of adults).

Serum bilirubin levels decrease as liver function returns. It is not necessary to wait until they return to normal to resume activity or for discharge as this may take as long as two months.

Enjoyable activities will help the patient avoid focusing on prolonged convalescence.

Some drugs are toxic to the liver; others are metabolized by the liver and should be avoided in severe liver diseases as they may cause cumulative toxic effects.

Prevent spread of disease.

Disease process may take several months to resolve.

DIAGNOSIS: Cirrhosis of the Liver

PATIENT DATA BASE

NURSING HISTORY

Patient complains of gradual onset of anorexia, weight loss/gain, abdominal enlargement, edema, jaundice, alteration in thinking process, bruises or accentuated blood vessels, change in bowel habits (diarrhea/constipation), abnormal bleeding, darkened urine, fatigue. Pruritus is often an early sign.

Patient history of viral hepatitis, drug use or toxic reactions, alcoholism, previous liver disease or chronic biliary obstruction, history of long-term congestive heart failure, pericarditis, or rheumatic heart disease may predispose patient to cirrhosis. Question patient about any history of infectious disease or exposure to recent infections, or chemicals.

Complete dietary history is essential as poor nutrition influences development of cirrhosis.

Current medications: patient may have taken hepatotoxic drug.

Bleeding tendencies may be aggravated by current medication.

Drinking habits: how long, how much, how often, and type of alcohol consumed.

More men than women are affected; the disease has a predominance in the middle years.

DIAGNOSTIC STUDIES

Bilirubin may be present in urine causing dark yellow/amber/mahogany urine with a yellow foam when shaken.

Serum bilirubin elevated causing jaundice; level of serum bilirubin and type can be helpful in diagnosis.

SGOT, SGPT, and LDH are usually elevated and useful in measuring the extent of liver damage. The SPGT is usually much lower than the SGOT if alcoholic hepatitis is the cause of the cirrhosis.

Abnormal flocculation tests.

Serum albumin is usually decreased in patients with chronic liver disease. The decrease in albumin causes loss of water intravascularly resulting in tissue edema.

Prothrombin time is prolonged; if the prothrombin time is not easily reversible with IM vitamin K, it usually indicates liver cell damage.

Anemia, leukopenia, or thrombocytopenia may be present.

Hypoglycemia may be seen in severe liver disease due to impaired gluconeogenesis.

Bromsulphalein (BSP) excretion test is used to indicate the extent of the damage to the liver.

Serum ammonia may become very elevated and is useful as a sign of impending hepatic coma.

Pancytopenia may be present.

Esophagoscopy may demonstrate presence of esophageal varices.

Liver scans can determine the size and shape of the liver and the location of abnormal tissue.

A liver biopsy is used to aid in differential diagnosis; fatty infiltration and cell necrosis are seen in patients with cirrhosis.

Paracentesis can aid in diagnosis; clear, straw-colored fluid with a decreased total protein is found in cirrhosis.

Arteriography may be used to show presence of collateral portal circulation.

PHYSICAL EXAMINATION

Evaluate liver status: height, recent weight gain/loss, fatigability, temperature, edema, ascites, jaundice, anorexia, spider telangiectasis, palmar erythema, asterixis (liver flap), abdominal tenderness may be present in liver disease, but the liver may be small and covered with bumps in chronic liver disease.

Observe for signs of tissue wasting.

Observe for signs of estrogen-androgen imbalances; regression of secondary sexual characteristics.

GI bleeding, esophageal varices may be present.

Mental status exam may reveal disturbances in thinking due to increased serum ammonia level.

In severe portal hypertension, splenomegaly, edema of the lower extremities, and distension of collateral circulation evidenced by esophageal varices, hemorrhoids, and caput medusae (dilated cutaneous veins around the umbilicus) occur.

NURSING PRIORITIES

1. Improve nutritional status and prevent fluid and electrolyte imbalance.
2. Promote comfort.
3. Observe for early signs of potential life-threatening complications, such as hepatic coma, hemorrhage, and renal failure.
4. Provide psychologic support.
5. Provide information about disease process and potential for prevention of further liver damage.

NURSING DIAGNOSIS:	**Nutrition, alteration in, less than body requirements.**
SUPPORTING DATA:	**Poor nutrition is influential in the development and progression of cirrhosis. Liver damage results in metabolic disturbances manifested by anorexia, nausea and vomiting, indigestion, abnormal bowel function, and associated muscle wasting.**
DESIRED PATIENT OUTCOMES:	**Nutritional intake is adequate for metabolic needs.**

INTERVENTIONS

Promote bed rest and/or rest periods.

Encourage patient to eat; explain reasons for the type of diet. Give small meals with supplemental snacks. Feed patient if tiring easily or have family assist patient. Consider patient preference in food choices.

RATIONALE

Conserving patient energy reduces metabolic demands on the liver and promotes cellular regeneration.

Proper diet is vital to recovery. Large meals may increase the nausea and anorexia. Patient may eat better if family is involved.

Discuss the deleterious affects of alcohol on nutrition.

Besides having a direct hepatotoxic effect, alcohol affects the patient's desire for foods.

Salt substitutes are given if allowed; avoid those containing ammonium. Suggest other flavoring agents, such as lemon juice and herbs.

Salt substitutes enhance the flavor of food and aid in increasing the patient's appetite.

MEDICAL MANAGEMENT

Tube feedings.

Patient may be too nauseated or anorexic to eat. Esophageal varices may make tube feeding necessary.

Increase protein in the diet, unless there is impending liver failure. Liquid supplementation may be necessary initially.

Increased protein helps in the regeneration of liver tissue if the disease is not too far advanced. Protein is important in synthesis and a decrease in albumin synthesis predisposes to edema formation. In liver failure, protein in the gastrointestinal tract is incompletely synthesized and forms ammonia and thus may be severely restricted or eliminated.

Increase carbohydrates in the diet. Total calories should range between 2000–3000/per day.

Increase calorie intake to sustain weight and spare use of protein for healing.

Soft diet may be necessary: avoid use of roughage foods.

Danger of hemorrhage from esophageal varices in advanced cirrhosis.

Vitamin supplements including thiamine and possibly iron and folic acid.

The patient is usually vitamin deficient due to previous poor diet. Also the injured liver is unable to store vitamins A, B complex, D, and K. There may be an iron or folic acid deficient induced anemia.

Pancreatin.

Promotes digestion of fats in the presence of steatorrhea and diarrhea.

NURSING DIAGNOSIS:	**Fluid volume, deficit, actual (failure of regulatory mechanisms).**
SUPPORTING DATA:	**Inappropriate levels of aldosterone may be excreted or not properly detoxified by the liver, causing retention of water and sodium and excretion of potassium. Ascites may occur as a result of portal hypertension, hepatic vein obstruction, a decrease in plasma colloid osmotic pressure due to decreased albumin synthesis, increased sodium retention or impaired water excretion. Use of diuretics may result in electrolyte imbalances.**

DESIRED PATIENT OUTCOMES: Normal serum electrolyte levels maintained. Fluid weight loss of not more than 1 kg per day with gradually decreasing abdominal girth measurement.

INTERVENTIONS	RATIONALE
Maintain accurate intake and output and report abnormalities.	Accurate record assists in evaluation of the management of diuretic therapy.
Record daily weights.	Weight gain may indicate fluid retention and is helpful in assessing fluid status.
Measure abdominal girth daily using guidelines marked in ballpoint ink.	Helpful in assessing status of ascites. Guidelines assure repeated measurement of same circumference.
Frequent mouth care; occasional ice chips.	Mouth care and ice chips decrease thirst.
Monitor serial serum electrolytes.	Helps to determine fluid needs as well as deficiencies due to diuretic therapy. Sodium imbalance may result from secondary hyperaldosteronism associated with ascites and edema. Magnesium may be decreased as a result of increased urinary loss and poor nutritional intake.
Be aware of nonfood items that contain sodium, including medications.	Products commonly used for indigestion, such as baking soda, and some mouth washes contain significant amounts of sodium.

MEDICAL MANAGEMENT

Diuretics.	Used to try to control edema and ascites. Controlled diuresis with a gradual weight loss of no more than 1 kg/day minimizes or prevents renal failure. When ascites is present without peripheral edema, diuresis must be slower with weight loss restricted to 0.2–0.3 kg/day minimizing the possibility of the development of encephalopathy.
Fluid restriction may be ordered in patients with ascites (1000 ml/day or less).	Used to decrease the edema and ascites when diuretics are inadequate.
Sodium restriction.	Aids in limiting the formation of ascites and edema and in the removal of excessive fluids from the body tissues.
Potassium replacement.	Total body potassium is usually decreased in liver disease; as well as losses from diuretics.
Aldactone, in addition to oral diuretics.	Aldosterone-blocking agent that reinforces effect of diuretic agents while minimizing potassium loss.
Daily urines.	To determine Na$^+$ and K$^+$.
Paracentesis.	See Nursing Diagnosis: Breathing patterns, ineffective.

NURSING DIAGNOSIS:	Skin integrity, impairment of, potential.
SUPPORTING DATA:	Edema of tissues decreases circulation to area. Ascites increases weight on supporting tissues. Lethargy decreases position changes. Bile salt accumulation in skin results in pruritus.
DESIRED PATIENT OUTCOMES:	Normal skin integrity without broken areas.

INTERVENTIONS

Use alternating pressure or egg carton mattress; frequent turning; massage to reddened areas, bony-prominences or areas of continued stress; lotions; restrict use of soap for bathing.

Place sheepskin under patient.

Change linens and patient's clothes frequently to keep them free of moisture. Limit the patient's activities to decrease perspiration.

Cut fingernails of patient short; patient may need to wear gloves at night to prevent scratching while asleep.

Calamine lotion with 1% phenol, cholestyramine, or baking soda baths can be used for pruritus.

MEDICAL MANAGEMENT

Cuemid with fruit juices. (Be alert for signs of bleeding.)

RATIONALE

Edematous tissue is more prone to breakdown and the formation of decubiti. Ascites may stretch the skin to the point of tearing. Soap has a drying effect and may increase itchiness of the skin.

Air spaces in wool help keep the patient's skin dry by allowing for circulation of air.

Moisture increases the chance of tissue breakdown. Pruritus is made worse by stretching of skin due to tissue edema.

Prevent the patient from inadvertently injuring the skin.

About 25% of patients with jaundice experience pruritus due to the bile pigment deposited in the skin.

May be given to prevent deposit of bile pigment in the skin. May prevent vitamin K absorption and may contribute to bleeding problems.

NURSING DIAGNOSIS:	Breathing patterns, ineffective.
SUPPORTING DATA:	General debilitated state places patient at risk for acquired infections. Pressure on the diaphragm due to ascites causes reduced lung volumes and hypoxemia may occur.
DESIRED PATIENT OUTCOMES:	Respiratory function maximized with ABGs within adequate range; free of respiratory infections.

INTERVENTIONS

Semi-Fowler's position, or high-Fowler's may be necessary.

Routine turn, deep breathing, and position changes.

Auscultate lung fields.

Monitor ABGs.

Monitor environment for potential sources of infection.

Monitor vital signs for spiking fever and chills.

RATIONALE

To allow maximal lung expansion.

Facilitates aeration to all areas of the lungs.

Listen for areas of congestion and other adventitious sounds (e.g., atelectasis).

Indicator of respiratory dysfunction.

Visitors, roommates, and staff may be sources of infection.

Signs of respiratory infection.

MEDICAL MANAGEMENT

Supplemental O_2.

Incentive spirometer.

Measures to correct anemia depending on etiology, such as iron and folic acid deficiency or hypovolemia.

Paracentesis.

Human blood albumin, salt poor.

Antibiotic therapy.

Increased inspired O_2 to offset decreased lung volumes and resultant hypoxemia.

To increase lung ventilation and enable patient to visualize respiratory effort.

Decreased RBCs for O_2 transport as well as arteriovenous shunting in the lung result in a ventilation perfusion imbalance.

For removal of small amounts of fluid, no more than 1L at a time. Considered as a last resort when respiratory embarrassment continues and other measures (Nursing Diagnosis: Fluid volume, deficit, actual) fail to control ascites. Hypovolemia, shock, and hepatic coma may occur with rapid fluid shifts. Protein and electrolyte losses may be minimized by removal of fluid in small amounts.

To counteract the loss of fluid and protein and increase osmotic pressure.

To combat infection.

NURSING DIAGNOSIS:	**Injury, potential for, hemorrhage.**
SUPPORTING DATA:	**In cirrhosis, blood flow from the liver can be obstructed, increasing pressure in the portal vein, resulting in the development of collateral circulatory channels within the gastrointestinal tract. As pressure increases, these fragile dilated vessels (most commonly esophageal varices) are subject to hemorrhage.**

┌───┐
│ **DESIRED PATIENT OUTCOMES:**   **Hemorrhage is controlled and re-** │
│   **currence is prevented.**   │
└───┘

INTERVENTIONS

Observe for signs of acute or subacute bleeding: hematemesis, melena, abdominal distention, signs of shock.

Monitor vital signs and lab studies, primarily Hct & Hb.

Keep patient NPO.

In upper GI bleed, maintain patency of NG tube.

Provide mouth care and keep nostrils clean and lubricated. Maintain proper positioning of the tube.

Place in semi-Fowler's position.

MEDICAL MANAGEMENT

IV fluids.

Cool saline/ice water lavage maintaining accurate I & O and recording nature and color of aspirant.

Vitamin K.

Transfusions.

Vasopressin IV or selected angiography of superior artery.

Magnesium sulfate and/or saline enemas.

Intestinal microbials, such as neomycin.

Endoscopy.

Sengstaken-Blakemore tube. (Refer to standard procedure manual for cautions and possible complications of use of this tube.)

RATIONALE

Varying degrees of bleeding may occur in various areas of the GI tract and early detection may prevent or minimize hypovolemia.

Signs of hemoconcentration or actual blood loss.

To rest GI tract.

Minimizes vomiting that might increase sites of hemorrhage. Removes large amounts of blood that may be present from the GI tract and lessens the possibility of encephalopathy.

Prevent patient discomfort and injury to the tissues due to pressure of the tube.

Minimizes gastroesophageal reflux and may minimize aspiration if vomiting occurs.

Maintain fluid balance.

May control bleeding temporarily through vasoconstriction. Indicator of continued bleeding.

Promote prothrombin synthesis and coagulation.

Fresh whole blood has a lower ammonia content and greater coagulation effect.

Constricts the splanchnic arterioles reducing portal pressure and blood flow. Because it reduces blood flow to the liver, caution should be exercised. Systemic administration may constrict coronary arteries and intraarterial infusion may be preferred.

Promote evacuation of blood from the GI tract to minimize ammonia intoxication and hepatic coma.

Minimizes bacterial breakdown of blood, which releases ammonia.

Identification of bleeding sites affects therapy choices. Risks need to be weighed, as these procedures present the danger of precipitating hemorrhage.

In uncontrolled hemorrhage from esophageal varices, tamponade may be effective.

Emergency surgical procedures, such as direct ligation of the varices, esophagogastric resection, splenorenal-portacaval anastomosis may be required.

With shunting, portal decompression results in a decrease in portal and collateral circulatory pressure and an increase in hepatic arterial flow and recurrence of bleeding is minimized.

NURSING DIAGNOSIS:	Injury, potential for, altered clotting factors.
SUPPORTING DATA:	Depression of clotting factors synthesized in the liver. The clearance of activated blood coagulation products is impaired. Fibrinolytic activity is increased to compensate for accelerated bleeding.
DESIRED PATIENT OUTCOMES:	Bleeding is minimized or does not occur.

INTERVENTIONS

Assist patient to minimize trauma by avoiding the use of harsh tooth brushes, forceful nose blowing, and so forth.

Observe for signs of bleeding from mucous membranes, in addition to ecchymotic areas of the skin.

Use small gauge needles for injections. Apply pressure to small bleeding sites and record site and cause. May also inform lab personnel re patient's bleeding pattern.

Monitor lab values for decrease in platelets and increased prothrombin time.

Test stools for occult blood.

MEDICAL MANAGEMENT

Vitamin K parenterally.

Heparin and antifibrinolytic drugs with replacement of factors and platelet concentrates.

Vitamin supplements of B complex, including thiamine.

RATIONALE

In the presence of clotting factor disturbances, minimal trauma can cause significant blood loss.

Occurs more readily due to the amount of surface blood supply and fragility of the mucous membranes (including genitourinary).

Minimizes damage to the tissues. Prolonged bleeding may indicate clotting factor disturbances.

Indicators of coagulation defect and may indicate increased risk of hemorrhage/developing DIC. Refer to Care Plan: Disseminated Intravascular Coagulation.

Bleeding may be subclinical.

When prothrombin level is decreased. (Will not be effective when the cause is liver cell damage.)

Activates anticlotting factors preventing further loss of clotting factors. Reestablish adequate levels of clotting factors. (Heparin is controversial.)

Deficiencies occur due to inadequate intake, decreased absorption, and decreased storage capacity. Essential in red blood cell enzyme activity.

Bile salts.	Aids digestion and absorption of fat-soluble vitamins. Use cautiously in marked hepatic dysfunction.
Vitamin C.	Lack of vitamin C is a factor in GI bleeding, increases susceptibility to irritation by other factors.

NURSING DIAGNOSIS: **Thought processes, alterations in.**

SUPPORTING DATA: **In the presence of cirrhosis, factors that further depress liver function and/or increase the circulating level of ammonia may precipitate hepatic coma.**

DESIRED PATIENT OUTCOMES: **Circulating level of serum ammonia is controlled and fluctuations in mentation are minimized.**

INTERVENTIONS

Observe for early changes in mentation, such as lethargy, confusion, drowsiness, and irritability; may be intermittent.

Note changes in behavior, such as untidy personal habits, note slowing and/or slurring of speech.

Have the patient write his/her name periodically and keep this record for comparison; report deterioration of ability. Have patient do simple arithmetic computations.

Provide continuity of care. If possible, assign same nurse over a period of time.

Monitor lab values for metabolic alkalosis, hypokalemia, ammonia levels, and signs of infection.

Eliminate or markedly restrict amount of protein in the diet. Provide calories in the form of carbohydrates by mouth, nasogastric, and/or IV. Provide adequate hydration.

Avoid use of narcotics or sedatives, tranquilizers, and ammonia products.

Protect the patient from injury. Leave siderails up and pad if necessary and provide close supervision.

RATIONALE

Ongoing assessment of the patient's behavior and mental status is important because of the fluctuating nature of impending hepatic coma.

Early intervention allows for treatment, which enhances the patient's chances for recovery.

This is an easy test of neurologic status and muscular coordination.

More accurate documentation of subtle changes is possible.

Serve as indicators of impending, potentiating, and precipitating factors in the development of hepatic coma.

Ammonia is a product of the breakdown of protein in the GI tract. Dietary changes may lead to constipation, which increases bacterial action and formation of ammonia.

Certain drugs are toxic to the liver and other drugs may not be metabolized quickly due to cirrhosis, causing accumulative effects that may precipitate coma or mask signs of developing encephalopathy.

Safety needs to be provided when confusion occurs.

Provide opportunities for significant others to ask questions and obtain information.

Patient's mental status may deteriorate rapidly and information can be helpful to patient's understanding.

MEDICAL MANAGEMENT

IV therapy and electrolyte replacement.

As indicated to correct imbalances.

Salt-poor albumin.

Often necessary as serum albumin levels decrease.

Stool softeners.

Aid in preventing constipation.

Colonic purges, such as magnesium sulfate and enemas. Lactulose.

Removes protein and blood from intestines. Acidifies the intestine and produces diarrhea, decreasing the production of nitrogenous substances.

Bactericidal agents such as neomycin and kanamycin.

Decreased intestinal bacterial production of ammonia.

NURSING DIAGNOSIS: **Tissue perfusion, alteration in.**

SUPPORTING DATA: **Tests reveal marked reduction in renal-cortical perfusion, decrease in renal plasma flow and glomerular filtration rate leads to diminished urine formation and subsequent renal failure. (Hepatorenal syndrome)**

DESIRED PATIENT OUTCOMES: **Renal filtration and satisfactory urinary output are maintained.**

INTERVENTIONS

See Care Plan: Acute Renal Failure

RATIONALE

MEDICAL MANAGEMENT

L-dopa, adrenergic amino, corticosteroids, salt-free albumin infusions.

Correct hemodynamic imbalances and may improve perfusion to the kidneys.

Portacaval anastomosis and hepatic transplantation.

Have been tried with some success but remain unproven.

NURSING DIAGNOSIS: **Self-concept, disturbance in.**

SUPPORTING DATA: **Serious illness may alter physical appearance and alcohol-induced disease may necessitate behavior and lifestyle changes leading to problems with self-esteem and role performance.**

DESIRED PATIENT OUTCOMES:	Patient verbalizes acceptance of self in the present situation.

INTERVENTIONS

Assist patient/significant others to cope with change in appearance, listen to patient ventilate feelings. Suggest clothing that does not emphasize altered appearance.

Assess need for referral(s) to drug and alcohol or other treatment programs.

(Refer to Care Plans: Psychosocial Aspects of Care in the Acute Setting; Chemical Dependency.)

RATIONALE

Patient will present unattractive appearance due to jaundice, ascites, ecchymotic areas.

Individual and family needs vary and may necessitate professional assistance.

NURSING DIAGNOSIS:	Knowledge deficit, of disease process, complications, and medical management.
SUPPORTING DATA:	Progressive nature of the disease process and severity of complications makes recovery difficult and relapses common.
DESIRED PATIENT OUTCOMES:	Patient/SO verbalize causes of disease and symptoms of complications that are immediately reportable to the physician. Participate in care with alterations in contributory behaviors and lifestyles.

INTERVENTIONS

Stress importance of avoiding alcohol. Give information about community services available to aid in alcohol rehabilitation, if indicated.

Inform the patient of the altered drug effects with cirrhosis and the importance of using only drugs prescribed or cleared by a physician who is familiar with patient's history.

Assist patient in identifying support person(s).

Instruct and emphasize the importance of good nutrition. Provide written instructions.

Provide information regarding sodium and salt substitute restrictions.

RATIONALE

Alcohol is currently the leading cause in the development of cirrhosis.

Certain drugs are hepatotoxic (especially narcotics, sedatives, and hypnotics); also the damaged liver has a decreased ability to metabolize drugs and they may accumulate and/or aggravate bleeding tendencies.

Due to length of recovery, potential for relapses, and slow convalescence, support systems are extremely important in maintaining behavior modifications.

Proper dietary maintenance will aid in recovery and help prevent further damage. Written instructions will be helpful for patient to refer to at home.

Minimize edema formation. Overuse of substitutes may result in other electrolyte imbalances.

Instruct patient/significant others in the importance of rest.

Promote diversional activities that are enjoyable to the patient.

Instruct patient and SO of signs and symptoms that warrant notification of physician, such as increased abdominal girth, rapid weight loss/gain, edema, fever, blood in stool or urine, bleeding of any kind in excess.

Instruct SO to notify physician of any confusion, untidyness, night wandering, tremors, or personality change.

Adequate rest is believed to shorten the length of illness by decreasing demands on the body, which increases the energy available for healing.

Prevent boredom and minimize anxiety and depression.

Prompt reporting of symptoms can avoid further hepatic damage and treat complication before it is life-threatening.

These changes may be more apparent to significant others and may indicate development of complications. Insidious changes may be noted by others with less frequent contacts with patient.

DIAGNOSIS: Pancreatitis

PATIENT DATA BASE

NURSING HISTORY

History of cholelithiasis; chronic, excessive alcohol consumption; recent history of duodenitis, bacterial disease, or opiate usage; recent abdominal surgery; trauma.

Note the type, severity, location, duration of pain and how relief is obtained.

Note effect of food, rest, activity, alcohol, and medication on the pain.

Note history of sudden onset of diabetes with no family history of the disorder.

Note history of food intolerances.

May occur as a side effect of drug therapy, such as steroid.

DIAGNOSTIC STUDIES

Leukocytosis may occur.

Serum enzymes (amylase and lipase) elevated due to the escape of pancreatic enzymes from necrotic pancreatic acini. Lipase level rises with the amylase level but tends to remain increased for approximately five days, whereas the amylase returns to normal in one or two days.

Serum bilirubin, alkaline phosphatase, and SGOT may be elevated if the biliary tract is also involved. If these are elevated, a complete diagnostic evaluation for biliary disease will be ordered. The same is also true when liver function tests are abnormal and the patient has a history of alcoholism.

Serum calcium may be decreased slightly. This may become more severe with tetany resulting. This is due to a fall in ionized calcium due to calcium deposition in fat necrotic areas in the abdominal cavity. These fat necrotic areas are due to the release of pancreatic lipase into the cavity. An increase of deposition of calcium from the serum to the bone may also be a cause. Total protein level may be decreased due to third space fluid loss.

In chronic pancreatitis the cause of decreased serum calcium may be due to poor absorption leading to vitamin D deficiency (fat-soluble vitamins have decreased absorption and digestion properties in the presence of decreased fat metabolism).

Serum glucose may be elevated and glucose tolerance impaired.

Transient hyperglycemia occurs in 25–75% of the patients due to release of glucagon from alpha cells and damage to the beta cells that secrete insulin. These signs usually disappear but occasionally diabetes mellitus may follow acute pancreatitis.

Diabetes mellitus is common after chronic pancreatitis and is considered a common delayed aspect of this disorder rather than a complication.

Urine amylase may be elevated. Amylase is taken up and excreted into the urine rapidly; therefore, it may be elevated for longer periods of time than serum amylase. It may remain elevated for two or three days. This is significant if the patient does not seek medical assistance for three or four days and the serum amylase is normal.

Glycosuria may occur in 10–35% of these patients.

Stool examination may be done for quantitative fat content. With failure of the pancreatic lipase to reach the intestine, fat remains undigested and unabsorbed.

X-ray to check for calcification of the pancreas.

Fiberoptic visualization of the ampulla of Vater may be done to differentiate obstructive biliary disease, or acute versus chronic disease.

PHYSICAL EXAMINATION

In acute pancreatitis:

Give special attention in regard to severe, prolonged, upper abdominal pain that may radiate to the back. Onset may be sudden but often occurring hours after heavy meals or excessive alcohol consumption.

Abdominal tenderness and muscle guarding rather than rigidity; distention may also appear due to localized or diffuse paralytic ileus. Nausea and vomiting may be present.

Hypotension, weakness, diaphoresis, tachycardia.

Temperature elevation, usually low grade.

In acute hemorrhagic pancreatitis:

Pain more severe, tenderness in epigastrium, usually without rigidity.

Respiratory distress may occur.

May have mental disturbances manifested by restlessness, hallucinations, coarse tremor.

Edema and ascites may be present, due to large third space fluid loss.

Symptoms of shock may be present due to decrease in circulating volume as great as 30% and the release of kinins, which dilate the vascular tree.

In chronic pancreatitis (during the acute stages, same as acute pancreatitis):

Loose, bulky, foul-smelling stools (steatorrhea and azotorrhea).

Minimal jaundice may be noted.

Pain may be chronic, dull, aching. May have tenderness in epigastrium on palpation.

Ecchymosis may be present.

Protein malnutrition with weight loss.

Fat-soluble vitamin deficiencies.

Symptoms of diabetes mellitus.

NURSING PRIORITIES

1. Control pain and promote comfort.
2. Prevent and treat shock and fluid and electrolyte imbalance.
3. Reduce pancreatic stimulation and maintain nutritional needs.
4. Prevent and/or minimize complications that may be immediate or long-term in nature resulting in permanent damage.

NURSING DIAGNOSIS:	Comfort, alteration in, pain.
SUPPORTING DATA:	Obstruction of pancreatic duct, destruction and interruption of blood supply.
DESIRED PATIENT OUTCOMES:	Pain is reduced to a manageable level.

INTERVENTIONS

Keep on bed rest. Allow patient to assume position of comfort.

Give medication as ordered after examination and assessment and before pain is severe.

MEDICAL MANAGEMENT

Meperidine rather than opiates. ·

Papaverine, nitroglycerin, barbiturates, or anticholinergics.

Sympathetic nerve blocks and epidural anesthesia.

For further measures related to reduction of pancreatic stimuli refer to Nursing Diagnosis: Nutrition, alteration in, less than body requirements.

RATIONALE

Decrease exertion, metabolic rate, and gastrointestinal secretions. Flexing the thighs on the trunk and rest with no sudden jarring will provide some relief.

If medication is given before examination, signs and symptoms will be relieved resulting in an inaccurate or late diagnosis of the true underlying problem. Relief of pain minimizes restlessness, which increases body metabolism and enzyme secretion.

Opiates produce spasm of the biliary and pancreatic ducts thus increasing pain.

Provides smooth muscle relaxation.

For persistent pain not relieved by other measures.

NURSING DIAGNOSIS:	**Fluid volume deficit, potential.**
SUPPORTING DATA:	**Vomiting, NG suctioning; restricted oral intake; third space fluid and blood loss; fever.**
DESIRED PATIENT OUTCOMES:	**Adequate hydration and electrolyte balance are maintained.**

INTERVENTIONS

Monitor and record accurate I & O and be aware of insensible losses. Note decreased urine output.

Monitor lab values; hematocrit and hemoglobin, BUN, serum protein, creatinine, electrolytes.

Take vital signs as necessary. Observe for tachycardia and hypotension. Monitor CVP as indicated.

RATIONALE

Provides information that serves as a guide for necessary volume replacement and renal function.

Hemoconcentration indicates the loss of plasma and/or blood as well as generalized fluid deficit into the peritoneal cavity.

Large losses of plasma into the pancreas and surrounding tissues leads to hypovolemia. The release of vasodilators, such as bradykinin and kallikrein, further alters capillary permeability contributing to hypotension. The resultant decrease in blood volume to the portal and circulatory system leads to compensatory tachycardia.

Observe for muscular twitching, jerking, or irritability.

Frequent vomiting and/or gastric suctioning may cause loss of electrolytes, with the possible development of tetany. Calcium is lost because it binds to the fatty acids and is lost in the stool.

Note changes in mental state.

Anorexia, toxicity to brain, withdrawal from alcohol, and pepsin may interfere with brain function.

MEDICAL MANAGEMENT

Glucose and Ringer's lactate with electrolytes.

Basic fluid/electrolyte replacement.

Plasma, dextran, albumin, and blood.

To correct losses from hemorrhage and/or large capillary fluid shifts.

Calcium gluconate IV.

For impending or occurrence of tetany.

Promazine.

For sedation.

NURSING DIAGNOSIS: Nutrition, alteration in, less than body requirements.

SUPPORTING DATA: Reflex irritation from inflamed pancreas, decreased intestinal peristalsis, and pain induce a stimulus to the vomiting center, loss of appetite, pancreatic enzymes unavailable for normal digestive process, presence of inflammatory process increases nutritional needs.

DESIRED PATIENT OUTCOMES: Gastrointestinal irritation is reduced. Nutrition is supported and returned to adequate levels.

INTERVENTIONS

Keep NPO.

Observe and record color, amount and nature of NG drainage as well as pH and if blood is present.

Alternate side positions.

Provide frequent oral care.

Monitor blood sugar levels.

Instruct patient in the importance of avoiding stimulants, such as coffee, alcohol, and nicotine.

RATIONALE

Food in the duodenum is the chief stimulus for enzyme secretion.

Suctioning removes hydrochloric acid from the stomach, reduces the amount of secretions, and relieves distention.

Minimize esophageal and/or gastric irritation.

Cleansing mouth decreases vomiting stimulus.

Serum sugar levels are more accurate than fractional urine tests.

Keep pancreatic secretions at a minimum.

MEDICAL MANAGEMENT

Anticholinergics.

Reduce pancreatic and gastric secretions with depression of the vagal mechanisms and decrease of motility. The decrease in volume and concentration of enzymes provides rest for the inflamed area. (These drugs are contraindicated in the presence of shock and paralytic ileus.)

Antacids.

May be used to neutralize gastric secretions.

Small amounts of clear liquids are allowed when the NG tube is clamped. The tube is removed as soon as liquids are tolerated with progression to a diet with carbohydrates the principal nutrient and protein added gradually.

With remission of symptoms, a careful resumption of oral intake is necessary to prevent exacerbation while meeting nutritional needs.

Eventually high-protein, high-carbohydrate, low-fat, bland diet with frequent small meals is recommended.

Restore nutritional balance. Will decrease steatorrhea.

Hyperalimentation.

In severe nutritional deficit, allows prolonged rest of digestive systems and/or supplement of inadequate oral intake. Refer to Care Plan: Total Parenteral Nutrition.

Replacement enzymes, such as pancreatin. (Check individual sensitivity to pork. Beef preparations are available.)

Correct deficiencies that prevent adequate nutritional absorption.

Bile salts.

Facilitate absorption of fat-soluble vitamins and decrease loss of fat in the stool.

Regular insulin, small doses.

Hyperglycemia may develop due to injury to beta cells and increased release of glucocorticoids.

Limit IV solutions containing glucose.

Although beta cell functioning is reduced, insulin production may still occur; therefore, long-acting insulin preparations are contraindicated.

NURSING DIAGNOSIS:	Injury, potential for, complications.
SUPPORTING DATA:	Secondary infections may occur with pancreatitis due to the inflammatory process. Pancreatic abscesses, cysts, fistulas, adynamic ileus and bacteremia may result.
DESIRED PATIENT OUTCOMES:	Afebrile. No infection present. Complications minimized.

INTERVENTIONS

RATIONALE

Observe rate and characteristics of respiratory breath sounds, occurrence of cough and sputum production.

Fluid accumulation and limited mobility predispose to respiratory infections and atelectasis. Retroperitoneal fluid accumulation may cause elevated diaphragm and shallow, abdominal breathing.

Observe for temperature elevation.

Lukewarm sponge baths may be used.

Monitor ABGs.

Assess peristaltic activity; note bowel sounds; check for passage of flatus; observe for abdominal distention and vomiting.

Observe for signs and symptoms of abscess or pseudocyst that may develop suddenly or over a period of several weeks or even months following acute attack, e.g., upper abdominal pain, mass or tenderness, fever, abdominal distention, leukocytosis, hyperglycemia, hypoalbuminemia, and sometimes elevation of serum/urine amylase.

When fistulas are present:
    Instruct patient in diet.

    Instruct patient to note amount of output from fistula.

Maintain meticulous skin care.

Indices for inflammatory/infectious processes.

Reduce temperature elevation and decrease metabolic rate.

Indicates level of respiratory functioning and early signs of failure.

Adynamic ileus may occur.

May result from extensive necrosis predisposing to a large fluid-containing cavity that is easily infected.

While external fistulas usually heal themselves in 6–12 months, careful nutritional balance needs to be maintained.

Fluids, enzymes, and electrolytes may be lost, leading to dehydration and acidosis.

Pancreatic enzymes can digest the skin and tissues of the abdominal wall.

MEDICAL MANAGEMENT

Broad spectrum antibiotics. Sulfonamides, kanamycin, and streptomycin.

IPPB treatment and O_2.

Surgical drainage of abscess or pseudocyst.

These antibiotics are excreted in the pancreatic secretions.

Improves respiratory functioning, mobilizes secretions, limits atelectasis.

Mortality from abscess is about 50%.

NURSING DIAGNOSIS: **Knowledge deficit, of disease process, treatment, and possible complications.**

SUPPORTING DATA: **Multiple etiology of disease process, possibility of development of chronic exocrine and/or endocrine deficiencies.**

DESIRED PATIENT OUTCOMES: **Progressive damage is prevented and complications are minimized.**

INTERVENTIONS

Review with patient/SOs specific cause of current episode, if known, and note other causative factors.

RATIONALE

Avoidance of predisposing factors may help to limit damage and prevent development of a chronic condition.

343

Explore availability of programs for treatment/rehabilitation of chemical dependency if indicated.

Assist patient in learning to identify changes in stool, such as the frothing, foul-smelling stools that indicate steatorrhea, and the importance of reporting to the physician. Other symptoms to note and report include pain, nausea and vomiting, abdominal distention, and low-grade fever.

Stress rationale and importance of initial continuation of bland, low-fat diet with frequent small feedings and restricted coffee usage, then gradual return to a normal diet as tolerated.

Instruct patient in usage of pancreatic enzyme replacements and bile salt therapy as indicated.

Explain signs/symptoms of diabetes mellitus, i.e., polydipsia, polyuria, weakness, polyphagia, and weight loss.

Drug usage is increasing as a factor, whether self-administered or prescribed. Pain can be severe and prolonged and may lead to the possibility of drug dependence. Alcohol abuse is currently the most common cause of recurrence.

May be signs of recurrent disease process or inadequate drug therapy.

Understanding the purpose of the diet in maximizing the use of available enzymes while avoiding overstimulation of the pancreas and thus steatorrhea may enhance patient cooperation.

If permanent damage has occurred, exocrine deficiencies will result.

Damage to the beta cells may result in a temporary or even permanent alteration of insulin production.

DIAGNOSIS: Hemorrhoids

PATIENT DATA BASE

NURSING HISTORY

May be internal or external, with or without complaints of pain/pruritus.

Dietary history: note fiber intake.

History of chronic constipation. Check use of laxatives.

History of cirrhosis/portal hypertension.

History of straining at stool with bleeding at defecation.

Pregnancy history.

May have family history of hemorrhoid problems.

Note whether patient has an occupation requiring long periods of sitting or standing.

Determine effect of symptoms on client, e.g., fear, anxiety, embarrassment.

DIAGNOSTIC STUDIES

CBC, may indicate anemia due to chronic or acute rectal bleeding.

Iron deficiency may also be present.

PHYSICAL EXAMINATION

Thorough examination of the gastrointestinal tract to r/o cancer of the colon.

Rectal examination: a visual and digital exam is done initially.

Proctoscopy is done, followed by a barium enema. The actual source of bleeding needs to be confirmed so other conditions that may exist are not overlooked.

NURSING PRIORITIES

1. Maintain patient comfort.
2. Restore normal bowel function.

MEDICAL TREATMENT

The patient who is being treated medically is usually able to care for oneself at home. With proper diet, fluid intake and regular exercise, the hemorrhoids are usually controlled.

NURSING DIAGNOSIS:	Comfort, alteration in, pain.
SUPPORTING DATA:	Congestion and edema result in pain and discomfort.
DESIRED PATIENT OUTCOMES:	Pain/discomfort is minimized/controlled.

INTERVENTIONS

Assess amount, character, and threshold of discomfort.

Allow patient to assume position of comfort.

Use flotation pad under buttocks.

Monitor for hypotension.

MEDICAL MANAGEMENT

Ice.

Warm compresses and sitz baths p.r.n.

Analgesic ointments, such as Nupercainal or witch hazel compresses.

Analgesics.

Hypnosis.

RATIONALE

Varies with patient and severity of individual case.

Will provide for less pain.

To distribute pressure.

May occur during sitz baths because of dilation of the pelvic blood vessels.

Local applications reduce congestion and edema.

Promote circulation. Soothing.

Control pain and itching.

Relieve pain.

Used by some physicians for pain control. Important to avoid the use of the word "pain" when talking to these patients.

NURSING DIAGNOSIS: Bowel elimination, alteration in, constipation.

SUPPORTING DATA: Constipation often leads to the development of hemorrhoids. Pain and bleeding lead to difficulty with defecation as the movement is restrained to prevent pain.

DESIRED PATIENT OUTCOMES: Stool is of normal consistency and is easily passed with little or no pain and bleeding.

INTERVENTIONS

Maintain intake of 2000 ml of fluid per day.

Maintain regular bowel habits and heed the defecation urge.

Instruct the patient in the importance of using high-fiber foods and low roughage in the diet.

Avoid opiates and their derivatives.

MEDICAL MANAGEMENT

Bulk laxatives, such as Metamucil; stool softeners and/or lubricants.

RATIONALE

Provides adequate hydration.

Regular evacuation helps maintain softer stool.

Helpful in maintaining soft formed stool.

These have a constipating effect.

Maintain soft stool. Medical supervision is helpful to prevent development of "laxative habit."

CARE PLAN: Hemorrhoidectomy

PATIENT DATA BASE

Refer to Care Plan: Hemorrhoids.

Hemorrhoids may be treated by injection, ligation, or surgical removal. Surgical excision with ligation is the treatment of choice when the hemorrhoids do not respond to more conservative methods.

Preoperative: Particular attention is given to cleansing of the lower bowel. No more than four enemas are usually given with normal saline solution the morning of surgery. A catheter may be used rather than the usual rectal tube if the hemorrhoids are severe or if the patient is experiencing pain.

Postoperative:

NURSING PRIORITIES

1. Maintain patient comfort.
2. Restore normal bowel function.
3. Prevent complications.
4. Provide information to assist in dealing with the illness.

NURSING DIAGNOSIS:	Comfort, alteration in, pain.
SUPPORTING DATA:	Edema and swelling in area postoperatively.
DESIRED PATIENT OUTCOMES:	Pain is controlled/minimized.

INTERVENTIONS	RATIONALE
Pad the bottom of the sitz tub or use a rubber ring.	Will be more comfortable.
Do not use soap in the tub.	May be irritating.

MEDICAL MANAGEMENT

Analgesics.	Helpful in reducing level of pain.
Restrict/limit use of analgesic/anesthetic ointments.	Helpful in reducing level of pain. Use of these products may result in secondary skin rashes due to allergy.
Ice packs.	Used initially to reduce congestion.
Sitz baths.	Usually begun the first postop day. Warm moist heat promotes comfort and healing with resorption of edema.
Hypnosis.	Used by some surgeons for pain control. Important to avoid the use of the word "pain" when talking to these patients.

NURSING DIAGNOSIS:	Bowel elimination, alteration in, constipation.

SUPPORTING DATA:	Dehydration, fear of pain on defecation may contribute to problems.
DESIRED PATIENT OUTCOMES:	Soft-formed stool is maintained and easily passed.

INTERVENTIONS

Encourage patient to have bowel movement as soon as the urge occurs.

Instruct patient in diet containing adequate fruit and roughage, importance of regular exercise and establishing a regular routine for defecation.

Avoid constipating foods and fluids.

RATIONALE

Prevents formation of strictures and preserves the normal lumen of the anus.

Helpful to avoid constipation.

Need to identify individually.

MEDICAL MANAGEMENT

Stool softeners.

Continue as before surgery.

NURSING DIAGNOSIS:	Urinary elimination, alteration in.
SUPPORTING DATA:	Retention may occur due to the proximity of the bladder and general tenderness in the area.
DESIRED PATIENT OUTCOMES:	Voiding in sufficient quantity in proportion to intake.

INTERVENTIONS

Keep accurate I & O for at least 24 hours.

Stand/sit patient to void.

Encourage to void while in sitz bath.

RATIONALE

Retention usually occurs during this period.

Normal position assists voiding.

Warm water relaxes bladder.

NURSING DIAGNOSIS:	Injury, potential for, hemorrhage.
SUPPORTING DATA:	Postoperatively, ligatures may slip and blood may collect unnoticed in the bowel. May occur up to ten days after surgery.
DESIRED PATIENT OUTCOMES:	If hemorrhage occurs, it is detected early and controlled effectively.

INTERVENTIONS

Monitor vital signs.

Gently observe perianal area and give explanation of actions.

Check stools for blood. Note frequent unrelieved sensation to defecate.

MEDICAL MANAGEMENT

Indwelling catheter.

Gelfoam.

RATIONALE

Early detection of hemorrhage.

Note signs of fresh bleeding. Area is sensitive and patient may be embarrassed.

Sequestered hemorrhage resulting in edema may cause feeling of fullness.

May be inserted in the rectum with the balloon inflated to provide pressure on the bleeding site.

Control bleeding by providing matrix for clot formation.

NURSING DIAGNOSIS:	**Knowledge deficit, postop management.**
SUPPORTING DATA:	**Patient may anticipate pain and fear defecation. Proper care after surgery will help prevent recurrence.**
DESIRED PATIENT OUTCOMES:	**Verbalizes understanding of the importance of proper perianal cleansing, adequate food and fluid intake, as well as recognition of complications that may arise and appropriate actions to take.**

INTERVENTIONS

Give explanation of expectations about defecation.

Discuss importance of avoiding straining at stool.

Reinforce previous information given about diet, exercise, and bowel regimen.

Instruct in necessity for observing occurrences of hematemesis and melena.

RATIONALE

Helpful in reducing anxiety.

Contributes to recurrence.

Repetition enhances learning.

Hemorrhoids may have functioned as a "pressure relief value" for portal hypertension and after surgery this pressure may be diverted to the esophageal circulation.

BIBLIOGRAPHY

Books and Other Individual Publications

BEYERS, M AND DUDAS, S.: *The Clinical Practice of Medical-Surgical Nursing.* Little, Brown & Co., Boston, 1977.
BOEDEKER, E. AND DAUBER, J.: *Manual of Medical Therapeutics,* ed 21. Little, Brown & Co., Boston, 1974.

BROOKS, F.: *Gastrointestinal Pathophysiology.* Oxford Univ. Press, New York, 1974.

BRUNNER, L. S. AND SUDDARTH, D. S.: *Lippincott Manual of Nursing Practice.* J. B. Lippincott, Philadelphia, 1978.

CONN, H. F. (ED.): *Current Therapy 1981.* W. B. Saunders, Philadelphia, 1981.

FREITAG, J. S., AND MILLER, L. W. (EDS.): *Manual of Medical Therapeutics,* ed. 23. Little, Brown & Co., 1980.

Gastroenterology in Clinical Nursing, ed. 3. C. V. Mosby, St. Louis, 1979.

GIVEN, B. A. AND SIMMONS, S. J.: *Nursing Care of the Patient with Gastrointestinal Disorders.* C. V. Mosby, St. Louis, 1971.

GREENBERGER, N.: *Gastrointestinal Disorders—A Pathophysiologic Approach.* Year Book Medical Publishers, Chicago, 1981.

GUYTON, A.: *Textbook of Medical Physiology.* W. B. Saunders, Philadelphia, 1971.

HARVEY, A. M., BORDLEY, J. III, AND BARONDESS. J. A.: *Differential Diagnosis: The Interpretation of Clinical Evidence,* ed. 3. W. B. Saunders, Philadelphia, 1979.

KIM, M. AND MORITZ, D. (EDS.): *Classification of Nursing Diagnosis.* McGraw-Hill, New York, 1981.

MINUCHEN, S., ROSMAN, B. L., AND BAKER, L.: *Psychosomatic Families.* Harvard Univ. Press, 1978.

NYHUS, L. M. AND WASTELL, C.: *Surgery of the Stomach & Duodenum,* ed. 3. Little, Brown & Co., Boston, 1977.

PHIPPS, W. J., LONG, B. C., AND WOODS, N. F.: *Medical-Surgical Nursing.* C. V. Mosby, St. Louis, 1979.

SMITH, D. AND GERMAIN, C.: *Care of the Adult Patient, Medical-Surgical Nursing,* ed. 3. J. B. Lippincott, Philadelphia, 1975.

TILKIAN, S. M., CONOVER, M. B., AND TILKIAN, A. G.: *Clinical Implications of Laboratory Tests,* C. V. Mosby, St. Louis, 1979.

TUCKER, S. ET AL.: *Patient Care Standards.* C. V. Mosby, St. Louis, 1975.

WILKINS, R. W. AND LEVINSKY, N. G. (ED.): *Medicine, Essentials of Clinical Practice.* Little, Brown & Co., Boston, 1978.

WILSON, H. S. AND KNEISL, C. R.: *Psychiatric Nursing.* Addison-Wesley, Menlo Park, CA, 1979.

WYNGAARDEN, J. B. AND SMITH, L. H. (EDS.): *Textbook of Medicine,* ed. 16. W. B. Saunders, Philadelphia, 1982.

Journal Articles

BARGMAN, F. J.: *Anorexia nervosa.* Family Practice Recertification, Vol. 3, No. 7, 47–59. July, 1981.

BECK, I. T. ET AL.: *Diffuse spasms & achalasis [letter].* J. of Clinical Gastroenterology, 1(3): 287, Sept. 1979.

CASTELL, D. O.: *Calling a halt to heartburn.* Emergency Medicine, Vol. 15, No. 13, 114–9, Feb. 1981.

CESEAUX, A., RICHARDSON, T. F., AND CLAGGETT, M. S.: *Anorexia nervosa: A view from the mirror; an overview; and a behavioral approach.* AJN, 1468–1472, Aug. 1980.

CHERRY, F. M.: *The Russian gun.* Nursing Times 74:28, 1601–2, Sept. 1978.

COYLE, N. ET AL.: *How to protect your patients against aspiration pneumonia.* Nursing 78, 8:50–1, Oct. 1978.

DOYEN, L.: *Primary anorexia nervosa: A review and critique of selected papers.* JPNMHS, 12–17, Vol. 20, No. 6, June 1982.

KAYE, M. D.: *Anomalies of peristalsis in idiopathic diffuse esophageal spasm.* Gut 1981, (22)3:217–22, Mar. 1981.

KORNGUTH, M. L.: *Nursing Management.* AJN 553–554, Mar. 1981.

McCREARY, C. S., AND WATSON, J.: *Pickwickian syndrome.* AJN, 555, Mar. 1981.

MILLER, B. K.: *Jejunoileal bypass: A drastic weight control measure.* AJN, 564–568, Mar. 1981.

MOJZISIK, C. M. AND MARTIN, E. W.: *Gastric partitioning: The latest surgical means to control morbid obesity.* AJN, 569–572, Mar. 1981.

When the anorectic patient challenges you—. Nursing 81, 46–49, Dec. 1981.

WHITE, J. H. AND SCHROEDER, M. A.: *Nursing assessment.* AJN, 550–553, Mar. 1981.

SUMMERFIELD, J. Y.: *Heller's operations for achalasia, a theatre of nursing care study.* Nursing Times 76:1470–3, 21 Aug. 1980.

350

CHAPTER 8

DISEASES OF THE BLOOD/ BLOOD FORMING ORGANS

DIAGNOSIS: Anemias

The blood system serves as the transport medium whereby the body cells receive the necessary nutrients to promote and to maintain life. The essential metabolic and chemical elements are exchanged at the capillary level and waste products are transported by the blood system for excretion. Alterations within the blood system, such as loss of blood components, inadequate elements or lack of required nutrients for the formation of blood cells, interfere with the nutritional needs of the body cells.

Anemia is a symptom of underlying disease that results in decreased oxygen-carrying capacity of the blood. This abnormality may be due to the quantity or quality of the red blood cells. In the majority of instances, anemia involves a reduction in the number of erythrocytes, the quantity of hemoglobin, and the volume of packed erythrocytes.

PATIENT DATA BASE

NURSING HISTORY

Note age, living and financial status.

History of decreased dietary intake.

May have had recent bleed, such as epistaxis, gastrointestinal tract, lung, hemoglobinuria.

May have history of celiac or other malabsorption diseases; intestinal resection, anticonvulsant or chemotherapy.

History of liver disease.

Regional enteritis, tapeworm infestation, polyendocrinopathies, which interfere with vitamin B_{12} production.

Chronic infection, rheumatoid arthritis, chronic granulomatous disease, and so forth may lead to secondary anemias.

May be on antibiotic therapy, which leads to bone marrow failure.

Leukemia or other cancer may be present.

Determine hereditary factors: such as thalassemia, sickle-cell anemia, and hemophilia.

May have had recent transfusion reaction.

Note environmental factors that may expose to lead poisoning.

May have had recent exposure to x-ray.

May have a heart valve prosthesis.

May complain of being tired, weak, easily fatigued, or aching of body or bones.

Note complaints of tinnitus, feeling faint, dimming of vision, numbness, and/or tingling of fingers or toes.

May have bladder or bowel incontinence or retention.

May have history of temperature elevation and weight loss.

Note complaints of shortness of breath, or "racing heart."

The majority of symptoms are related to tissue hypoxia and the severity is determined by the degree of anemia, the time span for development of the anemia and the patient's individual adaptive or compensating mechanisms.

DIAGNOSTIC STUDIES

The causes of anemia may be classified statistically, physiologically, and morphologically. In order to ensure an accurate diagnosis for the cause of anemia, the various approaches should be combined. Using the laboratory data, a morphological classification is based on the average red cell size and hemoglobin concentration. Because the anemias have various sizes and color patterns, they aid in identifying the specific type.

Complete blood count.

Stained red cell examination for inclusion of bodies in cell, change in color and shape, which may indicate particular type of anemia.

Differential white cell count: note increase or decrease in total cell count as well as specific white blood cells because each has a particular function.

Reticulocyte count helpful in differentiating hemolytic anemia from others.

Elevated plasma bilirubin may indicate hemolysis.

Serum iron and iron-binding capacities aid in diagnosing anemias caused by iron deficiency of chronic disease.

Hemoglobin electrophoresis identifies type of hemoglobin structure.

Erythrocyte indices noting relationship between the size of erythrocytes and number of and amount of hemoglobin.

Sickle cell preparation.

Red blood cell survival tests; shortened in certain types of anemia.

Bone marrow exam.

Sedimentation rate: indicates presence of inflammatory or malignant disease.

X-ray may show cardiac hypertrophy.

Check urine/stools for occult blood.

Studies to check for bleeding sites: sigmoid/colonoscopy, barium enema, upper GI series.

PHYSICAL EXAMINATION

General signs/symptoms:

Weakness, fatigue, feel cold.

Observe posture, energy level, tachypnea, dyspnea with exertion and/or at rest.

Dizziness, irritability, restlessness, headache, slowing of thought processes, lethargy, and depression.

Other symptoms may be more specific to certain anemias:

Pica, pagophagia, and spooning for finger nails are seen in iron deficiency.

Multiple GI complaints with loss of weight and beefy-red tongue are more frequently seen in pernicious anemia.

Infections with high fever and bleeding problems as noted by purpura, petechiae, and ecchymosis are reflective of aplastic anemia.

Observe skin pallor, lack of a "glow" in dark-skinned patient, yellow tint, or gray color. Is color in extremities different from other parts of the body? (Consider the effects of gravity.) Note presence of ecchymotic lesions (possible platelet disorder).

Determine the presence of edema, which will alter the true color. If edema precedes jaundice, the jaundice will not be seen because the fluid accumulation increases the distance between the surface and the vascular area thus obscuring the pigments that are normally reflected.

Note diaphoresis. Accumulation of sweat and sebum may interfere with color interpretation.

Observe for pallor in the mucous membranes, nail beds, lips, and palpebral conjunctiva. Observation of the conjunctiva is especially important in the dark-skinned person.

Note presence of thinning, prematurely gray hair.

Assess muscles: spastic or flaccid?

Note positive Romberg's sign.

Check for the presence of paresthesias.

Note presence of retinal hemorrhages; significant in leukemia, aplastic and pernicious anemias.

Note pain with pressure over the sternum; may indicate neoplastic disease.

Assess tachycardia, throbbing carotids, which might indicate compensatory mechanisms to provide the cell with required nutrients. Note systolic murmurs and bruits over carotid arteries. Note signs of congestive heart failure.

Note cracking at the corners of the mouth.

Check for amenorrhea, menorrhagia, loss of libido (men).

Note nodules, spleen enlargement, generalized lymphadenopathy, which may suggest lymphoma or leukemia.

NURSING PRIORITIES

(Because anemia is not a disease, but actually a manifestation of an underlying disorder, treatment will be initially aimed at identifying the cause of the anemia.)

1. Protect from injury.
2. Provide nutritional/fluid needs.
3. Relieve pain.
4. Support psychological well-being of patient/significant others.
5. Prevent/treat possible complications of treatment.

NURSING DIAGNOSIS:	Self-care deficit, ADL.
SUPPORTING DATA:	Weakness, fatigue, apathy attributable to anemia interfere with ability to function. The fatigue and weakness may be caused by a lack of sufficient oxygen for catabolic processes in the skeletal muscle cells, which leads to a decrease in the level of biochemical energy that is available for optimal functioning in daily activities.
DESIRED PATIENT OUTCOMES:	Tolerates existing anemia by temporary or permanent alteration of lifestyle. Completes activities of daily living without fatigue.

INTERVENTIONS

RATIONALE

INTERVENTIONS	RATIONALE
Assess patient's normal activities of daily living.	Maintaining as close to normal activities can help with necessary limitations.
Prioritize nursing care schedules to enhance rest.	Alleviate additional strain on the cardiac and respiratory systems and allow for maximum functioning as an increase in activities necessitates an increase in oxygen requirements by the cells.
Prevent disturbing noises, relocating patient if necessary.	Quiet environment can enhance rest.
Provide assistance with activities as necessary allowing patient to do as much as possible.	While help is necessary, self-esteem is enhanced when patients can do some things for themselves.

NURSING DIAGNOSIS:	Skin integrity, impairment of (actual or potential).
SUPPORTING DATA:	Poor wound healing occurs and the patient is at risk for the formation of decubiti due to circulatory and neurologic changes. Observation of skin eruptions can aid in diagnosis.
DESIRED PATIENT OUTCOMES:	Dermatologic signs/symptoms are improved/controlled.

INTERVENTIONS

Observe, record, and report:
- color changes in the skin, sclerae, mucous membranes, and nailbeds;
- bleeding, petechiae;
- complaints of pruritus, including signs of scratching, such as redness, marks, scabs.

Reposition frequently, pad bony prominences, and massage with lotion.

Trim fingernails short.

Limit use of soap.

RATIONALE

Alterations of the type and quantity of pigments in the circulatory system will affect the color that is reflected. Melanin deposits are reduced in the sclerae, mucous membranes, and nailbeds allowing for easier observation.

Promote circulation and prevent skin breakdown.

Prevent damage to skin.

May dry skin and increase irritation.

NURSING DIAGNOSIS: Mobility, impaired physical.

SUPPORTING DATA: Patient may have difficulty in ambulation and/or visual changes due to decrease in cellular oxygenation. Sudden movements further decrease blood supply to the brain, which aggravates dizziness.

DESIRED PATIENT OUTCOMES: Patient is coping with changes necessary to ensure safety. Alterations in lifestyle have been made to cope with changes.

INTERVENTIONS

Observe for dizziness or faintness.

Provide assistance with ambulation. Curtail activities as necessary.

Teach the patient to avoid sudden movements, such as bending, jumping out of bed.

Observe and record gait changes (droopiness), numbness and tingling of extremities, vision changes including dimness or diplopia.

Place necessary objects within reach of patient.

RATIONALE

Alteration in the oxygen-carrying capacity of the cells results in lack of nutrients necessary to function at an optimum level with side-effects, such as dizziness.

Prevent falls with possibility of injury.

Hypotensive effect may further decrease blood supply to the brain.

Neurologic changes, such as ataxia, paresthesias, or difficulty in walking are attributable to a lack of vitamin B_{12}, which is necessary to maintain an intact nervous system.

Prevent accidents by avoiding straining.

NURSING DIAGNOSIS:	Breathing patterns, ineffective.
SUPPORTING DATA:	Cardiac symptoms will vary with patients. If the anemia has developed within a short time the cardiovascular symptoms resulting from compensation may be apparent early. In contrast, if the anemia is insidious in onset, a patient may have a hemoglobin as low as 6 per 100 ml without being seriously handicapped.
DESIRED PATIENT OUTCOMES:	Cardiac, respiratory symptoms have decreased or abated.

INTERVENTIONS	RATIONALE
Note pulse rate, observe for weakness, threadiness, tachycardia, or periods of palpitations.	With increasing anemia, tolerance decreases resulting in tachycardia, and palpitations even in the resting state.
Observe respirations and related activity.	Dyspnea may occur with little or no activity.
Elevate head of bed.	To aid in breathing. The upright position will allow for greater lung expansion because it pulls the diaphragm down. Abdominal viscera are kept away from the lungs in this position, thus preventing undue pressure on the lungs.
Note complaints of chest pain.	May suggest angina. (Refer to Care Plans: Angina Pectoris; Myocardial Infarction.)
Avoid foods that are gas-forming.	Cause abdominal distention, which further interferes with the respiration process.

MEDICAL MANAGEMENT

Oxygen therapy.	May be needed to provide more available oxygen.

NURSING DIAGNOSIS:	Sensory perception, alteration in.
SUPPORTING DATA:	Blood supply shunted to vital organs resulting in decrease in peripheral cellular catabolism. Patient c/o feeling cold. Increase in body temperature may be a diagnostic clue to an underlying disorder that is causing the anemia. Fever may be due to an antigen-antibody reaction.

DESIRED PATIENT OUTCOMES:	Physical symptoms decrease or are abated.

INTERVENTIONS

Observe for complaints of feeling cold.

Provide extra clothing, blankets.

Avoid heating pads.

Monitor temperature, noting presence of fever and whether continual or intermittent and time of day it occurs.

Provide cool environment if fever is present, sponge baths and so forth.

Encourage fluid intake unless contraindicated.

MEDICAL MANAGEMENT

Antipyretic medications.

RATIONALE

Attributable to blood being shunted to areas of greater need.

Help retain body heat. Use cautiously as peripheral dilatation may result if patient is volume depleted.

Thermoreceptors in the dermal tissues may be dulled due to oxygen deprivation.

Fever may be attributable to the underlying disease. Time of day may be a diagnostic clue.

Provide relief and aid in reducing temperature.

Replace fluids in the presence of fever.

To reduce fever.

NURSING DIAGNOSIS:	Comfort, alteration in, pain.
SUPPORTING DATA:	Anemia is often secondary to another disease and pain may be an important diagnostic sign such as the anemia associated with joint pain is often secondary to a neoplastic disease.
DESIRED PATIENT OUTCOMES:	Pain is controlled/relieved.

INTERVENTIONS

Assess complaints of pain.

Record complaints of sore bones.

Use bed cradle or acceptable substitute.

MEDICAL MANAGEMENT

Analgesics.

Immobilize joints.

RATIONALE

Baseline data helpful in management.

May be a diagnostic sign.

Avoid pressure on joints and other sensitive areas.

To assist in pain management.

To reduce pain.

357

NURSING DIAGNOSIS:	Nutrition, alteration in, less than body requirements.
SUPPORTING DATA:	A wide variety of gastrointestinal symptoms, primary or secondary, may occur in the patient with anemia. Anorexia may interfere with nutrition.
DESIRED PATIENT OUTCOMES:	Weight is regained/maintained at an appropriate level.

INTERVENTIONS

Observe and record nausea, vomiting, flatus, and any other related symptoms.

Plan diet to the individual's needs and provide attractive, appetizing meals in a pleasant atmosphere.

Observe and record red and sore tongue, ulcerative lesions in mouth, and variations in gums.

Provide and assist with good oral hygiene; before and after meals use a soft-bristled toothbrush, gentle brushing (or substitute cotton balls if tissues bleed easily).

Use mouthwash.

Moisten lips with lubricant.

Provide bland diet, low in roughage, avoiding hot-spicy or very acid foods.

MEDICAL MANAGEMENT

Vitamin supplements.

Iron.

Nutritional supplements.

RATIONALE

Important to note the type of symptoms as some are specific to particular disease.

Alleviate, at least not aggravate, symptoms.

May need specific treatment to prevent infections as mouth is good media for growth of microorganisms.

Diminish bacterial growth.

May be only mouth care if tissue fragility is severe.

Maintain moist surface, prevent cracking, which permits access for bacterial invasion.

When lesions are present, pain will restrict type of foods patient can tolerate.

May be needed as replacement depending on type of anemia and/or the presence of poor nutrition and deficiencies.

May be useful in some types of iron-deficiency anemias.

Additional protein/calories.

| NURSING DIAGNOSIS: | Bowel elimination, alteration in (specify, diarrhea, constipation). |

SUPPORTING DATA:	Among the variety of GI symptoms that occur, diarrhea and constipation may be factors.
DESIRED PATIENT OUTCOMES:	Elimination is normal.

INTERVENTIONS

Provide for adequate fluid intake.

Observe and report diarrhea, constipation, abdominal distention, or flatus.

MEDICAL MANAGEMENT

Antidiarrheal drugs/stool softeners/laxatives.

RATIONALE

Assist in maintaining stool consistency.

May be due to anemia itself or be the result of drug therapy.

May be necessary for short-term control.

NURSING DIAGNOSIS:	Knowledge deficit, treatment and diagnosis of anemia resulting in anxiety and further stress.
SUPPORTING DATA:	Level of anxiety increases with concern over diagnosis and treatment.
DESIRED PATIENT OUTCOMES:	Able to verbalize accurate information about diagnosis and treatment, thus helping to allay anxiety. Patient states need for treatment if symptoms worsen or recur.

INTERVENTIONS

Plan nursing care to reduce stress for patient/SO.

Explain purpose and preparations for diagnostic studies.

Tell patient that loss of blood for laboratory studies will not make disease worse.

Encourage SO to participate in care as desired.

Restrict visitors who appear to annoy and upset the patient.

RATIONALE

Consider total patient, physical, emotional, fear of the unknown increases the stress level, which in turn increases the cardiac workload.

Can lower anxiety.

This is often an unspoken concern.

Promote lessened anxiety. Allow for assessment of potential support and evaluate postdischarge needs.

In the anemic patient, strain and fatigue must be prevented because the cardiac system is already compensating for the decrease in oxygen-carrying capacity of the cells.

Provide for education about specific anemia.

Information can allay anxiety and promote cooperation. In the presence of aplastic anemia, part of treatment is aimed at removal/avoidance of causative factors if possible.

NURSING DIAGNOSIS:	Injury, potential for, complications of treatment.
SUPPORTING DATA:	Patient may react to prescribed treatment on an individual basis.
DESIRED PATIENT OUTCOMES:	Blood studies within normal range for patient and side effects absent or under control.

INTERVENTIONS

Stress importance of taking only prescribed dosages.

Practice good oral hygiene measures.

Use Z-track method for parenteral administration.

Observe for systemic reaction, such as flushing, vomiting, nausea, myalgia.

Observe for signs of hypokalemia during initial B_{12} therapy.

Transfusion:

When administering blood, observe for dyspnea, cough, distended neck veins, or a raise in venous pressure.

Slow or stop transfusion, place patient in an upright position, and notify physician.

Observe for pruritus, wheezing, and laryngeal edema.

Observe for headache, fever, nausea/vomiting, and chills.

Observe for flushing, severe headache, vomiting, diarrhea, hypotension, shocklike symptoms.

Monitor for decrease in potassium and observe for cushinoid appearance.

Observe for alteration in growth, possible impotence, retention of salt and fluids.

RATIONALE

Overdose of iron medication can be toxic.

Iron supplements, such as Feosol, may deposit on teeth and gums.

Prevent extravasation (leaking) with pain.

Possible side effects of parenteral therapy.

During initial 48 hours after start of B_{12} serum K^+ may fall.

May be signs of circulatory overload.

Cardiac system is unable to accept the increased load. Refer to Care Plan: Congestive Heart Failure.

May be signs of allergic reactions thought to be attributed to the transfer of antibodies from the donor that react with the antigens of the recipient.

Febrile reaction is thought to be due to a sensitivity to leukocytes, platelets, or antigens.

Signs of bacterial reaction caused by administration of blood with toxins or bacteria.

May indicate side effects of steroid administration.

The administration of hormones interferes with fluid and electrolyte reactions.

Monitor for indications of increased susceptibility to fatal infection.

High rate of complications after removal of the spleen because of the problems that necessitated procedure.

Discuss required diet alterations.

May be necessary when deficiencies are present. Red meat, liver, egg yolks, green leafy vegetables, whole wheat bread, and dried fruits are sources of iron. Green vegetables, whole grains, liver, and citrus fruits are sources of folic acid.

Discuss the fact that therapy depends on the type and severity of the anemia.

Iron replacement is usually 3–6 months while B_{12} may be required for life.

Iron preparations and folic acid may be taken with orange juice.

Ascorbic acid enhances absorption of iron and the activity of folic acid in erythropoiesis.

Iron preparations are initially taken with meals then scheduled to be shifted to between meals.

Iron is absorbed best on an empty stomach but may cause multiple GI side effects that can be avoided/minimized by giving drug with meals until patient develops a tolerance.

Warn patient of the effects of iron preparations on the GI tract.

"Black" stools can be very frightening to the patient.

Avoid use of aspirin products.

Increases bleeding tendency.

MEDICAL MANAGEMENT

Digitalis and rotating tourniquets.

Emergency treatment may be used in circulatory overload.

Antihistamines.

Used to treat mild allergic reactions.

Parenteral epinephrine.

May be needed for severe respiratory distress in allergic reactions.

Antipyretics.

Treatment of febrile reaction.

Corticosteroids.

Given to stimulate regeneration of bone marrow. May need increased dosage during periods of stress.

Splenectomy.

Minimizes destruction of white cells and platelets.

Immunopressive drugs.

May induce remission of pure red cell aplasia.

Bone marrow transplants.

Treatment of choice in severe aplastic anemia.

DIAGNOSES: Sickle Cell Anemia (Hemolytic Anemias)

Hemolytic anemias are characterized by a reduction in the life span of the RBC. Anemia results when accelerated production can no longer compensate for the reduced span. Hemoglobinopathy, a type of hemolytic anemia, occurs when there is an abnormality in the hemoglobin structure. Sickle cell anemia is an example of this. Sickle cell anemia derives its name from the shape the cell assumes when oxygen tension is low.

PATIENT DATA BASE

NURSING HISTORY

See Care Plan: Anemia.

Occurs most frequently among blacks, and people from the Middle East, Mediterranean, Southern India, regions of South America, and the Carribbean.

Hereditary disease: may have sickle cell trait, or the actual disease.

Pregnancy may precipitate a crisis.

May have had history of previous episodes or this may be the initial episode.

Vaso-occlusive crisis: may complain of pain in extremities, chest, abdomen, and back.

Hypoplastic crisis: pallor and weakness will be apparent.

Hyperhemolytic crisis: may complain of pain, dark urine, and fever.

Sequestration crisis: abdominal pain and weakness will be present.

DIAGNOSTIC STUDIES

Vaso-occlusive crisis: laboratory values will be the same as in a steady state.

Hypoplastic crisis: reticulocytes will be low or absent in peripheral blood and bone marrow will be hypoplastic.

Hyperhemolytic crisis: reticulocytes are increased in peripheral blood, bone marrow will be hyperplastic.

Sequestration crisis: there will be massive, sudden erythrostasis.

CBC: moderate to severe anemia with anisocytosis, poikilocytosis, polychromasia, target cells, and particularly sickle-shaped cells. Immature cells are released to attempt to meet the oxygen needs of the body.

Reticulocyte count may vary from 5–30%.

Sickle cell test: false positive and negative testing may occur.

Erythrocyte sedimentation rate tends to be elevated.

X-rays may indicate thinning of the cerbral cortex as well as osteoporosis.

Lab studies noting survival rate of the cells indicate accelerated breakdown.

Because this disease resembles other hemoglobinopathies as well as other diseases, such as genitourinary tumors, tuberculosis, or vascular disease, differentiation is made on the basis of the sickle cell test, and hemoglobin electrophoreses.

PHYSICAL EXAMINATION

Symptoms are related to the specific crisis patient experiences.

Low-grade fever may be present.

Gallbladder exam: may reveal tenderness and pain.

Cardiac exam: may have signs of failure, circulatory collapse.

Examine skin and sclera for jaundice. May be pale and dry.

Sequestration crisis: the liver and spleen become congested from pooling of large amounts of blood.

NURSING PRIORITIES

1. Provide information to help patient/significant others to deal with disease and hereditary aspects/ genetic counseling.
2. Evaluate/treat complications.
3. Provide for relief of pain.
4. Provide psychologic support for patient/significant others.

Refer to Care Plan: Anemia.

NURSING DIAGNOSIS: Knowledge deficit, cause, treatment, and diagnosis of sickle cell anemia and trait.

SUPPORTING DATA: Patient level of anxiety increases with concern about diagnosis and treatment. Genetic counseling may be helpful in assisting families with decisions about having children when they have the disease/trait.

DESIRED PATIENT OUTCOMES: Patient verbalizes information about identified disorder and symptoms of crisis. Potential for being a carrier with sickle cell trait or having sickle cell anemia is identified.

INTERVENTIONS

Assess current level of knowledge and review signs/symptoms of crisis.

Review ways to avoid recurrences: avoid infections, dehydration, strenuous physical activity/ emotional stress, tight/restrictive clothing, and areas of decreased oxygen, such as air travel and high mountains.

Encourage adequate rest periods.

RATIONALE

Reduce/prevent complications by earlier identification of crisis and initiation of therapy.

Factors that may precipitate crisis by increasing sickling tendency.

Aid in maintaining level of resistance and decrease oxygen needs.

Encourage appropriate dental care and prompt treatment for breaks in skin integrity.

Review genetic implications and refer to counseling as necessary.

Provide information about possibility of trait developing into in vivo crisis.

Encourage wearing of medical identification tag.

Encourage participation in support groups.

Limit opportunity for bacterial invasion/sepsis.

Decision about having children may depend on knowledge of prospect of passing on disease.

In situations leading to severe hypoxia, sickling may occur in those with the trait.

Provide information in case of emergency.

Helpful in adjustment to long-term situation.

NURSING DIAGNOSIS:	Gas exchange, impaired.
SUPPORTING DATA:	Sickling in the pulmonary circulation may cause stasis, ischemia, and pulmonary infarct. This, combined with pulmonary congestion, may impair surface phagocytosis and predispose to bacterial pneumonia.
DESIRED PATIENT OUTCOMES:	Signs/symptoms of pulmonary complications are treated.

INTERVENTIONS

Assess complaints of chest pain and observe signs of increased fever and cough, tachypnea, use of accessory muscles and splinting, signs/symptoms of infection.

Maintain on bed rest and limit activities.

Obtain cultures of sputum.

Screen visitors/staff.

MEDICAL MANAGEMENT

Antibiotics.

Oxygen.

Transfuse with PRCs. Also experimental use of Buffy poor PRCs.

Immunization with polyvalent pneumococcal vaccines.

RATIONALE

Note signs of infection. Increased incidence of bacterial infections can increase the workload of the heart and oxygen requirements.

Reduction of the metabolic requirements of the body, reduces the oxygen needs.

Identify organism.

Protect from sources of infection.

As identifed by culture and sensitivities to combat infection.

Increase oxygen transport to tissues.

Increase number of oxygen-carrying cells. Minimizes isoimmune reactions.

Prevent occurence of pnemonias.

NURSING DIAGNOSIS:	Tissue perfusion, alteration in, decreased.

SUPPORTING DATA:	Myocardial damage from small infarcts, iron deposits, and fibrosis reduces function and lowers cardiac output. AV shunts in both pulmonary and peripheral circulation decrease arterial O_2 saturation. Vaso-occlusive nature of sickling crisis impedes blood flow.
DESIRED PATIENT OUTCOMES:	Perfusion is maintained.

INTERVENTIONS

RATIONALE

Monitor cardiovascular status.	Needs support during a crisis because of increased strain.
Place on bed rest and/or reduced activity.	The amount of hemoglobin that is able to effectively carry oxygen is reduced leading to signs/symptoms of cardiac/respiratory failure. The heart and lungs will attempt to compensate for the decrease in oxygen carrying capabilities.
Note chest pain, dyspnea, or fever.	Sickling of cells can lead to pulmonary infarct.
Note symptoms of CNS infarction.	Stagnant cells must be mobilized immediately to reduce further infarction.
Be alert for signs/symptoms of shock.	Sudden massive splenic sequestration of cells can lead to shock. Often no obvious precipitating cause noted.

MEDICAL MANAGEMENT

Antipyretics.	Reduce fever and tissue oxygen requirements.
Oxygen.	Decrease cardiac workload by increasing available oxygen.
Plasma expanders or blood.	Reverse damage and restore general circulation. Hemoglobin levels are usually stabilized at 6–8 g%. Patient will compensate. See Care Plan: Anemias.

NURSING DIAGNOSIS:	Fluid volume deficit, potential.
SUPPORTING DATA:	Sickling with stasis and vaso-occlusion may cause obliteration of vasa recta affecting the countercurrent mechanism and limiting the kidneys' ability to concentrate urine.
DESIRED PATIENT OUTCOMES:	Kidney function/fluid volume is maintained at desired level.

INTERVENTIONS

Note amount of urine and monitor specific gravity.

Maintain accurate I & O.

MEDICAL MANAGEMENT

IV fluids.

RATIONALE

Kidney loses ability to concentrate urine.

Patient may reduce fluid intake during periods of crises because of malaise and anorexia. May dehydrate easily, which predisposes to recurrent sickling crisis. Negative nitrogen balance occurs and with interference in renal concentration leads to excretion of large volumes of urine.

Replace fluids and reverse renal concentration. Must be given immediately in CNS involvement to decrease hemoconcentration and reduce further infarction.

NURSING DIAGNOSIS:	**Sensory perception, alterations in.**
SUPPORTING DATA:	**Sickled cells may become trapped in the vasculature of the eye causing interference with vision.**
DESIRED PATIENT OUTCOMES:	**Disturbances in vision are identified and treated.**

INTERVENTIONS

Observe for complaints of vision disturbances/pain.

MEDICAL MANAGEMENT

Photocoagulation.

RATIONALE

Early detection of problems may limit damage.

May prevent progression of damage if initiated early.

NURSING DIAGNOSIS:	**Comfort, alterations in, pain.**
SUPPORTING DATA:	**Intravascular sickling results in localized stasis and occlusion. May have migratory joint pain and effusions, especially of knees/elbows.**
DESIRED PATIENT OUTCOMES:	**Pain is treated/minimized.**

INTERVENTIONS

Assess location/type of pain.

Discuss with patient and significant others what works best for them.

Limit activities while encouraging ROM exercises.

Position/support affected joints.

Use localized heat and/or massage.

MEDICAL MANAGEMENT

Analgesics.

RATIONALE

Sickling of cells may lead to cardiac or pulmonary infarction.

Involves them in care and allows for identification of remedies they have already found for relief of pain.

Bed rest may be required to decrease pain when patient is in crisis.

Minimize stress and decrease pain.

Provide comfort and relief.

Reduce pain.

NURSING DIAGNOSIS:	Skin integrity, impaired.
SUPPORTING DATA:	**Stasis and vaso-occlusion often lead to obliterative vascular changes. Thrombosis and cellulitis may result. When bed rest is required, patient may be at risk for decubitus formation.**
DESIRED PATIENT OUTCOMES:	**Thrombosis/cellulitis do not occur.**

INTERVENTIONS

Observe for reddened and open areas.

Routine decubitis care and local measures to combat infection.

MEDICAL MANAGEMENT

Transfuse with packed red cells.

Skin grafts.

Zinc sulfate orally.

RATIONALE

Poor circulation may predispose to rapid skin breakdown.

Decreased circulation requires extra care to prevent breakdown. Refer to Care Plan: Long-Term Care, Nursing Diagnosis: Skin integrity, impairment of, actual, decubitus ulcer.

Increase oxygen delivered to tissues and decrease stasis and vaso-occlusion by diluting the concentration of sickle cells.

If other measures to heal lesion are unsuccessful.

Some success in accelerating healing.

NURSING DIAGNOSIS:	Mobility, impaired.
SUPPORTING DATA:	Multiple/recurrent infarctions, especially of weight-bearing bones may result in osteoporosis with fragmentation/collapse of femoral head or vertebra leading to compression deformities. In addition, these areas of bone infarction provide growth media for bacteria (osteomylitis). Pain and effusions, especially in knees/elbows, may limit movement.
DESIRED PATIENT OUTCOMES:	Mobility is maintained.

Refer to Care Plans: Fractures; Osteomylitis.

NURSING DIAGNOSIS:	Injury, potential for.
SUPPORTING DATA:	Vaso-occlusion of cerebral circulation may cause local infarctions with focal/generalized seizures/strokes.
DESIRED PATIENT OUTCOMES:	Seizures/strokes are treated.

Refer to Care Plans: Seizure Disorders; Cerbrovascular Accident/Hemorrhage.

DIAGNOSIS: Leukemias

The leukemias are a malignant disorder of the blood-forming organs of the body (spleen, lymphatic system, bone marrow). They are differentiated according to the leukocytic system that is involved. The common trait of all leukemias is the unregulated accumulation of a proliferation of white blood cells in the bone marrow that replaces the normal elements. There is an apparent lesion in the hematopoietic stem cell resulting in the inability to differentiate into the normal cells. As the normal cells are replaced by leukemic cells, anemia, neutropenia, and thrombocytopenia occur.

PATIENT DATA BASE

NURSING HISTORY

Symptoms will vary depending on the degree of the disease. (See Care Plans: Anemias; Cancer.)

May have chromosomal disorder, such as Down's syndrome or Franconi's aplastic anemia.

Note geographic factors that may show clusters of incidence.

History of exposure to chemicals, such as benzene, phenylbutazone, and chloramphenical, or excessive levels of ionizing radiation.

May complain of fatigue, malaise, weight loss, and tachycardia.

May have history of infection, bleeding, and/or pain.

May complain of headaches or vomiting in the mornings.

DIAGNOSTIC STUDIES

CBC will indicate a normocytic, normochromic anemia.

Hemoglobin may be less than 10 g/100 ml.

Reticulocyte count is usually low.

WBC may be >50,000/cm. A shift to the left will be reported as there is an increase in the immature WBC.

Neutropenia and thrombopoiesis may be present.

LDH may be elevated.

Serum uric acid may be elevated.

Serum muramidase (a lysozyme) is elevated in acute monocytic and myelomonocytic leukemias.

Bone marrow biopsy will indicate 60–90% of the cells are blast cells, with erythroid precursors, mature cells, and megakaryocytes reduced.

Chest x-ray and lymph node biopsy are done to indicate degree of involvement.

PHYSICAL EXAMINATION

Pharyngitis and gum hypertrophy may be present. (Gum infiltration may be a symptom of acute monocytic leukemia.)

Bruises, purpura, retinal hemorrhages, gum bleeding, or epistaxis may occur.

Lymph nodes, spleen, or liver may be enlarged due to tissue invasion.

Papilledema and exophthalmos may be present.

Note cranial nerve involvement and/or cerebral hemorrhage.

NURSING PRIORITIES

1. Protect patient from infection.
2. Promote optimal physical functioning.
3. Provide for relief of pain.
4. Provide psychologic support throughout treatment and resolution of the disease.

NURSING DIAGNOSIS:	**Injury, potential for, infection.**
SUPPORTING DATA:	**Due to the alterations in WBC from leukemia as well as the treatment, the patient is extremely susceptible to microorganisms and requires protection from infection.**
DESIRED PATIENT OUTCOMES:	**Infection is prevented/minimized.**

INTERVENTIONS

Place in reverse isolation in private room.

Provide sensory input of time, day, frequent visits, and other sensory stimulation techniques.

Provide for good oral hygiene. Use a soft brush for frequent mouth care.

Oral care may be limited to mouthwash. (May prefer mixture of hydrogen peroxide and water.)

Provide soft diet.

Observe for perirectal abscesses.

Avoid venipuncture and injections if possible.

MEDICAL MANAGEMENT

Antibiotics.

Sitz baths.

Stool softeners.

Obtain cultures and serial chest x-rays.

Granulocytes.

RATIONALE

Reduce contact with microorganisms.

Deprivation can occur with isolation.

The oral cavity is an excellent media for growth of organisms.

When severe bleeding is present.

May help reduce gum irritation.

Important to prevent infection.

Break in skin could provide an entry for organisms.

Appropriate to involved organism.

Promote cleanliness, circulation, and healing.

To reduce irritation.

For aerobes/anaerobes and to check pneumonia.

May be given to treat infection in severely neutropenic patient.

NURSING DIAGNOSIS:	**Injury, potential for, hemorrhage.**
SUPPORTING DATA:	**When moderate thrombocytopenia (count of <50,000) occurs there is danger of bleeding.**
DESIRED PATIENT OUTCOMES:	**Bleeding is prevented/minimized.**

INTERVENTIONS

Instruct patient to discontinue contact sports, alcohol intake, and shaving.

Withhold drugs, such as aspirin.

Monitor laboratory reports.

Observe for fatigue and weakness.

RATIONALE

Reduce the danger of bleeding.

Interfere with platelet function.

Patient will be receiving some form of transfusions (platelet and white blood cell transfusions are almost routine in acute leukemia). Granulocyte transfusions are helpful in periods of infections.

May be symptoms of anemia. See Care Plan: Anemias.

MEDICAL MANAGEMENT

Transfusion.

Platelet replacement.

Platelet/clotting factors.

May need RBC when anemia is severe.

May be used to prevent/treat hemorrhage.

May be necessary in DIC.

NURSING DIAGNOSIS:	Injury, potential for, uric acid nephropathy.
SUPPORTING DATA:	Uric acid is increased due to the increase in proliferation of blood cells and their destruction by antileukemic agents.
DESIRED PATIENT OUTCOMES:	Renal stones, gout prevented.

INTERVENTIONS

Encourage oral intake of up to 3–4 liters/day.

RATIONALE

Prevent uric acid percipitating in the urine.

MEDICAL MANAGEMENT

Allopurinal.

Potassium acetate or citrate, sodium bicarbonate.

May be given to reduce the chances of nephropathy.

May be used to alkalinize the urine.

NURSING DIAGNOSIS:	Injury, potential for, administration of chemotherapeutic agents.

Refer to Care Plan: Cancer

NURSING DIAGNOSIS:	Comfort, alteration in, pain.
SUPPORTING DATA:	Alterations in body, such as muscle wasting/edema, and treatment can be painful and anxiety about prognosis can affect comfort level.
DESIRED PATIENT OUTCOMES:	Pain is minimized/managed.

INTERVENTIONS

Observe for complaints of pain. Note changes in degree and site.

Provide for comfort measures and psychologic support.

MEDICAL MANAGEMENT

Analgesics.

Narcotics.

Tranquilizers.

For further information, refer to Care Plan: Cancer.

RATIONALE

Helpful in assessing need for intervention.

Minimize need for medication.

For mild pain not relieved by comfort measures.

When pain is severe.

May be given to enhance the action of analgesics/narcotics.

DIAGNOSIS: Lymphomas, Hodgkin's Disease

Lymphomas are a group of tumors with varying degrees of malignancy. Characterized by progressive and painless enlargement of lymphoid tissue. They are categorized histologically according to the presence or absence of nodules as well as the degree of cellular differentiation. Hodgkin's disease, lymphosarcomas, Burkitt's lymphoma, mycosis fungoides, and the leukemias fall into this category.

HODGKIN'S DISEASE

This disease is classified histologically into subgroups that are important in the prognosis. Paragranuloma has the more favorable outlook, with granuloma and sarcoma, in that order, having less favorable prognoses.

PATIENT DATA BASE

NURSING HISTORY

See Care Plans: Cancer; Anemias.

Tends to be more common in men that women; 2:1 in adults.

Young adults are affected most.

May have periods of unexplained fever.

May complain of generalized pruritus, night sweating, fatigue, weight loss, and malaise. Ask patient to identify onset and duration if possible.

May complain of nodal pain associated with alcohol ingestion.

May complain of dyspena, cough, and dysphagia.

DIAGNOSTIC STUDIES

Refer to Care Plan: Anemias.

CBC: anemia is usually not present in the initial stages, worsens as the disease progresses. WBC may be normal early, with slightly polymorphonuclear leukocytes.

Sedimentation rate: indicates presence of inflammatory or malignant disease.

Serum alkaline phosphatase and calcium levels; elevation may indicate liver or bone involvement.

Renal and liver function studies (IVP, excretory urograms, bone scans, SGOT, BUN, bilirubin, and uric acid) to detect organ involvement.

Chest x-ray, PA and lateral. Whole lung tomograms may be preferred if there is hilar adenopathy.

X-rays of thoracic, lumbar vertebrae, proximal extremities, pelvis, or areas of bone tenderness to determine areas of involvement and assist in staging.

Bone marrow biposy may be done if the alkaline phosphatase is elevated, there is unexplained anemia, other evidence of bone disease, or the disease appears to be in Stage 3.

Lymphangiography/inferior venacavography may be done to supplement other findings.

Lymph node biopsy: to diagnose disease and aid in staging.

The presence of a giant Reed-Sternberg cell on biopsy along with lymph node enlargement, pruritus and unexplained fever, and the pattern of mixed cellularity, lymphocyte depletion, nodular sclerosis, or lymphocyte predominance usually make the diagnosis.

Diagnostic laparotomy and splenectomy may be done.

PHYSICAL EXAMINATION

Symptoms presented will be related to the degree of the disease process.

Palpate for enlarged lymph nodes, particularly the cervical, axillae, or groin.

Temperature may be elevated, slightly or may have a pattern of elevation as high as 104°F from a few days to several weeks alternating with afebrile periods.

Vertebral compression, pain, and occasionally fractures may occur.

Neuralgias may occur due to pressure of enlarged lymph nodes.

Dyspnea may be noted.

Check for edema of the extremities.

Note presence of skin eruptions that might be herpes zoster. (Immune system is impaired in later stages.)

Disease is staged according to degree of involvement:
   Stage 1: involvement of a single lymph node or single site.

   Stage 2: two or more lymph node regions or localization to an organ or node regions on the same side of the diaphragm.

   Stage 3: involvement of lymph node regions on both sides of the diaphragm.

   Stage 4: Diffuse or disseminated disease involving one or more extralymphatic organs or tissue.

Prognosis for survival with treatment is estimated to be 90% for Stage 1 patients; 80% for Stage 2; with a drop in statistics for Stages 3 & 4.

NURSING PRIORITIES

1. Provide psychologic support during extensive diagnostic testing.
2. Provide physical support during chemotherapy and/or radiation therapy.
3. Provide appropriate interventions for complications.
4. Provide for relief of pain.

Treatment of Hodgkin's disease is radiotherapy and/or chemotherapy.

Refer to Care Plan: Cancer for nursing diagnoses and interventions.

DIAGNOSIS: Disseminated Intravascular Coagulation (DIC) (Consumptive Coagulopathy, Defibrination Syndrome)

PATIENT DATA BASE

NURSING HISTORY

Previous situation or disease known to precipitate DIC: rapid transfusion with stored units, severe dehydration, anaphylaxis, shock, hemolytic transfusion reaction, sepsis, abruptio placenta, amniotic fluid embolism, intrauterine fetal demise, liver disease, leukemia, disseminated malignancy, burns, hemorrhagic situation, such as GI bleed, extracorporeal circulation and snake bite.

Presence of blood in urine, stool, around gums, easy bruising or prolonged bleeding from open sites, menorrhagia.

Complains of dizziness, weakness, decreased urine output, increased thirst, chest pain, confusion, dyspnea, pallor, visual changes.

Evaluate current medications, such as anticoagulants or other medications, such as aspirin, which potentiate the action of anticoagulants or prolong clotting.

History of liver disease, bleeding problems, blood dyscrasias.

DIAGNOSTIC STUDIES

Serum K$^+$ level: decrease may cause muscle weakness.

CBC: may show increased WBC (sepsis), decreased Hct & Hb indicating bleeding.

Culture of nose, throat, urine, feces, blood: to identify causative sepsis organism.

Chest x-ray: shows interstitial edema characteristic of microemboli, may also show presence of enlarged heart or CHF.

ECG: arrhythmias due to abnormal K$^+$ level, hypoxia, altered pH; r/o myocardial damage.

ABG: decreased Po$_2$, increased Pco$_2$.

Peripheral blood smear: shows presence of fragmented RBCs.

Factor assay for II, V, VII, VIII, IX: may be reduced.

Platelets: usually low.

PT/PTT: may be prolonged or normal.

Thrombin time: usually prolonged.

Fibrinogen level: usually decreased.

Fibrin split products: increased, resulting from breakdown or degration of fibrin.

Protamine sulfate test: strongly positive.

PHYSICAL EXAMINATION

Petechiae, ecchymosis.

Pain and swelling of joints.

Decreased LOC, convulsions, coma, shock state.

Dyspnea, cyanosis, increased respiration rate.

Oliguria.

Congestive heart failure.

Bleeding from mucous membranes throughout body with guaiac positive urine, stool, NG aspirate/emesis.

N & V, severe abdominal/back pain.

NURSING PRIORITIES

1. Prevent/minimize further bleeding.
2. Maintain adequate perfusion of body tissues.
3. Minimize discomforts associated with bleeding.
4. Assist patient/significant others to deal with anxiety associated with uncontrolled or unpredictable bleeding that may be life-threatening.

NURSING DIAGNOSIS:	**Tissue perfusion, alteration in.**
SUPPORTING DATA:	**Excessive bleeding occurs, which results in loss of large amounts of fluids and proteins from the intravascular space and from the body. Loss of normal intravascular pressure reduces perfusion to non-essential and then essential body tissues. Minute fibrin deposits occur in capillaries throughout the body, decreasing or blocking flow to distal tissues. When the clotting mechanism is abnormally activated by a disease condition, clotting factors and platelets become depleted and bleeding occurs.**
DESIRED PATIENT OUTCOMES:	**Absence of evidence of active bleeding. Vital signs within normal limits, lying and standing. Normal laboratory coagulation studies. Adequate tissue perfusion.**

INTERVENTIONS

Monitor vital signs qh and p.r.n. If stable, and no signs of active bleeding, q2h.

RATIONALE

VS changes, especially increased pulse and decreased BP while standing, may indicate hypovolemia and rapidly changing condition. Document changes that may aggravate symptoms resulting from DIC or demonstrate cardiovascular strain.

Note significant changes and untoward reactions, such as pruritus.

Auscultate lungs q4h.

Provide gentle care.

Note all bleeding, petechiae, and changes in symptoms. Hematest all stools, urine, NG aspirant/emesis.

Keep accurate I & O qh, report if urine output decreased or below 30 ml/h.

Monitor platelet count, liver function studies.

Avoid giving IM injections, use IV, oral, rectal routes, if possible. Apply pressure to puncture sites for 5 minutes. Reinspect site for continued oozing and if present, apply pressure dressing. Inspect for increased size of bruise at puncture site.

Observe for increased bleeding.

May be more prone to transfusion reaction in debilitated state.

Determine occurrence of fluid shifts.

Even minimal trauma can be damaging.

Increase in number and size of such areas demonstrates continuing arterial bleeding. Occurrence of guaiac (+) excreta or stomach contents that were guaiac (−) signifies new bleeding.

Monitor renal perfusion, which may signal impending acute renal failure.

Influence clotting profile.

Injection sites may produce significant loss of blood via oozing interstitially and externally.

May occur if heparin therapy is used.

MEDICAL MANAGEMENT

Treatment of underlying disease process.

Anticoagulants.

Protamine sulfate for heparin-induced bleeding.

Fresh frozen plasma, fibrinogen, clotting factor concentrates, packed RBCs, platelet transfusions.

Epsilon aminocaproic acid (EACA).

Surgery to correct obstetrical problem and so forth.

Controversial but felt to interfere with clot formation and thereby, reduce consumption of clotting factors used in the coagulation process and prevent further deposit of fibrin and thrombi in the tissues. May be contraindicated in intracranial bleed or hepatic failure.

DIC may be erroneously diagnosied and heparin would accentuate bleeding.

Replaces depleted clotting factors, RBCs, plasma proteins to decrease bleeding and increase colloidal intravascular volume and perfusion pressure.

Inhibits fibrinolysis.

NURSING DIAGNOSIS:	**Comfort, alteration in, pain.**
SUPPORTING DATA:	**Bleeding associated with DIC may occur spontaneously anywhere to produce pressure, severe pain, gagging, choking, dyspnea, and so forth.**
DESIRED PATIENT OUTCOMES:	**Comfort is maintained.**

INTERVENTIONS

Evaluate discomfort, monitor for malaise, headache, vertigo, changes in vision, decreased vital signs, cyanosis, N & V, severe abdominal/back pain, chest pain, dyspnea, decreased LOC, hypothermia. Report occurrences and changes.

Provide comfort measures. Support joints in position of comfort with pads and pillows.

Provide frequent uninterrupted rest periods, interspersed with activity.

Give mouth care gently, use diluted mouthwash.

Note respiration and cardiovascular response to analgesics.

MEDICAL MANAGEMENT

Hot/cold compresses.

Analgesics.

Refer to appropriate care plans if hemorrhage occurs in specific organs, that is, brain, kidney, lungs.

RATIONALE

Information as base for interventions.

Decrease pain of movement. Joint pain usually caused by hemarthrosis.

Patient very weak and becomes easily exhausted. Pacing activity and rest helps patient conserve energy.

Oral mucous membranes are easily bruised and may bleed excessively.

Narcotics may depress these systems.

Used cautiously to provide comfort.

Help patient rest more easily.

NURSING DIAGNOSIS:	**Fear, of death.**
SUPPORTING DATA:	**Excessive bleeding and awareness of life threatening nature of the disease are anxiety producing. Life-threatening disease that patient/significant others are usually aware. Anxiety is potentiated by insufficient knowledge and fear of the unknown.**
DESIRED PATIENT OUTCOMES:	**Verbalizes knowledge of disease and treatment and demonstrates lessened anxiety.**

INTERVENTIONS

Assess level of anxiety and understanding of disease.

Discuss signs/symptoms in relationship to disease pathophysiology. Explain rationale for interventions related to alleviation of symptoms.

Encourage patient's/SO's verbalization and questions.

RATIONALE

Allows for identification of the individual need.

Allows patient to focus on specific causes of concern. Understanding of disease and diagnosis can alleviate fear of the unknown.

Provides atmosphere in which necessary questions can be asked and trust can be established.

378

Explain procedures, keep patient/SO aware of positive results and explain negative results.

Providing information can prevent anxiety about the unknown. Stress is linked to increased DIC, as it activates the fibrinolytic system.

Provide information and access to other counseling services, social worker, clergy, financial, as indicated.

May need additional assistance.

Encourage dealing with pain, verbalizing, relaxation, visualization, and so forth.

Pain increases anxiety and anxiety increases pain.

BIBLIOGRAPHY

Books and Other Individual Publications

BARNHART, M.I.: *Sickle Cell.* A Scope Publication, Upjohn Pharmaceutical, 1976.

BELAND, I. AND PASSOS, J,: *Clinical Nursing: Pathophysiological and Psychosocial Approaches,* ed. 3. MacMillan, New York, 1975.

BEYERS, M, AND DUDAS, S.: *The Clinical Practice of Medical-Surgical Nursing.* Little, Brown, & Co., Boston, 1977.

BRUNNER, L, AND SUDDARTH, D.: *The Lippincott Manual of Nursing Practice.* J. B. Lippincott, Philadelphia, 1974.

DAVIDSOHN, I. AND HENRY, J.: *Todd-Sanford Clinical Diagnosis by Laboratory Methods,* ed. 15. W. B. Saunders, Philadelphia, 1974.

GUYTON, A.: *Textbook of Medical Physiology,* ed. 3. McGraw-Hill, New York, 1973.

KIM, M. AND MORITZ, D. (EDS.).: *Classification of Nursing Diagnosis.* McGraw-Hill, New York, 1981.

PHIPPS, W. J., LONG, B. C., AND WOODS, N. F.: *Medical-Surgical Nursing.* C. V. Mosby, St. Louis, 1979.

TILKIAN, S. M., CONOVER, M. B., AND TILKIAN, A G.: *Clinical Implications of Laboratory Tests.* C. V. Mosby, St. Louis, 1979.

WILKINS, R. W. AND LEVINSKY, N. G. (EDS.): *Medicine, Essentials of Clinical Practice.* Little, Brown & Co., Boston, 1978.

Journal Articles

BRAKI, M. ET AL.: Non-Hodgkin's lymphoma: Weighing clues to possible lymphoma. Patient Care, Vol. 11, No. 4, 64–87, Feb. 1977.

COSTEA, N. AND RUBIN, A. (guest editor): *The differential diagnosis of hemolytic anemias.* Med. Clin. North Am. Vol. 57 No. 2, p. 289, W. B. Saunders, Philadelphia, March 1973.

GRAW, R, JR. AND YANKEE, R.: Principles of hematologic supportive care. Med. Clin. North Am. Vol. 57 No. 2, pp. 441–461, W. B. Saunders, Philadelphia, March 1973.

HIRSCH, J.: *New light on the mystery of neutrophil leukocyte.* Medical Times, Vol. 104, No. 11, pp. 88–109, Nov. 1976.

IHDE, D. AND DEVITA, V.: *Management of Hodgkin's disease. Continuing Education for the Family Physician.* Vol. 4, No. 5, pp. 37–45, May 1976.

ISLER, C.: *Blood: The age of components.* RN, Vol. 36, No. 6, pp. 31–41, June 1973.

KASS, L.: *The spectrum of chronic lymphocytic leukemia.* Postgrad. Med. Vol. 60, No. 4, 15 Oct. 1976.

KAHN, S.: *Recent advances in the nutritional anemias.* Med. Clin. North Am. Vol. 54 No. 3, 632–643, May 1970.

KEAVENY, M. AND WILEY, L: *Hodgkin's disease: The curable cancer—Part I: Diagnosis and treatment.* Nursing 75, Vol. 5, No. 3, 49–54.

MARINO, E. AND LEBLANC, D.: *Cancer chemotherapy.* Nursing 75, Vol. 5, No. 11, 23–33, Nov. 1975.

MCCREDIE, K. ET AL.: *Acute leukemia in adults.* Continuing Education for the Family Physician, Vol. 4, No. 5, 37–45.

MCGILLICK, K.: *DIC: The deadly paradox.* RN, 41–43, Aug. 1982.

REINHARD, E. *Anemia weakness and pallor.* In MACBRIDE, C. AND BLACKLOW, R. (EDS.): *Signs and symptoms: Applied pathologic physiology and clinical interpretation,* ed. 5. 599–631. J.B. Lippincott, Philadelphia, 1970.

ROACH, L.: *Assessment . . . Color changes in dark skin.* Nursing 77, Vol. 7, No. 1, 49.

RODMAN, M.: *Drug therapy today: Drugs that affect blood coagulation.* RN, Vol. 32, No. 6, 59–62, June 1969.

ROGERS, J.: *Hope is the key to nursing care—Part II: Nursing needs.* Nursing 75, Vol. 5, No. 3, 55–58, March 1975.

Signs and symptoms in the skin . . . Purpura. Roche Handbook of Differential Diagnoses, Vol. 2, No. 21, Roche Laboratories, Nutley, N.J., 1971.

WRIGHT, J.: *Staging of lymphoma: Prognostic and therapeutic significance.* Postgrad. Med. Vol. 59, No. 4, 95–99, April 1976.

CHAPTER 9

UROLOGY

DIAGNOSIS: Acute Renal Failure (ARF)

PATIENT DATA BASE

NURSING HISTORY

Abrupt loss of kidney function over a period of a few hours to a few days. Acute renal failure is usually reversible.

Assessment of patient to determine which of many possible conditions contributed to development of ARF.

Numerous causes of ARF can be categorized into 3 major areas:

PRERENAL: caused by interference with renal perfusion; decreased glomerular filtration rate (GFR).
  Examples of conditions causing decreased renal perfusion:
  volume depletion: vomiting, diarrhea, hemorrhage, excessive use of diuretics, burns, renal salt-wasting conditions, glycosuria, renal artery occlusion.
  volume shifts: "third space" sequestration of fluid, vasodilating drugs, gram-negative sepsis.
  volume expansion: cardiac pump failure, hepatorenal syndrome, severe nephrotic syndrome.

RENAL (or Intrarenal): refers to parenchymal changes caused by disease or nephrotoxic substances.
  Acute tubular necrosis (ATN) accounts for 90% of cases of acute oliguria;
  destruction of tubular epithelial cells results from (1) ischemia/hypoperfusion (similar to prerenal hypoperfusion except that in renal hypoperfusion, correction of the causative factor may be followed by continued oliguria for up to 30 days), and/or (2) direct damage from nephrotoxins. Other causes of ATN include the presence of heme pigments (such as myoglobin and hemoglobin liberated from damaged muscle tissue, and the toxins produced in gram-negative septicemia).
  Additional renal causes of acute renal failure include: glomerulonephritis; microvascular and large vascular occlusion (as in hemolytic-uremic syndrome); thrombosis; vasculitis; scleroderma; trauma; atherosclerosis; tumor invasion; and cortical necrosis (caused by prolonged vasospasm of the cortical blood vessels).

POSTRENAL: obstruction in the urinary tract anywhere from the tubules to the urethral meatus.
  Common sources of obstruction include prostatic hypertrophy, calculi, invading tumors, surgical accidents, and retroperitoneal fibrosis.

Iatrogenically-induced acute renal failure is of major concern and should be considered when other sources have been ruled out. It is also important to be aware of the most common factors associated with acute oliguria provoked by health care personnel in the course of therapy for other conditions so that such occurrences can be prevented. The most common causative factors include administration of potentially toxic agents, such as antibiotics, anesthetics, and radiographic contrast media; failure to adjust the dosage of drugs whose primary site for excretion is the kidneys; failure to use prophylactic preventive measures, such as adequate hydration and diuresis; surgical complications; and delay in recognizing and responding to the primary disease.

DIAGNOSTIC STUDIES

Values vary depending on whether the cause of ARF is prerenal, renal, or postrenal. All the processes result in the disturbed physiology of water and sodium metabolism in the body as well as accumulation of potassium.

PRERENAL

BUN and creatinine levels are elevated with a 20:1 or greater ratio, respectively, due to inability of kidneys to excrete nitrogenous wastes with resultant azotemia.

Urine specific gravity is usually greater than 1.020 because the kidneys are trying to concentrate the urine.

Elevation of urine osmolality above 450 Osm/Kg, and usually greater than plasma osmolality.

Urine sodium level less than 20 mEq/L; it may drop much lower than this if the patient has a sodium deficit, because the kidneys will retain sodium in the serum.

Hyperkalemia caused by inability of the kidneys to excrete potassium.

RENAL (Intrarenal or Intrinsic)

BUN and creatinine levels are elevated. In the presence of oliguria, BUN may rise as much as 20 points or more per day. A creatinine clearance test will often show a marked decrease before BUN and creatinine levels show significant elevation.

Urine specific gravity is less than 1.015, and urine osmolality is below 450 mOsm/Eq and is less than or near plasma osmolality. These findings reflect parenchymal damage with resultant loss of concentrating ability.

Urine sodium is above 40 mEq/L due to inability of the kidney to reabsorb sodium.

The ratio of urine urea nitrogen to BUN and of urine creatinine concentration to plasma creatinine concentration is less than 10:1.

In ATN, urinalysis shows presence of renal tubular cells, tubular cell casts, coarse granular casts, red blood cells, hemoglobin, and red blood cell casts.

In acute glomerulonephritis, urinalysis shows hematuria, proteinuria, and the presence of red blood cell and hemoglobin casts.

Hyperkalemia and elevated CPK are present if there has been significant renal tissue damage.

POSTRENAL

Urine may show a fixed specific gravity and elevated sodium concentration with little or no proteinuria. Urinalysis may also reveal scanty sediment, occasional white and red blood cells, and hyaline or fine granular casts.

X-rays may be taken to assess kidney size and to determine if renal stones or urinary tract obstruction are present.

PHYSICAL EXAMINATION

The most common overall sign of acute failure is alteration in the expected urine output. Usually there is a marked diminution of 24-hour output of less than 400 ml; less common is the nonoliguric or high-output failure when urine is dilute and nearly isomolar.

ARF symptomatology varies depending on the cause: Fluid volume deficit and/or decreased cardiac output support prerenal cause: thirst, tachycardia, hypotension, dry mucous membranes, confusion, listlessness, poor skin turgor.

Intrinsic renal failure: symptoms secondary to sodium and water overload: paroxysmal nocturnal dyspnea, dyspnea on exertion, weakness caused by anemia, peripheral edema, pulmonary edema, mild hypertension (glomerulonephritis).

Postrenal failure onset is usually quite sudden and painful. Symptoms include difficulty initiating and maintaining a urinary stream, and may include dysuria if infection intervenes. Depending on the degree of obstruction, there may be diminished or no urine output; fluid overload may result.

In obstruction with renal stones, the presenting symptoms include: excruciating flank pain radiating to the genital area; the pain is colicky in nature and requires potent analgesics for relief.

Prostate exam: may be enlarged

NURSING PRIORITIES

1. Maintain fluid and electrolyte balance.
2. Prevent secondary infection.
3. Minimize effects of azotemia.
4. Assist with emotional/psychologic needs of patient and significant others during prolonged stress of ARF.

NURSING DIAGNOSIS:	Fluid volume, alteration in, imbalance (potential).
SUPPORTING DATA:	Decreased glomerular filtration and/or obstruction to urinary outflow results in oliguria, fluid overload, and electrolyte imbalance. The course of ARF is marked by 4 stages: 1. **Oliguric-anuric phase:** urine output less than 400ml/day; may last one day to 8 weeks, (average 8–15 days). 2. **Early diuretic phase:** return of glomerular filtration and halting of BUN rise. 3. **Late (recovery) diuretic phase:** falling of BUN. 4. **Convalescent phase:** begins when BUN becomes stable and ends when patient has returned to normal activity; may take several months. Decreased urinary output, increasing daily weight, azotemia.

DESIRED PATIENT OUTCOMES:	Weight stabilized at normal level. BP stable; urine specific gravity usually between 1.010–1.025.

INTERVENTIONS

Assess fluid status. Maintain meticulous intake-output records.

Daily weight; same time, same scale, same clothing.

Observe skin turgor and mucous membranes.

Note orthostatic changes in BP, pulse, and respiratory rate.

Monitor vital signs.

Monitor central venous pressure readings.

Monitor urine specific gravity.

Monitor heart and breath sounds.

Monitor serum sodium concentration.

Note peripheral edema.

MEDICAL MANAGEMENT

Fluid replacement IV/po.

Diuretics.

Dialysis. Refer to Care Plan: Dialysis.

RATIONALE

Accurate assessment of fluid status will allow for effective fluid volume replacement.

Daily weight is a much more accurate parameter of fluid balance. Patients with well-managed acute renal failure lose 0.2–0.5 kg of body weight or more per day. This represents the usualy daily weight loss from protein catabolism.

Poor skin turgor and pale, dry mucous membranes indicate diminished fluid volume.

Positional changes in BP and pulse occur in the presence of intravascular volume deficit as a compensatory mechanism to maintain adequate cardiac output.

Hypertension can result directly from fluid overload, or from a disruption in the renin-angiotensin system.

Indicator of circulating fluid volume.

Reflects the kidney's ability to concentrate urine (value is negated by intrinsic renal disease).

Fluid retention and overload may lead to congestive heart failure and pulmonary edema.

Useful in detecting gross changes in water and salt balance. Hyponatremia generally reflects a relative excess of body water.

Fluid volume overload causes an increased hydrostatic pressure forcing fluid into the tissues.

One method used to calculate fluid replacement needs is to record the patient's total intake and output for eight-hour periods, add 200 ml to a negative balance (I < O) or subtract 200 ml from a positive balance (I > O), and replace that total over the next eight-hour period.

Remove fluid.

To correct overload if other measures fail.

NURSING DIAGNOSIS:	Fluid volume, alteration in, composition (electrolytes and blood buffers) related to acute loss of renal function.

SUPPORTING DATA:

The most serious potential electrolyte imbalance is hyperkalemia. In addition to the kidney's inability to excrete potassium, this electrolyte is released in greater quantities from the body cells when acidosis is present and is further increased by rapid tissue catabolism as in fever, severe infection, and trauma. The effects of hyperkalemia may be accentuated and potentiated by hypocalcemia and hyponatremia. The most common acid-base derangement in ARF is metabolic acidosis due to accumulation of acid waste products of protein catabolism and incomplete combustion of carbohydrates and lipids. Metabolic acidosis is aggravated by hyperkalemia, hyperphosphatemia, and loss of bicarbonates from diarrhea.

DESIRED PATIENT OUTCOMES:

Serum potassium level within normal limits. Normal cardiac rhythm with adequate cardiac output.

INTERVENTIONS

Monitor serum electrolytes, especially potassium.

Note symptoms of malaise, anorexia, paresthesias, and muscle weakness.

Continuous ECG monitoring.

Be aware of signs and symptoms of other common electrolyte disorders:

Hyponatremia.

Hypocalcemia.

RATIONALE

Progressing increase may herald life-threatening complications.

As diuresis occurs, K^+ levels may drop. Symptoms may be obscured by the preexisting clinical state.

Provides evidence of impending potassium intoxication in the presence of progressive hyperkalemia. The ECG initially shows peaked T waves with increased amplification, then prolonged QRS complexes, prolonged P–R intervals and diminishing P waves resulting in various degrees and types of heart block.

Refer to Care Plan: Fluid and Electrolyte Imbalances.

Usually an effect of hemodilution.

Etiology unclear; symptoms include circumoral and distal extremity paresthesias, painful carpopedal spasms, positive Chvostek's and Trousseau's signs, and tetany.

385

Hyperphosphatemia.	May occur as a result of dietary intake or catabolism.
Hypermagnesemia.	ECG mimics hyperkalemia. Symptoms of neuromuscular paralysis and respiratory depression.
Monitor blood gas levels.	Early detection of accumulation of acid/base imbalances.
Avoid the use of antacids containing magnesium.	Can contribute to the development of hyperphosphatemia.

MEDICAL MANAGEMENT

Kayexalate	Cation exchange resins may be administered orally or rectally to facilitate excretion of potassium.
with	
Sorbital.	Prevent impaction and to eliminate the sodium released by the exchange resins.
50% dextrose/regular insulin.	Emergency measure to drive K^+ into the cells.
Sodium bicarbonate or calcium gluconate IV.	Until other measures can reduce K^+ level. Use cautiously to correct severe acidosis and temporarily prevent cardiac arrest.
Fluids.	Replacement necessary in hyponatremia.
Phosphate binders with decreased dietary intake.	To treat hyperphosphatemia.
Physostigmine.	In hypermagnesemia may reverse respiratory depression and neuromuscular paralysis.
Oxygen.	Maintain arterial PO_2 while metabolic acidosis is being corrected.
Dialysis.	To filter excess fluid. Refer to Care Plan: Dialysis.

NURSING DIAGNOSIS:	**Nutrition, alteration in, less than body requirements.**
SUPPORTING DATA:	**Catabolism and prolonged starvation associated with common symptoms of anorexia and GI disturbances in ARF. Depressed sensorium, GI complications and symptomatology, such as nausea, vomiting, oral lesions, ulcers of the stomach and duodenum, and diarrhea contribute to the patient's risk of inadequate nutritional intake.**
DESIRED PATIENT OUTCOMES:	**Positive nitrogen balance is evidenced by wound healing, good muscle tone and strength, stable body weight.**

INTERVENTIONS

Maintain accurate record of dietary intake.

Assess response to prescribed diet therapy: appetite, daily weight, muscle mass and strength, wound healing.

Frequent mouth care, at least qid: brush teeth and gums with soft bristled brush; rinse with hydrogen peroxide or antiseptic mouthwash.

MEDICAL MANAGEMENT

Nutrition support team. Diet: usually high-calorie, low-protein, low-sodium, and low-potassium diet. Will probably have a fluid restriction also.

Nasogastric tube feedings and TPN.

RATIONALE

Diet history and daily record of intake may be used to calculate amount of calories, proteins, carbohydrates, and fats consumed.

Reflects state of protein metabolism and nitrogen balance.

Prevent stomatitis; promote salivation; maintain moistness and integrity of oral mucous membranes.

May need supplemental feedings and oral feedings may be impractical. Even in patients without severe complications, diets low in sodium and potassium and limited in protein and fluid prove unpalatable and therefore an unreliable source of nutrition.

Alternative methods of providing nutrition. (Refer to Care Plan: Total Parenteral Nutrition.)

NURSING DIAGNOSIS: Injury, potential for, secondary infection.

SUPPORTING DATA: Occurs as a result of complications of or conditions related to ARF. Catabolism and uremia lead to poor wound healing. CNS depression by uremia or oversedation promote development of respiratory tract infections. Indwelling urinary catheters are a common source of nosocomial infections. Stomatitis, often found in patients with ARF, can lead to parotitis.

DESIRED PATIENT OUTCOMES: No signs of infection are present.

INTERVENTIONS

Monitor oral temperature, leukocyte count and differential.

RATIONALE

Hypothermia in the ARF patient may mask the expected rise in temperature associated with infection; temperatures as low as 99°F may indicate serious infection. Leukocytosis may be present without infection, however, a shift to the left is a definite indication of infection. Secondary infections account for as many as 50–90% of the deaths from ARF.

Inspect skin for breaks in integrity: redress wounds using aseptic techniques; use aseptic technique during insertion and daily dressing changes of IV cannulas. Change IV tubing every 24 hours.

Skin care measures to prevent breakdown:
    antiembolic stockings;
    frequent position changes;
    extra mattress padding, alternating pressure, or egg mattress;
    lubrication and massage of skin; and
    careful manipulation of the patient's body.

The skin is the body's first line of defense. Prevention of skin breakdown is best, but when it occurs, aggressive wound care using strict aseptic techniques is essential. Intravenous catheters are a significant source of sepsis.

Facilitate mobilization of fluid.
Increase circulation to the area.
Prevent concentration of pressure over bony prominences.
Increase circulation, prevent dryness.
Prevent trauma.

Respiratory Tract:
Provide oral hygiene; encourage coughing and deep breathing; assist with incentive spirometry. Auscultate breath sounds.
Prevent aspiration when feeding or administering tube feedings.

The accumulation of bronchial secretions, immobility, aspiration of GI contents, and the inhibitory effect of peritoneal dialysis on ventilation promote bronchopneumonia, tracheitis, and tracheobronchitis.

Urinary Tract:
Avoid use of urethral catheter.

If catheterization becomes necessary use strict aseptic technique during insertion; thoroughly cleanse perineum at least q.i.d.

Tape catheter to the thigh in women and the abdomen in men.

Patients in ARF do not have the normal irrigating effect of urine.
Indwelling catheters are usually not necessary in the oliguric patient; unless a neurologic deficit is present, voiding will occur as renal function returns.
Decreases irritation from excessive movement in the urethra.

GI Tract:
Provide oral hygiene at least q.i.d.

Use soft rubber or small-bore rubber NG tubes.

Stomatitis most likely develops as a result of poor oral hygiene, dehydration, ammonia-producing bacteria that cause chemical irritation, and/or alteration of the normal flora by antibiotic therapy. Polyvinyl nasogastric tubes have been found to cause esophagitis by their constant irritating presence.

MEDICAL MANAGEMENT

Wound debridement and use of air-occlulsive dressings.

Uremia inhibits the proliferation of fibroblasts and the formation of granulation tissue, thus decreasing the effectiveness of the body's natural defenses once the skin integrity has been broken.

Antibiotic irrigating solutions.

The effectiveness of continuous bladder irrigation with an antibiotic solution is as yet undetermined. Use of this therapy is determined by the individual practitioner.

Antibiotic therapy.

Drug choice and dosage may be altered by degree of renal function.

Pulmonary toilet measures (e.g., postural drainage, percussion, incentive spirometry, and IPPB).

Mobilize secretions, prevent atelectasis/pneumonia.

NURSING DIAGNOSIS:	Cardiac output, alteration in, decreased.
SUPPORTING DATA:	Diminished contractility associated with cardiac tamponade. Pericarditis occurs in as many as 18% of patients with ARF. If not diagnosed and treated, pericarditis can lead to cardiac tamponade, cardiac failure, and death.
DESIRED PATIENT OUTCOMES:	Cardiac output remains stable.

INTERVENTIONS

Routinely assess cardiac status including auscultation of apical pulse.

Be aware of and observe for most common early symptoms of pericarditis:
Pleuritic chest pain relieved by upright position.
Fever.
Pericardial friction rub.
Unexplained tachycardia.

MEDICAL MANAGEMENT

Chest x-rays.

Echocardiography.

Steroids.

Pericardiocenteses and/or pericardiectomy.

RATIONALE

Pericardial friction rub may be the earliest sign of pericarditis.

Severity of symptoms depends on rate and quality of accumulation of fluid in the pericardium.

Initially negative for pericardial effusion.

Useful for detecting effusion.

Anti-inflammatory effect.

To drain accumulating fluid if cardiac function is compromised.

NURSING DIAGNOSIS:	Injury, potential for, neurologic dysfunction associated with uremic encephalopathy.
SUPPORTING DATA:	Uremic encephalopathy is less frequent with the advent of dialysis. The etiology is unclear, but the syndrome occurs more frequently with rapid onset of azotemia and in cases complicated by cerebral ischemia, hypoxemia, sepsis, or severe metabolic dysfunction. It is thought to be preterminal.
DESIRED PATIENT OUTCOMES:	Clear sensorium is maintained.

INTERVENTIONS

Be aware of and observe for signs and symptoms of uremic encephalopathy: apathy, defective recent memory, episodic obtundation, dysarthria, tremors, asterixis, myoclonus, frank convulsions, and coma.

If patient has convulsions, refer to Care Plan: Seizure Disorders.

RATIONALE

Detect and treat early signs of neurologic dysfunction.

May result in injury to the patient.

NURSING DIAGNOSIS:	Injury, potential for, anemia.
SUPPORTING DATA:	In patients with long-standing disease, severe anemia often develops from many causes.
DESIRED PATIENT OUTCOMES:	Anemia is recognized/treated.

Refer to Care Plan: Anemias.

CARE PLAN: Peritoneal Dialysis

PATIENT DATA BASE

NURSING HISTORY

Evidence of a clinical situation in which rapid return to normal blood values is desired. Examples of such situations include acute poisoning, acute/chronic renal failure, severe edema states, hepatic coma, metabolic acidosis, and extensive burns with prerenal azotemia.

History of diabetes is an indication for starting dialysis with lower creatinine levels than for nondiabetics in some clinical institutions.

Criteria for selection of patients for chronic intermittent hemodialysis may include:
1) The presence of terminal, irreversible renal failure for which conservative therapy is ineffective.
2) The absence of other chronic or incapacitating illnesses or problems that cannot be corrected.
3) Reasonable evidence that if the patient enters the program the patient will live more than one year.
4) Reasonable expectation of rehabilitation.
5) Patient and significant others having knowledge and understanding of the therapy and the willingness and ability to cooperate.

Patients need to:
1) have a degree of self-sufficiency;
2) understand the disease, as well as its treatment and effects; and
3) be able to adhere to a special regimen.

DIAGNOSTIC STUDIES

Evidence of uremia in patient's blood values caused by a loss of renal function:
Increased BUN, serum creatinine, uric acid, K^+, Na^+, phosphate and sulfate, and Mg^+.
Decreased creatinine clearance, Ca^{++}, Cl^-, Na^+, may be decreased or increased.
Acidosis.
Water metabolism imbalance.
Abnormal glucose tolerance as a result of impaired insulin secretion, use, and degradation.

Coagulation studies evaluate effects of disease process on clotting time as well as anticoagulation during the dialysis procedure.

Urinalysis: See Care Plan: Acute Renal Failure.

Blood levels of certain toxic substances based on patient's history.

Liver function studies to detect hepatitis.

Serum albumin protein levels may be decreased due to inappropriate loss via kidneys and catabolism.

Chest x-ray may show evidence of congestive heart failure secondary to fluid volume overload.

Arterial blood gases; metabolic acidosis.

WBC may indicate early inflammatory response in patients susceptible to infection.

Hemoglobin, hematocrit, red blood cell count diminished because of decreased erythropoietin production in patients with renal disease as well as disturbances in platelet function and clotting factors.

EEG may show neurologic changes resulting from uremia.

PHYSICAL EXAMINATION

Assess signs/symptoms associated with uremia.

Cardiovascular: evaluate BP, P, CVP, heart sounds, weight for evidence of: hypotension or hypertension, congestive heart failure, volume overload, arrhythmias, pericarditis (rub), edema, cardiomyopathy.

Respiratory: rate, breath sounds, pulmonary edema, hyperventilation.

Gastrointestinal: caloric intake, intake and output of fluids, stomatitis, anorexia, nausea, vomiting, diarrhea, constipation, melena, hematemesis, abdominal distention, hiccoughs.

Urinary: decreased output most common.

Hematopoietic: signs of bleeding (bruises, melena, petechiae, hematemesis) and weakness secondary to anemia.

Neurologic: assess orientation and level of consciousness, asthenia, myoclonus, mental aberration, drowsy to delerium, coma, convulsions, peripheral neuropathy, fatigue, sleep disturbance, headache, lethargy.

Skin: evaluate integrity, rashes, pruritus, purpura/ecchymosis, dryness, excoriation, Ca^{++} deposition, uremic frost, pallor caused by anemia.

Decreased resistance to infection, monitor temperature, urine, sputum, wounds.

Musculoskeletal: joint pains, osteodystrophy related to disturbance in calcium/phosphate metabolism.

Psychologic: depression, anxiety, denial, psychosis.

NURSING PRIORITIES

1. Promote fluid/electrolyte balance.
2. Provide adequate nutrition to maintain positive nitrogen balance and prevent protein catabolism.
3. Prevent infection.
4. Maintain cardiovascular and respiratory stability.
5. Maintain vascular access for hemodialysis.
6. Provide information and support to assist patient/significant others in dealing with illness/therapy/outcome.

NURSING DIAGNOSIS:	**Injury, potential for, associated with traumatic insertion of peritoneal catheter.**
SUPPORTING DATA:	**The peritoneal catheter is inserted via a trocar into the peritoneal cavity through a small incision 1 to 2 inches below the umbilicus; this location is close to the bladder and bowel.**
DESIRED PATIENT OUTCOMES:	**Atraumatic insertion with bowel and bladder intact.**

INTERVENTIONS

Have patient empty bladder prior to catheter insertion.

RATIONALE

Displace bladder away from abdominal surface; distended bladder more likely to be punctured during catheter insertion.

Monitor for signs/symptoms of bladder perforation:
>Intense urge to urinate.
>Large urine outputs.
>High urine glucose concentration.

Dialysate leaking into bladder.

Dialysate contains either 1.5% or 4.25% glucose and will test high for glucose if excreted via bladder.

If above signs/symptoms occur, stop dialysis and assist with catheter removal as needed.

Immediate action will prevent further damage.

Monitor for signs/symptoms of bowel perforation:
>Fecal material in dialysate returns.
>Urge to defecate.
>Stool mixed with large amounts of fluid.
>Hypotension/tachycardia.

Immediate action imperative.

Increased pressure from fluid leaking into bowel causing sensation of need to defecate.
Result of vasovagal stimulation.

Notify physician if above signs/symptoms occur; stop dialysis; monitor BP, pulse q 15–20 minutes.

Surgical repair of the perforation may be done immediately followed by several days of antibiotic lavage (via antibiotic added to dialysate).

Monitor for frank bloody drainage that continues past the first few runs.
If significant bleeding occurs; apply pressure dressing, ice packs, or sandbag; monitor BP, pulse.

Blood-tinged returns should subside after the first few runs.
Persistent bleeding may be due to arteriole laceration during catheter insertion.

NURSING DIAGNOSIS:	**Bowel elimination, alteration in, ileus.**
SUPPORTING DATA:	**Peritoneal cavity is used; catheter insertion and/or dialysate may cause physical and/or chemical irritation to the bowel resulting in a disturbance of bowel function.**
DESIRED PATIENT OUTCOMES:	**Normal bowel function maintained.**

INTERVENTIONS

Monitor for signs/symptoms persisting after the day of catheter insertion:
>Absence of bowel sounds.
>No bowel movements.
>Malaise, anorexia.
>Abdominal distention, tenderness.
>Large NG aspirates.

If ileus occurs:
>Patient should be NPO until bowel sounds return.
>Provide for adequate nutritional intake.
>Encourage ambulation if possible.

RATIONALE

Ileus may occur from bowel irritation/inflammation.

Prevent further distention.

MEDICAL MANAGEMENT

Medications, laxatives, stool softeners, and so forth.	To increase bowel activity.
Apply warm packs to abdomen.	Stimulate peristalsis.

NURSING DIAGNOSIS:	**Comfort, alterations in, pain.**
SUPPORTING DATA:	**Any or all of the following may be sources of pain or discomfort: Improper catheter placement in peritoneal cavity. Catheter irritation of bladder, vagina, root of penis. Cold or acidic dialysate. Peritoneal and/or abdominal distention with dialysate. Air infusion through administration tubing. Intraperitoneal infection.**
DESIRED PATIENT OUTCOMES:	**Absence of/or minimal discomfort during insertion, dialysis, and after discontinuation of dialysis.**

INTERVENTIONS

RATIONALE

Assess quality, location, duration, alleviation, and worsening of pain or discomfort.

Nature and location of pain helps in identifying source; pain may occur at point of catheter insertion into abdomen, at catheter tip inside peritoneum; generalized in the lower abdomen, perineal region; localized in bladder, vagina, or at root of penis.

Warm dialysate to body temperature before administration.

Cold dialysate can cause discomfort, lowering of core body temperature.

Monitor for pain that starts during inflow and continues during equilibration phase.

Acidic dialysate may be irritating.

Monitor for discomfort most pronounced toward end of inflow and beginning of outflow phases; assure patient, discomfort usually lessens after first few runs; position patient in semi-Fowler's.

This type of discomfort is most likely due to peritoneal and/or abdominal distention with dialysate.

Monitor for symptoms of air infusion (most commonly, pain in the shoulder blade area); prevent introduction of air into the system when making connections and infusing dialysate.

Irritation to diaphragm by free air results in referred pain.

Monitor for severe, continuing pain.

May indicate peritonitis.

MEDICAL MANAGEMENT

Analgesics.

Relieve discomfort and pain.

Smaller dialysate volumes.

If discomfort from distention worsens or is unrelieved, will reduce amount of fluid in abdomen.

Bicarbonate or procaine.

May need to add to dialysate when pain is present.

Aspiration.

If air infusion occurs, it is sometimes possible to remove it from the peritoneum through the catheter with the patient in the knee-chest or Trendelenburg position.

NURSING DIAGNOSIS:　**Injury, potential for, infection.**

SUPPORTING DATA:　**The major danger in the peritoneal dialysis procedure is the development of peritonitis; potential sources include contamination during catheter insertion, introduction of pathogens via dialysate or administration tubing, or infection through the catheter insertion site.**

DESIRED PATIENT OUTCOMES:　**Dialysate returns clear, patient painfree and afebrile.**

INTERVENTIONS

Monitor for signs/symptoms of peritonitis: fever, cloudy dialysate, leukocytosis, severe persistent abdominal pain.

Use strict aseptic technique during catheter insertion, insertion site dressing changes, and administration of dialysate.

If peritonitis occurs: send sample of dialysate returns for culture and sensitivity.

Monitor results of blood cultures.

Monitor renal function tests; BUN, creatinine.

RATIONALE

Provides for early intervention and enhances opportunity for successful treatment.

Peritonitis is associated with failure to observe sterile technique and to take necessary precautions.

Identify organism to initiate specific antibiotic treatment.

Choice of drugs based on culture and sensitivity tests.

Decreased renal function is considered in the choice of drugs.

MEDICAL MANAGEMENT

Antibiotics in dialysate. Systemic antibiotics.

Treatment includes systemic and intraperitoneal antimicrobial agents. The infection can often be eliminated without removing the catheter.

Note: Sterile peritonitis, an inflammatory response, may occur in reaction to the composition of the dialysate.

NURSING DIAGNOSIS:	Breathing patterns, ineffective.
SUPPORTING DATA:	Pressure resulting from the instillation of fluid may elevate the diaphragm and cause respiratory distress. Fluid in the abdomen may decrease the depth of respirations possible, causing dyspnea and contributing to development of atelectasis and pneumonia.
DESIRED PATIENT OUTCOMES:	Respiratory rate and ABGs within normal limits, lungs clear, and patient afebrile.

INTERVENTIONS

Place patient in semi-Fowler's position.

Instruct and assist patient with coughing, deep breathing, and use of incentive spirometry.

Monitor quality of respirations, breath sounds, quantity and quality of secretions, ABG results, chest x-rays, and temperature.

MEDICAL MANAGEMENT

Incentive spirometer.

RATIONALE

Use gravity to facilitate respiratory excursion.

Prevent atelectasis through maximum opening and clearing of the small airways.

Detect early signs of atelectasis, pneumonia.

Prevent atelectasis.

NURSING DIAGNOSIS:	Skin integrity, impairment of, potential.
SUPPORTING DATA:	Leakage of dialysate at the catheter insertion site can cause excoriation of the skin.
DESIRED PATIENT OUTCOMES:	Skin intact with absence of/or minimal leakage of dialysate around catheter insertion site.

INTERVENTIONS

Frequently assess insertion site dressing to determine need for changing and/or leakage.

If leakage occurs; weigh dressing and include in record of fluid loss, change dressing as frequently as needed.

RATIONALE

Early identification of leakage allows for appropriate intervention.

Inflow/outflow records are important in determining effectiveness of peritoneal dialysis.

Keep skin around catheter insertion site clean and dry; use protective skin barrier preparations as needed.

Prevent maceration and excoriation from irritating dialysate returns.

MEDICAL MANAGEMENT

Suture.

May be needed to tighten the catheter if leakage occurs at the insertion site.

NURSING DIAGNOSIS:	Fluid volume, deficit, potential.
SUPPORTING DATA:	Dialysis fluid contains either 1.5% or 4.25% glucose, both of which are hypertonic to normal plasma and will provide for an osmotic gradient for the passage of fluid through the peritoneal membrane into the dialysate and may result in too rapid removal of water from the intravascular space.
DESIRED PATIENT OUTCOMES:	Desired alteration in body fluid volume and weight with normal electrolyte levels and urinary output equal to or greater than patient's baseline.

INTERVENTIONS

Assess fluid volume status: weigh q6–10 runs when peritoneum is empty.

Take BP, pulse q15 min during first run and q1–2 hours thereafter.

Monitor central venous pressure and pulmonary artery pressures.

Monitor urine output with specific gravity; compare to patient's baseline data.

Monitor serum sodium and glucose levels.

Monitor carried K$^+$ levels closely.

RATIONALE

Too rapid fluid removal may be detected by comparing baseline body weights after dialysis has begun.

Decreased BP, increased pulse are early signs of compensatory response to hypovolemia.

Excellent indicators of fluid volume status; early changes can be detected and corrected.

Decreased urine output, in relation to patient's baseline status, may be early indication of decreased renal perfusion as a result of hypovolemia; urine will be more concentrated.

Hypertonic glucose solutions may cause hypernatremia by removing more water than sodium.

Hypokalemia can cause cardiac arrhythmias leading to death; it also enhances the effect of digitalis and can cause digitalis intoxication.

MEDICAL MANAGEMENT

Alternate 1.5% with 4.25% solutions.

Hyperglycemia is related to infusion of 4.25% glucose dialysate solution, which can lead to cellular dehydration, confusion, and eventually, coma (refer to Care Plan: Hyperglycemic, Hyperosmolar Nonketotic Coma).

NURSING DIAGNOSIS: Fluid volume, alteration in, excess (potential).

SUPPORTING DATA: Occlusion of the peritoneal catheter by omentum or fibrin clots will result in retention of dialysate within the abdomen. Sole use of 1.5% dialysate, particularly in adults, may not provide sufficient osmotic gradient to remove desired amount of fluid from the intravascular space. Inefficient dialysis may result from difficulties during the inflow or the outflow phases.

DESIRED PATIENT OUTCOMES: Efficient dialysis sufficient to achieve normovolemia and electrolytes to levels within normal limits.

INTERVENTIONS

Assess fluid volume status: serial body weights q6–10 runs.

Keep accurate I & O; monitor for positive fluid balance.

Monitor BP, P, CVP, and PAP (pulmonary artery pressure).

Monitor urine output.

Monitor serum electrolytes; assess for confusion, disorientation.

Monitor for signs of difficulty in both inflow and outflow phases; check for kinks in tubing, position of dialysate bottle; air in tubing; signs of peritonitis.

If difficulty in drainage occurs: turn patient from side to side; press hands against retroperitoneal spaces; sit up in bed, if able.

RATIONALE

Body weight gives a more accurate assessment of fluid volume status than does I & O.

Indicates patient is retaining fluid.

Elevations indicate hypervolemia.

Hyponatremia may result as dilutional effect of fluid volume overload.

Adhesions may cause obstruction of the catheter; may occur if patient has had previous abdominal surgery, peritonitis, or if catheter is in place several days. Drop chamber of dialysate administration tubing, should be 4 feet above the patient for optimum inflow.

These methods may enhance fluid drainage from the abdomen by use of gravity, and mechanical pressure. Useful if patient unable to turn.

MEDICAL MANAGEMENT

Increase proportion of runs using 4.25% glucose concentration.

Increased glucose concentration will create a higher osmotic gradient, causing rapid removal of water from the intravascular space into the dialysate.

NURSING DIAGNOSIS: **Nutrition, alteration in, less than body requirements.**

SUPPORTING DATA: **Patients undergoing peritoneal dialysis often have anorexia, nausea and vomiting, stomatitis, and decreased absorption of calcium and iron. Protein catabolism is a result of inadequate nutrition and the primary disease process itself.**

DESIRED PATIENT OUTCOMES: **Maintain positive nitrogen balance and ideal body weight.**

INTERVENTIONS

Assess patient's nutritional status and response to diet therapy: body weight; wound healing; muscle mass and strength.

Diet of low-sodium, moderate amount of high-quality protein, high-carbohydrate; potassium and sodium restriction will depend on BP and serum levels; small, frequent meals are generally most effective.

Mouth care, including brushing teeth and rinsing with antiseptic mouthwash, q2h.

RATIONALE

Provide a baseline of current status as compared with premorbid condition for evaluation of therapy.

Provide sufficient calories to maintain positive nitrogen balance and prevent muscle wasting.

Prevent stomatitis; clean and moisten oral membranes.

MEDICAL MANAGEMENT

Antiemetics.

Supplemental calories and feeding via a peripheral or central venous catheter.

Calcium, iron vitamin and iron supplements may be given.

Referral to nutritional support team or dietitian.

Testing of immunologic competency as indicated.

Relieve nausea and prevent vomiting.

If malnutrition occurs and patient is unable to ingest sufficient calories. (Refer to Care Plan: Total Parenteral Nutrition.)

Renal diets are frequently deficient and intake may be inadequate.

May need more accurate assessment of nutritional status and needs.

Related to protein balance.

NURSING DIAGNOSIS:	Fear, of unknown procedure.
SUPPORTING DATA:	Patient/significant others may have little experience with or knowledge of peritoneal dialysis. Patient may be too ill to inquire about procedures; SO may feel inadequate in foreign surroundings to provide comfort and support; may feel frustrated and alienated from the patient.
DESIRED PATIENT OUTCOMES:	Patient's/SO' behavior demonstrates understanding and acceptance of condition and treatment.

INTERVENTIONS

Assess level of fear, anxiety; evaluate family dynamic interrelationships.

Determine need for assistance from other resources including clergy, social worker, psychiatrist.

Explain disease process, dialylsis procedure, diagnostic tests.

Assess level of understanding and alleviation of anxiety.

Encourage and provide opportunities for patient/SO to ask questions and verbalize fears.

MEDICAL MANAGEMENT

Referral to social services, psychiatrist.

Antidepressant medications.

RATIONALE

Level of anxiety will determine level of nursing intervention to alleviate those fears. Understanding patient's family role will aid nurse in determining family/patient needs during illness and hospitalization.

May need additional support, counseling, and in depth discharge planning.

Enhances acceptance, decreases anxiety.

Provides for ongoing evaluation.

Create open, honest atmosphere in which exchange of information and feelings is enhanced.

Provide help for patient/significant others to cope with long-term aspects of disease/therapy.

May benefit from mood-elevating drug.

CARE PLAN: Hemodialysis

PATIENT DATA BASE

Refer to Care Plan: Peritoneal Dialysis.

NURSING DIAGNOSIS:	**Fluid volume deficit, potential.**
SUPPORTING DATA:	**Hemorrhage caused by needle dislodgement during hemodialysis. Accidental disconnection of shunt between treatments. Systemic heparinization during hemodialysis with resultant alteration in coagulation times. Repeated punctures of fistula through thin, dry skin resulting in erosion of fistula vessel walls. Puncture of external shunt. Tissue breakdown around cannula or fistula insertion sites. Patient taking antihypertensive medication.**
DESIRED PATIENT OUTCOMES:	**Closed system maintained during hemodialysis. Shunt remains intact. Coagulation times are moderately prolonged during dialysis. No bleeding from puncture sites. External shunt intact. No evidence of internal or external bleeding.**

INTERVENTIONS

Assess cannula or fistula for patency and intactness; check for signs/symptoms of external/internal bleeding after hemodialysis procedure.

Never take blood pressure measurements on the extremity used for hemodialysis; instruct patient to avoid tight clothing.

Permit no punctures of external shunt.

Monitor for signs/symptoms of hypovolemia: hypotension, tachycardia, oliguria.

If hypovolemia occurs: place patient in more horizontal position.

RATIONALE

Hemorrhage may occur in patients undergoing hemodialysis as a result of altered coagulation times from systemic heparinization, or erosion or aneurysm formation around cannula or fistula.

Prevent excessive pressure on the fistula or cannula, which may cause tissue damage and result in erosion or aneurysm formation.

May cause damage with resultant hemorrhage.

Fluid shifts may occur during dialylsis or in immediate post-run period.

Maximize venous return.

MEDICAL MANAGEMENT

Fluids/volume expanders.

Vasopressors.

Antihypertensive drugs may be withheld on the day of dialysis; check physician's order.

Replacement therapy.

Reduce size of vascular bed and maximize circulating volume.

These drugs prevent vascular reactivity to volume changes; severe postural hypotension can result.

NURSING DIAGNOSIS:	**Fluid volume, alteration in, excess, potential.**
SUPPORTING DATA:	**Inability of diseased kidneys to filter and excrete water results in body fluid overload. Cerebral edema as a result of the dialysis disequilibrium syndrome. Fluid overload occurring between dialysis treatments associated with high total body sodium and intake of fluids. Hypertension, peripheral edema, congestive heart failure, and pulmonary edema may occur.**
DESIRED PATIENT OUTCOMES:	**Normovolemia. BP, P within normal limits. Weight gain between treatments not more than 0.5kg/ 24hrs. Serum Na$^+$ within normal limits. Prevent or detect disequilibrium syndrome early.**

INTERVENTIONS

Monitor BP, P between treatments and q15–30 min during treatments.

Monitor serial body weights between dialysis.

Monitor serum sodium levels. Instruct patient/SO regarding control of sodium intake and its relationship to fluid balance; discuss fluid intake restrictions.

RATIONALE

Hypertension may result from fluid overload.

Changes in body weight reflect changes in fluid volume.

Usual fluid intake for adults is 500 to 800ml plus urine volume for previous 24 hours; intake of fluids will vary according to patient's residual kidney function, body weight, physical activity, type of food intake (fluids in food), ambient temperature, and tolerance to excess fluid accumulation between treatments.

Monitor for signs of dialysis disequilibrium syndrome: hypertension, headache, nausea and vomiting, agitation, twitching, confusion, seizures.

This syndrome may occur toward the end of dialysis or *following* it; it is related to the osmotic gradient produced via the bloodbrain barrier by efficient removal of urea from the blood but not from the brain tissue itself. The urea in the brain draws water from the plasma and extracellular fluid causing cerebral edema. Prevent by instituting dialysis in a severely uremic patient slowly; peritoneal dialysis may be used at first to reduce the urea levels more slowly.

Monitor for signs/symptoms of heart failure: dyspnea, orthopnea, fatigue, rales/rhonchi, peripheral edema.

Hypervolemia in heart failure results in low-cardiac output and venous congestion producing characteristic signs/symptoms. If detected early, complications may be avoided by altering dialysis treatment to remove excess fluid.

NURSING DIAGNOSIS:	**Cardiac output, alteration in, decreased.**
SUPPORTING DATA:	**Occurrence of cardiac arrhythmias because of abnormal potassium levels. Hyperkalemia results from inability of the kidneys to excrete potassium in renal disease. Potassium is removed by dialysis; the day before dialysis the potassium level may be dangerously high. Infection or excessive dietary intake may also contribute to hyperkalemia. Too rapid changes in potassium levels may cause cardiac arrhythmias. Digitalized patients are at risk for digitalis toxicity and cardiac arrhythmias related to rapid changes in potassium levels.**
DESIRED PATIENT OUTCOMES:	**Serum K⁺ levels within normal limits. Hemodynamic stability with adequate cardiac output.**

INTERVENTIONS

Monitor apical and radial pulses routinely.

RATIONALE

Pulse deficit (difference between apical and radial rates) may indicate presence of potentially serious, unperfused cardiac rhythms.

Instruct patient/SO regarding potassium intake prescription.

The dietary potassium restriction is usually 40 to 70 mEq/day for adults (or 1 mEq/kg of ideal weight/day).

Monitor electrolytes.

Note fluctuations in K$^+$ levels.

MEDICAL MANAGEMENT

Telemetry.

Identify arrhythmias and assess need for therapy.

NURSING DIAGNOSIS:	**Injury, potential for, hepatitis.**
SUPPORTING DATA:	**Dialysis-associated hepatitis is a serious public health problem. Potential modes of transmission include ingestion of infected blood through the oral-fecal route, inoculation by needle punctures and skin cuts, and possibly the inhalation of blood aerosols. There appears to be a vast reservoir for patients, staff, and presumably, the community in hemodialysis centers. Dialysis patients are often hepatitis-associated antigen (HAA) positive for prolonged periods. Home dialysis decreases exposure to sources of infection found in hospital or in-center settings.**
DESIRED PATIENT OUTCOMES:	**HAA-negative, SGOT, SGPT within normal limits.**

INTERVENTIONS

Monitor serial liver function tests monthly: SGOT, SGPT, and hepatitis-B antigen.

If hepatitis occurs:
    Isolate patient.
    Administer supportive care as indicated.
    Monitor liver function tests.

RATIONALE

HAA or hepatitis-B antigen is thought to be evidence of either an active or carrier state; liver enzymes will elevate in hepatitis.

Extreme precaution must be taken to avoid cross-contamination.

MEDICAL MANAGEMENT

Consider transfer to home dialysis.

Patients on home dialysis and following transplantation appear to have a lower incidence of hepatitis than in-hospital or satellite dialysis.

NURSING DIAGNOSIS: Gas exchange, impaired.

SUPPORTING DATA: Anemia associated with the effects of uremia and/or the hemodialysis procedure itself. Hemolysis may occur from dialysate that is too warm or too cold, or of wrong concentration or composition. Decreased erythropoietin production by diseased kidneys results in decreased red blood cell production and fragile red blood cells. Turbulent blood flows in dialysis machine can cause destruction of fragile RBCs. Patients with renal disease may have splenomegaly with shortened RBC survival. Transfusion reaction.

DESIRED PATIENT OUTCOMES: Hemodialysis without hemolysis or excessive loss of blood. Hct, Hb, platelets stable. Blood administered without hemolysis.

INTERVENTIONS

Monitor serial Hct, Hb, and platelet levels before, during, and after hemodialysis.

Avoid unnecessary blood tests.

Minimize number of dialysis runs by dietary control of protein intake.

Minimize blood loss during hemodialylsis: connection and disconnection of blood lines, blood samplings, dialyzer leak or rupture, residual blood in dialyzer, gastrointestinal hemorrhage or menorrhagia that may be associated with anticoagulation.

Carefully check for compatibility and monitor closely for early signs of transfusion reactions.

Observe for signs/symptoms of a severe transfusion reaction: fullness in the head, severe pain in the back, chest tightness, tachycardia, hypotension.

Clamp off the blood and immediately notify the physician.

RATIONALE

It has been found that patients can tolerate Hct levels of less than 14%.

Decreasing laboratory studies to a every three months in stable patients eliminates a very real source of blood loss.

Reducing catabolism of protein will minimize uremia and limit need for dialysis runs which cause anemia.

Anemia is one of the problems that continue on dialysis.

Blood is no longer necessary to prime the dialyzers, so transfusions are used only for patients who are seriously symptomatic from anemia or in preparation for surgery.

Signs start immediately; rapid hemolysis occurs with administration of incompatible blood.

MEDICAL MANAGEMENT

Benadryl.

Helpful for minor transfusion reaction.

NURSING DIAGNOSIS: **Injury, potential for, shunt malfunction and/or infection.**

SUPPORTING DATA: **The vascular access for hemodialysis is subject to malfunction and/or infection. A subcutaneous AV fistula is a surgically created opening between an artery and vein (most commonly the radial artery and cephalic vein); fistula life is 3–4 or more years. The external AV cannula is easy to insert and can be used immediately; because it is an external device made of foreign material, it is more prone to infection, clotting, and hemorrhage than is the fistula; cannula life averages 7–10 months. Ischemia of the hand may result from the "steal" phenomenon; the nondominant arm is used whenever possible.**

DESIRED PATIENT OUTCOMES: **Patent shunt/fistula is maintained.**

INTERVENTIONS

Monitor for patency frequently following placement of a shunt or fistula: listen for bruit.
Palpate for thrill by lightly depressing fistula or lightly pressing shunt.
> For shunts: monitor color of blood; normal: uniform medium red color. Dark purplish red may indicate sluggish flow or beginning clot formation. Dark reddish black next to clear yellow fluid indicates full clot formation with separation of red cells from serum.

Feel shunt for warmth.

Instruct patient in precautions following:
Do not allow cuff BP readings or venipuncture in extremity with shunt or fistula.
Instruct patient not to sleep on affected extremity.
Avoid wearing tight clothing on affected extremity.
Avoid lifting or carrying heavy objects.
Bathing and swimming are possible with a cannula but extremity must not be immersed.

RATIONALE

The rerouting of the arterial blood flow with its increased pressure causes the vein and its branches to dilate; an arterialized vein results. The bruit and thrill result from the turbulent flow in the usual low-pressure vein.

Indication blood flow at body temperature.

Prevent shunt/fistula closure caused by clotting.

Carry cannula clamps at all times.

Limit hemorrhage in the event of accidental separation.

Use aseptic technique for daily shunt dressing change as well as thorough cleaning pre/post dialysis.

Prevent contamination with subsequent infection.

Monitor for signs of local infection: swelling, redness, warmth in skin temperature around shunt or fistula site; drainage from shunt insertion sites; decreased circulation to extremity, fever.

Detect early and treat to prevent systemic infection.

Monitor for systemic sepsis: fever, shaking, chills, hypotension, peripheral vasocontriction.

Local infection may become systemic if not treated effectively and kept localized; patients undergoing hemodialysis are particularly susceptible to infection (accounts for 20% of deaths). Unexplained fever in a patient on dialysis should suggest infection in the cannula.

Monitor BUN, serum K$^+$.

Infection increases metabolism and thus the load of nitrogenous wastes and potassium.

Monitor for signs of "steal" syndrome; pain with use of the hand, discomfort with elevation of the hand.

The ulnar arterial circulation must be adequate if the radial artery is used, to avoid subsequent arterial insufficiency to the hand.

MEDICAL MANAGEMENT

Culture and sensitivity.

In the presence of suspected infection, the specific organism can be identified from the drainage so effective antibiotic therapy can be instituted.

Antipyretics and/or antibiotics.

As indicated to decrease temperature/infection.

Dry heat to the extremity.

Helps dilate the vessels and increase blood flow.

Clot removal.

If fistula/shunt clots.

Surgical removal and placement of new shunt/fistula.

May need to replace if occluded.

NURSING DIAGNOSIS:	**Nutrition, alteration in, less than body requirements.**
SUPPORTING DATA:	**Protein losses occur from catabolism, dietary restrictions, and hemodialysis procedure. Adequate protein intake is needed to build, repair, and maintain body cells and tissues.**
DESIRED PATIENT OUTCOMES:	**An adequate protein intake as reflected by a BUN to serum creatinine ratio of 10:1. Maintain positive nitrogen balance, and ideal body weight.**

INTERVENTIONS

Assess patient's nutritional status and response to prescribed diet therapy: body weight, percentage of lean muscle mass, muscle strength, wound healing, appetite activity level.

Instruct and reinforce prescribed dietary regimen with patient/SO; individualize diet based on usual dietary habits and budget; assess home situation regarding food preparation.

Monitor BUN, serum creatinine.

MEDICAL MANAGEMENT

Have the dietitian do a complete nutritional assessment. Include measurement of immunologic competency.

RATIONALE

Diet restrictions depend on the frequency and efficiency of treatments; intake of protein, sodium, potassium, and fluids may be regulated depending on the patient's needs and responses.

Eating is one of the most important social events; individualizing dietary prescriptions to more closely fit with patient's lifestyle and expectations may enhance compliance with the regimen.

Assess adequacy of dietary regimen.

More accurate assessment of nutritional status; immunologic competence is directly related to protein balance.

NURSING DIAGNOSIS:	**Coping, ineffective, individual/family, potential.**
SUPPORTING DATA:	**Hemodialysis causes a change in body image and role in family dynamics. With dependence on a machine to perform what was previously a normal function the patient experiences loss of control and enforced inactivity in living with a chronic illness that can be controlled but not cured, and is terminal without treatment.**
DESIRED PATIENT OUTCOMES:	**Patient/SO verbalize realistic expectations and acceptance of hemodialysis as a mode of treatment. Progress through stages of grieving to acceptance of illness and treatment. Participate in self-care activities and administer treatment regimen as ordered. Financial needs met and relationships preserved.**

INTERVENTIONS

Assess adjustment to life on dialysis: physical well-being; cognitive functioning, psychologic well-being, family dynamics.

RATIONALE

Adjustment varies considerably among individuals. Patients who are self-confident, extroverted, motivated to live, and who have the strong emotional support of their spouses and SO are more likely to live successfully in dialysis.

Assess stage of grieving process.	Excessive mourning is a sign of severe depression that may result in lack of cooperation with medical regimen and eventually, suicide.
Observe patient's self-care activities related to aspects of prescribed regimen: dietary cooperation, administration of medications, care of fistula or shunt.	Improper care of the cannula and excess weight gain are common; suicide may result from deliberately drinking excessive water, eating excess amounts of foods containing potassium, and from separation of the cannula.
Arrange for financial or marital counseling as needed, support family and mobilize psychosocial resources.	Professional counseling may be helpful in dealing with stresses of illness and treatment.
Encourage questions and expression of feelings.	Listening is therapeutic as well as a means of identifying problems.
Assess and discuss (as needed) sexual desire/performance.	Often decreased by uremia and does not return even with adequate hemodialysis. Both impotence in men and decreased orgasm in women are reported.
As much as possible, have patient make decisions regarding scheduling and process of care.	Restore independence, autonomy within prescribed regimen.
Assess level of anxiety on an ongoing basis.	Anxiety reduces ability to concentrate and learn. Usual outlets for release of tension and anxiety, alcohol, sex, exercise, food, or withdrawal are not practical for these patients.
Assess understanding of disease process and need for dialysis; provide information in terms at patient's level of understanding as needed.	Although understanding treatment regimens has been shown to have little effect on cooperation, it has been effective in reducing anxiety, and may help in terms of learning.

DIAGNOSIS: Urinary Tract Infection

PATIENT DATA BASE

NURSING HISTORY

Clinical manifestations differ depending on location of infection in urinary tract:

ACUTE PYELONEPHRITIS
Severe constant ache over one or both kidneys. Pain may radiate to lower abdomen. Nausea, vomiting.

ACUTE CYSTITIS
May follow initiation of sexual activity in women; ''Honeymoon Cystitis''
Burning on urination, urgency, frequency, nocturia, mild low backache, suprapubic discomfort.

CHRONIC PYELONEPHRITIS
Major cause is refluxing vesicoureteral valves. If not reflux, obstruction is likely cause. Mild discomfort over kidney. Vesical irritability. Generally, very few symptoms except during acute excerbations.

CHRONIC CYSTITIS
May be associated with chronic infection of upper tract, obstruction or reflux. Vesical irritability.

Incidence of cystitis increases with age, peaking in women over age 60 when the bladder, ureters, and urethra have become less elastic, resulting in decreased muscle tone, which impairs complete emptying of the bladder.

Cystitis is rare in children and men: rarely occurs between the ages of 10 and 20, with the exception of the sexually active female adolescent, where the incidence is very high.

Four major factors that promote urinary tract infections are:

1. Structural and functional abnormalities of the urinary tract (e.g., congenital malformation, Foley catheter).
2. Obstruction of the flow of urine (e.g., benign prostatic hypertrophy).
3. Impaired bladder innervation (e.g., neurogenic bladder).
4. Reduced general body resistance (e.g., chronic illness, malnutrition, steroid therapy).

The major predisposing cause of nosocomial (hospital-acquired) infection is urethral instrumentation, particularly, urinary catheterization.

Women are more predisposed to urinary tract infections than men; possibley contributing factors are a shorter urethra (3–5cm compared to 15cm in men) and close proximity of urethra to anus and vagina in women (permits bacteria on rectal or vaginal mucosa to be transferred to urethra). Sexual intercourse seems to play a significant role in moving bacteria along the perineum to the urethra.

Pregnant women are at increased risk for vesicoureteral reflux, predisposing them to pyelonephritis.

Acute cystitis in men is usually associated with urinary retention caused by an obstruction from an enlarged and/or infected prostate gland.

Most urinary tract infections affect the bladder only; majority of UTIs are asymtomatic and clear spontaneously.

DIAGNOSTIC STUDIES

White blood cell count: will be elevated, with shift to the left in acute infection.

Sedimentation rate: will be elevated, indicating acute infection.

Anemia may be found in chronic pyelonephritis.

Urinalysis: specific gravity may be low (1.001–1.003) in pyelonephritis if tubular damage has affected kidney's ability to concentrate urine.
Color may be cloudy due to white cells or smoky due to red blood cells.

Heavily infected urine has a particularly unpleasant odor.

Urine is generally alkaline (pH greater than 7) in urinary tract infections.

Appears cloudy or turbid because of presence of red blood cells, white blood cells, or bacteria.

Proteinuria, if present, may indicate renal disease.

Hematuria.

White cells.

White cell casts (pyelonephritis).

Bacteriuria (greater than 100,000 organisms/ml in a properly obtained and stored midstream specimen).

Cystoscopy: check for obstruction in the lower urinary tract.

Intravenous pyelogram: to rule out upper urinary tract disease.

PHYSICAL EXAMINATION

ACUTE PYELONEPHRITIS
Intermittent high fever with chills. Acutely ill. Tachycardia. Tenderness over kidney (at costovertebral angle). May develop abdominal distention with rebound tenderness.

CHRONIC PYELONEPHRITIS
Low grade fever. Mild hypertension.

ACUTE CYSTITIS
Low grade fever. Bladder spasm. Tenderness over bladder. Tender urethra.

CHRONIC CYSTITIS
May be asymptomatic except for laboratory findings.

NURSING PRIORITIES

1. Alleviate discomfort.
2. Assist patient in identifying causative factors; teach preventive measures
3. Provide for follow-up care as indicated.
4. Prevent complications.

NURSING DIAGNOSIS:	Comfort, alterations in, pain.
SUPPORTING DATA:	Dysuria (burning), urgency, frequency associated with cystitis. Flank pain, abdominal discomfort associated with pyelonephritis.
DESIRED PATIENT OUTCOMES:	Discomfort relieved.

INTERVENTIONS

Encourage bed rest in acute phase.

Encourage increased fluid intake.

MEDICAL MANAGEMENT

Apply heating pad to abdomen or flank as needed. Local heat to perineum via sitz bath.

Antispasmotics (belladonna or atropine with phenobarbitol).

RATIONALE

Assists healing.

Relieves pain/discomfort by flushing bladder.

Promotes circulation, which assists in healing and encourages muscle relaxation.

For bladder spasms.

411

Phenazopyridine hydrochloride, such as Pyridium and Azodine.

Azo dyes are believed to have an anesthetic effect. Will color the urine. If using Clinistix/Testape will alter result. Clinitest may be used without alteration.

NURSING DIAGNOSIS:	**Knowledge deficit, recurrence, inadequate treatment.**
SUPPORTING DATA:	**UTI recurs in approximately 35% of patients. Patients may stop taking their antibiotics as their symptoms subside. The infection will keep recurring unless the cause is determined and eliminated.**
DESIRED PATIENT OUTCOMES:	**Full course of prescribed medication is taken and recurrence is minimized.**

INTERVENTIONS

Instruct patient in the importance of taking ALL prescribed medication, even after the symptoms disappear.

Instruct women in preventive measures:
After intercourse, empty bladder and drink two glasses of water.
After a bowel movement, wipe from front to back.
Wear cotton, not nylon, panties; avoid pantyhose, tight slacks.
Notify physician if vaginal discharge occurs, treat promptly.

Avoid use of strong cleansing powders and bleaches in laundry.

Instruct in proper technique for collection of urinary specimens; deliver specimen to lab immediately, or store in refrigerator as directed by hospital laboratory.

Instruct uncircumcised men in proper cleansing under foreskin.

RATIONALE

Full course of antibiotic therapy is needed to eradicate bacteria in urine.

Prevent recurring infections.
Flushes bladder and minimizes opportunity for ascending infection.
Avoid fecal contamination of urethra.
Prevent excessive moisture that may lead to maceration of perineum.
Opportunistic infection may occur.

May cause perineal irritation from clothes and lead to maceration and breakdown.

Obtaining sterile midstream urine specimen for determination of infecting organism is crucial step in treatment.

Accumulation of exudate may provide media for bacterial growth.

NURSING DIAGNOSIS:	**Injury, potential for, associated with urinary catheterization.**
SUPPORTING DATA:	**The major predisposing cause of nosocomial infection is urethral instrumentation, particularly urinary catheterization.**

DESIRED PATIENT OUTCOMES:	Catheterization done only when necessary. Asepsis and closed system maintained. Urine flow remains unobstructed and infection is prevented.

INTERVENTIONS

Use catheterization as means to facilitate urinary elimination only when absolutely necessary.

Insert catheter using strict aseptic technique.

Maintain closed drainage system; i.e., never disconnect the catheter-tubing junction.

Obtain urine specimens by aspiration with sterile needle and syringe from self-sealing catheter or drainage port.
Tape drainage tubing and suspend bag.
"Milk" the catheter as needed.

Use strict aseptic technique when irrigating via two-lumen catheter:
   Cleanse catheter-tubing junction before disconnecting it.
   Use a new sterile syringe with each irrigation.
   Don't touch the sides of the syringe plunger.

   Don't store irrigating solution in opened bottles, or at room temperature. Any solution remaining should be refrigerated and discarded after 24 hours.

Observe urine flow for significant changes or if output is less than 30ml/hour.

MEDICAL MANAGEMENT

Irrigate three-lumen catheter with antibiotic solution.

RATIONALE

Use sparingly as a mode of treatment because of associated risks:
Abdominal surgery to prevent accidental injury to distended bladder.
Postoperative urinary retention.
Critically ill patients who require hourly monitoring of urinary output.
Incontinent patients who require precise measurement of urine output.

Prevent contamination of the urinary tract.

Closed drainage has been shown to be vastly superior to open drainage (i.e., any disconnection of the catheter from the drainage tubing).

Maintain the closed system.

To prevent accidental disconnection.
Maintains patency and reduces need for irrigation.
Prevent contamination of open drainage system.

It will come in contact with irrigating solution on refilling.

Limits growth of bacteria.

Foreign object (catheter) in the bladder predisposes to bacteriuria; and urinary stasis promotes bacterial growth.

Irrigation with an antibiotic solution may delay onset of bacterial invasion for up to 10 days in closed system, but it will not cure infection; long-term antibiotic irrigation may actually result in colonization of resistant organisms. Irrigation is indicated when urine flow is sluggish. The three-lumen catheter permits continuous or intermittent irrigation without ever disconnecting the catheter-tubing junction.

NURSING DIAGNOSIS:	Urinary elimination, alteration in pattern.
SUPPORTING DATA:	Frequency, urgency, incontinence, nocturia.
DESIRED PATIENT OUTCOMES:	Voiding adequate amounts of clear, yellow, odorless urine.

INTERVENTIONS

Observe pattern and frequency of urinary elimination; monitor I & O.

Observe quality of urine.

Give information to patient that altered elimination pattern is temporary and will return to normal when infection is cleared.

Encourage patient to verbalize fears/concerns.

RATIONALE

Help verify diagnosis.

Distinctive odor and color to infected urine.

Alleviate anxiety.

May have created other problems in the patient's life, such as disruption in sexual activity with resultant marital problems; inability to continue working. Talking about problems enables appropriate and therapeutic interventions to be instituted.

NURSING DIAGNOSIS:	Injury, potential for, infection.
SUPPORTING DATA:	Potential complications from untreated or ineffectively treated infections include septicemia, calculus formation, hypertension, renal insufficiency, and renal failure.
DESIRED PATIENT OUTCOMES:	Complications are avoided and/or minimized.

INTERVENTIONS

Encourage fluids to 3L/day if patient physiologically able to tolerate this amount, otherwise to patient's ordered limit. Include cranberry juice in intake. Acid-ash diet may also be helpful.

Cleanse and dry perineum q8h; observe for vaginal discharge.

RATIONALE

Promote urinary flow, mechanical movement of bacteria out of bladder (vesical defense mechanism). Of particular importance when patient is taking sulfonamide drugs because of potential for crystaluria. Assists in acidifying the urine, which decreases the rate of bacterial growth.

Monilia is a common side effect following prolonged use of antibiotics.

MEDICAL MANAGEMENT

Acidifying agents.

Acidification alone does not lower the colony count, but is believed to retard bacterial growth; ascorbic acid is most effective acidifying agent.

Broadspectrum antimicrobials.

Initially used until urine C & S results are known. Drug therapy may be altered when organism is identified and sensitivity to drug is established.

Sulfonamides; Gantrisin.

Urinary antiseptic.

Soda bicarbonate.

May be given to alkalize urine when sulfa drugs are being used.

DIAGNOSIS: Benign Prostatic Hyperplasia

PATIENT DATA BASE

NURSING HISTORY

In early cases, the patient usually has minimal symptoms because the detrusor musculature is capable of compensating for increased resistance to urinary flow.

With increased obstruction of the urethra, symptoms of prostatism occur: decreased force of urinary flow, hesitancy in initiating voiding, inability to empty bladder completely, urgency and frequency of urination, nocturia, dysuria, urinary retention, mass in lower abdomen, overflow urinary incontinence, and hematuria. Suprapubic, flank, or back pain may be present. This may be caused by acute urinary tract infection, acute urinary retention, or renal colic with resulting hydronephrosis.

Prostatic hyperplasia is characteristically a disease of men over age 45. It is not related to occupation, hobbies, or diet.

Urinary elimination is altered in some ways. There may be evidence of weight loss or edema, pallor, and tenderness in renal areas.

History may include renal hypertension and chronic urinary tract infections.

Family history of cancer, hypertension, kidney disease.

Medication: antihypertensive and urinary antibiotics or antibacterial agents.

DIAGNOSTIC STUDIES

Urinalysis: Color: yellow to bloody. Appearance may be cloudy, pH 7. Bacteria may be present. Blood 0–4 + . WBC, RBC may be present microscopically.

Urine culture: may present with staphylococcus aureus, proteus, klebsiella, pseudomonas, or E. coli.

BUN >20/per 100 ml, serum creatinine >1.0 mg%: indicating secondary renal failure; seen only in advanced stages.

Acid phosphatase: increased because of cellular growth and hormonal influences in cancer of the prostate and may indicate metastasis to the bone.

WBC: may be greater than 11,000, indicating infection.

IVP with post voiding film: shows delayed emptying of bladder, varying degrees of upper urinary tract obstruction, and the presence of prostatic enlargement.

VCU may be used instead of IVP, because it does not use systemic dye.

Cystoscopy: to view degree of prostatic enlargement and bladder wall changes.

PHYSICAL EXAMINATION

Evaluate general condition: height, weight, temperature, blood pressure, pulse, overall cardio-respiratory status, skin turgor and condition.

Catheterize to determine residual after voiding.

Evaluate the patient's voidings to document decrease in size and force of urinary flow.

Palpate for suprapubic mass, bladder distention, and presence of tenderness in renal areas.

Identify symptoms of distress.

Rectal exam to determine enlarged prostate, i.e., firm with smooth edges.

NURSING PRIORITIES

1. Relieve acute urinary retention.
2. Relieve pain and promote comfort.
3. Maintain adequate renal function and tissue perfusion.
4. Prevent complications, monitor for postobstructive diuresis.
5. Assist patient to deal with psychosocial concerns.

NURSING DIAGNOSIS:	**Urinary elimination, alteration in pattern.**
SUPPORTING DATA:	**Inability to empty bladder completely because of decompensation of detrusor musculature and inability of bladder to contract adequately. Acute urinary retention because of enlarged prostate that leads to bladder outlet obstruction and distended bladder.**
DESIRED PATIENT OUTCOMES:	**Return proper function of detrusor musculature. Relief of obstruction with complete bladder emptying. Patient free of urinary tract infection.**

INTERVENTIONS

Observe urinary stream and document size and force.

Monitor and document time and amount of each voiding.

Percuss suprapubic area to determine bladder distention.

Meatal care.

Force fluids to 3000ml/daily, if cardiac status permits, and keep accurate I & O.

Irrigate catheter as indicated.

MEDICAL MANAGEMENT

Catheterize for residual urine. Leave indwelling catheter in place.

Urinalysis and culture.

RATIONALE

May help differentiate cause of prostatism due to compensatory hypertrophy of the detrusor muscle.

Provides information about the patient's inability to void adequately.

A distended, overloaded bladder may be felt in the suprapubic area.

Clean area decreases chance of infection.

Increased fluid flushes kidneys and bladder of bacterial growth. Important to have accurate record of fluid balance.

Maintain patency.

Normally there should be no urine left in the bladder after voiding. Indwelling catheter will prevent urinary stasis.

When residual urine is present there is usually some degree of urinary tract infection.

Antibiotics and antibacterials.	Combat infection.
Antispasmotics; rectal suppositories (B & Os).	Spasms may occur due to irritation of the catheter. Suppositories are absorbed easily into bladder tissue to produce relaxation.

NURSING DIAGNOSIS:	**Sleep-pattern disturbance.**
SUPPORTING DATA:	**Nocturia and frequency contribute to sleeplessness and irritability.**
DESIRED PATIENT OUTCOMES:	**Patient well-rested; nocturia minimized or relieved.**

INTERVENTIONS

RATIONALE

Determine patient's ideal sleep pattern.	Helpful in setting goal.
Document sleep intervals.	Information about how much sleep patient is getting. Reduction in sleep may contribute to deterioration in patient's general condition.
Discourage ingestion of large amounts of fluid before bedtime.	Reduces need to void during night.

NURSING DIAGNOSIS:	**Comfort, alteration in, pain.**
SUPPORTING DATA:	**Urinary obstructions may lead to urinary infection and/or renal colic. Distended bladder is painful.**
DESIRED PATIENT OUTCOMES:	**Relieve obstruction and secondary pain.**

INTERVENTIONS

RATIONALE

Document and report pain.	Necessary information for relief of pain.
Tape catheter to the abdomen.	Prevent pull on the catheter and erosion of the penile-scrotal junction.

MEDICAL MANAGEMENT

Narcotics.	Induce mental and physical relaxation.
Indwelling catheter to straight drainage.	Reduced bladder tension reduces bladder irritability.
Antibacterials.	Reduces bacteria present in urinary tract and those introduced by drainage system.
Antispasmodics & bladder sedative.	Relieve bladder irritability.
Prostatic massage.	Aids in evacuation of ducts of gland and decreases inflammation. Has limited use.

NURSING DIAGNOSIS:	Fluid volume, alteration in, excess, potential.
SUPPORTING DATA:	Bladder decompensation may produce ureteral dilatation and hydronephrosis. Generalized cardiovascular symptoms result from fluid overload.
DESIRED PATIENT OUTCOMES:	Maintain adequate kidney functioning. Normal fluid volumes are maintained.

INTERVENTIONS

Monitor serum creatinine, BUN, and electrolytes as well as specific gravity.

Monitor vital signs closely. Observe for edema. Weigh daily. Accurate intake and output.

RATIONALE

Prostatic enlargement (obstruction) eventually causes dilatation of upper urinary tract, potentially impairing kidney function and leading to uremia. If resultant fluid imbalance due to decreased kidney function is left untreated, certain electrolytes, BUN and creatinine levels become elevated.

Loss of kidney function results in decreased fluid elimination, may progress to complete renal shutdown. Indicators of fluid retention.

NURSING DIAGNOSIS:	Fluid volume deficit, potential.
SUPPORTING DATA:	Postobstructive diuresis. Onset of bleeding from sudden filling and rupture of mucosal blood vessels can be a complication from rapidly emptying of a chronically overdistended bladder.
DESIRED PATIENT OUTCOMES:	Maintain adequate fluid levels. Control bleeding.

INTERVENTIONS

Monitor output carefully, hourly outputs if indicated (100–200ml/hr).

Monitor blood pressure, pulse; hourly.

Observe for symptoms of shock.

Position patient to decrease cardiac workload.

Monitor electrolytes.

RATIONALE

Too rapid diuresis causes the patient's total fluid volume to become depleted, insufficient amounts of Na^+ are resorbed in renal tubules.

Assess systemic hypovolemia and enables early intervention.

Enables early intervention.

Circulatory homeostasis must be maintained.

Fluid is pulled from extracellular spaces and Na^+ may follow the shift.

419

MEDICAL MANAGEMENT

Intravenous fluid as needed.

Replace fluid losses to prevent hypovolemia.

NURSING DIAGNOSIS: Tissue perfusion, alteration in.

SUPPORTING DATA: Increased ureteral pressure leads to decreased renal blood flow, cellular atrophy, and necrosis.

DESIRED PATIENT OUTCOMES: Normal renal pressure gradients.

INTERVENTIONS

Monitor for diminished urinary output.

Observe for lethargy, pallor, and edema. Record and report changes in level of consciousness.

RATIONALE

Any deficit in blood flow to the kidney impairs its ability to filter and concentrate substances.

Toxic wastes accumulate and circulating fluid volume increases, causing central nervous system symptoms.

NURSING DIAGNOSIS: Fear, outcome of illness.

SUPPORTING DATA: Possible surgical procedure, anxiety about prognosis and possibility of malignancy can create a fearful situation.

DESIRED PATIENT OUTCOMES: Relief of anxiety. Patient demonstrates calm attitude and verbalizes lessened fear.

INTERVENTIONS

Prepare patient for diagnostic tests by giving needed information.

Allow patient to verbalize fears. Reinforce physician's preoperative teaching.

Be aware of how much information the patient wants.

Involve significant others in teaching.

Be available to the patient.

Answer questions realistically.

RATIONALE

Helps patient understand purpose of procedures and increases rapport between nurse and patient.

Identifies more specifically what the individual is afraid of. Helpful for patient to hear information from more than one source.

Overload of information will not be helpful and may increase anxiety.

Provides opportunity to enhance support system.

Demonstrates concern and willingness to help.

Realistic information allows the patient to deal with reality and strengthens trust in caregivers and information presented.

NURSING DIAGNOSIS:	Knowledge deficit, discharge planning.
SUPPORTING DATA:	Prostate is in sensitive area that people do not readily have knowledge of or ask questions about. Concern regarding sexual functioning.
DESIRED PATIENT OUTCOMES:	Verbalizes understanding of sexuality and how the condition may affect him. Demonstrates effective coping skills in dealing with existing problems.

INTERVENTIONS

Establish trusting relationship with patient and SO.

Include discussion of basic anatomy during teaching session(s). Be honest in answers to patient's questions.

Encourage verbalization.

Avoid spicy foods, coffee, and alcohol. Avoid long automobile rides.

During acute episodes of prostatitis, intercourse is avoided, but may be helpful in treatment of chronic condition.

Give information that the causative agent of prostatitis is not venereal.

Reinforce importance of medical follow-up for at least 6 mos-1 year.

RATIONALE

Helpful in discussing sensitive subject.

The nerve plexus that controls erection runs posteriorly to the prostate through the capsule. In procedures that do not involve the prostatic capsule, impotency and sterility usually are not a consequence.

Helping patient work through feelings can be vital to rehabilitation.

May cause prostatic irritation with resulting congestion.

Increases pain in acute; serves as massaging agent in chronic.

May be an unspoken fear.

Recurrence of infection caused by same or different organisms is not uncommon.

SURGICAL INTERVENTIONS: PROSTATECTOMY

1. *Transurethral Resection (TUR)*
   Obstructive prostatic tissue of the medial lobe that surrounds the urethra is removed by means of a resectoscope introduced through the urethra.
2. *Suprapubic Prostatectomy*
   Removal of large amount of obstructing tissue through a low midline incision made through the bladder.
3. *Retropubic Prostatectomy*
   Hypertrophied prostatic tissue mass located high in the pelvic region is removed through a low abdominal incision without opening the bladder.
4. *Perineal Prostatectomy*
   Prostatic tissue is removed through an incision between the scrotum and the rectum. A radical procedure is done for cancer. This procedure usually results in impotence.

421

NURSING PRIORITIES

1. Maintain fluid balance and adequate kidney functioning.
2. Promote comfort.
3. Minimize complications.
4. Promote rehabilitation.

NURSING DIAGNOSIS:	Fluid volume, deficit, potential.
SUPPORTING DATA:	Patients may restrict intake because of discomfort and frequency.
DESIRED PATIENT OUTCOMES:	Adequate hydration is maintained.

INTERVENTIONS

Monitor I & O.

Weigh daily.

Force fluids to 3000ml/day unless contraindicated.

Observe for restlessness, confusion, changes in behavior.

RATIONALE

Indicator of adequacy of intake and fluid balance.

Indicates fluid retention.

Flush kidneys/bladder of bacteria and debris but may result in water intoxication if not monitored closely.

Cerebral edema may result from excessive solution absorbed into the venous sinusoids during surgery (TUR).

MEDICAL MANAGEMENT

IV therapy.

May need fluids IV if oral intake inadequate.

NURSING DIAGNOSIS:	Injury, potential for, infection and hemorrhage.
SUPPORTING DATA:	Insertion of catheter carries potential for introduction of bacteria and development of infections. Vascular nature of surgical area makes it difficult to control all the bleeding points.
DESIRED PATIENT OUTCOMES:	Infection does not occur. Hemorrhage is minimized and/or controlled.

INTERVENTIONS

Note excessive bleeding in urinary drainage.

RATIONALE

Urine will show bright blood in the beginning decreasing to pink and then clear.

Differentiate type of bleed:
    Bright red, increased viscosity and bright red clots.
    Dark, burgundy drainage with dark clots.

Note absence of clots.

Monitor vital signs, as indicated by condition.

Irrigate catheter, only if not draining well, with isotonic solutions.

Maintain accurate I & O.

Anchor catheter to prevent dislodging. Document period of application and release of traction, if used.

Maintain a sterile catheter system, with catheter care every shift.

Ambulate with drainage bag dependent.

Meatal care with soap and water, applying antibiotic ointment around catheter.

Be sure patient has accurate information about catheter, drainage, and bladder spasms.

Instruct patient to avoid tub baths after discharge.

Avoid the use of enemas.

Usually arterial and may require aggressive therapy.
Usually venous and will subside on its own.

May indicate blood dyscrasias or hemolysis of blood.

Identify potential problems early.

Avoids clot formation and obstruction of the catheter, but may increase bleeding if done unnecessarily. "Milking" catheter will not increase bleeding. Isotonic solutions will not cause hemolysis.

With repeat bladder irrigations, it is essential in order to esimate blood loss and urine output.

Excessive manipulation may cause bleeding, clot formation, plugging of the catheter, and distention. Therapy could result in injury.

Prevent introduction of bacteria.

To avoid reflux.

Prevent infection.

Allay anxiety and promote cooperation with necessary procedures. Presence of catheter and bladder spasms cause urge to void.

Decrease the possibility of infection.

May result in referred irritation to prostatic bed and increase bleeding.

MEDICAL MANAGEMENT

Catheter (taped to inner thigh).

Release traction within 4–5 hours.

Antibiotics.

Continuous bladder irrigation.

If balloon inflated in bladder, traction will create pressure on the arterial supply to the prostatic capsule as it passes through the bladder neck.

Prolonged traction may cause permanent problems with urinary control.

Promote urinary antisepsis.

Flush bladder of debris and maintain patency of catheter.

NURSING DIAGNOSIS:	Comfort, alteration in, pain.
SUPPORTING DATA:	Painful bladder spasms occur following transurethral and suprapubic surgery because of irritation of the bladder mucosa.

DESIRED PATIENT OUTCOMES:	Bladder spasms are minimized/controlled.

INTERVENTIONS

Promote intake of large amounts of fluid.

Maintain continuous bladder drainage.

MEDICAL MANAGEMENT

Belladonna and Opium suppositories.

Pro-Banthine.

RATIONALE

Decrease irritation by maintaining constant flow of water over the bladder mucosa.

The catheter balloon puts pressure on the internal sphincter, creating constant pressure to void. A properly draining catheter allows this feeling to pass. When the patient tries to void around the catheter, spasms result.

Provide relief of spasms. Will usually decrease by the end of 24–48 hours.

Anticholinergic to relieve bladder spasms.

NURSING DIAGNOSIS:	Urinary elimination, alteration in pattern.
SUPPORTING DATA:	Obstruction has interferred with elimination and normal pattern will need to be reestablished.
DESIRED PATIENT OUTCOMES:	Patient verbalizes understanding of normal process and a normal pattern is reestablished.

INTERVENTIONS

Note time and amount of voiding (after catheter is removed).

Instruct patient in perineal exercises.

Advise patient that "dribbling" is to be expected after catheter is removed.

RATIONALE

The catheter is usually removed 2–5 days after surgery and voiding may be a problem due to urethral edema.

To help regain urinary control.

Information is helpful in dealing with the problem.

NURSING DIAGNOSIS:	Fear, loss of male identity and sexual functioning.
SUPPORTING DATA:	Incontinence, leakage of urine after catheter removal, areas involved evoke concern about sexual functioning and adequacy.

DESIRED PATIENT OUTCOMES:	Sexual functioning is maintained at a satisfactory level. The patient has information about individual expectations of return of function.

INTERVENTIONS

Provide openings for patient to talk about concerns of incontinence and sexual functioning.

Give accurate information about physical expectation of return of sexual function (usually in 6–8 weeks).

Give information about retrograde ejaculation.

Instruct in exercises to be done to promote urinary control: perineal and interruption/continuation of urinary stream.

RATIONALE

Most patients will have anxieties and questions about the effects of surgery. May be hesitant about asking necessary questions.

Physiologic impotence occurs only when the perineal nerves are cut during radical procedures. In other procedures, sexual activity can usually be resumed in 6–8 weeks.

Seminal fluid goes into the bladder and is excreted with the urine, but does not interfere with sexual functioning.

May be helpful in regaining urinary control.

NURSING DIAGNOSIS:	Skin integrity, impairment of, potential.
SUPPORTING DATA:	With suprapubic, retropubic, and perineal incision dressings present, urine leakage may cause excoriation.
DESIRED PATIENT OUTCOMES:	Skin remains intact.

INTERVENTIONS

Change dressings frequently, cleaning and drying skin thoroughly.

May use ostomy-type skin barriers.

RATIONALE

Promote integrity.

Provide protection for surrounding skin.

DIAGNOSIS: Urolithiasis

PATIENT DATA BASE

NURSING HISTORY

Pain may occur anywhere along course of the ureters or in kidney area. May present as an acute episode of colicky pain occurring initially in the flank in the region of the costovertebral angle and may radiate around the abdomen and down to the genitalia.

Patients may describe pain as acute, severe, moving irritation not relieved by positioning or anything else. May have nausea and vomiting with pain, fever, diarrhea, hematuria, alterations in voiding pattern and grunting respirations.

Occupation: calculi have a higher incidence in people with sedentary occupations and those occupations that are exposed to high environmental temperatures.

Note geographic location/water supply.

Sex: calculi occur more frequently in men than women (3:1) and typically from age 30–60.

Hobbies give insight into activity levels. Active vs. sedentary habits.

Diet: ingestion of excessive amounts of purines, oxalate, calcium, and phosphates. Insufficient fluid intake. Vitamin A deficiency or vitamin D excess may be a factor.

Elimination patterns may suggest urinary tract infection and/or intestinal disturbances.

Past history of chronic urinary tract infections, or obstruction with urinary stasis, calculi, metabolic disease, dietary excess or insufficiency, hypertension, gout, small bowel disease, and previous abdominal surgery may predispose to development of urinary tract stones. Patient who has been on bed rest or immobilized, e.g., fracture with traction.

Medication history may include use of antibiotics, antihypertensives, sodium bicarbonate, allopurinal, phosphates, thiazides.

Family history of calculi, hypertension, cystinuria, renal tubular acidosis, gout, chronic UTI, kidney disease.

DIAGNOSTIC STUDIES

Urinalysis: color, yellow to bloody. Appearance may be cloudy. Bacteria, pus, and crystals may be present, (cystine, uric acid, calcium oxalate). Blood, 0 to 4 + . WBC, RBC may be present microscopically. pH, determines acidity/alkalinity.

Urine culture: may reveal staphylococcus aureus, proteus, klebsiella, pseudomonos as cause of UTI, which may occur with urolithiasis.

Urine calcium: may indicate increased amounts of calcium as predominant ingredient in stone content.

24 hour urine for uric acid and calcium may be elevated.

Biochemical survey: may show elevated levels of magnesium, calcium, uric acid, phosphates.

Parathyroid hormone: may be increased indicating hyperparathyroidism. (PTH stimulates reabsorption of calcium from bones increasing circulating serum calcium and urine calcium.)

CBC: WBC may be increased indicating secondary infection or septicemia; r/o leukemia. RBC, usually normal. Hemoglobin, hematocrit only abnormal if severely dehydrated (encourages precipitation of solids), anemia owing to hemorrhage, polycythemia.

BUN-creatinine: may be abnormal secondary to high obstructive stone in kidney causing ischemia/necrosis.

KUB: shows radiodense calculi in the area of the kidneys or along the course of the ureter.

IVP: shows delayed presence of contrast media in lower urinary tract. Delayed films are usually done at 20, 30, and 60 minutes, and as late as one day.

Cystoscopy: stone demonstration and manipulation.

PHYSICAL EXAMINATION

Evaluate general condition: height, weight, temperature (may be elevated), blood pressure, pulse (may be elevated due to pain and anxiety).

Respirations may be grunting due to pain.

Evaluate general cardiovascular status to rule out atherosclerotic, cardiovascular problems that may aggravate kidney function.

Assess gastrointestinal disturbances and association with pain.

Assess genitourinary disturbances, hematuria, and so forth.

Evaluate pain intensity, location plus course of pain radiation, and if positioning relieves pain.

Palpate for tenderness in renal areas.

NURSING PRIORITIES

1. Relieve pain due to renal colic.
2. Maintain adequate renal functioning.
3. Maintain adequate fluid and electrolyte balance (control GI disturbances).
4. Retrieval of calculi.
5. Reduce or correct factors predisposing to calculi formation.

NURSING DIAGNOSIS:	**Comfort, alteration in pain.**
SUPPORTING DATA:	**Interference with normal peristalic action of the ureter by calculi.**
DESIRED PATIENT OUTCOMES:	**Pain controlled/pain free. Spasms controlled.**

INTERVENTIONS

Document intensity, location, duration, and areas of pain radiation.

Document increased abdominal pain.

Explain cause of pain and importance of notifying staff of pain.

Give medication on initial complaint of pain and at regular intervals p.r.n.

RATIONALE

Symptoms may rule out other causes of pain. Accurate documentation of location may help evaluate progress of calculi movement. Pain may radiate due to proximity of nerve plexus and blood vessels supplying other areas, such as the testicles.

Extravasation may occur due to increased ureteral pressure. Urine in perirenal spaces produces discomfort and predisposes to infection.

Pain is usually caused by movement of the calculi and if understood can be helpful in enhancing the patient's coping ability, and alerts staff to possibility of passing of stone.

Severe pain becomes worse if not alleviated promptly.

MEDICAL MANAGEMENT

Narcotics.

Decrease ureteral colic and promote mental and physical relaxation.

Antispasmotics, p.r.n.

Decreasing renal spasm usually will decrease renal colic and pain.

NURSING DIAGNOSIS:	**Fluid volume deficit, potential.**
SUPPORTING DATA:	**Renal or ureteral colic causes a generalized abdominal and pelvic nerve irritation causing GI symptomatology.**
DESIRED PATIENT OUTCOMES:	**Cause of GI disturbance identified. Fluid volume is maintained. Patient able to tolerate food. Mucosal irritation and breakdown is prevented.**

INTERVENTIONS

Document incidence of vomiting, diarrhea. Note characteristics, frequency, as well as accompanying or precipitating events.

Increase fluid intake to 3000ml/day.

Monitor Hct & Hb, electrolytes, urinary output.

Give frequent oral care.

Give clear liquids, bland foods as tolerated.

RATIONALE

Documentation may help rule out abdominal disturbances and pinpoint urinary calculi and colic as causes of symptoms.

Dehydration and electrolyte imbalance may occur secondary to excessive fluid loss due to vomiting and diarrhea. Maintain fluid balance for homeostasis as well as "washing" action that may flush the stone(s) out.

These parameters help to assess hydration.

Eliminate tastes that may cause anorexia, nausea & vomiting. Decreases oral mucosal irritation caused by dehydration and stasis of secretions.

Easily digested foods decrease GI activity and helps maintain fluid and nutritional balance.

MEDICAL MANAGEMENT

IV fluids.

May need IV fluid replacement if oral intake is insufficient.

Antiemetics.

Relax smooth muscles and enhance ability to enjoy food.

NURSING DIAGNOSIS:	**Urinary elimination, alteration in pattern.**

SUPPORTING DATA:	Urgency and frequency may be caused by stimulation of the bladder by calculi. Hematuria may be due to renal or ureteral irritation caused by calculi.
DESIRED PATIENT OUTCOMES:	Normal voiding pattern is resumed.

INTERVENTIONS

Determine patient's normal voiding pattern. Document variations in voiding pattern.

Send urine for analysis and culture.

Force fluids.

Strain all urine for calculi.

Describe any stones expelled and send to lab for analysis.

Monitor voidings for changes in color or excessive bleeding.

Monitor vital signs, Hct & Hb.

RATIONALE

Calculi may cause nerve excitability. Usually frequency and urgency increase as calculi nears uretervesical junction.

Rule out UTI as cause of symptoms.

Increasing fluids decreases ureteral colic and flushes bacteria, blood, and debris and may progress calculi.

Retrieval of calculi is important.

Analysis gives insight into possible cause of stone formation.

Increased bleeding may indicate increased obstruction or irritation of ureter. Hemorrhage due to ureteral ulceration is rare.

Vital signs, Hct & Hb variations may indicate hemorrhage/dehydration.

NURSING DIAGNOSIS:	Tissue perfusion, alteration in.
SUPPORTING DATA:	Renal or ureteral obstruction produces buildup and back pressure against renal tissues, decreasing renal blood flow, urine output, and stimulating renin production.
DESIRED PATIENT OUTCOMES:	Urine output appropriate to intake.

INTERVENTIONS

Monitor laboratory studies of electrolytes, BUN, creatinine, Hct & Hb.

Monitor intake & output.

Monitor for increased blood pressure.

RATIONALE

Elevated BUN, creatinine, and certain electrolytes indicate kidney dysfunction. Decreased Hct & Hb may reflect dilution due to overhydration.

Any deficit in blood flow causes cellular atrophy and necrosis, which interferes with the kidney's ability to filter and concentrate substances. Decreased GFR stimulates production of renin, which acts to raise BP in an effort to increase renal blood flow.

Observe for changes in level of consciousness; decreased movement, response to verbal commands, painful stimuli, change in pupillary responses.

Decreased glomerular filtration with accumulation of wastes and electrolytes causes body levels that are toxic to the CNS.

NURSING DIAGNOSIS:	**Fluid volume, alteration in, potential overload.**
SUPPORTING DATA:	**Obstructive calculi may produce hydronephrosis.**
DESIRED PATIENT OUTCOMES:	**Adequate kidney functioning with balanced intake and output.**

INTERVENTIONS

Monitor increased BP, respirations, rales/rhonchi, dependent tissue edema.

Monitor output qh.

Weigh daily.

Record changes in responses/orientation.

RATIONALE

Impaired kidney functioning, decreased output resulting in higher circulating volumes. Fluid overload commonly presents with signs/symptoms of CHF.

Diminished output can be a sign of renal failure or decreased cardiac output in response to advent of CHF.

Rapid weight gain may be related to water retention.

CNS symptoms may be in response to water retention or decreased cerebral perfusion secondary to decreased cardiac output of CHF.

NURSING DIAGNOSIS:	**Fear, possible surgery.**
SUPPORTING DATA:	**Stone basket, ureterlithotomy; calculi >1cm in diameter will not readily pass spontaneously.**
DESIRED PATIENT OUTCOMES:	**Anxiety is reduced and patient is dealing realistically with treatment regimen.**

INTERVENTIONS

Explain reasons for GI disturbances and pain.

Listen to patient's concerns.

RATIONALE

Celiac ganglion serves both kidneys and stomach so nausea, vomiting, and diarrhea are commonly associated with renal colic. Knowledge of cause helps reduce anxiety.

Allowing patient to verbalize helps establish trusting relationship, helpful in reducing anxiety.

Prepare patient for surgical procedure, uretero-lithotomy; ureter may be left open, or loosely sutured. Urine drains via rubber tissue drains. Drainage should stop after 10–14 days if no obstruction is present.

Helps patient cope with surgery and enhances postoperative recuperation.

Frequent dressing changes weigh for I and O if necessary.

Drainage may be significant.

NURSING DIAGNOSIS:	**Knowledge deficit, cause of condition and possible alterations in lifestyle.**
SUPPORTING DATA:	**Calculi recurrence, underlying cause of stone formation, may be hyperthyroidism, and so forth. Possibility of dietary restriction and/or alterations.**
DESIRED PATIENT OUTCOMES:	**Verbalizes knowledge of cause of problem and measures necessary for treatment and control.**

INTERVENTIONS

Discuss importance of increased fluid intake and following prescribed therapy.
As much as 6–8 L of water/day may be needed. Include cranberry juice in intake.

Encourage activity within physical limitations.

Discuss disease process.
Prepare for work-up.
Reinforce restriction and/or alterations in lifestyle, importance of medications, and so forth.

Discuss need to decrease precursors of calculi.

RATIONALE

Understanding of stone formation and preventive measures may give patient a sense of control.
When cystine stones are present.
Acidifies the urine.

Inactivity contributes to stone formation.

Being truthful with patient and showing concern helps patient work through feelings and gain control.

Knowledge of dietary alteration can be an important aspect of disease control.

MEDICAL MANAGEMENT

Diet order.

Depends on the type of stone, usually moderately reduced calcium and phosphorus. Over 90% of stones contain calcium combined with phosphates and/or other substances.

Low-purine diet.

Decreases oral intake of uric acid precursors.

Shorr regimen: Low Ca^{++}/phosphorus diet with Aluminum carbonate gel 30–40 ml 30 min pc/hs (watch for constipation).

Prevents phosphatic calculi by forming an insoluble precipitate in the GI tract, reducing the load to the nephron. Also effective against other forms of calcium calculi.

Appropriate drugs; Ammonium chloride and Mandelamine.	Maintain proper urine pH. Acidify the urine. Phosphate, oxalate, and carbonate stones form in alkaline urine.
Potassium acetate or citrate, sodium bicarbonate.	Alkalize the urine. Uric acid, urate, and cystine stones form in acid urine.
Allopurinal.	Use with uric acid stones.

BIBLIOGRAPHY

Books and Other Individual Publications

BEYERS, M. AND DUDAS, S.: *The Clinical Practice of Medical-Surgical Nursing.* Little, Brown & Co., Boston, 1977.

BRUNDAGE, D. J.: *Nursing Management of Renal Problems.* C. V. Mosby, St. Louis, 1976.

BRUNNER, L. S. AND SUDDARTH, D. S.: *Lippincott Manual of Nursing Practice.* J. B. Lippincott, Philadelphia, 1978.

JOHANSON, B. C. ET AL.: *Standards for Critical Care.* C. V. Mosby, St. Louis, 1981.

KIM, M. AND MORITZ, D. (EDS.): *Classification of Nursing Diagnosis.* McGraw-Hill, New York, 1981.

KEUHNELIAN, J. G. AND SANDERS, V. E.: *Urological Nursing.* MacMillan, New York, 1970.

LUCKMAN, J. AND SORENSEN, K. C.: *Medical-Surgical Nursing: A Psychophysiological approach,* ed. 2. W. B. Saunders, 1980.

PHIPPS, W. J., LONG, B. C., AND WOODS, N. F.: *Medical-Surgical Nursing.* C. V. Mosby, St. Louis, 1979.

TILKIAN, S. M., CONOVER, M. B., AND TILKIAN, A. G.: *Clinical Implications of Laboratory Tests.* C. V. Mosby, 1979.

WILKINS, R. W., LEVINSKY, N. G. (EDS.): *Medicine, Essentials of Clinical Practice.* Little, Brown & Co., Boston, 1978.

Journal Articles

METHANY, N.: *Renal stones and urinary pH.* AJN, pp. 1372–1375, Sept. 1982.

REED, S. B.: *Giving more than dialysis.* Nursing 82, pp. 58–63, April.

CHAPTER 10

ENDOCRINOLOGY

CARE PLAN: Hypophysectomy

Surgical approaches are dictated by causative factor and/or tumor extension.
1. Craniotomy: transfrontal approach if tumor extends upward involving the optic chiasm.
2. Transsphenoidal approach if tumor is confined to sella turcica. (Most frequently used.)
3. Destruction by stereotaxic (heat) or cryosurgery (freezing).

PATIENT DATA BASE

NURSING HISTORY
May have a pituitary tumor.

Diabetic retinopathy may be present.

May have metastatic disease due to ovarian/testicular cancer.

May be a primary pituitary problem.

DIAGNOSTIC STUDIES

Skull x-ray reveals enlarged sella turcica.

Angiography to r/o aneurysm and evaluate extension of tumor.

Pneumoencephalogram to r/o other possible diagnoses and evaluate extension of tumor.

CT scan.

PHYSICAL EXAMINATION

Evaluate visual fields to note compresion of optic chiasma.

NURSING PRIORITIES

1. Provide for alleviation of anxiety.
2. Provide for treatment of postoperative consequences and complications.
3. Assist patient in dealing with sexual/psychologic aspects of procedure.

NURSING DIAGNOSIS:	Fear, brain surgery.
SUPPORTING DATA:	Surgery on the brain has especially fearful connotations for most people with ideation of "brain damage" and death.
DESIRED PATIENT OUTCOMES:	Fear and anxiety are discussed/allayed.

INTERVENTIONS

RATIONALE

INTERVENTIONS	RATIONALE
Encourage patient to verbalize fears.	May have fear of serious consequences of brain surgery. When discussed openly, anxiety may be decreased.
Emphasize positive aspects of procedure.	Limited postoperative problems and minimal pain.
Educate re the possibility of diabetes inspidus, which may occur postoperatively.	Most patients are not aware of the difference between diabetes mellitus and diabetes insipidus.

MEDICAL MANAGEMENT

ACTH.	Given preoperatively, assists in management of stress.

NURSING DIAGNOSIS:	Injury, potential for, increased intracranial pressure. Refer to Care Plan: Increased Intracranial Pressure.

NURSING DIAGNOSIS:	Injury, potential for, cerebral spinal fluid (CSF) leak/infection.
SUPPORTING DATA:	Surgical area prone to leak with subsequent infection.
DESIRED PATIENT OUTCOMES:	Prevent/control CSF leak/infection.

INTERVENTIONS

RATIONALE

INTERVENTIONS	RATIONALE
Instruct patient to avoid vigorous cough/sneeze.	Increases intracranial pressure and may cause leak to occur.
Observe for rhinorrhea and/or postnasal drip.	May be sign of CSF leak.

Test clear drainage with glucose test strip (Diastix).

Positive glucose indicates drainage is cerebral spinal fluid.

Assess character of pain.

Severe generalized or supraorbital headache may indicate developing meningitis.

If leak occurs:
Elevate head of the bed, bed rest, and notify physician.

Usually resolves within 72 hrs.

MEDICAL MANAGEMENT

Gelfoam saturated with antibiotics placed in anterior sella turcica intraoperatively.

Packing minimizes chance of infection and CSF leak.

Systemic antibiotics.

Prevent meningitis.

Lumbar puncture every day/p.r.n.

If severe leak occurs, taps will reduce CSF pressure and allow fossa to heal.

NURSING DIAGNOSIS:	Fluid volume deficit, potential.
SUPPORTING DATA:	Loss of ADH stores can result in inadequate hormonal regulation of kidney functioning.
DESIRED PATIENT OUTCOMES:	Fluid balance is maintained.

INTERVENTIONS

RATIONALE

Monitor I & O every hour and urine specific gravity as indicated.

If urine output >800 ml/2 hours or >7000 ml in 24 hours or specific gravity <1.004, drug intervention is indicated.

If Pitressin is used:
evaluate for drowsiness, headache, listlessness, convulsions, coma.

Water intoxication is a potential side effect of Pitressin therapy.

Encourage intake of 1–2 glasses of water with drug administration.

Minimizes side effects of nausea and abdominal cramping that may occur with Pitressin.

Instruct patient in usage of nasal vasopressin (may be long-term therapy).

Drug is regulated according to degree of polydipsia/uria.

MEDICAL MANAGEMENT

IV fluid replacement.

Maintain adequate hydration if loss is severe.

Pitressin p.r.n.

Form of ADH that signals the kidney to retain fluid.

NURSING DIAGNOSIS:	Comfort, alteration in, pain.
SUPPORTING DATA:	Surgical procedure accompanied by pain, pressure on sella turcica.
DESIRED PATIENT OUTCOMES:	Pain is minimized/controlled.

INTERVENTIONS

Raise head of bed 30°

Assess pain.

MEDICAL MANAGEMENT

Low dose Demerol/Codeine.

ASA/Tylenol.

Skull x-rays

RATIONALE

Decreases pressure on sella turcica and may reduce headache secondary to surgical approach and nasal packing.

If character of pain changes and headache becomes sharp, may indicate presence of intracranial air.

Usually pain is not severe enough for high dosage and do not want to mask symptoms that need medical attention.

As pain lessens in 3–4 days, narcotics are no longer required.

May be necessary to diagnose the presence of intracranial air. (This will usually be absorbed within 1–2 weeks without any intervention.)

NURSING DIAGNOSIS:	**Knowledge deficit, postoperative/long-term care.**
SUPPORTING DATA:	**Hormonal changes may include adrenal insufficiency if cortisol levels are decreased, hypothyroidism, hypogonadism, and decrease in ADH resulting in diabetes insipidus. In addition, required drug therapy may result in side effects of "hyper" function.**
DESIRED PATIENT OUTCOMES:	**Verbalizes necessary lifestyle changes and medication schedules.**

INTERVENTIONS

Instruct patient/significant others in signs/symptoms of hypo/hyper function.

Teach patient/SO stress management techniques and to recognize when they need to contact the physician.

Present drug information in both oral and written format.

Encourage patient to wear medical identification at all times.

RATIONALE

Alert patient to need for medical followup.

Stress may increase hormonal needs and necessitate changes in drug therapy.

Multiple long-term drug therapy must be taken as ordered. Retention is enhanced when given in more than one form and written material provides for reference at home.

Sudden withdrawal of hormone therapy may be fatal.

Avoid any activity that could increase intracranial pressure, e.g., bending over to tie shoes, pick up objects, shampoo hair, or straining at stool.

May take up to 2 months for fossa to heal and increased pressure can cause CSF leak.

Increase fluid, fruit/fiber intake in diet.

To promote bowel functioning and minimize straining.

Use mouthwash and dental floss for oral care and avoid tooth brushing.

Approximately 10 days are required for suture line to heal.

MEDICAL MANAGEMENT

Long-term drug therapy may include: Pitressin, ACTH, thyroid, testosterone/estrogen.

Dependent on deficiencies that exist.

Stool softeners/laxatives.

May be necessary for a short period to avoid straining at stool.

NURSING DIAGNOSIS:	**Sexual dysfunction.**
SUPPORTING DATA:	**If anterior pituitary is removed, gonadal functioning is affected. In men, sterility, decreased libido, and impotence may occur. In women, atrophy of the vaginal mucosa and infertility may occur.**
DESIRED PATIENT OUTCOMES:	**Sexual functioning is maintained at a desired level.**

INTERVENTIONS

Provide for counseling for sexual problems.

RATIONALE

Helpful to develop new skills for managing sexual relationships.

Give information that, changes in sexual functioning may indicate tumor growth/regrowth.

Important to inform physician of problems as they arise.

MEDICAL MANAGEMENT

Hormonal replacement therapy.

Testosterone/estrogen can be given to prevent development of dysfunction.

Refer to Care Plan: Psychosocial Aspects of Care in the Acute Setting.

DIAGNOSIS: Addison's Disease: Primary Adrenal Insufficiency

PATIENT DATA BASE

NURSING HISTORY

Complains of weakness, malaise (tiring quickly), muscle aches, and/or progressing to paresthesia/paralysis.

Increasing pigmentation of the face, neck, hand, knuckles, knees, and skin creases.

Weight loss and muscle wasting may be evident.

Complains of anorexia, nausea and vomiting, food idiosyncracies (may crave salt), abdominal cramps and diarrhea, steatorrhea.

May complain of dizziness.

May have heart palpitations.

May have recently experienced a period of stress, such as trauma, surgery, infection, history of diabetes mellitus, or premature menopause.

May have had episodes of hypoglycemia with headaches, diaphoresis, and trembling.

History of recent anticoagulant therapy or changes in steroid therapy.

DIAGNOSTIC STUDIES

Blood studies reveal hypoglycemia, hyponatremia, hyperkalemia, and low-fasting plasma cortisol levels.

BUN/creatinine: may be moderately elevated.

24-hour urine specimen for 17-ketosteroids, 17-hydroxycorticoids, and 17-ketogenic steroids: all values will be decreased.

PHYSICAL EXAMINATION

Skin has bronze pigmentation, especially in areas exposed to the sun and often in areas of pressure, such as knees, elbows, and under belt (waistline).

Neurologic exam will reveal muscle weakness and decreased reflexes.

Blood pressure will be low.

Loss of axillary/pubic hair may be noted.

Mental changes may be noted; depression, irritability, and anxiety.

NURSING PRIORITIES

1. Maintain fluid and electrolyte balance for optimal tissue perfusion.
2. Prevent complications, i.e., addisonian crisis.
3. Provide information and assist patient/significant others in accepting and dealing with necessity for lifelong therapy psychologic manifestations.

438

NURSING DIAGNOSIS:	Tissue perfusion, impaired.
SUPPORTING DATA:	Electrolyte imbalance and volume depletion impair cardiac function and occurence of related arrhythmias and further decrease tissue perfusion. The vasoconstriction response is blocked and hypotension/shock may occur. The heart may decrease in size and may not be able to increase it's stroke volume to adapt to stress.
DESIRED PATIENT OUTCOMES:	Adequate tissue perfusion/cardiac output is maintained.

INTERVENTIONS

Monitor changes in mentation.

Monitor vital signs, including apical/radial pulses and postural blood pressures.

Observe for nervous system signs of hyperkalemia: weakness, paresthesia or paresis, possible paralysis.

Minimize stressful situations and promote rest.

Assist with activity.

Monitor I & O.

Monitor ABGs and electrolytes.

Observe for signs of infection, avoid exposure to cold.

Tepid water/alcohol sponge bath.

MEDICAL MANAGEMENT

Normal saline IV.

Glucocorticoids IV × 24–36 hrs, then by mouth.

Plasma expanders.

Vasopressors.

Antibiotics.

RATIONALE

Decreased cerebral perfusion and severe hypoglycemia may lead to coma.

Pulse deficit may reflect cardiac arrhythmias secondary to increased potassium. Orthostatic hypotension may occur due to decreased sodium and extracellular fluid volume.

Potassium clearance decreases because decreased aldosterone level blocks exchange of K^+ for Na^+ in distal tubules.

Vascular collapse may occur. Conserve patient energy.

General weakness, orthostatic hypotension and possibility of syncopal episodes may result in patient injury.

Reflect changes in fluid balance.

Note imbalances and guide for replacement therapy.

May precipitate crisis.

Reduce fever, which also may act as a stressor.

To replace sodium and fluid losses.

Increase cortisol level and reverse shock state.

Emergency therapy in face of vascular collapse.

Reverse severe hypotension.

Used when infection is the "stressor."

439

NURSING DIAGNOSIS:	Nutrition, alteration in, less than body requirements.
SUPPORTING DATA:	Decreased GI enzymes result in N/V, anorexia, abdominal cramps and diarrhea. Prone to severe hypoglycemia.
DESIRED PATIENT OUTCOMES:	Nutritional needs met and weight is maintained.

INTERVENTIONS

Determine which foods are tolerated.

Create mealtime environment conducive to eating.

Encourage adequate rest periods.

Monitor daily weights.

Provide regular meals and snacks.

Avoid fasting even for test preparation, if possible.

RATIONALE

Patient will take and retain more.

Promote nutritional intake.

Lack of muscle/hepatic glycogen stores cause patient to tire easily.

Weight loss and muscle wasting occur because of GI disturbances.

Maintain adequate blood glucose levels.

Increased insulin sensitivity and inability to maintain blood glucose levels can result in severe hypoglycemia if regular calorie intake is not maintained.

MEDICAL MANAGEMENT

Glucose IV. Increased glucocorticoid dosage.

Increased sodium diet.

High-protein, low-carbohydrate diet.

Meet metabolic needs if fasting/stress occur.

Oral replacement for sodium losses secondary to lack of reabsorption in distal tubules.

Prone to hypoglycemia.

NURSING DIAGNOSIS:	Knowledge deficit, long-term therapy.
SUPPORTING DATA:	Deficiency requires lifelong replacement therapy to avoid symptoms and to live a normal life.
DESIRED PATIENT OUTCOMES:	Balance is maintained and patient is free of symptoms.

INTERVENTIONS

Discuss need for lifelong medication and how patient feels about disease. (Rreplacement therapy will depend on general medical condition.)

Instruct patient in selfadministration of steroids; dosage, expected effects and side-effects. Include information about the need for adjustment of dosage when under undue stress and importance of taking daily dosage AM and PM.

Discuss stress identification and reduction.

Discuss signs/symptoms of recurrence or need for consultation with physician as well as need for regular appointments, at least twice a year.

Instruct in obtaining/wearing of a medical identification tag. May also carry a water-soluble synthetic analog of cortisol and sterile syringe.

RATIONALE

Information and discussion of feelings can be helpful to the patient in making decisions and co-operating with necessary lifestyle changes. May not require replacement of mineral corticoids, especially if hypertensive.

May be oral or IM replacement. Knowledge of drugs will enable patient to manage drug regimen well. Emotional upsets, dental care, minor surgery, or trauma, and infections may alter body need.

Individual situations will differ and when patient identifies own stressors and appropriate management techniques the patient will be able to exercise more control of body responses.

Diaphoresis, fever, nausea/vomiting, weight gain, and so forth. Even when patient is doing well, it is important to maintain contact with the physician as drug dosage must be assessed and tailored to the individual patient.

To identify therapy needs in an emergency. May need readily available hormone supply when unplanned trauma/stress occur.

DIAGNOSIS: Cushing's Syndrome: Excessive Glucocorticoids

Cushing's syndrome refers to increased cortisol secretion that can be attributed to various causes: adrenocortical tumors, may be adenoma or carcinoma; hyperplasia of both glands by nonpituitary tumors that stimulate excess secretion; exogenous administration of ACTH; and Cushing's disease.

Cushing's disease is caused by a pituitary tumor, usually an adenoma.

Diagnostic evaluation is aimed at identification of the underlying cause. Treatment is determined by the cause.

PATIENT DATA BASE

NURSING HISTORY

Patient complains of weight gain, feeling puffy, rounding shoulders, easy bruising with minor trauma.

History of adrenal hyperplasia, adrenocortical neoplasms, extrapituitary tumors, or excessive administration of exogenous glucocorticoids (steroid therapy, note drug and dosage).

Also may have insulin-resistant diabetes.

Diet and weight history may be beneficial as to possible causes of extracellular fluid accumulation.

May demonstrate emotional instability.

Occurs in women 10:1.

DIAGNOSTIC STUDIES

Cortisol plasma levels are elevated. Need to be drawn at the same time each day because of circadian rhythms.

Blood sugar is elevated due to anti-insulin effect of cortisol.

LDH, CPK levels elevated; protein catabolism and muscle wasting.

Na^+ levels may be increased (Na^+ and H_2O retention).

Lymphocytes may be decreased; anti-inflammatory response to glucocorticoids.

Depressed antibody formation; same as above.

RBC may be increased, eosinophils decreased.

Gastric acid and pepsin production increased because of parasympathetic stimulation.

Urine: increased 17-hydroxycorticoids and 17-ketogenic steroids.

Increased plasma ACTH in presence of pituitary tumors.

PHYSICAL EXAMINATION

Evaluate areas of edema; face, backs of hands, scapular area, abdomen.

Observe for signs of protein catabolism in muscle, dermal and collagen-supporting networks: loss of muscle mass, osteoporosis, cutaneous striae, and ecchymosis after minor trauma.

Observe for androgen imbalances in women; fine coating of hair on face, oligomenorrhea, amenorrhea, atrophy of breasts, decreased libido.

Assess body response to blood sugar levels; cortisol levels are increased having an anti-insulin effect.

Assess mental status for effects of hormone imbalances.

NURSING PRIORITIES

1. Prevent injury and infection.
2. Maintain fluid balance.
3. Maintain mental functioning and provide psychologic support.
4. Instruct patient and SO re disease process and treatment.

NURSING DIAGNOSIS: **Injury, potential for, infection.**

SUPPORTING DATA: **Immune system is suppressed decreasing resistance to infection. May have few symptoms and when infection does develop, healing process may be slower.**

DESIRED PATIENT OUTCOMES: **Remains infection-free.**

INTERVENTIONS	RATIONALE
Place in reverse isolation and restrict visitors who have obvious infections.	Remove known sources of infection.
Monitor temperature on a regular basis.	Temperature elevation may not occur, or may have low temperature when other symptoms of infection are present.
Observe for signs of infection and/or nonhealing.	May be masked because steroids decrease pain, redness, temperature and swelling. Early intervention extremely important.
Instruct patient in importance of avoiding sources of infection as well as early identification and treatment.	Awareness of problem can enhance cooperation in avoiding infection.

NURSING DIAGNOSIS: **Fluid volume, deficit, potential.**

SUPPORTING DATA: **With excessive secretion of the glucocorticoids, an exaggeration of the normal functioning occurs, resulting in hyperglycemia, potassium depletion, sodium and water retention, changes in cardiac functioning and metabolic acidosis.**

DESIRED PATIENT OUTCOMES: **Fluid and electrolyte balance is maintained.**

INTERVENTIONS	RATIONALE
Explain diet restrictions of low sodium and high potassium.	Control development of edema and prevent hypokalemia.

Observe for vomiting, abdominal pain and tarry stools.	Increased hydrochloric acid production can cause gastric ulceration and hemorrhage.
Monitor serum potassium levels closely.	May be an increase in K^+ excretion; which may precipitate digitalis toxity.
Monitor blood pressure on a regular basis.	Hypertension may develop.

MEDICAL MANAGEMENT

Digoxin.	Congestive heart failure may develop.
Potassium supplements.	May be necessary to correct depletion.
Antacids p.r.n., and/or Cimetidine ac/hs.	Counteract hyperacidity and minimize gastric irritation.

NURSING DIAGNOSIS:	**Nutrition, alteration in, less than body requirements.**
SUPPORTING DATA:	**Carbohydrate, fat, and protein metabolism are disturbed. Pancreatic secretions are decreased, necrosis of pancreatic tissue and increased resistance to insulin occur. Overt diabetes may occur. Excess fat formation is deposited in a typical pattern.**
DESIRED PATIENT OUTCOMES:	**Weight is maintained at a stable level and fat deposits are minimized.**

INTERVENTIONS

RATIONALE

Discuss diet restrictions with patient/significant others.	Helpful to understand that excess cortisol increases the appetite.
Note complaints of loss of taste.	Senses of taste and smell may be impaired.
Consult dietitian.	To aid in preparation of palatable food. May use nonirritating herbs and spices to enhance tests.
Weigh daily at a given time.	Weight may vary at different times of the day.
Monitor intake and output.	Polydipsia/polyuria may indicate problems of diabetes.
Monitor Clinitest and acetone before meals and bedtime.	Be aware of development of diabetic symptoms. See care Plan: Diabetic Ketoacidosis.

MEDICAL MANAGEMENT

Provide low-sodium, low-carbohydrate, high-protein, high-potassium diet. Calories may be limited.	Control metabolism and weight gain.

NURSING DIAGNOSIS:	Self-concept, disturbance in, body image.
SUPPORTING DATA:	Body changes with fat deposits in the neck "buffalo hump," trunk area, and cheeks "moon face," and disturbances in protein metabolism resulting in muscle wasting, making the extremities extremely thin. Purple striae may occur on the abdomen, breasts, and buttocks, and the patient may have a florid complexion. Increased androgen secretion may cause amenorrhea in women and increased body hair may be noted.
DESIRED PATIENT OUTCOMES:	These side effects are minimized and patient verbalizes understanding of body changes and effective ways of dealing with them.

INTERVENTIONS

RATIONALE

Assess patient's emotional state.

Different situations are upsetting to different people. Depression may lead to suicide. Masculinization creates stress for most women.

Record emotional changes.

Personality changes, emotional lability, psychosis, delusions, insomnia, and irritability may occur.

Provide accurate information about treatment and the possibility of controlling body changes.

Treatment may remove the cause but hormone replacement therapy will be necessary for the rest of the patient's life.

Refer to Care Plan: Psychosocial Aspects of Care in the Acute Setting.

MEDICAL MANAGEMENT

Hormone replacement.

As indicated by the cause.

Surgery.

Adrenalectomy, hypophysectomy (see related care plans including Surgical Intervention).

Irradiation.

Effective against some tumors.

Psychologic counseling.

May be indicated by severity of condition.

NURSING DIAGNOSIS:	Skin integrity, impairment of, potential.

SUPPORTING DATA:	Skin becomes fragile due to breakdown in connective tissue and is susceptible to bruising.
DESIRED PATIENT OUTCOMES:	Skin remains intact.

INTERVENTIONS

Protect from bumping and bruising.

Change position, pad bony prominences, provide skin care.

RATIONALE

Keep skin damage to a minimum.

Measures to prevent skin breakdown.

NURSING DIAGNOSIS:	Injury, potential for, fractures.
SUPPORTING DATA:	Increased protein breakdown creates a negative nitrogen balance resulting in muscle weakness; awkward, poorly coordinated movements; loss of calcium from the bones. Weakened muscles and bones along with increased weight create a potential for falls and fractures.
DESIRED PATIENT OUTCOMES:	Fractures and other injuries do not occur.

INTERVENTIONS

Instruct patient to call for help when getting out of bed and to assist with walking.

Check environment for hazards.

Be alert to evidence of frustration.

Promote adequate rest periods.

Maintain a nonstressful environment.

MEDICAL MANAGEMENT

Sedatives.

RATIONALE

Prevent falls and possible injuries.

Remove objects that might cause accidental injuries.

Weakness can be difficult for the formerly active person.

May have difficulty sleeping at night because cortisol may cause restlessness and insomnia secondary to the fact that cortisol levels are circadian in nature.

Promote rest.

May be required to ensure adequate rest.

DIAGNOSIS: Conn's Syndrome (Primary Aldosteronism, Increased Mineral Corticoids)

PATIENT DATA BASE

NURSING HISTORY

Patient complains of feeling bloated, generalized weakness with decreased reflexes, flabby muscles without tone.

Pulse can be weak though blood pressure is high.

Note diet history with special attention to Na^+ and K^+ intake.

May complain of polyuria and polydipsia.

Frequent severe headache secondary to increased blood pressure.

History of adrenal adenoma, adrenocortical nodular hyperplasia, and adrenal carcinoma, which may cause hypersecretion of aldosterone; congestive heart failure, nephrosis and cirrhosis can also lead to Conn's syndrome due to poor cardiac function or disproportionate extracellular fluid shifts into interstitium and peritoneal spaces.

Usually seen in women > men, ages 30–50.

DIAGNOSTIC STUDIES

Sodium may be increased but is not always followed by water retention due to severe potassium depletion.

Potassium is decreased due to wasting effects of aldosterone. Hypokalemia can be severe enough to cause kidneys to ignore the ADH effects.

Increased hematocrit and hemoconcentration because of polyuria, even though Na^+ is increased in levels that should cause H_2O retention.

Urine specific gravity is low.

Metabolic alkalosis and hypokalemia.

ECG: S-T wave depression and asymmetry of T waves.

PHYSICAL EXAMINATION

May have complaints of nausea, vomiting, and abdominal distention.

Evaluate fluid status: blood pressure may be increased, edema, weight gain, increased heart rate, urine output.

Observe for reflex changes in relation to potassium-wasting and lowered calcium levels: muscle hypertonicity and weakness, tetany, Chvostek's and Trousseau's signs may be positive.

Urine output will also increase greatly if K^+ levels go low enough to cause kidneys not to respond to ADH.

Assess cardiac status as signs of hypokalemia and alkalosis develop: S-T wave depression and asymmetric T waves as seen in left ventricle enlargement.

Alkalosis results in tetany and paresthesia.

NURSING PRIORITIES

1. Maintain fluid balance to prevent related complications.
2. Provide for safety related to alteration in muscle strength.

3. Prevent skin breakdown.
4. Maintain adequate nutritional status.

NURSING DIAGNOSIS:

SUPPORTING DATA:

DESIRED PATIENT OUTCOMES:

Fluid volume deficit, potential.

Aldosterone occuring in excess affects electrolyte and fluid balance with resulting renal failure and hypertension.

Potassium levels are normal, symptoms of hypertension are reversed.

INTERVENTIONS

Monitor intake and output, daily weight.

Monitor electrolytes.

Monitor blood pressure frequently.

Auscultate lungs; note increased JVD, and development of systemic edema.

RATIONALE

To establish fluid therapy and monitor effects of replacement.

Alterations in aldosterone levels may result in electrolyte fluctuation.

Will be lower and fluctuations may occur postoperatively.

Reflects fluid overload/heart failure.

MEDICAL MANAGEMENT

Spironolactone and potassium for 3–5 weeks before surgery.

Surgery.

Epinephrine IV.

Steroid replacement therapy.

Aldosterone antagonist given to reverse the suppression of the renin-angiotensin feedback system and increase potassium levels before surgery.

Removal of the adenoma, if present, and/or adrenalectomy (removal of the adrenal glands, one or both). In early stages, symptoms may be reversed by surgical intervention. In later stages, changes in the renal and cardiovascular systems may be permanent. See appropriate care plans as indicated including Surgical Intervention; Adrenalectomy.

May have an abrupt fall of blood pressure when the tumor vessels are ligated.

Will be required prior to and following surgery and when both glands are removed, lifetime replacement is necessary. Refer to Care Plan: Addison's Disease: Primary Adrenal Insufficiency, Nursing Diagnosis: Knowledge deficit for steroid therapy.

NURSING DIAGNOSIS:	Mobility, impaired physical.
SUPPORTING DATA:	Hypokalemia results in muscle weakness, tetany, and paresthesias.
DESIRED PATIENT OUTCOMES:	Symptoms are reversed and mobility is maintained.

INTERVENTIONS

Observe for muscle irritability, jerky and uncontrollable movements.

Provide a safe environment and assist with moving when out of bed.

Provide information about condition/therapy.

Refer to Care Plan: Cushing's Syndrome: Excessive Glucocorticoids for further interventions and nursing diagnoses prior to surgical treatment.

RATIONALE

Signs of tetany.

Protect from injury.

Treatment will reverse symptoms.

DIAGNOSIS: Pheochromocytoma

PATIENT DATA BASE

Clinical signs/symptoms depend upon intermittent or consistent secretion of catecholamines and whether epinephrine or norepinephrine is secreted.

NURSING HISTORY

May complain of headaches, palpitations, weight loss, anxiety, excessive perspiration.

May present with hyperventilation, tremulousness and/or psychosis and the initial diagnosis may be masked.

History of persistent or intermittent hypertension.

Episodes may be precipitated by allergic reaction, emotional stress, or physical activity.

DIAGNOSTIC STUDIES

Excessive production of norepinephrine and/or epinephrine (spontaneously or after stimulation).

Pressor test has a number of false positives/negatives.

Urine testing: for metabolites; VMA, metanephrines, catecholamines.

Increased serum glucose and free fatty acids.

Arteriography, ultrasound and/or CT scan may assist in localizing tumor.

PHYSICAL EXAMINATION

Does not reveal much unless it is a familial form of disease: café au lait pigmentation, diaphoresis, orthostatic hypotension, thyroid tumors/neurofibromas.

NURSING PRIORITIES

1. Maintain control of blood pressure.
2. Prepare for surgery.

NURSING DIAGNOSIS:	**Tissue perfusion, alteration in.**
SUPPORTING DATA:	**Stimulation of the sympathetic nervous system by the tumor produces hypertension, hypermetabolism, and hyperglycemia. Effective control is necessary prior to surgery. Potential for paroxysmal hypertensive crisis.**
DESIRED PATIENT OUTCOMES:	**Patient is stabilized and ready for surgery.**

INTERVENTIONS

Assess signs/symptoms of headache, dizziness, nausea/vomiting, palpitations, diaphoresis, chest/abdominal/back pain, dyspnea, tremors, and pallor.

Monitor vital signs and maintain frequent contact with patient.

Place in semi-Fowler's position.

Promote rest and quiet, nonstressful environment, avoid activities that may increase bood pressure.

Avoid the use of beverages, such as coffee, tea and so forth.

Observe for signs/symptoms of CHF and renal failure.

Document effectiveness of sedation, if used.

MEDICAL MANAGEMENT

Phentolamine, (Regitine).

Sedatives.

Propranolol.

Surgery.

RATIONALE

Occur suddenly and usually lasts 15–30 minutes but may last hours and can cause blindness/stroke.

Diastolic over 110 increases possibility of MI and/or CVA; arrhythmias may occur. Helpful to allay anxiety.

Decrease intracranial pressure.

Reduce sympathetic nervous system stimulation that may potentiate occurrence of crisis.

Caffeine has a stimulating effect.

Frequently occuring complications, secondary to hypertension.

May be physiologically resistant to sedatives and require increased dosage because of hypermetabolism.

Long-acting beta-adrenergic blockers to control blood pressure.

To promote rest.

To control arrhythmias, if present.

To remove tumor. Refer to Care Plan: Adrenalectomy.

CARE PLAN: Adrenalectomy

May be done for removal of adrenal tumor, Cushing's disease, or as treatment for breast/prostate cancer. Preoperative: may need to correct hyperglycemia and protein deficiency. For surgical care refer to Care Plan: Surgical Interventions.

NURSING PRIORITIES

1. Maintain tissue perfusion/fluid and electrolyte balance.
2. Provide for steroid replacement.
3. Provide information and assist patient in dealing with postoperative care and rehabilitation needs.

NURSING DIAGNOSIS:	**Tissue perfusion, alteration in.**
SUPPORTING DATA:	**Sudden alteration in the production of catecholamines following manipulation of the tumor during surgery can cause vascular collapse due to vasodilation and pooling of blood. Acute adrenal insufficiency may decrease circulating volume through dehydration. Hemorrhage may occur as adrenal glands are highly vascular organs and proximity to the vena cava, aorta, and renal vessels may result in intraoperative trauma. Patient suffering from Cushing's disease may require an increased amount of anesthetic agents, prolonging the recovery phase and potentiating the incidence of shock.**
DESIRED PATIENT OUTCOMES:	**Blood pressure and tissue perfusion are maintained.**

INTERVENTIONS

Monitor vital signs, CVP, intake and output, and level of consciousness frequently.

Monitor serum electrolytes and urine sodium.

Turn, do leg exercise and pulmonary hygiene on a regular basis.

Clinitest/acetest.

RATIONALE

Monitor changes in circulating volume and signs of impending shock.

Altered renal perfusion and function may affect fluid and electrolyte balance.

Promote circulation, prevent stasis, and minimize atelectasis.

Release of catecholamines may result in glycosuria and osmotic diuresis.

MEDICAL MANAGEMENT

Hypertonic saline IV.

Replace sodium losses.

IV fluids, glucose, blood, plasma, dextran.

Maintain circulating blood volume and prevent shock. Adrenals are highly vascular and hemorrhage may occur.

Norepinephrine. Dopamine.

Maintain/stabilize BP and increase renal blood flow.

Cortisone.

Prevent/treat adrenal insufficiency.

Insulin, sliding scale coverage.

To correct glycosuria.

NURSING DIAGNOSIS:	**Knowledge deficit, postoperative care.**
SUPPORTING DATA:	**When bilateral adrenalectomy is done, patient will have to be on corticosteroids for life. Information will be helpful to postoperative adjustment.**
DESIRED PATIENT OUTCOMES:	*Verbalizes reasons for replacement therapy, medications regimen, and symptoms of recurrence that require medical attention.*

Refer to Care Plan: Addison's Disease: Primary Adrenal Insufficiency, Nursing Diagnosis: Knowledge deficit, long-term therapy.

DIAGNOSIS: Hypothyroidism, Myxedema

PATIENT DATA BASE
NURSING HISTORY

PRIMARY: Thyroid gland does not secrete a sufficient amount of hormone.
   May have history of thyroidectomy or irradiation treatments; thyroiditis, Hashimoto's disease; or iodine deficiency.

SECONDARY: Pituitary gland does not secrete an adequate amount of thyroid-stimulating hormone (TSH).
   May have pituitary infarct or tumor, or a head injury.

TERTIARY: Hypothalmus does not secrete thyroid-releasing hormone (TRH).

Signs/symptoms depend on extent of the deficiency.

Can occur in men and women any age including neonates; generally seen in women ages 30–60. Can be common in advanced old age with symptoms that mimic "senility."

Numbness/tingling of extremities.

Intolerance of cold.

Complains of headaches and syncope, slowing of speech and mental functions.

Complains of weakness and fatigue, may have mental apathy, depression, or paranoia.

May complain of nausea/vomiting, gastric distention, constipation, fecal impaction.

History of weight gain.

Note history of allergy to iodine, as it may be used in testing.

DIAGNOSTIC STUDIES

Normocytic or normochromic anemia secondary to decreased erythrocyte mass.

Thyroid scan; aids in detecting thyroid nodules and active tissue.

Increased serum cholesterol.

Decreased radioactive iodine uptake (T3) done with scan; measures ability of thyroid to accumulate ingested iodine. Drugs and contrast media (from x-rays) can alter results from 1 week to 1 year: oral contraceptives, large doses of aspirin, topical betadine, dilantin, estrogen, androgens.

Thyroid-stimulating hormone: elevated in hypothyroidism.

Urine creatinine decreased.

Cardiac enlargement may be noted on x-ray/ECG.

PHYSICAL EXAMINATION

Complains of weakness and fatigue, may have mental apathy, depression, or paranoia.

Movements may be slow and clumsy.

Achilles reflex time prolonged.

Mental processes become dulled and neurologic signs, such as polyneuropathy, and cerebellar ataxia, may develop.

On palpation, note size, shape, and consistency of the gland and the presence of nodules. Do not palpate if thyrotoxicosis exists.

Pemberton's sign may be positive if retrosternal goiter is present. (When the arms are raised straight up along the head, congestion of the face and respiratory distress occur.)

Skin is dry and coarse, may have a yellowish cast.

Facial edema may be present.

Hair is thin, coarse, and brittle and may fall out.

Nails thicken and become brittle.

Temperature and pulse are subnormal, blood pressure is low.

Menorrhagia may occur.

NURSING PRIORITIES

Based on the extent or progression of the disease: early signs/symptoms to myxedema coma.
1. Recognize metabolic slowdown and support organ/system functioning.
2. Provide for safety when muscular weakness and ataxia are present.
3. Improve nutritional status.
4. Provide information re disease process and lifelong therapy.

NURSING DIAGNOSIS: Cardiac output, alteration in, decreased.

SUPPORTING DATA: Low levels of thyroid hormone increase blood lipids, such as cholesterol and lipoproteins. Chronic hypothyroidism predisposes patient to ischemic heart disease, arteriosclerosis, and coronary artery disease. Oxygen demands of the heart remain the same even though metabolism slows. Cardiac output decreases because of decreased heart rate and stroke volume. Pericardial effusions can occur, which can cause bradycardia, increased diastolic pressure and distant heart sounds. Potential for cardiac tamponade is present.

DESIRED PATIENT OUTCOMES: Patient will have heart rate >60, baseline BP, no evidence of ischemic heart pain.

INTERVENTIONS

Note decreasing urinary output; increasing heart rate; hypotension; cool, clammy skin; and changes in mentation.

RATIONALE

Signs of developing vascular collapse.

Monitor heart rhythm by ECG strips and report arrhythmias.	T waves are inverted and Q-T intervals are prolonged. Ischemia or pericardial effusions may cause arrhythmias, which may result in ventricular tachycardia.
Ascultate heart tone, monitor pulse rate and blood pressure.	Note developing pericardial effusion and tamponade.
Monitor for pain.	Can be manifested when ischemic heart disease and/or pericardial effusion are present.
Monitor drug therapy carefully.	Vasopressors are synergistic with thyroid medications.

MEDICAL MANAGEMENT

Vasopressors.	Treat vascular collapse.
Refer to Care Plans: Angina Pectoris; Myocardial Infarction.	

NURSING DIAGNOSIS: Gas exchange, impaired.

SUPPORTING DATA: Potential for hypoventilation and respiratory acidosis because of obesity, decreased vital capacity and ventilatory flow rates, pleural effusion, upper airway obstruction by enlarged tongue or edema of vocal cords or glottis dysfunction. Ventilatory assistance may be needed as CO_2 retention, hypoxia, and respiratory acidosis occur.

DESIRED PATIENT OUTCOMES: Hypoventilation and respiratory acidosis are prevented.

INTERVENTIONS

RATIONALE

Monitor rate, depth, quality, of breath sounds.	Snoring, crowing, decreased breath sounds can indicate obstruction from vocal cords, tongue, or glottis. Rales and rhonchi may indicate effusions of the pleura that need immediate attention.
Stimulate patient to increase respiratory rate and promote deep breathing.	Increase tidal ventilation and O_2/CO_2 exchange.
Monitor ABGs periodically, especially when restlessness and agitation are present.	Direct assessment of ventilatory function. Necessary to evaluate respiratory status.
Monitor for increased respiratory effort, decompensation respiration >28/min, shallow, minimal air movement.	Treatment necessary before respiratory collapse occurs.

MEDICAL MANAGEMENT

Avoid sedatives, hypnotics, and tranquilizers.

These drugs depress respirations.

Treat pulmonary infections aggressively.

Interfere with respiratory functioning.

Ventilatory assistance.

For severe hypoxia, until patient can breathe adequately on own. Refer to Care Plan: Ventilatory Assistance (Mechanical).

NURSING DIAGNOSIS:	Tissue perfusion, alteration in, metabolic functioning.
SUPPORTING DATA:	Decreased thyroid hormone circulation in peripheral tissues. As a result, chemical reactions at the tissue level are slow. Patient is hypersensitive to narcotics, barbiturates, anesthetics, and drugs that require breakdown. Temperature is lower and patient is intolerant of the cold due to decreased metabolism. Response to infection is impaired due to adrenal function alterations.
DESIRED PATIENT OUTCOMES:	Afebrile, no signs/symptoms of infection are present, and desired drug levels are maintained.

INTERVENTIONS

Monitor individual response to drugs closely.

RATIONALE

Many drugs are potentiated and must be monitored when used. Smaller doses of narcotics, barbiturates, anesthetics, vasopresors, insulin, and heart drugs (digitalis) are given initially and gradually increased as the patient becomes euthyroid. Metabolism is slow, affecting drug therapy, which may result in toxic symptoms that do not respond well to treatment.

Monitor temperature.

If temperature was previously low or baseline, a rise may indicate infection. Adrenal function is altered and body may not be able to respond to infection stress appropriately.

Use caution in warming patient, allowing temperature to rise gradually, protect from chilling.

Temperature may be subnormal and slow warming is necessary. If done quickly, a massive vasodilation could occur, causing heart problems, and circulatory collapse. Chilling increases the metabolic rate, which can strain the heart.

MEDICAL MANAGEMENT

Thyroid replacement therapy.

Antibiotics.

Corticosteroid replacement therapy.

Vasopressors.

Regain/maintain normal level.

To treat infection. May be used prophylactically.

Until adrenal function returns to normal.

For vascular collapse.

NURSING DIAGNOSIS: **Fluid volume, alteration in, excess, potential.**

SUPPORTING DATA: **Adrenal insufficiency and metabolic complications. Impaired renal diluting capacity because of inappropriate secretion of ADH, changes in osmoreceptors or cortisol insufficiency, leads to hyponatremia, causing impairment in water excretion, Na$^+$ is diluted. Hypoglycemia is seen due to metabolic complications of the adrenal cortex.**

DESIRED PATIENT OUTCOMES: **Fluid and electrolytes are maintained within normal limits.**

INTERVENTIONS

Mouth care, ice chips, wet sponges may be used.

Monitor serum electrolytes.

Keep accurate I & O and daily weight.

RATIONALE

Provide comfort when fluid intake is restricted.

Detect fluid needs or deficiencies caused by water retention. Hyponatremia caused by dilutional effect of fluid retention

Assist in management of total body fluid levels and Na$^+$ retention and excretion.

MEDICAL MANAGEMENT

Fluid restriction.

Sodium replacement.

Control hypervolemia.

For severe hyponatremia as seen in myxedema coma. Patient is volume expanded, therefore Na$^+$ level <115 mEq/L is usually treated with small amounts of hypertonic saline. Serum Na$^+$ >120 mEq/L is not treated to avoid compromising the cardiac status. Fluid restriction is the normal treatment with concurrent serum electrolyte monitoring.

Glucose replacement.

For severe hypoglycemia caused by metabolic slowdown. High concentration glucose is used to avoid expanding blood volume.

Steroid replacement therapy.

Adrenal insufficiency may occur secondary to increased plasma thyroxine levels.

NURSING DIAGNOSIS:	**Thought processes, impairment in.**
SUPPORTING DATA:	**Edema throughout the body develops as mucopolysaccharides and mucin deposits invade the interstitial spaces. Signs/symptoms develop: decreased hearing, hoarseness, enlargement of tongue. In addition, water retention occurs because of adrenal gland changes and presents in patient as headaches, drowsiness, fatigue, lethargy, and forgetfulness, although mental alertness may be intact. May be easily confused and have cerebral ataxia. Paranoia and delusions have also been observed as well as grand mal seizures. Lastly, coma may develop.**
DESIRED PATIENT OUTCOMES:	**Edema is minimized/prevented and mental processes remain intact.**

INTERVENTIONS

Observe for increase in lethargy, forgetfulness, drowsiness, irritability. Note paranoia and delusions, hallucinations that occur.

Monitor these signs/symptoms, after treatment begins.

Take seizure precautions and keep accurate documentation: Refer to Care Plan: Seizure Disorders.

Provide for psychologic comfort; continuity of care, daily routines, listening, and being available to patient.

Discuss with significant others, changes in patient's mental status, and encourage tolerance of mood changes and slowness.

RATIONALE

May indicate impending myxedema coma. May be prevented by early treatment with thyroid replacement.

Reflect effectiveness of drug therapy.

Provides for patient safety as seizure activity may precede coma.

Usually retain mental alertness, so even though patient appears slow and confused, it is helpful for staff to remain tolerant and understanding.

Helpful for SO to treat the patient the same as before the symptoms appeared.

MEDICAL MANAGEMENT

Thyroid hormone replacement therapy.

Mentation and nervous system return to normal within a few days to 2 weeks after therapy has begun.

NURSING DIAGNOSIS:	**Bowel elimination, alteration in, constipation.**
SUPPORTING DATA:	**Appetite is decreased, motility of GI tract is decreased due to myxedema fluid buildup in peritoneal sac. Constipation, flatulence, abdominal distention, and fecal impactions are frequent. Often associated with ascites, ileus, and bowel obstruction. Megacolon and paralytic ileus usually accompany coma.**
DESIRED PATIENT OUTCOMES:	**Normal bowel function as evidenced by active bowel sounds, passing flatus, soft, formed bowel movements, and soft abdomen.**

INTERVENTIONS

Maintain dietary regimen with sufficient roughage and fluids in the early stage.

Provide for exercise, such as walking.

Instruct patient not to strain at stool.

Avoid enemas, rectal temperatures, suppositories.

Listen to bowel sounds and record.

Maintain record of bowel movements and flatulence.

Measure abdominal girth and palpate abdomen for distention and hardness.

RATIONALE

Prevent bowel impaction, constipation, and obstruction.

If able to be up, assists in bowel functioning.

Potential danger to heart.

Decreases potential for vagal stimulation.

Indicate changes in bowel function.

Evidence of working bowel.

Indicators of obstruction/ileus.

MEDICAL MANAGEMENT

Stool softeners and laxatives may be ordered.

Thyroid replacement therapy.

Assist/facilitate bowel functioning.

Will increase/decrease motility and remove ascites that interfere with motility.

NURSING DIAGNOSIS:	Mobility, impaired physical.
SUPPORTING DATA:	Weakness, fatigue, cramps, muscle soreness occur. A diagnostic symptom is the prolonged relaxation phase of tendon reflexes, even though contraction phase is normal. Seen best in Achilles or biceps tendons. Signs/symptoms are due to mucinous deposits in joints and interstitial spaces.
DESIRED PATIENT OUTCOMES:	Patient will exhibit normal gait, normal muscle movement, and little or no pain and fatigue when moving.

INTERVENTIONS

Provide for safety; depending on degree of muscular impairment, walking aids, rest periods, hand rails, wheel chair, and possibly restraints.

RATIONALE

Has less control of movement due to pain and slow reflexes. Providing aids will assist patient in independence and comfort as well as provide for patient's safety.

MEDICAL MANAGEMENT

Begin thyroid replacement.

Aspirin and other antiarthritic drugs may be useful.

Signs/symptoms of muscle involvement will disappear within first few days.

To relieve arthritic symptoms until thyroid levels return to normal.

NURSING DIAGNOSIS:	Nutrition, alteration in, less than body requirements.
SUPPORTING DATA:	As signs/symptoms increase, metabolism and the gastrointestinal tract slow, causing malabsorption and poor digestion of food. Appetite decreases as well. Consequently, low-protein synthesis from dietary deficiency leads to anemia; hypoglycemia, hyponatremia, hyperkalemia, and hyperlipedema present as a result of the nutritional imbalances, aggravating hypothyroidism and leading to myxedema coma.

461

DESIRED PATIENT OUTCOMES: Patient becomes nutritionally balanced by maintaining balanced diet, supplementation, and replacement therapy.

INTERVENTIONS

Provide low-calorie diet, with increased protein, and moderate Na$^+$ content.

Maintain adequate fluid intake, 6–8 glasses/day (don't overload), and increase roughage.

Avoid goitrogens, i.e., cabbage, soybean, peanuts.

Encourage patient to eat; explain diet and include patient preferences.

MEDICAL MANAGEMENT

Supplementary diets.

Give vitamin supplements.

RATIONALE

Patient is usually overweight with poor appetite. Increased protein will help prevent anemia.

Helps eliminate or prevent impactions and constipation. In acute stages may need to restrict water to correct hyponatremia.

Although not proven as a cause of hypothyroidism, they do interfere with production of thyroid hormone.

When the patient is involved, appetite and intake may be improved.

To correct deficiencies. Usually has difficulty tolerating large amounts of food. Supplementation can provide necessary electrolytes and so forth without bulk.

Correct deficiencies when dietary intake is insufficient.

NURSING DIAGNOSIS: Skin integrity, impairment of, actual.

SUPPORTING DATA: Persons in hypothyroid state exhibit characteristic dry, flaky, cool skin. Flaking with hyperkeratosis is usually over flexures in skin. Skin usually has a faint yellow color due to impaired conversion of carotene to vitamin A. Hair is coarse and dry, nails are dry and brittle, and thinning of eyebrows can occur. Skin can appear coarse and has subcutaneous swelling seen easily in eyelids, periorbital tissue, nose, and the backs of the hands. May bruise more easily due to increased capillary fragility.

DESIRED PATIENT OUTCOMES: Normal skin color and texture without flaking, roughened, or edematous areas.

INTERVENTIONS

Use soap sparingly, use oils or creams to lubricate, massage. Instruct patient in skin care.

Turn patient often, check pressure points often, protect bony prominences with padding. Place on sheep skin, egg crate or alternating pressure mattress.

Handle patient gently, arrange for and teach safety to avoid bumps/trauma.

RATIONALE

Treat dry flaky skin before several skin layers are lost and breakdown occurs. Increase circulation to skin.

Edema makes skin prone to breakdown because of decreased circulation.

Capillary fragility leads to easy bruising.

NURSING DIAGNOSIS:	Sexual dysfunction.
SUPPORTING DATA:	Alteration in levels of sexual hormones may result in decreased sexual drive and infertility. In addition, women may experience prolonged menstrual cycles.
DESIRED PATIENT OUTCOMES:	Return to normal/previous levels of sexual functioning and activity.

INTERVENTIONS

Tell patient that normal sexual functioning can be expected to return after treatment has begun.

Assess need for counseling referral.

RATIONALE

Information may be all that is needed.

May be necessary in individual situations. Refer to Care Plan: Psychsocial Aspects of Care in the Acute Setting.

NURSING DIAGNOSIS:	Knowledge deficit, medication regimen and prevention of complications.
SUPPORTING DATA:	Patient undergoes various changes as hypothyroidism progresses. Patient needs information that signs/symptoms will disappear with treatment. The neurologic and muscular changes are often the most unsettling. Psychologic support is essential for well-being. Because thyroid replacement therapy is lifelong, a thorough education program is helpful to give patient and SO the information they need to follow therapy regimen.

DESIRED PATIENT OUTCOMES:	Will verbalize understanding of therapy regimen and healthy functioning will be maintained.

INTERVENTIONS

Instruct in lifelong need for medication on a regular routine, with checkups as necessary.

Give information about the s/s of hyper/hypothyroidism and when to seek medical attention. Refer to Care Plan: Hyperthyroidism (Thyrotoxicosis).

Give information more than once and in different forms; written, verbal and by requesting repetition to evaluate understanding.

Include significant others in teaching.

RATIONALE

Circulating thyroid hormone is essential for life. Stressful events may precipitate need for alteration in medication.

Patient is responsible for own self and can assume this when sufficient information is available. Excessive thyroid hormone may lead to hyperthyroidism.

Impaired memory during hypothyroid periods may interfere with understanding and retention.

Helpful to understanding and acceptance of patient's behavior as well as being helpful to patient in recovery process.

DIAGNOSIS: Hyperthyroidism (Thyrotoxicosis)

PATIENT DATA BASE

NURSING HISTORY

Complaints of nervousness, increased irritability, muscle weakness, rapid and hoarse speech.

History of recent weight loss, >20 lbs.

May relate improved appetite.

May complain of heat intolerance and diaphoresis.

Complaints of palpitations and angina.

May have history of hypothyroidism, thyroid hormone replacement therapy, or antithyroid therapy.

May have had a recent thyroidectomy.

May have history of cardiac disorders; recent illness, such as pneumonia; or surgery.

May have recently experienced a stressful situation, such as infection, trauma (emotional/physical), or surgery.

Women are affected 7:1 with familial tendencies, 30–50 years old.

Patient with history of a nodular toxic goiter, overtreatment with thyroid drugs, a functioning thyroid carcinoma, and pituitary adenoma that secretes excess TSH can be in thyrotoxic crisis.

Other precipitators are: insulin-induced hypoglycemia, vascular accidents, pulmonary emboli, x-ray contrast studies, premature withdrawal of antithyroid drugs.

Complains of increased gastric motility with stool changes.

Note history of allergy to iodine, as it may be used in testing.

DIAGNOSTIC STUDIES

Abnormal radioimmunoassay (RIA) test.

Serum thyroxine (T4) and triiodothyronine (T3) are increased.

Thyroid ^{131}I uptake is increased.

Increased erythrocyte mass.

Blood sugar increased because of adrenal involvement: increased adrenal activity causes impaired insulin secretion. Thyroid hormone increases glycogenolysis and increases absorption; therefore, elevating blood sugar.

Low-plasma cortisol levels from less adrenal reserve.

Alkaline phosphatase increased.

Increased serum calcium levels.

Serum cholesterol decreased.

Abnormal liver function tests.

Urine creatinine increased.

Lab values can be altered (especially the RIA) if patient: ingests excessive thyroid hormone; has subacute thyroiditis; has acute hepatitis (releases hepatic bound thyroid hormone).

ECG: cardiac systole is shorter; cardiomegaly, heart is enlarged with fibrosis and necrosis.

Achilles reflex time shortened.

PHYSICAL EXAMINATION

Skin smooth, warm, and flushed, may have excessive sweating.

Hair is fine, silky, straight.

Complains of nausea, vomiting, diarrhea, and urinating in large amounts.

Blood pressure is elevated with widened pulse pressure, tachycardia at rest, and patient may be dyspneic.

Temperature may be elevated, >100°F.

ECG may show atrial fibrillations.

May have signs/symptoms of exophthalmia.

Thyroid gland may be enlarged with oversecretion of hormone.

Alterations in mental status may be apparent; nervousness, irritability, and tremors or psychotic behavior.

In thyrotoxic crisis, patient may be in delerium, frank psychosis, or stupor, coma, circulatory collapse, shock, pulmonary edema, with possibility of death.

Fine tremor may be apparent when hand is outstretched as well as purposeless, quick, jerky movements of other body parts. Leg extension may be hindered.

NURSING PRIORITIES

1. Promote comfort.
2. Provide psychologic support.
3. Observe for complications.
4. Provide patient with information about disease process and therapy.

NURSING DIAGNOSIS: **Rest-activity pattern, ineffective.**

SUPPORTING DATA: **Increased metabolic rate results in irritability; nervous, tense, and jittery behavior. Extent of the disease and the effect on the patient needs to be determined for decision about medical or surgical treatment. Emotional lability may result from increased irritability of the CNS.**

DESIRED PATIENT OUTCOMES: **Activity is controlled and adequate rest is obtained.**

INTERVENTIONS

Instruct patient in signs of toxicity from use of thiourea derivative drug use.

Provide for quiet environment; cool room, decreased sensory stimuli, soothing colors, quiet music.

RATIONALE

Toxic reactions, such as fever, sore throat, skin eruptions, may occur and it is important to report them as they may indicate agranulocytosis.

Reduce stimuli that may increase hyperactivity.

Provide for diversional activities that are calming.

Allows for use of nervous energy in constructive manner.

Avoid topics that irritate or upset the patient.

Increased irritability of the CNS may cause patient to be easily excited, agitated, and prone to emotional outbursts.

Discuss with SO reasons for emotional lability.

Understanding that the behavior is physically based, can allow for different responses/approaches.

MEDICAL MANAGEMENT

Sedatives (phenobarbital), tranquilizers (chlordiazepoxide).

Promote relaxation.

Radioactive iodine.

Destroys functioning gland tissue. Results take 6–8 weeks, 2–3 treatments may be necessary.

Antithyroid drugs, most commonly, propylthiouracil and methimazole.

Inhibit synthesis of thyroid hormone. May be definitive treatment or used to prepare patient for surgery.

Iodine and iodine preparations may be used.

Rapid action reduces metabolic rate quickly. May interfere with radioactive iodine treatment and may exacerbate the disease in some people. May be used as surgical prep to decrease size and vascularity of the gland.

Adrenergic blocking agents.

Given as adjunctive therapy to control side effects of tachycardia, tremors, and nervousness.

Surgery.

Subtotal thyroidectomy with 5/6 of the gland removed may be done. Refer to Care Plan: Thyroidectomy.

NURSING DIAGNOSIS:	**Nutrition, alteration in, less than body requirements, potential.**
SUPPORTING DATA:	**Increased metabolism leads to increased appetite and food intake with loss of weight.**
DESIRED PATIENT OUTCOMES:	**Weight is stabilized at normal level.**

INTERVENTIONS

Increase number of meals and snacks, using high-calorie foods that are easily digested.

RATIONALE

Maintain weight and meet energy requirements.

Avoid foods that increase peristalsis, such as tea, coffee, fibrous and highly seasoned foods.

Increased motility of the GI tract may result in diarrhea.

Weigh daily and report losses.

Continued weight loss may indicate failure of therapy.

Increase fluid intake. Avoid fluids that cause diarrhea, such as apple/prune.

Increased perspiration, polyuria, and increased metabolic wastes can create problems of dehydration.

NURSING DIAGNOSIS:	Injury, eye, potential for.
SUPPORTING DATA:	Alteration of protective mechanisms of the eyes due to exophthalmos.
DESIRED PATIENT OUTCOMES:	Progression of the condition is halted. Eyes remain moist and free of ulcerations.

INTERVENTIONS

RATIONALE

Protect exposed cornea by using dark glasses when awake and taping the eyelids shut during sleep.

May be unable to close eyelids completely due to edema and fibrosis of the fat pads.

Elevate the head of the bed and restrict salt intake.

Decrease edema.

Instruct the patient in the use of extraocular muscle exercises.

Improve circulation and maintain mobility of the eyelids.

Provide opportunity for patient to discuss feelings about altered appearance and measures to enhance self-image.

Protruding eyes may be viewed as unattractive. Appearance can be enhanced with proper use of makeup, overall grooming, and the use of dark glasses.

MEDICAL MANAGEMENT

Methylcellulose drops.

To lubricate the eyes.

ACTH, prednisone.

Decrease inflammation.

Antithyroid drugs.

Decrease signs/symptoms and prevent worsening of the condition.

Eyelids may need to be sutured shut.

To protect cornea until edema resolves.

NURSING DIAGNOSIS:	Tissue perfusion, alteration in. Thyroid crisis and cardiac decompensation.
SUPPORTING DATA:	Uncontrolled hyperthyroidism with increased amounts of hormone in the bloodstream and increased metabolism with abrupt rise in temperature, respiratory distress, and cardiac failure; may be precipitated by infection, stress, surgical procedures, and dental work in patients with preexisting disease.

DESIRED PATIENT OUTCOMES:	Thyroid activity is controlled, and cardiac functioning is maintained.

INTERVENTIONS

RATIONALE

Cool cloth on head and lukewarm sponge bath.

Decrease temperature.

Monitor vital signs.

For shock and hypotension.

Monitor for increased temperature, >100°F (37.8°C); tachycardia greater than normally anticipated with increased temperature; diaphoresis; emotional lability leading to delirium and coma; history of recent weight loss of 18–20 lbs.

Signs of exaggerated state of thyroid crisis/storm.

Sputum culture and sensitivities may be indicated.

Pulmonary infection is the most frequent precipitating factor.

Observe for diarrhea, jaundice, CHF, hepatic necrosis, psychosis.

May be signs of impending crisis.

Monitor for hyperglycemia.

Increased adrenergic activity can cause impaired insulin secretion/resistance.

MEDICAL MANAGEMENT

Hypothermia blanket.

Decreases temperature and metabolic needs.

Avoid giving ASA.

Increases free thyroxine levels.

Fluids, electrolytes as indicated.

Replacement to prevent dehydration.

Vitamin B-complex, glucose.

Meet nutritional requirements, if hypoglycemia is not present.

Insulin, small amounts.

To aid in controlling serum glucose if elevated.

Glucocorticoids and vasopressor drugs.

Adrenal insufficiency may be present and Decadron (dexamethasone) reduces peripheral conversion of thyroxine rapidly and combats shock and hypotension.

Propylthiouracil (PTU), orally.

Blocks synthesis of hormone as well as peripheral conversion of thyroxine.

Sodium iodide IV one hour after loading dose of PTU.

Inhibit release of thyroid hormone.

Supportive therapy for CHF (Inderal).

Arrhythmias are usually refractory until hyperthyroid is controlled. Beta-adrenergic blocking effect may decrease tachycardia.

Barbiturates may be given IV.

To control agitation.

Antibiotic therapy.

Indicated if precipitating factor is infection.

Dialysis and hemoperfusion.

May be used occasionally to remove excess hormone.

NURSING DIAGNOSIS:	Knowledge deficit, disease, cause, course, treatment, and prognosis.

SUPPORTING DATA:	Many factors, such as adenomas, infection, may be involved in precipitating this disease and recurrences are common.
DESIRED PATIENT OUTCOMES:	Patient/significant others will verbalize the cause of the patient's illness, anticipated treatment, and prognosis.

INTERVENTIONS

Assess current level of knowledge.

Give information appropriate to individual situation.

Assess level of anxiety. May need referral to professional therapy.

Provide information about drug therapy regimen.

Give information about the signs/symptoms of side effects, particularly agranulocytosis.

Patient who has been treated for hyperthyroidism needs to be given information about the signs/symptoms of hypothyroidism and the need for follow-up care.

RATIONALE

More helpful to build on existing information.

Severity of condition, cause, age, and concurrent complications determine treatment. Review of signs and symptoms as there can be as high as 50% chance of recurrence.

May interfere with accessing information. Refer to Care Plan: Psychosocial Aspects of Care in the Acute Setting. Psychogenic factors are often of prime importance in the occurrence of this disease.

Inhibits hormone production and may be necessary on a long-term basis.

Agranulocytosis is the most serious side effect that can occur and alternate drugs may be given.

Can occur immediately after treatment or as long as five years later, needs to be aware of possible complications.

CARE PLAN: Thyroidectomy

PATIENT DATA BASE

Refer to Care Plan: Hyperthyroidism (Thyrotoxicosis).

Total Thyroidectomy: The gland is removed completely, usually done in the case of malignancy. Thyroid replacement therapy is necessary for life.

Subtotal Thyroidectomy: Up to 5/6 of the gland is removed when antithyroid drugs do not correct hyperthyroidism and radioactive-iodine therapy is contraindicated.

NURSING PRIORITIES

1. Reverse hyperthyroid state preoperatively.
2. Prevent postoperative hemorrhage/airway obstruction.
3. Maintain comfort.
4. Provide information re postoperative care.

PREOPERATIVE

NURSING DIAGNOSIS:	**Injury, potential for, hyperthyroid state.**
SUPPORTING DATA:	**Thyrotoxicosis symptoms of weight loss, tachycardia, and irritability need to be reversed before surgery is done.**
DESIRED PATIENT OUTCOMES:	**Weight is gained, pulse rate is slowed, existing heart damage is identified, and CNS irritability is diminished.**

INTERVENTIONS

Promote dietary intake; may need 4000–5000 calories/day.

Avoid foods/fluids containing caffeine.

Promote restful environment.

Routine preop teaching to include safety measures for incision, need for voice rest, and need for assessing airway patency.

Note development of rash; excessive tearing of the eyes, nasal discharge, and salivation; and swelling of the buccal mucosa.

RATIONALE

Regain lost weight as indicated and prevent depletion of glycogen stores due to increased metabolism.

Has a stimulating effect.

Limit external stimuli and reduce metabolic needs.

Helpful in alleviating anxiety and increases patient cooperation.

Indications of iodine toxicity requiring discontinuance of the drug.

MEDICAL MANAGEMENT

Antithyroid drugs and iodine administration 1–2 weeks preoperatively.

Depletion of stores of thyroid hormone in the gland to achieve a euthyroid state. Iodine provides a reduction in vascularity to decrease risk of thyroid storm or postoperative hemorrhage.

ECG.

To determine status of cardiac functioning.

POSTOPERATIVE

NURSING DIAGNOSIS: **Injury, potential for, hemorrhage.**

SUPPORTING DATA: **Increased vascularity from the hyperthyroidism increases the risk of postoperative hemorrhage.**

DESIRED PATIENT OUTCOMES: **Hemorrhage is minimized/controlled.**

INTERVENTIONS

Monitor vital signs frequently.

Note signs of upper airway obstruction and difficulty swallowing.

Check dressing frequently, especially posterior portion.

RATIONALE

Increased pulse, decreased blood pressure are indicators of possible bleeding.

May indicate developing sequestered bleeding.

If bleeding occurs, anterior dressing may appear dry as blood pools dependently.

MEDICAL MANAGEMENT

Return to surgery.

For ligation of bleeders.

NURSING DIAGNOSIS: **Airway clearance, ineffective.**

SUPPORTING DATA: **Operative area around trachea, swelling, bleeding, as well as other causes can result in obstruction of the airway.**

DESIRED PATIENT OUTCOMES: **Airway is maintained with effective respirations.**

INTERVENTIONS

Assess for dyspnea, stridor, "crowing," and cyanosis.

RATIONALE

Symptoms of respiratory obstruction.

Encourage voice rest, but do assess speech and swallowing periodically.

Hoarseness and sore throat secondary to edema or damage to laryngeal nerve may last several days. Increased difficulty may indicate impending obstruction.

Suction mouth/trachea.

May have difficulty clearing own airway due to edema/pain.

Keep trach tray at bedside.

Emergency tracheostomy may be necessary.

MEDICAL MANAGEMENT

Steam inhalation.

Provides added humidity and promotes expectoration of secretions.

Tracheostomy.

May be necessary to maintain airway if obstructed by edema of glottis or hemorrhage. Nerve damage can cause paralysis of vocal cords and/or compression of the trachea.

NURSING DIAGNOSIS:	Injury, potential for, tetany.
SUPPORTING DATA:	Thyroid storm and tetany may occur as a complication of the surgery.
DESIRED PATIENT OUTCOMES:	Complications are minimized/controlled.

INTERVENTIONS

Monitor for temperature increase, tachycardia, arrhythmias, developing pulmonary edema/CHF.

Monitor serum calcium levels and observe for neuromuscular irritability with twitching, cramping, numbness, paresthesia, positive Chvostek's and Trousseau's signs.

Avoid use of cholinergic blockers, for example, atropine or adrenergics, such as epinephrin/norepinephrine.

RATIONALE

Early indicators of thyroid storm. See Care Plan: Hyperthyroidism (Thyrotoxicosis). Manipulation of gland during surgery may result in increased hormone release.

Hypocalcemia with tetany may occur 1–7 days postop and indicates hypoparathyroidism. See Care Plan: Hypoparathyroidism.

Sensitivity to these drugs is increased.

MEDICAL MANAGEMENT

Calcium IV, followed by oral dosage.

Deficiency may occur 1–7 days postoperatively and may be temporary or permanent.

NURSING DIAGNOSIS:	Comfort, alteration in, pain.
SUPPORTING DATA:	Delicate tissues, weight of head creates stress on operative area.
DESIRED PATIENT OUTCOMES:	Pain is minimized/controlled.

INTERVENTIONS

Place in semi-Fowler's position with support of head/neck with sandbags or small pillows.

Support head/neck during position changes.

Cool liquids by mouth or soft foods, such as ice cream/popsicles.

MEDICAL MANAGEMENT

Narcotics.

RATIONALE

Prevent hyperextension of neck and protects integrity of suture line.

Prevent stress on the suture line.

Soothing to sore throat but soft foods may be tolerated better if patient experiences difficulty swallowing.

Provide relief of surgical pain.

NURSING DIAGNOSIS:	**Knowledge deficit, postoperative care.**
SUPPORTING DATA:	**May need hormone replacement for hypothyroidism. This drug therapy is important to the satisfactory recovery of the patient and adequate knowledge can enhance cooperation.**
DESIRED PATIENT OUTCOMES:	**Verbalizes expectations of postoperative needs and cooperates with necessary regimen.**

INTERVENTIONS

Discuss need for adequate rest.

Discuss necessity for well-balanced, nutritious diet.

Provide information about possibility of changes in voice.

Give information about the use of loose fitting scarves to cover the scar. Avoid the use of jewelry.

Apply cold cream after sutures have been removed.

Observe for signs of hypothyroidism.

RATIONALE

Promote healing.

To regain/maintain adequate weight and promote healing.

Possible alteration in vocal cord function may cause changes in pitch and quality of voice, which may be temporary or even permanent.

Covers the incision without aggravating healing or precipitating infections of the suture line.

Moistens tissues and may help to minimize scarring.

Possibility of occurrence increases with time. See Care Plan: Hypothyroidism, Myxedema.

DIAGNOSIS: Hypoparathyroidism

PATIENT DATA BASE

NURSING HISTORY

Secondary to other conditions, such as removal during thyroidectomy, or damage to the vessels that supply the glands.

May complain of muscle weakness, fatigue, numbness, tingling, and paresthesia of the extremities.

May appear anxious and apprehensive, depressed, or exhibit neurotic behavior.

Note allergy to iodine, as may be used in testing.

DIAGNOSTIC STUDIES

Serum blood calcium is decreased.

Hyperphosphatemia is present.

Alkaline phosphatase is either normal or low.

Calcium tolerance test: may be done to determine the response to changes in the feedback cycle of calcium and parathyroid hormones.

Renal calculi may be present.

ECG: Q-T interval prolonged and T wave inverted.

PHYSICAL EXAMINATION

Neurologic exam reveals general dystonia; voluntary movements result in uncoordinated movements.

Laryngeal stridor and dyspnea may be present.

Spasms may occur and in severe cases, grand mal seizures may occur.

Trousseau's and Chvostek's signs may be positive.

Carpopedal spasm common.

Epidermal lesions, coarse, rough skin, thinning hair, and brittle fingernails.

Calcium deposits may be found in the lens resulting in lenticular cataract.

NURSING PRIORITIES

1. Restore calcium balance to normal.
2. Assist the patient in controlling anxiety.
3. Provide for safety of the patient.

NURSING DIAGNOSIS:	**Injury, potential for, tetany.**
SUPPORTING DATA:	**Decreased amounts of parathyroid hormone leads to decreased calcium levels causing neuromuscular symptoms of hyperexcitability, tremors, and the spasmodic movements of tetany.**

Tetany will be identified early, treated and/or controlled.

INTERVENTIONS

Monitor for hypercalciuria.

Monitor blood serum calcium levels.

Note anorexia, N & V, diarrhea, polyuria, polydipsia, and headache. Alert patient to awareness of these signs.

Observe for renal colic.

Provide opportunity for patient to discuss feelings of anxiety and for sharing of information.

MEDICAL MANAGEMENT

Calcium per IV push, give every 10 minutes slowly. Continue calcium IV by slow drip until tetany is controlled, then give IM or orally.

Vitamin D.

Antacids (aluminum hydroxide gel), ALternaGel, Amphojel.

RATIONALE

Important to identify early to treat and prevent convulsions.

Decreased or increased levels indicate need for alteration in calcium therapy.

Signs/symptoms of hypercalcemia. Need to monitor to minimize excess accumulation of vitamin D and calcium.

May have stone formation.

Patient may be concerned about symptoms and information about the reversability of the symptoms may help alleviate the anxiety.

Rapid availability in the presence of severe tetany. Highly irritating to the veins, may cause thrombosis, and too rapid administration can cause cardiac arrest.

Increases absorption of the calcium.

Binds phosphate and decreases intestinal absorption.

DIAGNOSIS: Hyperparathyroidism, Primary

PATIENT DATA BASE

NURSING HISTORY

May have no signs/symptoms or may manifest in kidney stones, polyuria, hypertension, renal failure, fractures, bone pain, anorexia, constipation, ulcer disease, pancreatitis, hypotonic muscles, lethargy, weakness, decreased reflexes, mood swings, personality changes, depression, apathy, confusion, coma, puffy eyes, gout, and deafness.

Hypercalcemia: nausea, vomiting, constipation, reddened eyes, pruritus, irritation of conjunctiva.
Crisis stage: $Ca^{++} > 115/100$ ml represents severe condition. Usually has history of previous problems.

Women ages 35–65 predisposed after menopause.

Check history of allergy to iodine, as diagnostic tests may use iodine preparations.

Rule out other causes of hypercalcemia: Cushing's syndrome, hyperthyroidism, malignancy, vitamin D excess, sarcoidosis, and so forth.

DIAGNOSTIC STUDIES

Dilute urine, low specific gravity.

Increased urine acidity.

Electrolyte imbalance may be present.

Increased serum calcium levels (hypercalcemia). Test must be run three times to verify consistency of results as these normally vary.

Alkaline phosphatase may be moderately increased with hypercalcemia and normal liver function tests.

Hypophosphatemia.

Phosphate deprivation test may be done.

Decreased K^+, bicarb and phosphate in urine.

Urinary alkalosis.

Metabolic acidosis.

May have kidney stones in the urine (strained).

Radioimmunoassay or CT scan may be done to locate adenomas.

X-ray for bone changes. May present with fractures; skeletal changes, decalcification. May have an overgrowth of osteoclasts.

Cortisone administration: has no effect on hypercalcemia if it is caused by hyperparathyroidism.

Administration of IV calcium may be used diagnostically, as there is no effect on phosphate excretion in hyperparathyroidism.

PHYSICAL EXAMINATION

Hyperplasia of two or more of the parathyroid glands.

Enlarged parathyroid gland, may be benign adenoma.

Hypertension may be present.

May complain of pain if kidney stones are present.

May have renal failure if severe.

Sluggish, neuromuscular exam may reveal hypotonic muscles.

May have red, swollen joints suggestive of gout.

NURSING PRIORITIES

1. Maintain adequate fluid intake.
2. Monitor diet.
3. Provide safe environment.
4. Monitor for complications and prepare for surgery if indicated.

NURSING DIAGNOSIS:	**Fluid volume deficit, potential.**
SUPPORTING DATA:	**Vomiting, diarrhea, and renal dysfunction can result in dehydration. GI bleed, secondary to ulcers may occur.**
DESIRED PATIENT OUTCOMES:	**Fluid balance is restored/maintained and dehydration does not occur.**

INTERVENTIONS	RATIONALE
Promote oral intake.	If able to retain liquids, is route of choice for replacement.
Monitor serum calcium.	Decreasing level indicates dehydration is being corrected; increasing level may indicate increasing dehydration.
Observe for hypotension.	When phosphate is being administered may potentiate hypotension if present.

MEDICAL MANAGEMENT

IV glucose, fluids, and electrolytes.	Replace as necessary to provide adequate hydration.
Inorganic phosphate.	Given to reduce calcium levels when severe hypercalcemia is present. (Needs to be corrected preoperatively.)
Antacids, aluminum hydroxide. Avoid milk.	Neutralize gastric acidity. Must restrict calcium intake.

NURSING DIAGNOSIS:	**Urinary elimination, alteration in.**
SUPPORTING DATA:	**The kidneys are sensitive to an excessive amount of parathyroid hormone. Kidney stones may develop, calcification of the parenchyma and renal shutdown may occur.**

DESIRED PATIENT OUTCOMES:	Stone formation is minimized/ prevented and renal shutdown is avoided.

INTERVENTIONS

Provide diet low in calcium and alkalies, such as milk and dairy products.

Promote oral fluid intake.

Monitor serum calcium and BUN daily.

MEDICAL MANAGEMENT

Diuretics (avoid thiazides).

Oral phosphate and IV saline.

RATIONALE

Potentiate stone formation.

Flush renal system.

Observe for changes in renal clearance.

Promote renal clearance of clacium, however thiazides decrease renal excretion of calcium and result in increased serum calcium.

Inorganic phosphate can decrease serum calcium.

NURSING DIAGNOSIS:	Injury, potential for, pathologic fractures.
SUPPORTING DATA:	Calcium is pulled from the bones resulting in osteoporosis and fragile bones are subject to fracture.
DESIRED PATIENT OUTCOMES:	Calcium balance is maintained and no fractures occur.

Refer to Care Plans: Urolithiasis; Ulcers; Gastric Resection.

The treatment of primary hyperparathyroidism is surgery. Frequently a single adenoma is found to be the cause.

CARE PLAN: Parathyroidectomy

PATIENT DATA BASE

Refer to Care Plans: Thyroidectomy; Hypoparathyroidism; Hyperparathyroidism, Primary.

NURSING PRIORITIES

1. Maintain fluid balance.
2. Prevent injury from tetany/convulsions.

POSTOPERATIVE CARE

NURSING DIAGNOSIS:	**Fluid volume deficit, potential.**
SUPPORTING DATA:	**Parathyroid hormone regulates the level of calcium and phosphate ions in the body fluids. Disturbances that result in decreased serum calcium levels, increased excitability of the nervous system, lead to tetany and convulsions. The metabolic disturbance needs to be stabilized before surgery.**
DESIRED PATIENT OUTCOMES:	**Electrolyte balance is restored and maintained. Blood pressure is normal, tetany is not present, and serum sodium and phosphorus levels are within normal range.**

INTERVENTIONS

Monitor vital signs.

Monitor hourly urine output. Avoid overhydration. In initial postop period.

Observe for tetany.

Monitor serum sodium and potassium and observe for diuresis.

RATIONALE

Hypotension may occur.

May retain fluid with resulting low output.

May be transient, or may be permanent depending on the amount of tissue removed and/or the edema present. See Care Plan: Hypoparathyroidism.

Normally occurring diuresis may result in loss of electrolytes and it is important to initiate therapy promptly.

MEDICAL MANAGEMENT

Electrolyte replacement as indicated.

Radical neck is usually done.

Ca gluconate IV.

Oral calcium and vitamin D.

Serum levels will provide guide.

To examine glands in mediastinal area.

For emergency use if severe tetany occurs.

Given to prevent mild/recurrent tetany. Vitamin D increases absorption of calcium.

Refer to Care Plans: Thyroidectomy; Surgical Intervention; Cancer of the Larynx: Radical Neck.

DIAGNOSIS: Diabetic Ketoacidosis

PATIENT DATA BASE

NURSING HISTORY

Undiagnosed diabetic with or without family history of diabetes.

Insulin-dependent diabetes (out of control).

Patient reduced insulin dosage, omitted one or more doses.

History of hyperthyroidism.

Recent symptoms of infection: urinary, respiratory, skin, and so forth.

Recent increase in insulin need, i.e., pregnancy, trauma, surgery, and/or emotional stress.

Change in dietary habits, increased intake.

Acute myocardial infarction.

Taking and/or increased dosage of medications, such as phenytoin, phenobarbital, diuretic, or steroids.

Symptoms may develop over several weeks or just a few hours (as in a young juvenile diabetic): polydipsia, polyuria, muscle weakness, fatigue, headache, nausea and vomiting, weight loss, abdominal pain, anxiety, confusion, or unconsciousness.

Symptoms of decreasing consciousness, such as drowsiness or somnolence, may go unnoticed by the person or family members.

DIAGNOSTIC STUDIES

Serum glucose increased: 300–600 mg/100ml or more.

Plasma ketones may be increased to 4 + in a 1:2 dilution.

Bicarbonate decreases with an increase in acidity (pH), 7.3–7.2 or less.

BUN may be normal or as high as 100 mg/ml.

Urine: positive for sugar and ketones.

Culture and sensitivities: possible UTI, respiratory, or wound infections.

Serum lipids, hematocrit, BUN, and WBC are all elevated.

Serum insulin levels: may indicate insulin insufficiency or inability to use endogenous insulin efficiently.

Sodium: normal or decreased.

Serum amylase: elevation may indicate acute pancreatitis.

Cardiac enzymes: r/o acute MI.

Thyroid function tests: dysfunction may increase insulin needs.

Potassium: normal or elevated at first, then decreased.

Phosphorus: frequently decreased.

Arterial blood gases: metabolic acidosis with compensatory respiratory alkalosis.

PHYSICAL EXAMINATION

Motor weakness, paralysis and paresthesias, memory loss, and lethargy progressing to coma.

Hypotension, tachycardia, decreased or absent peripheral pulses, signs of possible hypovolemic shock.

Kussmaul's respirations and acetone breath may be present.

Rales and/or rhonchi are suggestive of infection.

Presence of abdominal pain or rigidity, gastric dilatation, and vomiting.

Polyuria is an early sign, but oliguria or anuria may be present in severe dehydration and shock.

Skin: may be flushed, warm and dry; dry mucous membranes, poor skin turgor, soft eyeballs, cracked lips.

Rectal temperature: elevation may indicate possible infection. More accurate rectally, especially when Kussmaul's respiration and/or decreased sensorium exists.

NURSING PRIORITIES

1. Correct fluid and electrolyte imbalances.
2. Shift fat and protein metabolism to carbohydrate metabolism.
3. Correct factors that precipitated the development of diabetic ketoacidosis.

NURSING DIAGNOSIS:	**Fluid volume deficit, actual.**
SUPPORTING DATA:	**Hyperosmolar effect of glucose pulls water out of the body. The patient develops a thirst and drinks to compensate for the fluid loss. If the patient becomes debilitated, and does not drink enough fluids, dehydration quickly occurs.**
DESIRED PATIENT OUTCOMES:	**The patient will be optimally hydrated.**

INTERVENTIONS

Monitor blood glucose, K$^+$ and other electrolytes, I & O, daily weights, and CVP closely.

Monitor serum osmolality, BUN, Hct and Hb.

Monitor for cracked lips, decreased skin turgor, soft eyeballs, weight loss, abdominal pain and rigidity, sensorium changes, and paresthesias leading to paralysis.

RATIONALE

Alterations in K$^+$ can be life-threatening. Sodium and chloride tend to be low or normal in ketoacidosis. Sodium can be excreted in the urine. Urinary output should be at least 30 ml/hour. Less than this indicates decreased kidney perfusion. Decreased output and severe hypotension, tachycardia, and decreased CVP precede hypovolemic shock.

These values will be increased secondary to hemoconcentration.

These signs and symptoms are associated with dehydration and/or electrolyte imbalances. Abdominal pain and rigidity may be associated with sodium deficit, as well as dehydration. Level of consciousness can decrease due to worsening acid-base abnormalities or coma may result from cerebral edema related to decreased serum glucose and fluid shifts.

MEDICAL MANAGEMENT

IV is administered at a rate based on factors, such as age and degree of dehydration. 5–10 liters can be given over 24 hours. Isotonic saline, followed by a glucose solution when the blood sugar has dropped.

Isotonic saline is used to restore volume quickly and possibly restore normal sodium balance. Restriction of glucose in the IV is desired until the blood sugar has begun to drop.

NURSING DIAGNOSIS:	**Cardiac output, alteration in, deficit.**
SUPPORTING DATA:	**Cardiac arrhythmias occur secondary to hyper/hypokalemia. In acidosis H$^+$, ions enter the cells in exchange for K$^+$, which is then eventually excreted in the urine. In addition to the ion exchange, hemoconcentration contributes to the high serum K$^+$. As the patient is treated with fluids and insulin, the serum becomes hemodiluted and K$^+$ is driven back into the cells causing hypokalemia. Both extremes can cause cardiac arrhythmias.**
DESIRED PATIENT OUTCOMES:	**Cardiac output and tissue perfusion are maintained. BP and pulse remain stable.**

INTERVENTIONS

Check BP and pulse frequently.

Monitor K$^+$ levels and ECG continuously.

Check for peaked T waves, loss of P wave, and disrupted Q-R-S.
Check for inverted or flattened T waves and prolonged Q-T interval.

Assess level of consciousness, color and temperature of skin, pedal pulses, and urinary output.

Monitor CVP, daily weight, serum osmolality, electrolytes, CBC, BUN, and I & O.

RATIONALE

BP is one means of estimating cardiac output. Pulse increases suggest increased effort of the heart to maintain cardiac output.

Arrhythmias may compromise cardiac output, or cause cardiac arrest.

These changes could be an indication of hyperkalemia.
Changes indicative of hypokalemia.

Help monitor the degree of tissue perfusion.

Indicators of the level of hydration. Active fluid replacement may lead to overhydration. The presence of rales, lab data indicative of hemodilution, and increased weight and CVP can signal fluid excess.

MEDICAL MANAGEMENT

IV fluids.

By increasing blood volume with IV, cardiac output and tissue perfusion may improve, as long as the heart is an effective pump.

Potassium replacement.

Though patient may appear to be hyperkalemic, as acidosis is corrected potassium returns to the cell and severe hypokalemia may result.

Sodium bicarbonate.

Used cautiously to correct severe acidosis.

Dextran, blood, or plasma.

May be required for severe vascular collapse.

Indwelling catheter.

Necessary to provide the most accurate measurement of output if there are sensorium changes.

Lidocaine and/or other drugs.

Need to have available to decrease ventricular irritability and life-threatening arrhythmias.

NURSING DIAGNOSIS:	**Breathing patterns, ineffective, potential.**
SUPPORTING DATA:	**Paralysis of the respiratory musculature and cessation of breathing, secondary to hypo/hyperkalemia.**
DESIRED PATIENT OUTCOMES:	**Adequate ventilation maintained.**

INTERVENTIONS

Monitor respirations closely, for increased rate, dyspnea, and decreasing tidal volume.

Monitor K⁺ levels closely.

Monitor for a deteriorating sensorium.

RATIONALE

Quality of respirations can deteriorate rapidly to respiratory arrest.

Potassium depletion may cause muscle weakness interferring with respiratory function.

As the pH rises with sodium bicarbonate, the Kussmaul respirations cease. Carbon dioxide can still accumulate and cross the blood-brain barrier, causing cellular damage and a deteriorating sensorium.

MEDICAL MANAGEMENT

Potassium replacement.

May be needed to replace renal losses.

Ventilator assistance.

May be necessary if paralysis occurs. Refer to Care Plan: Ventilatory Assistance (mechanical).

NURSING DIAGNOSIS:	**Nutrition, alteration in, less than body requirements.**

SUPPORTING DATA:	Glucose is needed to produce energy for cell metabolism. When glucose is not available, fats and proteins are broken down for energy and ketoacidosis occurs.
DESIRED PATIENT OUTCOMES:	Adequate amounts of glucose will be available for cellular metabolism.

INTERVENTIONS

Monitor for Kussmaul's respirations. Check urine ketones.

Monitor sensorium.

Monitor for nausea and/or vomiting.

Observe for flushed skin.

Closely monitor serum glucose, urine, ABGs, ketones, and electrolytes.

Review diet prescription and compare patient intake prior to current episode.

MEDICAL MANAGEMENT

Short-acting insulin IV (may be continuous IV infusion).

Begin glucose infusion after insulin therapy is begun and blood sugar starts to drop.

Sodium bicarbonate.

ADA diet.

RATIONALE

Rapid, deep respirations indicate alkaline reserves are decreasing due to ketoacidosis. Carbon dioxide and acetone are being excreted with these breaths, decreasing excess acids in the body and causing the pH to rise.

The patient can switch quickly from diabetic ketoacidosis to insulin shock if too much insulin is given too rapidly.

Nausea occurs because of the electrolyte imbalance caused by glucosuria and ketonuria. If vomiting occurs when the level of consciousness is decreased, aspiration can easily occur.

Vasodilation occurs with acidosis.

The blood sugar should begin to decrease with insulin therapy. With fat and protein breakdown in ketoacidosis, metabolic acidosis will be present. In addition, electrolytes, such as potassium, are affected by acidosis and should decrease with insulin and fluid therapy.

Irregularities/imbalances of intake and/or changes in activity level may have contributed to development of DKA.

Insulin promotes transport of glucose into the cells and promotes fat and protein storage. Given initially to insure uniform absorption. When circulation is compromised, as in volume depletion, absorption may be erratic through the subcutaneous route.

As carbohydrate metabolism accelerates; blood glucose levels drop and hypoglycemia and cerebral edema may occur.

If insulin and fluids do not raise the pH, this base can decrease the metabolic acidosis.

May need revisions.

NURSING DIAGNOSIS:	Injury, potential for, infection.
SUPPORTING DATA:	The patient may have a CVP and/or peripheral IV and indwelling catheter that could predispose to infection and other complications. Diabetics are especially susceptible to infections due to high glucose levels in the blood, and compromised circulatory and hematopoietic systems.
DESIRED PATIENT OUTCOMES:	Infiltration, phlebitis, or infection will be prevented.

INTERVENTIONS

Change IV, tubing, and dressings aseptically per hospital policy.

Monitor for puffiness around the IV site; a warm, hard pink streak above the site (in line with the vein) and/the presence of purulent drainage.

Apply warm compresses.

Monitor temperature closely, WBC count periodically.

Routine aseptic catheter care every shift.

Monitor for the appearance of cloudy, odoriferous urine, elevated temperature, increased WBC count in the serum and urine or increased RBCs in the urine.

MEDICAL MANAGEMENT

Culture and sensitivities.

Antibiotics.

RATIONALE

Detect early signs of complications. Prevent infection from occurring by maintaining sterile equipment and field.

Fluids may be entering the tissue rather than the vein. Potassium and antibiotics are particularly irritating to the veins. A pink streak can indicate infection/phlebitis.

Increase circulation/assist in resolution of infection/phlebitis.

Fever and elevated WBC count can indicate infection.

Organisms can enter via the external portion of the catheter and encrustations can develop around the catheter, predisposing to infection.

Signs of infection.

Identify causative organism(s).

Treat infection.

NURSING DIAGNOSIS:	Urinary elimination, alteration in patterns.
SUPPORTING DATA:	The patient could have an indwelling catheter to straight drainage.

DESIRED PATIENT OUTCOMES:	Urine output will be maintained with no signs of bladder discomfort or infection.

INTERVENTIONS

Maintain careful I & O.

Monitor for the presence of bladder spasms.

Secure the catheter tubing to the body as indicated for women and men.

RATIONALE

Greatly decreased or lack of urine output may indicate renal shutdown.

Reaction to the balloon or obstruction could cause bladder spasms and prevent output.

Reduces the friction and subsequent tissue irritation. Taping the tubing on the abdomen helps prevent urethral strictures in men.

NURSING DIAGNOSIS:	Mobility, impaired physical.
SUPPORTING DATA:	The patient may be weak and/or confused due to electrolyte imbalances and dehydration.
DESIRED PATIENT OUTCOMES:	Strength gradually increases and no injury occurs.

INTERVENTIONS

Monitor fluids and electrolytes closely.

Provide safety as necessary.

Promote a gradual increase in activity. Assist the patient with ambulation, as needed.

RATIONALE

Detect imbalances.

Assistance helps prevent injury; bed siderails up may be necessary during coma or decreased sensorium.

As strength increases, activity levels may be advanced.

NURSING DIAGNOSIS:	Self-care deficit, ADL.
SUPPORTING DATA:	Fatigue and weakness associated with electrolyte imbalances.
DESIRED PATIENT OUTCOMES:	The patient will gradually become independent in ADL.

INTERVENTIONS

Assist as necessary with bathing, feeding, dressing, grooming, and toileting.

Gradually increase patient's involvement in care.

RATIONALE

Patient's state of fatigue will necessitate assistance. Will also preserve strength while recovering.

As strength increases, independence is encouraged. Will hasten recovery and discharge from the hospital.

NURSING DIAGNOSIS:	Knowledge deficit, management of diabetes.
SUPPORTING DATA:	Understanding the complexities of the disease, effects on other body systems, resulting complications, and lifestyle changes that may be required is essential to proper management of this disease.
DESIRED PATIENT OUTCOMES:	Diabetes will be controlled, infections will be absent or minimized. Patient verbalizes the importance of maintaining routine on a daily basis as well as how the patient is going to maintain treatment regimen during times of emotional and/or physical stress.

INTERVENTIONS

Explore the reasons for the ketoacidotic episode.

Encourage verbalization of feelings about disease and how it affects the patient's life.

Assess need for referral to psychosocial counseling.

Assess and/or review with patient, insulin administration, urine testing, importance of dietary regulation, and recognizing symptoms that require medical attention.

Review onset, peak, and duration of prescribed insulin.

Review briefly the role of diet consistency and regularity in diabetes control and insure initiation of diet. Consult with dietitian if further instruction or review of diet is necessary.

Review and observe patient in insulin drawing, administration, site choice and rotation. If insulin pump is being used, instruct in care.

Advise keeping bottle of insulin in use at room temperature.

RATIONALE

Knowledge of the precipitating factors will enable the patient to avoid recurrences.

Provides opportunity for venting feelings and looking at changes that may be necessary in patient's lifestyle.

May need additional help in coping with chronic illness and/or how to manage stress adequately.

Important to determine the patient's level of knowledge. Self-esteem and control of disease is more effectively maintained when information is available and patient is in charge of own life.

Important information for anticipating reactions.

Control depends on matching the daily dietary intake, exercise, and insulin prescription. Understanding diet exchanges is essential. Consistency and adherence is one of the more important cornerstones of diabetes care, prevention of complications, and recurrence of diabetic ketoacidosis.

Correct procedure insures accurate insulin dosage and use. Pumps are implanted devices that inject small amounts of insulin at regular intervals and before meals and more closely approximate the normal insulin pattern.

To avoid development of lipodystrophy.

Instruct and observe patient in urine testing and/or home glucose monitoring.

Urine testing may be very inaccurate secondary to differing renal thresholds per patient. Some patients may not spill glucose into the urine until serum levels of 200–300 mg/dl are reached. Therefore, patients are being instructed on home glucose monitoring with various techniques, e.g., Chemstrip or Dextrostix with digital reading by the glucometer or Dextrometer. Blood is obtained by fingerstick. These techniques usually have an error factor of only 10–30 mg/dl. This allows more accurate home monitoring and with close physician instruction, allows patients to alter insulin, diet, or exercise prescription on their own when necessary.

Review the roles exercise, stress, and illness play in diabetes control.

Exercise decreases glucose levels and should be engaged in daily to insure consistent diabetic control. Too great an increase in exercise may necessitate a snack beforehand to compensate for the decreased serum glucose level that will arise and to prevent an insulin reaction. Stress/illness can alter diet/insulin needs.

Discuss ways to manage stress. May need to learn new ways of stress management. Instruct in importance of contacting physician.

Chronic stress and/or illness can increase glucose levels and therefore increase insulin requirements. When stress/illness occurs, consultation with the physician can often prevent further complications.

Review symptoms of hypoglycemia (insulin reactions), their causes, prevention, and therapy. Stress need for additional protein if glucagon is used to treat hypoglycemia.

Strictly controlled diabetic patients will periodically experience mild to moderate insulin reactions secondary to slightly decreased food intake, a delay in mealtime, slightly increased exercise, and so forth. Rapid onset of symptoms requires early identification and treatment. Glucagon uses stored protein to meet energy needs.

Instruct patient to notify physician if hypoglycemia occurs frequently.

May need to make alterations in therapy regimen.

Review symptoms of hyperglycemia, causes, prevention, evaluation, and the necessity to seek a change in treatment.

Patient has experienced the extreme results of hyperglycemia (DKA) and needs to understand the possible causes, how self-monitoring and improved self-care can usually prevent hyperglycemia leading to DKA. Close patient/physician rapport and intervention is essential.

Review and insure knowledge of Sick Day Rules.

Will experience occasional acute illnesses and understanding of the rules as provided by the patient's physician is essential to prevent DKA. It is important to always take the usual insulin prescription even if one is unable to eat because illness usually increases insulin needs. If unable to eat secondary to vomiting/diarrhea, diet must be converted to clear liquid as prescribed. Urines, or preferably, home blood glucose must be monitored qid (before meals and at bedtime) and recorded. Increasing values may necessitate an addition of a sliding scale of increased quick-acting insulin as directed by physician, or an office evaluation, depending on severity.

Stress the importance of routine physician follow-up.

Maintain control and evaluate for possible complications of diabetes. Routine evaluation of eyes (fundoscopy); kidneys, (renal function tests); heart, auscultation, BP, and lab for routine check of electrolytes, cholesterol, triglylcerides, and HgbA (glycosalated hemoglobin indicates blood sugar control over the past 45–90 days). Their value should be normal or close to normal, which indicates good control.

Instruct in the importance of routine examination and care of the feet. Avoid injury to feet.

Look for corns, calluses, breaks in the skin, redness, or nail problems. Bathe feet daily and dry thoroughly, using lotion to massage the skin. Wear sturdy, well-fitting shoes. Diabetic patients are prone to stasis ulcers and poor wound healing.

Discuss the possibility of long-term complications of vascular changes leading to atherosclerosis, retinopathy, and neuropathy.

While complications may occur in spite of good disease management, major vessel occlusions can lead to strokes, MIs, and gangrene. Yearly eye examinations can identify retinal changes. Diet control and vitamin supplements may help prevent peripheral nerve damage.

Discuss sexual functioning and concerns. Assess need for further counseling, if indicated.

Impotence occurs in a significant number of men and may be the initial symptom leading to a diagnosis of diabetes.

Instruct in the importance of wearing a medical identification bracelet.

Provides information for identification of condition.

Refer to Care Plan: Psychosocial Aspects of Care in the Acute Setting.

Research is being done in the areas of genetic engineering to create bacteria that manufacture insulin as well as beta-cell transplants and other methods of controlling this disease.

DIAGNOSIS: Hyperglycemic Hyperosmotic Nonketotic Coma (HHNK)

PATIENT DATA BASE

NURSING HISTORY

Noninsulin dependent diabetics.

Elderly patients, usually age 60 or older who have cardiovascular or renal disease.

History of acute stress conditions: possible infection or stress; i.e., pneumonia, pancreatitis, hyperalimentation, dialysis when high amounts of glucose are used; also use of diabetogenic drugs; GI hemorrhage; uremia; burns; glucocorticoid therapy.

Nausea and vomiting, diarrhea.

Polyuria, polydipsia, progressing to decreased urinary output.

NPO for 12 hours before surgery or diagnostic tests.

DIAGNOSTIC STUDIES

Serum glucose: 600 to as much as 2800mg/100ml.

Serum osmolarlity: 350–475 mOsm/kg.

Serum sodium: about half of all HHNK patients are hypernatremic, with levels as high as 160 mEq/L.

Ketosis: absent or mild.

Increased BUN frequently occurs secondary to dehydration/stress/protein catabolism and/or glucocorticoids.

PHYSICAL EXAMINATION

Same as for diabetic ketoacidosis, except Kussmaul's respirations and acetone breath are not present. (Metabolic acidosis does not occur unless there is lactic acidosis associated with shock.)

NURSING PRIORITIES

1. Give fluid replacement.
2. Monitor insulin therapy judiciously.
3. Provide potassium replacement.
4. Maintain patient safety.

If this condition is occurring in a nondiabetic patient, correction of the underlying cause; e.g., infection, hyperalimentation, fluid replacement and brief insulin therapy may be all the treatment that is indicated. The mortality for nonketotic hyperosmolar coma has been reported to be up to 44%.

NURSING DIAGNOSIS:	**Fluid volume deficit, actual.**

SUPPORTING DATA:

Elevated blood glucose levels cause an osmotic diuresis, which can result in severe dehydration. As a result of reduced body fluid, the cardiac output and tissue perfusion decreases. In addition, hemoconcentration may create abnormally high potassium levels. When hydration is begun, the blood becomes diluted and K$^+$ levels can fall extremely low. Abnormally low or high K$^+$ levels can paralyze the respiratory and cardiac muscles. Dangerous ventricular arrhythmias, cardiac and/or respiratory arrest may occur.

DESIRED PATIENT OUTCOMES:

Optimal fluid and potassium balance. Adequate cardiac output and tissue perfusion.

INTERVENTIONS

Monitor Na$^+$ and K$^+$, as well as other electrolytes; I & O, daily weights, and CVP closely.

Monitor BP, pulse, serum osmolality, BUN, Hct & Hb, blood and urine sugar levels.

Observe for cracked lips, decreased skin turgor, soft eyeballs, weight loss, abdominal pain and rigidity, sensorium changes, and paresthesias leading to paralysis.

Monitor for pulmonary edema.

MEDICAL MANAGEMENT

IV replacement of ½ normal saline, with CVP monitoring.
Normal saline. Four to six liters of fluid should be replaced within the next 12 hours.

RATIONALE

See rationale in Care Plan: Diabetic Ketoacidosis, Nursing Diagnosis, Fluid volume, deficit, actual. Special attention should be given to replacing K$^+$ as soon as renal function is assured.

Reflect level of hydration, tissue perfusion, and renal clearance.

Signs and symptoms associated with dehydration and/or electrolyte imbalances. Abdominal pain and rigidity may be associated with sodium deficit, as well as dehydration.

Presence of rales and lab data indicative of hemodilution can signal fluid excess that may occur with rehydration. Daily weight increase, intake significantly greater than output, as well as increasing CVP levels can signal overload.

A patient with HHNK may be hypernatremic. Therefore, ½ normal saline may be given instead of normal saline. However, if the patient is severely hypotensive, normal saline will be given to rapidly increase the intravascular fluid volume and increase osmotic gradient to prevent fluid shifting into the intracellular compartment and perpetuating the hyperosmolality.

NURSING DIAGNOSIS:	**Nutrition, alteration in, less than body requirements.**
SUPPORTING DATA:	**In HHNK, there is an inadequate amount of glucose reaching the cells. However, there is enough glucose to prevent fat and protein breakdown.**
DESIRED PATIENT OUTCOMES:	**Blood sugar will reach optimal levels.**

INTERVENTIONS

Monitor blood sugar closely.

Monitor nausea/vomiting.

RATIONALE

Identify fluctuations to avoid further hyperglycemia or hypoglycemia.

When level of consciousness is decreased, may aspirate vomitus. Nausea occurs because of the electrolyte imbalance caused by glucosuria and ketonuria.

MEDICAL MANAGEMENT

Insulin; small doses of perhaps 10 u/hour or less. IV or subcu doses can be used.

Reduce insulin dosage when approaching normal glucose levels.

People with HHNK tend to be very sensitive to insulin. The subcutaneous route may be used provided circulation is not impaired.

Avoid further hyper/hypoglycemia.

Refer to Care Plan: Diabetic Ketoacidosis, Nursing Diagnoses: Injury, potential for, infection; Urinary elimination, alteration in patterns; Mobility, impaired physical; and Self-care deficit, ADL.

NURSING DIAGNOSIS:	**Knowledge deficit, potential, prevention of complications.**
SUPPORTING DATA:	**Infections, such as pneumonia; pancreatitis; GI hemorrhage; uremia; burns; excessive glucose intake from peritoneal dialysis or IV fluids can predispose to HHNK. Twelve hours of NPO prior to surgery/diagnostic tests can lead to dehydration and HHNK.**
DESIRED PATIENT OUTCOMES:	**Patient will verbalize knowledge of etiology, preventive measures, diagnosis, treatment, and complications of HHNK.**

INTERVENTIONS

Instruct in general health measures, such as, consistent, nutritious diet; adequate fluids; exercise; and rest.

If the patient is diabetic, assess knowledge and practices re treatment protocol.

Discuss problem areas and set goals for achieving.

RATIONALE

Optimal health will aid in prevention of HHNK.

May identify areas of lack of knowledge and/or factors that interfere with practices. See Care Plan: Diabetic Ketoacidosis, Nursing Diagnosis: Knowledge deficit, management of diabetes. If patient is not diabetic, patient will not need diabetic teaching.

Enhance patient's control of treatment regimen.

DIAGNOSIS: Hypoglycemia (Fasting, Postprandial)

PATIENT DATA BASE

NURSING HISTORY

History of pancreatic disease (cancer), hepatic disorder, enzyme defect, Addison's disease, or cancer.

History of steroid usage (withdrawal can cause drug-induced hypoglycemia).

History of diabetes in the family.

With postprandial, usually complains of feeling ill about four hours after eating; cold sweats, headache, jittery, blurred vision, speech problems, numbness of lips/fingers, unilateral weakness, and racing pulse.

History of gastric pyloroplasty.

Note dietary history: eating habits, length of time between food ingestion. With fasting hypoglycemia, low-ebb period is between midnight and 6 AM.

Age: most prediabetic hypoglycemic patients are middle-aged.

May have previous complaints of manic behavior, hemiplegia, convulsions (symptoms of fasting hypoglycemia).

DIAGNOSTIC STUDIES

Give high-carbohydrate diet (300 gm) for three days, followed immediately by 10 hour overnight fast. Take fasting blood specimen, followed by ingestion of 100 gm of glucose in 400 ml water within 15 minutes. Take serum glucose and insulin samples every 30 minutes × 5 hours.
In postprandial: blood sugar is normal, never low and insulin level is within normal fasting range and appropriately related to glucose level.
In fasting: blood sugar is usually low at the beginning and end of the test, peaking in the middle.

During the fast: glucose concentrations in men is 60–65 mg/100 ml; for women it is 30–35 mg/100 ml. (Levels of 40–50 ml should not be diagnosed as hypoglycemia unless associated with symptoms of epinephrine discharge, neurologic dysfunction, and evidence of biologic response, i.e., increased serum cortisol and glucagon. Autonomic symptoms include tachycardia, anxiety, sweating, and tremors. CNS symptoms include confusion, bizarre behavior, seizures, and coma).

Immunoreactive assay: measure insulin during glucose tolerance test: note relationship and alterations in the relationship between glucose and insulin.

Glucose tolerance test: blood sugar decreased 45 mg% serum, decreased 50% plasma level.

CBC: rule out anemia as cause of fatigue.

72-hour-fasting trial: test for ketones may be done to document adherence to fast. Ketonuria usually appears 12–24 hours into the fast.

Pancreatic function tests: adenoma may be present.

Liver and pituitary/adrenal function tests; to rule out as causative factor.

Drug assessment.

PHYSICAL EXAMINATION

Evaluate cold sweats, jitteriness during a period of hypoglycemia, complaints of vision disturbances, numbness of extremities, tachycardia, speech disturbances present, complaints of headaches. Note time of occurrence of symptoms.

CNS evaluation: in fasting hypoglycemia. Unilateral weakness, manic behavior.

NURSING PRIORITIES

1. Maintain homeostasis in metabolism.
2. Provide information and support in making necessary lifestyle changes to maintain optimal functioning.

NURSING DIAGNOSIS:	Nutrition, alteration in, potential.
SUPPORTING DATA:	Alteration in the metabolic balance between the rate at which glucose is used in the tissues and the rate at which glucose is released from the liver results in hypoglycemia.
DESIRED PATIENT OUTCOMES:	Hypoglycemic state does not occur.

INTERVENTIONS

Provide small, frequent (6×/day) meals.

Discuss symptoms that the individual experiences.

Discuss importance of having a rapid-acting oral carbohydrate available at all times. Stress that this does not take the place of regular meals.

Discuss use of alcohol.

RATIONALE

Maintain steady glucose level.

Will help patient identify when attack is beginning and avoid severe reaction that could lead to coma or convulsions.

A candy with nuts is most helpful as the nuts provide protein for longer effect. Because glucose can stimulate hypoglycemia, it is important to use it only on an occasional emergency basis.

Can deplete glycogen stores because alcohol causes increased insulin levels but does not replace glycogen.

MEDICAL MANAGEMENT

50% glucose IV injection or 10% glucose IV over 6 hour period.

Glucagon 1–3 mg IM or subcu.

Hydrocortisone sodium succinate.

Anticholinergics.

Antihypoglycemic agent (Diazoxide or streptozotacin).

High-protein, low-carbohydrate meals with simple sugars.

When vomiting, unconscious, or uncooperative and unable to take by mouth.

To maintain blood sugar level above 100mg%.

May be added to IV to attain hyperglycemic state.

To slow gastric emptying when the problem is one of food being expelled too rapidly from the stomach.

May be beneficial in patients with islet cell tumors.

Carbohydrates precipitate postprandial hypoglycemia.

NURSING DIAGNOSIS:	Knowledge deficit, disease management.

SUPPORTING DATA:	Lack of recognition of symptoms and actions related to onset of problem can lead to recurrences. Control of hypoglycemia may require changes in lifestyle.
DESIRED PATIENT OUTCOMES:	Patient verbalizes symptoms related to the onset of own situation and actions the patient can take to avoid recurrences.

INTERVENTIONS

Discuss signs/symptoms of hypoglycemia.

Teach use of Dextrostix and acceptable glucose levels.

Alert to symptoms that might require physician care.

Discuss food choices that will enable control of condition:
Allowed: such as, fresh fruit, canned fruit (water pack), low-calorie soda, saccharine.
Avoid: cake, pie, ice cream, honey, potatoes, pasta, grapes, raisins, plums, figs, dates, coffee, cherries, strong tea, wine, beer, and other alcohol.
Never: sugar, candy, colas, grape/prune juice.

RATIONALE

Aid in early recognition of onset and appropriate action to take.

Enables patient to maintain control over own care and enhances cooperation.

Hemiplegia, blurred vision, persistent dizziness, slurring of speech, hypo/hyperglylcemia not controlled by diet may need further evaluation.

Knowledge of foods will enable patient to manage own life with little or no hypoglycemic episodes.

Candy is only permissible as an emergency for severe hypoglycemic reaction.

BIBLIOGRAPHY

Books and Other Individual Publications

BEYERS, M. AND DUDAS, S.: *The Clinical Practice of Medical-Surgical Nursing.* Little, Brown & Co., Boston, 1977.

BELAND, I. L. AND PASSOS, J. Y.: *Clinical Nursing: Pathophysiological and Psychosocial Approaches,* ed. 3. MacMillan, New York, 1975.

BONAR, J. R.: *Diabetes, A Clinical Guide.* Medical Examination Pub. Flushing, New York, 1977.

BRUNNER, L. AND SUDDARTH, D. S.: *Lippincott Manual of Nursing Practice.* J. B. Lippincott, Philadelphia, 1978.

ISSELBACHER, K. J. ET AL. (EDS.): *Harrison's Principles of Internal Medicine.* McGraw-Hill, New York, 1980.

KIM, M. AND MORITZ, D. (EDS.): *Classification of Nursing Diagnosis.* McGraw-Hill, New York, 1981.

LUCKMANN, J. AND SORENSEN, K.: *Medical-Surgical Nursing: A Psychophysiologic Approach.* W. B. Saunders, Philadelphia, 1980.

Nursing '77 Books, (A Skillbook Series):*Managing Diabetics Properly.* Intermed Communications, Horsham, Pennsylvania, 1977.

PESTANA, C.: *Fluids & Electrolytes in the Surgical Patient,* ed. 2. Williams & Wilkins, Baltimore, 1981, pp. 85–89.

PHIPPS, W., LONG, B., AND WOODS, N.: *Medical-Surgical Nursing.* C. V. Mosby, St. Louis, 1979, pp. 568–594.

SKILLMAN, T. G.: *Endocrinology, A Review of Clinical Endocrinology.* Med. Exam. Pub., New York, 1974.

TILKIAN, S. M., CONOVER, M. B., AND TILKIAN, A. G.: *Clinical Implications of Laboratory Tests.* C. V. Mosby, St. Louis, 1979.

WAIFE, S. O. (ED.): *Diabetes Mellitus.* Eli Lilly & Co., Indianapolis, 1980.

WILKINS, R. W. AND LEVINSKY, N. G. (EDS.): *Medicine, Essentials of Clinical Practice.* Little, Brown & Co., Boston, 1978.

Journal Articles

Bacterial hypoglycemia. Emergency Med. 12:171, Oct. 15, 1980.

BOLLNGER, R. E.: *Hypoglycemia.* Critical Care Quarterly, 3:99–109, Sept. 1980.

CAVALIER, J. P.: *Crucial decisions in diabetic emergencies.* RN 10:32–37, 1980.

GRENSHAW, J. F.: *Hypoglycemia . . . what's causing it?* Consultant, 20–163, Nov. 1980.

HALLAL, J. C.: Thyroid disorders. AJN, Vol. 77, No. 3:418–432, Mar. 1977.

HOFFMAN, J.T.T. AND NEWBY, T. B.: Hypercalcemia in primary hyperparathyroidism. Nursing Clinics of North America, Vol. 15, No. 3:435–498, Sep. 1980.

JONES, S. G.: *Adrenal patient, proceed with caution.* RN, 66–72, Jan. 1982, Vol. 45, No. 1.

JONES, S. G.: *Kid-glove care in pheochromocytoma.* RN, 67–74, Feb. 1982, Vol. 45, No. 2.

JONES, S. G.: *Bilateral adrenalectomy: Post-op dangers to watch for.* RN, 66–68, Mar. 1982, Vol. 45, No. 3.

LAVINE, R. L.: *How to recognize . . . and what to do about . . . hypoglycemia.* Nursing '79, 52–55, April 1979, Vol. 9, No. 4.

NEMCHIK, R.: *Diabetes today, a startling new body of knowledge.* RN, 31–36, Oct. 1982, Vol. 45, No. 10.

Never let sleeping drunks lie . . . check for hypoglycemia and ketoacidosis. Emerg. Med., 13:160–161, Feb. 28, 1981.

SANFORD, S. J.: *Dysfunction of the adrenal gland: Physiologic considerations and nursing problems.* Nursing Clinics of North America, Vol. 15, No. 3:481–498. Sep. 1980.

SCHIMKE, R. N.: *Adrenal insufficiency.* Critical Care Quarterly, Vol. 3, No. 2:19–27. Sep. 1980.

URBANIC, R. AND MAZZAFERRI, E.: *Thyrotoxic crisis & myxedema coma.* Heart & Lung, Vol. 7, No. 3:435–447, May–June, 1978.

WAKE, M. AND BRENSINGER, J., III,: *The nurse's role in hypothyroidism.* Nursing Clinics of North America, Vol. 15, No. 3:453–467, Sep. 1980.

WALESKY, M. E.: *Adult diabetes: Diabetic ketoacidosis.* AJN, Vol. 78, No. 5, May 872–874, 1978.

CHAPTER 11

REPRODUCTIVE

DIAGNOSIS: Epididymitis

PATIENT DATA BASE

NURSING HISTORY

May have had recent episode of prostatic infection (most common cause), venereal disease, especially gonorrhea; urinary tract infection; or surgery, prostatectomy, cystoscopy, herniorraphy.

Complains of malaise.

DIAGNOSTIC STUDIES

WBC is elevated, may be as high as 20,000–30,000.

If discharge is present, urethral stain may show gonococcus or other organisms.

Urinalysis may show pyuria and/or bacteriuria.

Rule out infection from tubercle bacilli.

PHYSICAL EXAMINATION

Pain, swelling, and severe tenderness in the groin and scrotum.

May walk with a waddle.

Elevated temperature, chilling may occur.

Edema, redness of the scrotum, may feel hot to the touch.

NURSING PRIORITIES

1. Control and treat infection.
2. Minimize pain and discomfort.
3. Prevent complications.

NURSING DIAGNOSIS:	Injury, potential for, infection.
SUPPORTING DATA:	Most common infection of the male reproductive tract, usually descends from the prostate or urinary tract. Usually is pyogenic, may be a complication of gonorrhea or tuberculosis of the urinary tract. Untreated infection can cause sterility due to scarring.
DESIRED PATIENT OUTCOMES:	Infection will be controlled without complications.

INTERVENTIONS

Push fluid intake to at least 3 L/day. Include acid/ash juices, such as cranberry.

Observe for continued temperature elevation and pain.

MEDICAL MANAGEMENT

Antibiotics.

Local heat/sitz baths.

Incision and drainage.

RATIONALE

Prevent dehydration and flush urinary system. Acidifying the urine will decrease bacterial count.

Possible abscess formation.

Combat infection.

To hasten resolution of inflammatory process.

If abscess occurs.

NURSING DIAGNOSIS:	Comfort, alteration in, pain.
SUPPORTING DATA:	In an area that contains numerous nerve endings, swelling and irritation from infection produces pain and discomfort.
DESIRED PATIENT OUTCOMES:	Pain/discomfort is managed/minimized.

INTERVENTIONS

Keep the patient on bed rest and elevate the scrotum with a scrotal support, (Bellevue bridge).

Wear scrotal support when out of bed.

RATIONALE

Promote healing. Scrotal support relieves edema, discomfort, and pressure on the cord.

Prevent pull on cord and consequent discomfort.

MEDICAL MANAGEMENT

Analgesics.

For pain relief.

Intermittent cold compresses, ice bag may be applied.

Reduce swelling and relieve pain. Do not use continuously, to avoid ice burn. Heat is usually contraindicated because of the possibility of damage to spermatic cells.

Spermatic cord may be injected with a local anesthetic within the first 24 hours after onset.

To relieve severe pain.

NURSING DIAGNOSIS:	**Knowledge deficit, complications.**
SUPPORTING DATA:	**Recurrence is common. Sterility and septicemia can occur if infection is left untreated or treatment is not completed.**
DESIRED PATIENT OUTCOMES:	**Infection does not recur and there are no complications.**

INTERVENTIONS

Instruct patient in the importance of continuing the full course of antibiotics.

Avoid straining in lifting and defecation as well as sexual activity.

Discuss concerns about the possibility of sterility and give necessary information.

Give information about the expected length of recuperation.

Discuss concerns about sexual activity, and possibility of sharing infection with partner.

Refer to Care Plan: Sexually Transmitted Diseases.

RATIONALE

To ensure best opportunity for clearing up the infection completely.

Until infection is under control. Prostate is close to the rectum. Straining increases pressure and may force infection further into ducts.

Patient often has unspoken fears about what is happening and accurate information and the opportunity to discuss these fears can be helpful.

It may take 4–6 weeks for the epididymis to return to normal.

Intercourse is usually contraindicated while pain is severe. Can be resumed when comfortable to do so. Sharing of infection is dependent on the cause; if the organism is sexually transmitted, treatment will be necessary before resuming sexual activity.

DIAGNOSIS: Hysterectomy

Subtotal Hysterectomy: Removal of the body of the uterus, cervical stump remains.

Total Hysterectomy: Removal of the uterus and cervix.

Total Hysterectomy With Bilateral Salpingo-oophorectomy: removal of uterus, cervix, tubes, and ovaries.

Abdominal procedure may have a vertical or transverse incision.

Vaginal route may be used in certain conditions, such as prolapse, carcinoma in situ, and extreme obesity. It is contraindicated if the diagnosis is obscure.

PATIENT DATA BASE

NURSING HISTORY

May have history of endometriosis.

May have recent diagnosis of cancer.

Age and marital (relationship) status note pregnancy/gravida history: may influence outlook and have implications for projected self-concept.

DIAGNOSTIC STUDIES

See Care Plan: Surgical Intervention.

PHYSICAL EXAMINATION

See Care Plan: Surgical Intervention.

NURSING PRIORITIES

1. Provide preoperative counseling.
2. Prevent postoperative complications.
3. Provide information postoperatively for uneventful convalescence.

NURSING DIAGNOSIS:	**Self-concept, disturbance in.**
SUPPORTING DATA:	**For optimum result from surgery, the patient's mind as well as body must be prepared. Concerns about the inability to have children, religious conflicts, femininity, and how it will affect her sexual relationship/s may all be concerns associated with this procedure.**
DESIRED PATIENT OUTCOMES:	**Verbalizes concerns and indicates ways of dealing with them.**

INTERVENTIONS

Assess emotional stress the patient is experiencing.

Provide time to listen to concerns and fears.

Provide information, reinforcing and interpreting physician's information.

Refer to professional counseling as necessary.

Refer to Care Plan: Psychosocial Aspects of Care in the Acute Setting.

RATIONALE

Determine individual response to the procedure.

Conveys interest and concern.

Preoperative teaching is very important for this patient.

May need additional help to resolve feelings about loss.

NURSING DIAGNOSIS:	Urinary elimination, alteration in pattern.
SUPPORTING DATA:	Presence of edema, hematoma, or nerve paralysis may interfere with bladder functioning.
DESIRED PATIENT OUTCOMES:	Bladder is emptied/problems recognized/resolved.

INTERVENTIONS

Monitor intake and output.

Give sterile catheter care.

MEDICAL MANAGEMENT

Catheterize after 8 hours.

Catheterize for residual.

RATIONALE

May indicate urine retention if voiding frequently in small amounts.

May have indwelling catheter because edema or interference with nerve supply may cause bladder atony. May have a suprapubic catheter.

If have not voided and indwelling catheter is not present.

May not be emptying bladder completely and retention of urine increases possibility for infection.

NURSING DIAGNOSIS:	Bowel elimination, alteration in, potential.
SUPPORTING DATA:	Abdominal surgery, handling of bowel may cause ileus and interfere with bowel functioning.
DESIRED PATIENT OUTCOMES:	Peristalsis and elimination are resumed.

INTERVENTIONS

Observe for abdominal distention and change or absence of bowel sounds.

Assist patient with sitting on the edge of bed and walking.

Abdominal binder may be used.

Restrict fluids and foods.

Auscultate bowel for return of peristalsis.

Begin fluids and diet as tolerated.

MEDICAL MANAGEMENT

Nasogastric tube.

Rectal tube, heat to the abdomen.

RATIONALE

Indication of ileus.

Early ambulation is helpful to return of peristalsis.

Support during ambulation may be helpful.

For 1–2 days until peristalsis begins.

Guide to resumption of oral intake.

When peristalsis begins.

May be inserted in surgery to decompress stomach.

To promote passage of flatus.

NURSING DIAGNOSIS:	**Tissue perfusion, alteration in.**
SUPPORTING DATA:	**Respiratory and vascular disorders, such as phlebitis, thrombosis, or edema, may occur.**
DESIRED PATIENT OUTCOMES:	**Respiratory or vascular complications are prevented/minimized/treated.**

INTERVENTIONS

Turn, cough, and deep breath frequently.

Avoid high-Fowler's position and pressure under the knees.

Monitor blood loss.

Check for Homan's sign.

Assist with leg exercises and ambulate as soon as able.

MEDICAL MANAGEMENT

Antiembolis stockings.

Incentive spirometer.

RATIONALE

Prevent stasis and respiratory/vascular complications.

Creates stasis and pooling of blood in the extremities.

Weigh pads and compare with dry weight.

Tenderness, pain in calf indicative of thrombophlebitis.

Movement enhances circulation and prevents stasis.

Aid in venous return.

Promote lung expansion/minimize atelectasis.

NURSING DIAGNOSIS:	Knowledge deficit, convalescence.
SUPPORTING DATA:	Patient needs to know which type of operation was performed and what, if any, limitations/restrictions may be imposed.
DESIRED PATIENT OUTCOMES:	Verbalizes type of surgery and schedule for recuperation.

INTERVENTIONS

Begin giving information immediately postop.

Instruct in resumption of activity. Stress importance of individual response in recuperation. Avoid heavy lifting and strenuous activities, such as vacuuming, for at least 6 weeks. (Check with physician for individual instructions.)

Avoid tub baths until physician allows.

Instruct patient to note amount/character of vaginal discharge or temperature elevation.

Discuss emotional lability and expectation of feelings of depression and sadness.

Discuss physician's recommendations for resuming sexual intercourse.

Provide for and listen to patient's expressions of concern about resumption of sexual activity.

Stress importance of followup care.

Refer to Care Plans: Surgical Intervention; Cancer.

RATIONALE

Patient needs to know she will no longer menstruate and whether surgical menopause will occur with the possible need for hormonal replacement.

Sitting too long is contraindicated because of possibility of thromboembolus. Do not drive a car until the third postop week. Patient can expect to feel tired when she goes home and needs to plan a gradual resumption of activities. Returning to work is an individual matter.

Showers are permitted but tub baths may cause vaginal irritation as well as be a safety hazard for getting in and out of the tub.

May indicate presence of infection.

Loss of a part of the body is accompanied by a process of grieving.

It is best to resume sexual activity easily and gently at first. May use other coital positions and express sexual feelings in other ways.

May have feelings of inadequacy. See Nursing Diagnosis: Self-concept, disturbance in.

Provides for opportunity to ask questions and clear up misunderstandings as well as detect any beginning complications.

DIAGNOSIS: Pelvic Inflammatory Disease

PATIENT DATA BASE

NURSING HISTORY

May or may not have history of past infection; vaginitis, gonorrhea, salpingitis and/or oophoritis.

May have had recent abortion or be postpartum.

May have used an intrauterine device.

Complains of malaise and lethargy. If acute, pain may be severe and described as a "bearing down" discomfort in the lower abdominal quadrants and pelvic area.

DIAGNOSTIC STUDIES

WBC is elevated.

Gonococcal smear may be positive.

Streptococcus, staphyloccus, Escherichia coli may be identified on culture of discharge.

Nonspecific urethritis (NSU), Chlamydia may be infectious agent. In 25 percent of cases, more than one infectious agent is present.

PHYSICAL EXAMINATION

Temperature will be elevated.

Abdominal palpation will reveal pain and tenderness.

Nausea and vomiting may be present.

Purlent, foul-smelling discharge may be present (malodorous leukorrhea). Will be helpful to r/o appendicitis.

Ectopic pregnancy must be ruled out.

NURSING PRIORITIES

1. Control infection.
2. Assist patient in dealing with complications and psychologic implications.
3. Prevent infection spreading to others. Refer to Care Plan: Sexually Transmitted Diseases.

NURSING DIAGNOSIS:	**Injury, potential for, current infection.**
SUPPORTING DATA:	**Infectious process produces an acute debilitating illness.**
DESIRED PATIENT OUTCOMES:	**No signs of infection are present, discharge is absent.**

INTERVENTIONS

Encourage increased fluid intake.

Provide nutritious, well-balanced diet in attractive manner.

Provide for rest and quiet environment.

Place in semi-Fowler's position.

Do not catheterize or allow patient to use tampons.

Use isolation techniques in handling of linen and equipment.

Give information and enlist patient cooperation in prevention of contamination of self and others.

MEDICAL MANAGEMENT

Parenteral fluids.

Antibiotics.

Heat to abdomen and/or hot douches.

RATIONALE

Flush toxins from the body.

Necessary to aid body in combating infection. Appetite may be poor.

Promote healing.

Facilitate drainage.

Prevent spread of infection.

Prevent contamination of others.

Important to ensure that patient will not reinfect herself and others.

If unable to take sufficient amount orally.

Appropriate to causative organism.

Improve circulation and enhance healing.

NURSING DIAGNOSIS:	**Comfort, alteration in, pain.**
SUPPORTING DATA:	**Acute illness with swelling, edema of structures and surrounding tissues.**
DESIRED PATIENT OUTCOMES:	**Pain is controlled/absent.**

INTERVENTIONS

Provide for comfort measures of rest and relaxing environment.

MEDICAL MANAGEMENT

Analgesics.

RATIONALE

Helpful to reduce pain.

May be necessary when pain is acute.

NURSING DIAGNOSIS:	**Self-concept, alteration in, self-image.**
SUPPORTING DATA:	**Social aspects of venereal disease as causative factor, possibility of sterility as complication and possibility of chronic condition.**
DESIRED PATIENT OUTCOMES:	**Verbalizes improved self-esteem.**

509

INTERVENTIONS

Assess level of patient's distress.

Provide opportunities for listening and discussion.

Refer to Care Plan: Psychosocial Aspects of Care in the Acute Setting.

RATIONALE

May differ according to varying causative factors and individual coping abilities.

Can provide for support and acceptance.

NURSING DIAGNOSIS:	**Knowledge deficit, disease management and complications.**
SUPPORTING DATA:	**Social aspects of venereal disease that may be responsible for infection; possibility of reinfection; complications of untreated or recurrent infection make it extremely important for the patient to have information about the condition.**
DESIRED PATIENT OUTCOMES:	**Verbalizes cause of disease, knowledge of and necessity for completion of treatment regimen.**

INTERVENTIONS

Assess level of knowledge and anxiety.

Discuss possibility of complications of chronic pain, sterility and/or ectopic pregnancy, and total hysterectomy.

RATIONALE

High-anxiety level may interfere with processing of information.

Discussion is helpful in allowing patient to assimilate information in a nonthreatening manner. Recurrent/residual infections can result in scarred/compromised tissues, which predispose to further/other infections.

Refer to Care Plan: Sexually Transmitted Diseases for further nursing diagnoses and interventions.

DIAGNOSIS: Mastectomy

PATIENT DATA BASE

NURSING HISTORY

Usually a woman, although can be a man.

Usually in menopausal years (50 +).

Cancer of the breast is the leading cause of cancer death among women in the United States.

Frequently a family history of breast cancer.

Usually no pain associated with a lump that is found by the patient. (95% of all patients find a lump on their own.)

Increased incidence among childless women or women who had first child after 30 and did not breast-feed.

History of previous cancer.

Note history of weight loss.

Note history of changes in breast tissue as reported by the patient.

Note type of mastectomy to be performed.

Determine menstruation history.

Note anxiety about the diagnosis and treatment/surgery.

DIAGNOSTIC STUDIES

Usually a breast biopsy, with histologic classification and estrogen receptors noted.

Mammography, usually positive.

Thermography or xeroradiography. In thermography, circulation deviations are reflected by temperature changes. Positive results show increased circulation where tumors are present.

Transillumination: cyst or neoplasm is easily demonstrated.

PHYSICAL EXAMINATION

Note asymmetry of the breast, elevation, bloody discharge from the nipple, and skin changes around or on the breast.

Check weight, edema of limbs, history of infections.

General health status.

Note classification of cancerous tumors.

Refer to Care Plans: Surgical Intervention; Cancer.

NURSING PRIORITIES

1. Assist patient/significant other to deal with anxiety and fears regarding surgery, cancer, and postcare.
2. Prevent postsurgical complications.
3. Assist with establishing individualized rehabilitation program.
4. Provide support for maintenance of self-concept.

NURSING DIAGNOSIS:	Fear (specify).
SUPPORTING DATA:	Patients undergoing mastectomy often fear findings of the extent of the disease; anxiety over extent of the surgical scar; change of body image; loss of body part, sexual attractiveness as perceived by self/others, femininity.
DESIRED PATIENT OUTCOMES:	Verbalizes type of surgical procedure, potential cure rates, and postoperative care. Support of others will be evident.

INTERVENTIONS

Explain purpose of preop tests and preparation; for example, shaving the axilla, removing areola hairs.

Provide an atmosphere of concern, openness, and availability as well as privacy.

Provide information about available support groups, such as Reach for Recovery.

Provide opportunity for patient/significant other to discuss situation.

RATIONALE

Clear understanding of the surgical procedure and what is happening can increase feelings of control and self-esteem.

Often require time and privacy to discuss feelings of anticipated loss and other concerns. Therapeutic communication skills; open questions, listening, and so forth allows for patient/significant other to express/discuss concerns.

Can be a helpful resource when patient is ready; a peer who has experienced the same process can provide validity to the comments.

Provides for assessment of degree of support available to the patient.

NURSING DIAGNOSIS:	Injury, potential for, infection.
SUPPORTING DATA:	Postmastectomy patients can have lymphedema of the affected arm due to transection of the axillary lymph nodes (depending on type of procedure) and have an increased risk for infection.
DESIRED PATIENT OUTCOMES:	Free of infection, minimal edema postmastectomy.

INTERVENTIONS

Instruct patient to splint operative area when coughing and deep breathing.

RATIONALE

Prevents atelectasis and pneumonia and encourages expelling of secretions.

Place in semi-Fowler's position, on back, or unaffected side with arm raised and supported by pillow.

Monitor vital signs.

Do not take BP on affected side.

Assess dressing for drainage; type, amount, and content. Note edema, redness of the area. Dressings will differ depending on the extent of surgery and the type of wound closure. (Pressure dressings are usually applied and are reinforced not changed.)

If hemovac or other suction is used, note patency of tubing, color, amount, and type of contents. Drain and measure every 4–6 hours. (Tubes are removed between the third and fifth days or when drainage ceases.)

Check color of hand on affected side and have patient move fingers, noting sensations.

If skin graft is done, monitor donor site for unusual drainage.

Assess for complaints of pain.

Assists with drainage of fluid through the use of gravity. Support relieves tension on the arm and increases venous return.

Tachycardia or decreased BP could be sign of hemorrhage or shock.

Increase potential of constriction and lymphodema on affected side.

Early signs of hemorrhage, infection, or lymphedema and treatment can be instituted. Drainage occurs because of the trauma of the procedure and manipulation of the numerous veins and arteries in the area.

Drainage of exudate encourages skin flap to adhere to the chest wall, reduces the susceptibility to infection, maintains negative pressure, and promotes healing.

Discoloration can indicate problems of circulation; movement can identify problems with the intercostal brachial nerve.

Early identification of infection and to note healing.

The amount of tissue, muscle, and lymphatic system removed can affect the amount of pain experienced.

MEDICAL MANAGEMENT

Narcotics and analgesics.

Antibiotics.

To relieve pain.

Prophylactically and to treat infection.

NURSING DIAGNOSIS:	**Mobility, impaired, potential.**
SUPPORTING DATA:	**When a radical procedure is performed, muscles are removed, nerves are damaged, and the lymph system impaired; interfering with mobility of the affected limb.**
DESIRED PATIENT OUTCOMES:	**Mobility is maintained in the affected arm.**

INTERVENTIONS

After 48 hours postop, begin passive range of motion, advancing to swinging arm with straight back.

RATIONALE

Prevents shoulder stiffness and increases circulation and muscle strength of the shoulders and arm. If back is not straight, may defeat exercise by not using musculature.

INTERVENTIONS	RATIONALE

Do hand exercises.

Increase circulation and prevent contractures, maintain strength and function of the hand.

Start hand climbing and full abduction exercises after the seventh day.

This group of exercises can cause excessive tension of the incision if begun early.

Discuss types of exercises to be done at home to reestablish strength and encourage circulation in the affected arm.

Necessary to continue with exercise program to regain function of the affected side.

Coordinate exercise program with home activities.

Patient is usually more willing and it is easier to maintain a program that fits into own lifestyle, such as dressing self, washing, swimming, dusting.

Emphasize importance of doing bilateral activities.

Encourage greater use of the affected arm.

Massage healing site with cream, i.e., lanolin or cocoa butter.

Increases circulation to the site and elasticity of the area.

Assess degree of pain and joint mobility.

May need to postpone increasing exercises and wait until further healing occurs.

MEDICAL MANAGEMENT

Analgesics.

May need to treat pain prior to exercise. Incentive to exercise is decreased and patient does not exercise as fully when pain is present.

Refer to physical/occupational therapist.

Provide individual exercise program. Assess limitations/restrictions regarding employment requirements.

NURSING DIAGNOSIS:	Self-concept, disturbance in.
SUPPORTING DATA:	Mastectomy is a surgical procedure that is disfiguring to an area of the body that is identified with femininity in our society. Concerns of masculinity may be an issue when the patient is male.
DESIRED PATIENT OUTCOMES:	Verbalizes awareness of effect of surgery on self-concept and participating in social activities.

INTERVENTIONS

RATIONALE

Encourage questions about incision, scar, and future.

May feel disfigured and afraid of viewing scar by self/significant other.

Allow patient to express and discuss anger and grief.

Loss of body part engenders grieving process that needs to be dealt with so patient can deal with the future.

Discuss signs/symptoms of depression with patient/significant other.

Common reaction to this type of procedure.

514

Discuss use of prosthesis, exercises, and realistic expectations.

Provides social acceptance and allows patient to feel more comfortable about body image. Prosthesis may be implanted or worn in bra.

Discuss and refer to support groups.

Provide a place to exchange concerns and feelings with others who have had a similar experience.

MEDICAL MANAGEMENT

Reconstructive surgery, implant of prosthesis.

If feasible, reconstruction provides a less disfiguring cosmetic result.

NURSING DIAGNOSIS: **Knowledge deficit, postoperative management.**

SUPPORTING DATA: **Removal of the axillary lymphatics necessitates continued monitoring to ensure maximal movement and avoid injury.**

DESIRED PATIENT OUTCOMES: **Verbalizes exercise routine to follow at home and symptoms to be aware of that indicate impending complications.**

INTERVENTIONS

Instruct patient about signs/symptoms of lymphedema and infections.

Avoid taking blood, giving IV fluids, medications, and taking BP on the affected side.

Instruct patient to protect hands and arms when gardening; use thimble when sewing; use potholders when handling hot items; and plastic gloves when doing dishes, and so forth. Do not carry purse or wear jewelry/wristwatch on affected side.

Discuss ordering and wearing of a Medic Alert device.

RATIONALE

Lymphangitis can occur as a result of an infection causing lymphedema.

May restrict the circulation as the lymphatic system is compromised.

Compromised lymphatic system more susceptible to infection and/or injury.

To avoid accidental injury when problem is not initially detected.

MEDICAL MANAGEMENT

Antibiotics.

Treat infection.

Diuretics.

Reduce fluid to aid in treating and preventing fluid accumulation.

Intermittent compression.

Massage/mechanical device aid in treating lymphedema by assisting with venous return.

Refer to Care Plan: Cancer.

Other treatment may be required as adjunct therapy, such as radiation.

BIBLIOGRAPHY

Books and Other Individual Publications

A Cancer Source Book for Nurses. American Cancer Society, 1970.

BEYERS, M. AND DUDAS, S.: *The Clinical Practice of Medical-Surgical Nursing.* Little, Brown & Co., Boston, 1977.

BRUNNER, L. AND SUDDARTH, D. S.: *Lippincott Manual of Nursing Practice.* J. B. Lippincott, Philadelphia, 1978.

KIM, M. AND MORITZ, D. (EDS.): *Classification of Nursing Diagnosis.* McGraw-Hill, New York, 1981.

KINNEY, J., EGDAHL, R., AND ZUIDEMA, G.: *Manual of Preoperative and Postoperative Care.* Committee on Reconstructive and Postoperative Care, American College of Surgeons. W. B. Saunders, Philadelphia, 1971.

LUCKMANN, J. AND SORENSEN, K.: *Medical-Surgical Nursing: A Psychophysiologic Approach.* W. B. Saunders, Philadelphia, 1980.

PHIPPS, W., LONG, B., AND WOODS, N.: *Medical-Surgical Nursing.* C. V. Mosby, St. Louis, 1979.

STRAX, P.: *Early Detection Breast Cancer is Curable.* Harper & Row, New York, 1974.

TILKIAN, S. M., CONOVER, M. B., AND TILKIAN, A. G.: *Clinical Implications of Laboratory Tests.* C. V. Mosby, St. Louis, 1979.

WILKINS, R. W. AND LEVINSKY, N. G. (EDS.): *Medicine, Essentials of Clinical Practice.* Little, Brown & Co., Boston, 1978.

Journal Articles

CADY, B.: *Current philosophy in treatment of primary cancer of the breast.* Medical Clinics of North America, Vol. 59, No. 2, March, 285–292. W. B. Saunders, Philadelphia, 1975.

BULLOUGH, B.: *Emotional support for the patient with breast cancer.* Health Values, Mar./Apr., 6:19–22, 1982.

CLOUGH, J.: *Mastectomy: The operation that every woman dreads.* Case Study, Nurs. Mirror, Jan. 6:154–48–50, 1982.

MILLER, M.: *Mastectomy case study: Adding years to life . . . the emotional pitfalls on the way to full recovery.* Community Outlook, May, 119–120 +, 1982.

STOLAR, G. E.: *Coping with mastectomy: Issues for social work.* (research) Health & Social Work, National Assoc. of Social Workers, Feb., 7:26–34, 1982.

STUMM, D.: *Rehabilitation of the breast cancer patient.* Clinical Management in Physical Therapy, Spring, 2:20–22, 1982.

CHAPTER 12

ORTHOPEDIC AND CONNECTIVE TISSUE DISORDERS

DIAGNOSIS: Fractures

PATIENT DATA BASE

NURSING HISTORY

Immediate severe pain at the time of injury due to trauma may continue until bone fragments are immobilized. Nerve damage may cause pain to disappear immediately after the injury.

Recent history of trauma or accident. A detailed account of what transpired provides insight as to possibility, site, and type of fracture.

May have loss of function of affected part.

History of malnutrition, previous fracture, bone disease, which may predispose patient to fracture.

Occupation: type of work and activity involved.

DIAGNOSTIC STUDIES

CBC provides baseline for determination of blood loss. Increased WBC with increased neutrophils indicates bacterial infection.

Calcium and phosphorus levels are useful in differentiating diseases that affect the bones.

ABGs as needed to assess respiratory status.

X-rays: taken in two planes and to include the joint above and below the suspected fracture. May also show filling defects or disruption of bone integrity.

Arthroscopy, shows derangement of joint.

Bone biopsy, may show pathologic processes.

PHYSICAL EXAMINATION

Symptoms of fracture depend on: site, severity, type of fracture, and amount of damage to other structures. There are over 150 fracture classifications, five major ones are as follows:
1. Complete: fracture line involves entire cross section of the bone; usually displaced.
2. Incomplete: a fracture involving only a portion of the cross section of the bone; one side breaks, the other usually just bends (greenstick).

3. Open (compound): bone fragments extend through the muscle and skin, potentially infected.
4. Closed (simple): the fracture does not extend through the skin; infection is not introduced at the time of injury.
5. Pathologic: a fracture that occurs in diseased bone (such as cancer); trauma may be absent.

Expose the injured part. Cut clothing along seams as necessary.

Inspect and palpate for deformities or changes in shape and alignment of body parts.

Inspect for: lacerations, localized swelling, discoloration of skin, angulation (bending), shortening, and/or rotation. Redness may be present in affected area.

Note: weakness and any loss of function or sensation in the affected part; any abnormal movement of joints or limbs by the patient; and crepitation or grating sensation felt upon palpation.

Observe for muscle spasms near the fracture site; limb length and circumference may be altered.

Assess for type of pain and radiation, pulses, coolness, and blanching distal to the affected site.

NURSING PRIORITIES

1. Prevent further injury.
2. Relieve/prevent pain.
3. Minimize complications and maintain maximum function of limb.

NURSING DIAGNOSIS:	Comfort, alteration in, pain.
SUPPORTING DATA:	Movement of the fracture site, edema, and injury to the soft tissue may cause severe pain.
DESIRED PATIENT OUTCOMES:	Pain is minimized/controlled.

INTERVENTIONS

Continue immobilization of part by splinting, traction. Be sure splint is properly padded.

Elevate injured part.

If the fracture is open, apply a sterile dressing before splinting. Obtain a culture and sensitivity of the wound.

Investigate and document any pain or pressure.

Remove jewelry from affected limb.

MEDICAL MANAGEMENT

Analgesics including narcotics. Muscle relaxants.

RATIONALE

Relieves pain, prevents displacement and extension of injury. Prevents hemorrhage and helps decrease muscle spasm. Proper padding protects soft tissue from injury.

Promotes venous return and prevents the development of edema.

Piercing the skin allows easy entry for bacteria. Exudate at a wound opening promotes bacterial growth.

Continuing pain may indicate poor alignment or impaired circulation. Pressure may indicate increasing edema, hemorrhage, or improperly applied splint.

May restrict circulation when edema occurs.

Relieve pain and muscle spasms. Pain may induce shock and/or signal impending or actual tissue damage.

External immobilization by casting, traction, or surgery.

Maintain proper alignment for healing in a functional position. Refer to Care Plan: Traction.

NURSING DIAGNOSIS:	Tissue perfusion, alteration in.
SUPPORTING DATA:	**Decreased circulation, distal to affected part. Generalized shock. Heavy blood loss may occur with fracture due to vascularity of bone (especially with fracture of pelvis or femur). Cardiopulmonary alterations produce decreased O_2 supply to the tissue and circulatory collapse. Trauma, secondary to fracture, may cause extensive damage to surrounding nerves, vessels, and body organs.**
DESIRED PATIENT OUTCOMES:	**Maintain adequate tissue perfusion. Prevent or minimize neurologic deficit.**

INTERVENTIONS

Monitor blood pressure and apical pulse.

Remove constricting clothing and/or jewelry.

Assess and document capillary return, color, sensation, and warmth distal to the fracture qh. Document presence and quality of pulses. Compare to unaffected limb, if possible.

Monitor temperature, pulses, color, sensation, movement distal to the fracture site postsurgical repair.

Exercise the joints above and below the immobilized area.

Monitor output.

MEDICAL MANAGEMENT

Patent IV.

RATIONALE

Decreased blood pressure and a rapid, thready pulse are indicators of impending shock.

Constricting objects impair circulation and reduce tissue perfusion.

Return of color should be rapid (3–5 sec). White, cool skin indicates arterial impairment. Cyanosis indicates venous impairment. Absence of pulses necessitates immediate evaluation of circulatory status. Impaired feeling, perception (numbness, tingling) occurs when there is inadequate circulation to peripheral nerves or nerve damage and may be a surgical emergency.

Impaired circulation, nerve damage, infection, and tissue necrosis are the most common postoperative complications following orthopedic surgery.

Promotes bone healing. Decreased muscle tone results from interrupted nerve function immobilization, and insufficient tissue nutrition. Minimize loss of calcium from bone.

30ml/hour urinary output is indicative of adequate kidney perfusion.

May be necessary as ready route for medications replacing loss of circulating volume.

IV, plasma, plasma expanders, blood.

Systolic blood pressures below 80 mmHg (or a significant drop from patient normal), produce inadequate tissue perfusion.

Urinary retention catheter.

Monitor urinary output and assess kidney perfusion and adequacy of fluid therapy.

NURSING DIAGNOSIS:	**Injury, potential for, alteration in bone continuity.**
SUPPORTING DATA:	**Necessity for closed manipulation or open (surgical incision) reduction. Fracture reduction is an attempt to restore normal bone alignment. May also require traction (see Care Plan: Traction).**
DESIRED PATIENT OUTCOMES:	**Restore limb to maximum functioning with best cosmetic result. Prevent infection and neurovascular complications.**

INTERVENTIONS

Handle fracture extremity as gently as possible.

When surgery is pending, prep skin areas thoroughly in a nontraumatic manner.

Refer to Care Plan: Traction.

RATIONALE

Closed fracture may cause open wound with improper handling.

Bone is more susceptible to infection than soft tissue and will not heal properly with infection present.

NURSING DIAGNOSIS:	**Breathing pattern, ineffective.**
SUPPORTING DATA:	**Multiple fractures and fractures of the pelvis, tibia, and femur increase the chances of fat or thromboemboli occuring. Thromboembolism is a common complication following hip fractures and may occur without clinical signs.**
DESIRED PATIENT OUTCOMES:	**Prevent circulatory or respiratory collapse.**

INTERVENTIONS

Use incentive spirometer, promote coughing, deep breathing, and so forth.

RATIONALE

To clear secretions and promote good ventilation.

Encourage active/passive ROM to extremities. Have patient fully extend toes distal to the fracture.

Pooling of blood in the lower extremities predisposes to clot formation, which can then be dislodged and travel throughout the body causing severe complications.

Ambulate as soon as possible. Alternate with periods of elevation of affected limb.

Encourages venous return and minimizes stasis. Prolonged dependent position may result in edema.

Observe for tachycardia, tachypnea, petechiae, signs of hypoxemia, and substernal pain.

Beginning signs of onset of emboli. Appearance of petechia on the upper trunk and axilla is a hallmark of fat embollus.

Assess mentation.

Changes in mental status and personality, such as confusion and anxiety, are early clinical indicators of hypoxia.

Draw ABGs and send urine specimen for free fat.

Arterial blood gases indicate tissue oxygenation and help determine treatment modalities. Presence of free fat is indicative of fatty emboli.

Assess pain symptoms as possible respiratory problem. Avoid overmedication.

Respiratory distress often presents with restlessness, and vague complaints of discomfort.

MEDICAL MANAGEMENT

O_2 per nasal cannula.

Supplemental oxygen may be helpful in mild cases of hypoxia.

Endotracheal intubation with volume ventilator and PEEP.

May be needed as respiratory failure is the most common cause of death. Refer to Care Plan: Ventilatory Assistance (mechanical).

Corticosteroids.

Steroid therapy reduces cerebral edema, increases breakdown of fatty acids, suppresses inflammation, inhibits release of adrenocorticotropins, and minimizes capillary leak.

Heparin therapy.

Reduces platelet aggregation and minimizes clot formation. May be contraindicated as it increases free fatty acid formation in the lungs by increased lipase activity.

Diuretics.

To decrease pulmonary edema.

Elastic stockings.

Encourage venous return.

NURSING DIAGNOSIS:	**Injury, potential for, healing impairment.**
SUPPORTING DATA:	**Possibility of delayed union or nonunion of fracture and/or avascular necrosis. In adults, fractures usually heal in 10–18 weeks. Healing time is affected by the type of bone involved, the type of injury, and the patient's general nutritional status.**

DESIRED PATIENT OUTCOMES:	Bone union and consolidation occur with little or no complications.

INTERVENTIONS	RATIONALE
Keep affected extremity elevated.	Elevation promotes circulation and reduces edema.
Observe for any interference with circulation.	Impaired circulation interferes with healing and may result in nonunion.
Begin mobilization of the affected part as early as possible.	Mobilization promotes tissue oxygenation and prevents thromboembolism.
Provide for overall exercise, active and passive ROM.	Especially important in the bedfast patient to minimize calcium shifts and prevent the formation of renal calculi.
Insure adequate fluid intake.	To flush renal system and assist in prevention of renal calculi.
Provide dietary intake high in protein, iron, calcium, and vitamins.	Bone healing is facilitated by a nutritional diet. Deposition of calcium salts is mandatory for permanent bony callus formation.

MEDICAL MANAGEMENT

Braces and/or crutches.	Ancillary support may be needed indefinitely until healing occurs.
Surgical repair.	May be required if nonunion occurs.

NURSING DIAGNOSIS:	Injury, potential for, infection.
SUPPORTING DATA:	Compound fractures and contused, lacerated wounds are susceptible to invasion by bacteria, including gram-positive clostridia (gas gangrene).
DESIRED PATIENT OUTCOMES:	Infection does not occur/is treated successfully.

INTERVENTIONS	RATIONALE
Observe for signs of infection at the wound site; redness, swelling, pain.	Indicators of infections. Gas and edema in the tissues causes pain.
Monitor for rapid, feeble pulse; anemia; prostration; apprehension; delirium; and stupor.	May indicate progression to circulatory collapse. Toxemia may develop with gas gangrene.
Observe appearance of skin: white, tense, crepitus, vesicles filled with red, watery fluid and gas bubbles coming from tissues.	Signs of developing gangrene.

Monitor urinary output.

Observe wound and skin isolation measures as indicated.

Oliguria/anuria indicative of decreased renal perfusion and developing septic shock.

Drainage may be infectious.

MEDICAL MANAGEMENT

IV fluids.

Maintain fluid and electrolyte balance.

Invasive monitoring.

Assess perfusion and circulatory volume.

Surgical debridement.

Remove necrotic tissue; preventive and curative.

Antibiotics.

Assist in prevention and/or spread of infection.

Hyperbaric oxygen chamber.

May interrupt toxin formation and reproduction of anaerobic organism.

NURSING DIAGNOSIS:	**Knowledge deficit, activity limitations and routine for healing.**
SUPPORTING DATA:	**Injury creates limitation of and interferes with normal activity. Complications may develop that require intervention.**
DESIRED PATIENT OUTCOMES:	**Complications are limited or do not occur.**

INTERVENTIONS

Instruct the patient regarding active exercises for the joints above and below the fracture.

Discuss signs and symptoms that are important to report to the physician; severe pain, coldness, blueness, foul odors, and changes in sensation.

Discuss importance of clinical appointments for followup.

Instruct patient in methods of proper ambulation as indicated by individual situation.

RATIONALE

Active exercise prevents joint stiffness, contractures, and muscle wasting promoting earlier return to activities of daily living.

Participation in health monitoring increases patient responsibility in health maintenance.

Fracture healing may take as long as a year for completion and patient cooperation with the medical regimen is helpful for proper union of bone to take place.

Most fractures require casts, splints, or braces during the healing process. Further damage and delay in healing could occur secondary to improper use of ambulatory devices.

CARE PLAN: Casts

GENERAL DATA BASE

A cast is a temporary immobilization device usually made of plaster of Paris bandages, fiber glass (light cast), or resin impregnated plaster of Paris bandages.

Casts are used to prevent or correct deformities; maintain, support, and protect realigned bone fragments; and to promote early weight-bearing.

Usually, the joints above and below a fracture are immobilized.

Usually weight-bearing occurs after 48 hours.

A green cast refers to a newly applied cast that has not fully dried. Evaporation of all water in the cast may take as long as 72 hours but is usually accomplished within 36 hours.

Green casts should always be handled with the palms of the hands as fingertips may cause indentations.

The warmer the water (not hot), the faster plaster "sets." "Setting" refers to the chemical process when water reacts with the plaster. Casts are usually considered to be "set" within 2–8 minutes depending on the type of plaster used.

A cast attains its full strength after complete drying.

Know the location of cast cutter or how to obtain it.

NURSING PRIORITIES

1. Provide knowledge base for patient.
2. Maintain position and integrity of the cast.
3. Maintain adequate circulation to and neurologic function of the affected area.
4. Prevent complications.

NURSING DIAGNOSIS:	Fear, anxiety re treatment for injury.
SUPPORTING DATA:	Casting frequently occurs in an emergency situation when hurried activities are occurring with little opportunity for questions.
DESIRED PATIENT OUTCOMES:	Verbalizes purpose of the cast and has information about the location of the area to be enclosed.

INTERVENTIONS	RATIONALE

Explain the purpose for the cast. Include a discussion of the following:
    Exact location of area to be enclosed.
    Size of cast.
    Heat during application.
	Understanding of a procedure usually increases cooperation and reduces anxiety.
	
	The rehydration of gypsum produces heat. The amount of heat produced is affected by the temperature of the immersion H_2O and the amount of plaster applied.

No movement during application and setting stage.
Weight of the cast.
Length of time of immobilization.
Position changing after cast application.

Movement during the setting process weakens the cast.

Post Cast Application

NURSING DIAGNOSIS:	Skin integrity, impairment of, potential.
SUPPORTING DATA:	Skin area under a cast is subject to injury, by pressure of the cast on bony prominences causing ulcerations, necrosis, and/or nerve palsies.
DESIRED PATIENT OUTCOMES:	Skin is prepared for casting and integrity is maintained under the cast. A dry, intact cast is maintained.

INTERVENTIONS

Examine the skin for breaks in continuity, rashes, or unremovable particles and record.

Cleanse area with soap and water. Rub gently with alcohol and/or dust with small amount of a borate or stearate of zinc powder.

Cut a length of stockinette to cover the area and extend several inches beyond the cast.

After the cast has set, elevate the extremity on pillows covered with a folded sheet.

Trim excess plaster from edges of cast as soon as casting is completed.

Cleanse excess plaster from skin while still wet, if possible.

Leave the cast uncovered, open to air to dry.

Reposition the patient every two hours, maintaining body and cast alignment with soft pillows.

RATIONALE

Open wounds increase the risk of infection. Foreign bodies may lead to pressure sores.

Provides a dry, clean area for cast application. Too much powder may cake when it comes in contact with water/perspiration.

A soft knit material used for padding bony prominences, protecting the skin, and finishing cast edges.

A hard surface may cause flattening or indentation of the cast. Placing a "cooling" cast directly on rubber or plastic pillows traps heat and increases drying time.
An improperly shaped or dried cast is irritating to the underlying skin and may lead to circulatory impairment.

Uneven plaster is irritating to the skin and may result in abrasions.

Dry plaster may flake into completed cast and cause skin damage.

Premature drying of the outside of the cast may leave moisture inside the cast, which causes mildew.

Frequent position changes prevent flattening of the cast at pressure points and promotes drying.

525

Inspect the cast every eight hours for drying, cracks, or excessive flaking.

May be indication of improper casting or drying.

Instruct patient not to place objects down inside edges of the cast.

Sharp objects used for scratching may cause breaks in skin continuity providing a source for infection.

Apply heel or elbow protectors as needed. Use foam mattresses, sheepskins, floatation pads, or air mattress as indicated.

Due to immobilization of body parts, bony prominences other than those affected by the casting may suffer from decreased circulation.

Document patient's exact description, localization, and quality of pain before administration of analgesics.

Pain may indicate impaired circulation, and/or excessive pressure on soft tissue or bony prominences. Pain may result from surgical repair or trauma incurred prior to casting.

Petal the edges of a cast with waterproof tape (if "stockinette" petal was not provided).

Petaling refers to the application of tape to cast edges providing an effective barrier to flakes and moisture. Helps prevent breakdown of cast material at edges and reduces skin irritation.

Massage the skin around the cast edges with alcohol q8h.

Has a drying effect, which toughens the skin. Creams and lotions are not recommended secondary to excessive oils sealing cast perimeter, not allowing the cast to "breathe." Powders are not recommended due to excessive accumulation inside the cast. Lotions also tend to cause the cast to become sticky.

If cast is cut, petal cut edges and tape pieces together.

To protect skin.

MEDICAL MANAGEMENT

Monovalve, bivalve, or cut a window in the cast.

Allow the release of pressure and provide access for wound and skin care. May be done on an emergency basis.

NURSING DIAGNOSIS:	Tissue perfusion, alteration in.
SUPPORTING DATA:	Swelling secondary to bone hemorrhage or tissue edema may reduce blood supply to the extremity and result in vascular insufficiency.
DESIRED PATIENT OUTCOMES:	Maintain adequate tissue perfusion.

INTERVENTIONS

Assess and document capillary return, color, sensation, warmth distal to and above the cast, presence and quality of pulses qh × 8 hours, then q4h. Compare both injured and uninjured extremities.

RATIONALE

A tight cast can impair tissue circulation, cause tissue necrosis, and produce severe pain. May lead to amputation. See Care Plan: Fractures.

Apply half-filled ice packs beside the casted area after setting for 24–48h.

Cold application decreases heat, pain, and swelling of soft tissue. Might cause indentation if placed directly on the cast.

Exercise the joint above and below the immobilized area qh × 8h then q4h.

See Care Plan: Fractures.

NURSING DIAGNOSIS: Injury, potential for, infection.

SUPPORTING DATA: Compound fracture with drainage or traumatic wounds and abrasions may act as growth media for bacteria when covered with a cast.

DESIRED PATIENT OUTCOMES: Prevent infection.

INTERVENTIONS

RATIONALE

Monitor temperature and WBC.

A wet cast with bleeding provides an opening for the entry of pathogenic organisms.

Observe for foul odor, document, and notify physician.

Infection or tissue necrosis may be manifested by an unpleasant odor.

Inspect cast for wound drainage or blood stains, circle area, and mark with date and time.

Helpful indicator of increased bleeding or drainage. Allows for noting enlarging area of drainage.

Feel the cast for excessively warm areas.

May indicate infectious process.

MEDICAL MANAGEMENT

Change dressings, maintaining sterile technique.

Prevent or lessen opportunity for infection.

Antibiotics.

May be given prophylactically or in the presence of infection.

NURSING DIAGNOSIS: Mobility, impaired physical.

SUPPORTING DATA: Any injury to the body requiring immobilization of a part will interfere with the patient's ability to manage ADL.

DESIRED PATIENT OUTCOMES: Performs activities of daily living within the limitations of the cast. Performs muscle strengthing exercises on a regular basis as permitted.

INTERVENTIONS

RATIONALE

List activities the patient can perform independently, and which require assistance.

Activities need to be organized around who is available to provide needed help.

Teach crutch walking, if indicated.	May be done by physical therapy. Nurse needs to reinforce and assist.
A backpack may be substituted for a purse.	Leaves hands free to manipulate crutches.
Elevate the casted leg when not ambulatory. Elevate the casted arm with a sling when the patient is out of bed. Teach the proper use of the sling.	Intermittent weight bearing alleviates venous pooling. At rest a dependent extremity develops venous pooling, which causes pain and swelling.
Use plastic bags to protect the cast during wet weather or while bathing.	Moisture weakens a cast.
Use a blowdryer to dry small areas of dampened casts.	Cautious use can hasten drying.
Actively exercise the joints above and below the cast:	Exercise prevents complications, promotes healing, and aides in rehabilitation process post cast removal.
Raise the casted arm over the head.	
Move each finger and thumb or toes.	Moving fingers and toes stimulate circulation and promotes venous return.
Raise and lower wrist. Quadriceps setting: tightening and relaxing of muscles. Gluteal setting. Abdominal tightening. Deep breathing. Opening and closing the hand.	
Teach isometric exercises starting with the unaffected limb.	Isometric exercises cause muscles to contract without bending joints or moving limbs and help maintain muscle strength and mass.
Teach patient to put unaffected joints through full range of motion four times daily.	Performing full ROM of the uncasted structures helps maintain muscle tone and mobility.

NURSING DIAGNOSIS:	**Knowledge deficit, potential for complications.**
SUPPORTING DATA:	**Damaged cast may interfere with proper healing.**
DESIRED PATIENT OUTCOMES:	**Will maintain a whole, dry, intact cast, and will notify physician if complications occur.**

INTERVENTIONS

RATIONALE

Give patient information re signs and symptoms of complications to watch for: e.g., severe pain; burning; numbness; tingling; swelling; skin discoloration; paralysis; white, cool toes or fingertips; foul odor; warm spots; soft areas; cracks.

May be signs of infection/impaired circulation. Some darkening of the skin and swelling may occur normally when walking on the casted extremity or using casted arm; however, this should resolve with rest and elevation.

Instruct patient and SO how to care for "green" or wet cast.

Some patients are sent home with wet casts. Inclusion of significant others in teaching, provides reference person for patient whose anxiety level may inhibit retention of instructions. Written instructions for cast care and observations provides a reference for remembering details.

Cover toes with stockinette or soft socks.

Will help to keep warm.

Clean a soiled cast with a slightly dampened cloth and some scouring powder.

Important to avoid getting the cast wet.

NURSING DIAGNOSIS: Injury, potential for, compartmental syndrome or paralysis.

SUPPORTING DATA: Volkmann's contracture most commonly occurs in the forearm and hand from elbow injuries, but may be seen in the lower leg and foot.

DESIRED PATIENT OUTCOMES: Circulation, sensation, and movement proximal and distal to the cast will be maintained.

INTERVENTIONS

Observe hourly for color, pulses, temperature, capillary filling, movement, and sensation above and below the cast for 48 hours.

Have cast cutter available.

Turn and position the patient q2h.

RATIONALE

Edema that occludes the arterial blood supply results in ischemic myositis or muscle necrosis.

For emergency removal of cast.

May feel comfortable but poor alignment may cause painless obstruction.

POST CAST REMOVAL

NURSING DIAGNOSIS: Self-concept, disturbance in.

SUPPORTING DATA: Muscle atrophy occurs, skin becomes pale, dry, and scaly looking under a cast.

DESIRED PATIENT OUTCOMES: Patient accepts appearance of affected part. Increases muscle strength and ROM, and prevents new injuries.

INTERVENTIONS

Inform the patient that the skin under the cast is commonly mottled and covered with scales or crusts of dead skin.

Wash the skin gently with soap, Betadine, or pHisoHex, and water. Lubricate with a protective emollient.

Inform the patient that muscles may appear flabby and atrophied (less muscle mass).

Support the joint above and below the affected part when removing the cast. Continue support as necessary with pillows, elastic bandages, splints, braces, crutches, walkers, or canes.

Elevate the extremity.

Instruct the patient in the importance of continuing exercises as permitted by the physician.

Assist physical therapist to perform prescribed activities; such as whirlpool baths, massage, paraffin baths, and ultrasound.

RATIONALE

It is several weeks before normal appearance returns.

New skin is extremely tender because it has been protected beneath a cast.

Muscle strength will be lessened and new or different aches and pains may be manifested secondary to loss of support.

Sudden movement of disused joints may cause pain or injury.

Swelling and edema tend to occur after cast removal.

To reduce stiffness and improve strength and function of extremity.

Teamwork is important to satisfactory outcome.

SPICA OR BODY CAST SPECIFICS

NURSING DIAGNOSIS:	**Bowel elimination, alteration in, constipation.**
SUPPORTING DATA:	**Immobility predisposes to constipation.**
DESIRED PATIENT OUTCOMES:	**Normal bowel functioning is maintained. Bowel obstruction or adynamic ileus prevented.**

INTERVENTIONS

Encourage fluids unless ileus suspected. Auscultate bowel sounds, as able.

Increase the amount of roughage in the diet. Avoid gas-forming foods.

MEDICAL MANAGEMENT

Stool softeners, enemas, and laxatives.

RATIONALE

Provides information about bowel activity. Maintain consistency of stool. If bowel sounds are absent, may cause gastric distention and emesis.

Assists in prevention of constipation. Gas-forming foods may cause abdominal distention.

May need assistance, pressure of the cast on the peritoneal cavity may cause a change in bowel habits.

NURSING DIAGNOSIS:	Urinary elimination, alteration in pattern.
SUPPORTING DATA:	Immobilization contributes to the formation of urinary calculi and stasis in the bladder.
DESIRED PATIENT OUTCOMES:	Urinary tract infections and/or calculi are prevented.

INTERVENTIONS

Force oral fluid intake, including acid/ash juice.

Perform perineal hygiene daily and after each stool.

Use fracture bedpan.

Report any complaints of back or flank pain to the physician.

Encourage complete emptying of the bladder by nursing measures.

RATIONALE

To flush kidneys and minimize opportunity for stone formation.

Prevent opportunity for contamination of meatus.

Limits elevation of hips and lessens pressure on lumbar region and cast.

May indicate presence of stone.

Prevents stasis.

NURSING DIAGNOSIS:	Fluid volume deficit, potential.
SUPPORTING DATA:	May develop hypokalemia, alkalosis, and hypovolemia, which may lead to death.
DESIRED PATIENT OUTCOMES:	"Cast-syndrome" does not occur.

INTERVENTIONS

Observe for prolonged nausea and vomiting and report to physician.

Place in prone position.

MEDICAL MANAGEMENT

NG tube.

Cut an opening (window) over the abdominal area. (Total cast removal may be necessary.)

IV fluid and electrolyte replacement.

Duodenaljejunostomy.

RATIONALE

Gastric and duodenal dilitation occur secondary to compression of the fourth portion of the duodenum by the superior mesenteric artery.

May relieve pressure symptoms.

May be necessary to relieve gastric distention.

Relieve pressure over duodenum.

Maintain normal levels.

Surgical intervention may be required if obstruction is not relieved. Refer to Care Plan: Surgical Intervention.

NURSING DIAGNOSIS:	Injury, potential for, infection.
SUPPORTING DATA:	Contaminated, dirty cast provides environment for the growth of bacteria.
DESIRED PATIENT OUTCOMES:	Cast remains free from contamination.

INTERVENTIONS	RATIONALE
Line the perineal cast edges with plastic wrap.	Damp soiled casts can weaken and may cause skin irritation and/or promote growth of bacteria.
Petal the edges of the cast with waterproof tape.	Maintain integrity of cast/prevent crumbling of edges and trauma to skin.
Slightly raise the head of the bed when using the bedpan.	Prevents urine from running back underneath the cast.

NURSING DIAGNOSIS:	Breathing patterns, alteration in.
SUPPORTING DATA:	Cast may restrict chest movement. Pain on inspiration may be present.
DESIRED PATIENT OUTCOMES:	Pulmonary complications do not occur.

INTERVENTIONS	RATIONALE
Turn/reposition, cough and deep breathe q2h × 24 hours, then q4h.	Promotes adequate ventilation, and varies pressure of cast on chest.
Auscultate exposed areas of the chest for breath sounds.	Early identification of congestion.

MEDICAL MANAGEMENT

Incentive spirometry.	Assists ventilation and minimizes atelectasis.

NURSING DIAGNOSIS:	Injury, potential for, alteration in cast continuity.
SUPPORTING DATA:	Improper handling may damage cast and interfere with healing.
DESIRED PATIENT OUTCOMES:	Cast integrity maintained.

INTERVENTIONS

Place a bedboard under the mattress.

Place a pillow crosswise of the bed at the patient's waist and two pillows lengthwise under each leg.

Turn frequently to include the uninvolved side and prone position with patient's feet over the end of the mattress.

Use sufficient personnel for turning. Do not use the abduction bar for turning. Support the casted limb inside the thigh and at the knee and ankle with the hands during the turn. Can use a heavy stockinette sling attached to overhead frame for turning.

Instruct the patient in the use of the trapeze bar.

Place a folded towel between the arm and the cast prior to turning.

RATIONALE

Soft or sagging mattress may deform a green cast or crack a dry cast.

Pillows under the head and shoulders of the patient in a green spica cast produces pressure on the chest and abdomen deforming the cast.

Alternating position assists in maintaining respiratory functioning and varies pressure areas. Minimizes pressure on feet and around cast edges.

Hip or body casts can be extremely heavy and cumbersome. Failure to support these areas may cause the cast to break. Help support limb in hip spica when turning from side to side.

Aids in movement and allows the patient to assist.

Sometimes the arm is pinched between the bed and the cast during turning.

CARE PLAN: Traction

GENERAL DATA BASE

Traction is force or pull exerted in one direction. *Countertraction* is a pull in the opposite direction. Force is applied through the use of various systems of ropes, pulleys, pins, and weights.

Traction may be applied manually or mechanically. *Mechanical traction* is accomplished through the use of ropes, pulleys, casts, or braces.

Traction is used to reduce or eliminate muscle spasms; correct or prevent deformities; and to reduce pain.

A Balkan frame is a metal rectangular frame supported on four corners above the patient's bed. This serves as the base for other parts of the traction setup.

Balanced or suspension traction allows patient movement without a change in the pull of traction.

Running traction exerts a direct pull in one plane unilaterally or bilaterally.

NURSING PRIORITIES

1. Prevention of complications.
2. Assist patient to develop effective coping behaviors to deal with current situation.

Problems encountered with traction are essentially the same as those for a fracture or cast. Some nursing measures specific to traction patients are delineated.

SKIN TRACTION

NURSING DIAGNOSIS:	**Skin integrity, impairment of.**
SUPPORTING DATA:	**The use of tape to anchor the traction can be irritating as the traction exerts a pull on the skin. In addition, immobility may lead to skin breakdown in other areas of the body.**
DESIRED PATIENT OUTCOMES:	**Traction remains constant with the desired pull and the skin remains intact.**

INTERVENTIONS

Inspect the skin for preexisting irritation or breaks in continuity.

Cleanse the skin with warm soapy water.

Apply tincture of benzoin.

Apply commercial skin traction tapes (or make some with strips of moleskin or adhesive tape) lengthwise to opposite sides of the affected limb. Extend the tapes beyond the length of the limb.

RATIONALE

Provides a source of entry for pathogenic organisms.

Reduce level of contaminants on skin.

"Toughens" the skin for tape application.

Traction tapes encircling a limb may compromise circulation.

Traction is exerted in line with the free ends of the tape.

Palpate over area of tapes daily and document any tenderness or pain.

If area under tapes is tender, suspect skin irritation and prepare to remove the bandage system.

Place protective padding under the leg and over bony prominences.

Minimize pressure on these areas.

Mark the line where the tapes extend beyond the extremity.

Marking the tapes allows for quick assessment of slippage.

Wrap the limb circumference including any tapes or padding with elastic bandages.

Be careful to wrap snugly but not so tight that circulation is compromised.

Observe pulley and weight system to:
    Secure knots holding weights.
    Maintain ropes and weights freely moveable and in straight alignment.
    Prevent excessive motion of weights.
    Maintain position of weights off the floor or bed.

To maintain degree of traction. Counter-traction can be broken as ordered.

Remove skin traction every 24 hours, if allowed; inspect and give skin care.

Maintains skin integrity.

Provide good skin care to rest of body. Change position as allowed. Alternating air or foam mattress should be used.

Inactivity and movement limitations may lead to decubitus formation.

MEDICAL MANAGEMENT

Place weights per order (usually 5–7lbs).

The tolerance of the skin determines the amount of traction to be applied.

SKELETAL TRACTION

NURSING DIAGNOSIS:	Injury, potential for, infection, thrombus formation, and nerve damage.
SUPPORTING DATA:	Skeletal traction is applied to bones through the skin using metal; Kirschner wires, Steinmann pins, or Crutchfield or Barton tongs. Break in skin integrity provides entry for bacteria. Immobility contributes to stasis of circulation and potential for thrombophlebitis. Prolonged pressure can lead to nerve damage.
DESIRED PATIENT OUTCOMES:	Infection does not occur. Thrombophlebitis and/or nerve damage do not occur.

INTERVENTIONS

Inspect the skin for preexisting irritation or breaks in continuity.

Monitor neurovascular stability during skeletal traction application.

Observe and document skin conditions around tongs, pins, or wires q8h. Note especially, odors or signs of inflammation.

Instruct the patient not to touch the insertion sites.

Cover ends of wires/pins with rubber/cork protectors or needle caps; or bend wires.

Inspect traction apparatus q8h for the following:
Proper alignment and maintenance of proper weights. Loose pins, wires, or tongs.

Do not remove weights, even when repositioning the patient.

Provide support, splints or footboard for hands or feet.

Note presence of positive Homann's sign.

Check peripheral pulses to extremities, skin color, temperature.

Observe for complications of immobility.

MEDICAL MANAGEMENT

Cleansing solution.

Hoffman traction.

RATIONALE

Pins or wires should not be inserted through skin infections, rashes, or abrasions as compromised skin barrier may lead to bone infection.

Skeletal traction is usually applied under local or general anesthesia. Pins or wires are inserted through skin, subuctaneous tissue, and bone only (muscles, tendons, arteries, and nerves are avoided).

Insertion sites may become infected, and may result in osteomyelitis.

Minimize opportunity for contamination.

To prevent injury to other body parts.

Insure that optimal position for healing is maintained. Loose pins, wires, or tongs may cause tissue damage and aid in the introduction of infection.

Countertraction must be maintained.

Prevent nerve damage with subsequent wrist/foot drop.

Evidence of thrombus formation.

Indication of adequate blood flow.

There is some degree of immobility with skeletal traction. Refer to Care Plan: Casts.

Daily removal of old drainage and crusts decreases chances of infection.

An external type of traction that does not require ropes, pulleys, or weights, allowing for greater mobility.

NURSING DIAGNOSIS:	**Coping, ineffective, individual.**
SUPPORTING DATA:	**Patient in traction for extended period may have difficulty dealing with prolonged inactivity.**
DESIRED PATIENT OUTCOMES:	**Patient spends time with diversional activities and verbalizes acceptance of situation.**

INTERVENTIONS

Provide time for talking and listening to concerns.

Assess need for referral to social services.

Provide diversional activities compatible to the situation.

Assess sexual needs and provide for privacy.

Refer to Care Plan: Psychosocial Aspects of Care in the Acute Setting.

RATIONALE

Identify areas of concerns and ideas for resolving problems.

May need help with handling personal matters/maintaining home/dealing with employment concerns.

Dependent upon individual preferences and degree of immobilization.

Individual needs, desires, and the degree of mobility will need to be taken into consideration.

CARE PLAN: Amputation

PATIENT DATA BASE

NURSING HISTORY

Amputations are classified as upper or lower extremity. There are two types of amputations:
1. Open; requires strict aseptic technique and later revisions.
2. Closed or "flap."

Indications include: trauma, vascular insufficiency, osteomyelitis, and cancer.

Patients are usually fitted with a prosthetic device immediately or within several weeks.

NURSING PRIORITIES

1. Preparation of the patient psychologically and physiologically.
2. Relieve pain.
3. Promote early ambulation.
4. Prevent complications and prolonged disability.

NURSING DIAGNOSIS:	**Self-concept, disturbance in.**
SUPPORTING DATA:	**Loss of a body part creates a change in body image, and results in a grieving process.**
DESIRED PATIENT OUTCOMES:	**Open communication is established. Patient verbalizes understanding of treatment process and "phantom limb" pain.**

INTERVENTIONS

Encourage expression of fears, negative feelings, and grief over loss of body part.

Confirm and support information given to the patient by the surgeon. Review the following:
 Location of amputation.
 Type of prosthetic fitting (immediate, delayed, not a candidate for prosthesis).
 Initial postoperative course including discussion of phantom limb sensations.

Introduce the patient to the physical therapy and/ or occupational staffs (the entire team in your particular institution).

RATIONALE

Knowing what to expect reduces anxiety and promotes cooperation.

Provides opportunity for patient to begin to deal with change in body image and facilitate postoperative recovery.

Patients who have phantom limb pain sometimes think they are losing their sanity.

Involvement with these groups will provide opportunities to learn ways of handling the new problems the patient will be facing.

Involve with other amputee patients.	The support of other amputee patients may provide courage and hope for the future.
Prepare for surgery.	See Care Plan: Surgical Interventions.
Correct underlying infections, nutritional and fluid imbalances.	Promote optimal healing.
Prepare for postoperative ambulation. Instruct in exercise program, mobility training, and transfer techniques.	Instruction in these skills preoperatively facilitates postoperative functioning.

Refer to Care Plan: Psychosocial Aspects of Care in the Acute Setting.

NURSING DIAGNOSIS:	**Comfort, alterations in, pain.**
SUPPORTING DATA:	**Nerves that have been severed, continue to send messages of pain and the feeling of having the limb still there.**
DESIRED PATIENT OUTCOMES:	**Pain is controlled and/or minimized. Phantom pain is understood and managed.**

INTERVENTIONS

RATIONALE

Keep patient active physical/mental diversions.	Decreases occurrence of phantom limb pain.
Give patient information about phantom limb sensations and that it is not permanent.	Knowing about these sensations allows the patient to understand this is a normal phenomenon. Some individuals continue to experience the sensation that the missing limb is still there for long periods.
Assess pain characteristics.	May indicate developing necrosis/infection.

MEDICAL MANAGEMENT

Analgesics.	As required for pain/discomfort.

NURSING DIAGNOSIS:	**Injury, potential for, hemorrhage, infection.**
SUPPORTING DATA:	**Extensive trauma predisposes to possibility of these complications.**
DESIRED PATIENT OUTCOMES:	**Hemorrhage and infection do not occur.**

INTERVENTIONS

Keep tourniquet at bedside.

Elevate stump by elevating foot of bed. Do not use a pillow. (Pillows or slings may be used for upper limb amputations.)

Note and record amount of wound drainage per Hemovac.

Maintain aseptic technique when changing dressings.

Cover dressing with plastic when using the bedpan, or if patient is incontinent.

When dressings are discontinued, expose stump to air; wash with mild soap and water.

RATIONALE

Immediately available if hemorrhage occurs.

Promotes venous return and decreases edema without causing hip flexion contractures.

Indicator of hemorrhage and reduces need for dressing changes. Removes drainage, which can be a growth media for infection.

Minimize infection.

Prevent contamination in lower limb amputation.

Skin is sensitive, tender, and fragile.

PROSTHESIS

Immediate/early: allows ambulation and permits more positive self-image. *Immediately postop,* a rigid plaster of Paris dressing is applied to the stump. A pylon and artificial foot may then be attached. Weight-bearing begins within 24–48 hours. In *early postop* fitting, weight-bearing does not occur until 10–30 days postop.

Delayed: More common in areas that do not have facilities available for immediate/early application. Also the condition of the stump and the patient will affect this choice.

NURSING DIAGNOSIS:	Mobility, impaired physical.
SUPPORTING DATA:	Loss of a limb, particularly a lower extremity, results in a change in the sense of balance.
DESIRED PATIENT OUTCOMES:	Deformities are prevented and a prosthesis is used with ease.

INTERVENTIONS

Cleanse and inspect area, dry thoroughly; may use cornstarch. Measure circumference.

Do ROM exercises with the stump, early postop.

Instruct patient to lie in prone position b.i.d. with pillow under abdomen and stump.

Continue preop muscle strengthening exercises as soon as allowed out of bed, e.g., while holding on to chair for balance; knee bends, hop on foot, stand on toes.

RATIONALE

Routine stump care to note healing, infection. Measurement to estimate shrinkage.

Deformities develop rapidly and may delay prosthesis usage.

Stretches flexor muscles and prevents contracture of hip.

Contributes to maintaining sense of balance.

If "immediate/early" cast is accidently dislodged, rewrap stump immediately with an elastic bandage, elevate, notify physician, and prepare for reapplication of cast.

Edema will occur rapidly and rehabilitation will be delayed.

Preparation for prosthesis, "delayed:"

Wrap stump with elastic bandage or air splint. A stump shrinker also may be used (heavy stockinette socks).

Prevents edema and helps to shrink stump. Provides uniform compression of stump. Air splint permits visual inspection of the wound.
Hardens the stump.

Instruct patient in stump-conditioning exercises of pushing the stump against a pillow.
Massage the stump.

Decreases tenderness, softens the scar, and improves vascularity.

Instruct in care of the stump after discharge.

Activities allowed, exercises, skin care, further shrinkage are some of the topics to be discussed.

DIAGNOSIS: Rheumatoid Arthritis

Patient Data Base

NURSING HISTORY

Symetrical joint pain, warmth, tenderness, stiffness, swelling, and redness of the involved joint.

More common in women, 3:1 (increased incidence in young women who have just given birth). Age group: 25–45.

Disease may be polycyclic with series of exacerbations and remissions or monocyclic.with acute episode and spontaneous remission.

History of morning stiffness, early afternoon fatigue, anorexia and weight loss, systemic malaise, and low-grade fever.

May become candidate for joint replacement; most notably the ankle, hip, and knee.

DIAGNOSTIC STUDIES

ASO titer to r/o streptococcal infection as cause of arthritis symptoms.

C-reactive protein test (CRP) positive.

Serum protein electrophoresis indicates increased globulins (gamma and alpha) and decreased albumin.

Increased ESR indicate active inflammatory disease.

Synovial fluid abnormal, viscosity poor. Analysis will identify inflammatory, traumatic, or degenerative disease.

WBC: elevation indicative of inflammation.

CBC: anemia may be present.

X-rays of involved joints to determine extent of disease.

Arthroscopy may be done to permit direct visualization of area.

PHYSICAL EXAMINATION

Joints show edema, increased vascularity, increased synovial fluid.

Subcutaneous nodules over bony prominences; enlarged lymph nodes, especially those that drain inflamed joints.

Subsequent difficulties include crepitation, dislocations, ankylosis, and muscle contractions with ambulation.

Deformity of the joints may be present; in hands, ulnar drift of the fingers and swan-neck and boutonniere deformities of the proximal interphalangeal (PIP) joints and distal interphalanageal (DIP) joints are frequently present.

Possible muscle atrophy adjacent to affected joints.

Contractures subluxation, gross local distortion of joints, and rheumatic nodules may be seen.

Decreased subcutaneous fat.

Distal phalanges are hyperextended, the proximal are flexed, and ulnar deviation of the fingers.

Skin covering fingertips is thin, pale, smooth, and shiny; the nails are rough and brittle; and intrinsic muscles of the hand are wasted.

NURSING PRIORITIES

1. Control pain.
2. Increase mobility of affected joints.
3. Assist in developing coping behaviors to deal with illness and debilitating effects.
4. Increased independence, and ADL.

NURSING DIAGNOSIS:	Comfort, alteration in, pain.
SUPPORTING DATA:	Synovitis is manifested by warm, red, swollen joints resulting from distention of tissues by the accumulation of fluid, and inflammatory cells producing pain by pressure on sensory nerve endings.
DESIRED PATIENT OUTCOMES:	Maximal/optimal relief and/or control of pain.

INTERVENTIONS	RATIONALE
Assess type of pain, location, duration, and severity.	Helpful in determining pain management program.
Observe for salicylate overdose, tinnitus, gastric intolerance, GI bleeding, purpuric tendencies.	Tinnitus usually indicates high, therapeutic blood levels. If tinnitus occurs, the dosage is usually decreased by 1 tablet/q 2–3 days until it stops.
Instruct patient to have blood tests every few months, especially checking prothrombin time.	Aspirin prolongs prothrombin time.
Have patient assume position of comfort while in bed or sitting in chair.	
Maintain bed rest as indicated.	In severe disease, total bed rest may be necessary until objective and subjective improvements are seen. Important during periods of inflammatory process.
Assist patient to move in bed, supporting affected joints, above and below the joint.	To avoid increase in pain.
Instruct patient to take warm bath or shower upon arising to relieve morning stiffness.	Heat increases muscle relaxation and mobility and decreases pain.
Warm moist application to affected joints may be used several times daily. Be sure temperature of compress is not too hot, watch for tissue damage.	May not be sensitive to degree of heat, and damage may occur.
Use ice or cold packs when indicated.	Heat may be contraindicated in the presence of hot, swollen joints. Cold relieves pain and swelling.
Use gentle massage.	For relaxation.
Discuss alternative therapies, such as relaxation, Therapeutic Touch, biofeedback, and visualization. May benefit from referral to pain clinic.	Often helpful in long-term, painful illness, which can be discouraging.

MEDICAL MANAGEMENT

Acetylsalicylic acid q3h as well as 1½ hours before arising.

To maintain optimum blood level. ASA exerts anti-inflammatory and mild analgesic effect. Exact mechanism is unknown, but may be due to salicylate induced reduction of capillary permeability, inhibition of mucopolysaccharide syntheses, and oxidative phosphorylation. ASA must be taken regularly in order to sustain a blood level between 18–25 mg/percent. Will decrease stiffness and increase mobility.

Antacid with ASA, enteric coated or buffered aspirin.

To minimize gastric irritation.

Paraffin tub baths for painful fingers and hands. Check temperature before applying.

Provides sustained heat to affected joints.

Splints.

To rest painful joints. A variety of splinting arrangements are available dependent on the individual need.

NURSING DIAGNOSIS:	Mobility, impaired physical.
SUPPORTING DATA:	Joint swelling, inflammation, pain, and decreased mobility.
DESIRED PATIENT OUTCOMES:	Increased mobility of affected joints.

INTERVENTIONS

Assist with range of motion exercises, passive/active. Useful after heat treatments.

Maintain proper body alignment while in bed, use footboard; firm mattress; bedboard; avoid external rotation of extremities, using sandbags and trochanter rolls.

Instruct patient in regular schedule of exercises within individual limitations.

Instruct patient to avoid excessive exercise. If pain lasts more than ½ hr after exercise, it is too vigorous.

Isometric exercises may be beneficial.

Resistive exercises.

RATIONALE

Passive ROM exercises help to prevent contractures, mobilize edema, maintain muscle strength, lessen the severity of the generalized stiffness and weakness caused by myositis and disuse.

Proper maintenance of body alignment while the patient is immobile will help to prevent contractures of muscles that are needed for ambulation and activities of daily living.

A regular program maintains mobility.

Patient may become impatient and go beyond personal limits without understanding this may lead to rapid joint destruction.

Preserve muscle strength when the patient has swollen and painfully inflamed, or severely damaged joints.

Used to develop strength, performed primarily in nonweight-bearing positions to avoid additional trauma to the joint.

Observe patient's tolerance to the exercise program.

Provides opportunity for necessary adjustments. Increased pain and/or fatigue may indicate too much exercise.

Instruct patient to lie in prone position at least 2 × / day.

Will help to prevent hip flexion and knee contractures.

May wear nylon stretch gloves at night.

Relieves numbness and tingling of the fingers.

Maintain proper body weight, provide diet instruction; decreased calories, increased nutritional value foods as indicated.

Will decrease stress on affected joints. May need to lose weight.

NURSING DIAGNOSIS:	Self-concept, disturbance in.
SUPPORTING DATA:	Joint deformity, awkward gait. Possible confinement to wheelchair and changes in usual ADL.
DESIRED PATIENT OUTCOMES:	Verbalizes increased confidence in ability to deal with illness, changes in lifestyle, and possible limitations.

INTERVENTIONS

RATIONALE

Encourage verbalization about fears of disease process. Take time to sit down and talk with the patient. Do not appear rushed or in a hurry.

Opportunity to identify fears and/or misinformation and deal with directly. Constant pain is wearing and feelings of anger and hostility are common.

Deal with behavioral changes. Tell patient what behavior is acceptable. Reinforce positive changes. Be supportive, but firm in dealing with patient.

Setting limits is helpful in maintaining self-esteem.

Give positive reinforcement for tasks accomplished.

Allows patient to feel good about self. Reinforces positive behavior. Enhances self-confidence.

Reinforce explanations of disease process, expectations, and limitations.

Having information helps allay fear of the unknown and identify realities that need to be dealt with.

Discuss patient's perception of how significant others perceive limitations.

May have significant impact on how patient views self.

Refer to Care Plan: Psychosocial Aspects of Care in the Acute setting.

MEDICAL MANAGEMENT

Tranquilizers and mood-elevating drugs.

May be prescribed when depression is severe.

NURSING DIAGNOSIS:	Self-care deficit, personal hygiene, feeding, dressing, sexual performance.

SUPPORTING DATA:	**Decreased mobility, increasing stiffness of joints, joint deformity, pain. Pain and difficulty with movement may interfere with sexual performance.**
DESIRED PATIENT OUTCOMES:	**Increased independence in spite of existing disabilities.**

INTERVENTIONS

Discuss usual ADL prior to onset of illness and potential changes now anticipated.

Maintain mobility, pain control, and exercise program.

Modify personal hygiene items: large grips on combs, brushes, and so forth; raised toilet seats; safety bars in the bathroom; special aids to assist in dressing. Assist in learning to use new/changed devices.

Assist significant others by giving instructions on how to modify the environment and assist the patient to be independent.

Allow patient sufficient time to complete tasks.

Provide for sexual counseling if necessary.

Arrange visiting nurse home evaluation prior to discharge with follow-up afterward.

Arrange for consultation with other agencies as necessary.

RATIONALE

May be able to incorporate much of usual activities in necessary adaptations to limitations.

Keeping patient ambulatory and pain within control will greatly aid in physical/emotional independence.

The ability of the patient to do self-care will greatly increase self-confidence.

Allows for increased independence and enhances opportunity for improved relationships.

May need more time. More helpful to complete tasks by self than to have others do tasks on a regular basis. Provides an opportunity for greater sense of self-confidence and self-worth.

Information re different positions and techniques and/or other options for sexual fulfillment may be needed.

Identify problems that may be encountered with current level of disability. Provides for more successful team efforts with others who are involved in care, e.g., occupational therapy team.

May need additional kinds of assistance, such as Meals-on-Wheels, homemaking.

DIAGNOSIS: Degenerative Joint Disease (Osteoarthritis)

PATIENT DATA BASE

NURSING HISTORY

Age and Sex: usually occurs in individuals over age 50, more often in women, although there is an increase in the incidence in younger age group.

Family history of joint disorders.

Determine level of activity.

Check regarding employment: is there constant wear and tear on a particular joint, causing injury or excessive use.

History of systemic diseases (diabetes mellitus, acromegally): especially a history of inflammatory type of arthritis.

History of single, major injury, or repetitive, minor injuries to involved joint/s, such as in sports, football and motorcycling.

Presents with complaints of pain in joints (dull, persistent), which is worsened on movement.

May c/o stiffness, which is usually greater in the morning or after a period of inactivity, especially in distal joints of the fingers, knees, hips, vertebrae, and occasionally ankles.

Note nutritional status, especially obesity.

DIAGNOSTIC STUDIES

Usually tests show no abnormalities. RBC and sedimentation rate should be normal for age group.

Rheumatoid factor usually negative.

Radiologic changes are most helpful for diagnostic purposes.

Synovial fluid analysis usually will not reveal any signs of inflammation.

Arthroscopy may reveal degenerative changes and r/o other causes of joint pain.

PHYSICAL EXAMINATION

Evaluate involved joint/s:
 ROM limitations.
 If fingers are involved, note presence of Heberden's nodes, bony enlargements, small effusions, crepitus.
 Erythema and heat over involved joint are unusual in osteoarthritis.
 Most commonly involved joints are distal joints of fingers, base of thumb, weight-bearing joints, such as knees, hips, vertebrae. Occasionally, elbows, shoulders, ankles involved, usually caused by occupational trauma.

Assess nutritional status, excess body weight has deleterious effect on weight-bearing joints, especially the knees.

Assess posture and position of body parts. When patient is walking, obese thighs may cause the patient to walk in a bowlegged manner, causing abnormal wear and tear on the bones of hips and knees.

NURSING PRIORITIES

1. Protect joints from undue strain and trauma.
2. Control pain.
3. Improve, maintain patient's functional capacity.

NURSING DIAGNOSIS:	Mobility, impaired physical.
SUPPORTING DATA:	Range of motion is usually decreased and accompanied by pain, which is commonly worsened on use and movement of involved joint.
DESIRED PATIENT OUTCOMES:	Optimal functioning at acceptable level for patient.

INTERVENTIONS

Help patient protect joints from undue strain and trauma; keeping joints and muscles warm; resting involved joints with splints, braces, traction.

• Canes, crutches, and other mechanical devices may be helpful.

• Instruct in correct posture and body mechanics.

• Give information about and encourage the use of ROM and isometric exercises to maintain function. Discourage vigorous activity.

RATIONALE

Wear and tear on involved joints causes initial disorder. Overuse should be avoided. Gloves, warm clothes helpful to maintain mobility and prevent pain. Traction may help relieve compression on nerve roots.

• Local support when weight-bearing joints are involved.

• Abnormal wear and tear, anatomical abnormalities, malalignment predispose one to degeneration of cartilage.

Maintain mobility and muscle tone/strength and lessens deformities.
Minimizes damage and further degeneration.

NURSING DIAGNOSIS:	Comfort, alteration in, pain.
SUPPORTING DATA:	Cardinal presenting complaint is of dull, persistent pain in involved joint/s, accompanied by limited ROM and stiffness, especially after a period of inactivity. Heberden's nodes (if fingers are involved) may be painful early in development.
DESIRED PATIENT OUTCOMES:	Pain decreased.

INTERVENTIONS

Apply heat to affected joints, try cold if heat is ineffective.

Elasticized gloves may be worn at night.

Provide patient with realistic assessment of the situation.

RATIONALE

Relieves muscle spasm, stiffness, and pain.

Provide warmth and relieve pain.

Can be reassuring, symptoms will probably improve either spontaneously or with treatment.

- Assess for imposing psychologic or emotional factors.

- May alter patient's perception and acceptance of pain. Psychologic and/or emotional factors may reduce pain threshold.

MEDICAL MANAGEMENT

Analgesics.

Relieve pain. Use of medications in controlling pain should be minimal. Joint disease in fingers and thumbs is rarely incapacitating and is usually painless or will probably become so.

Local steroid injection.

Used on an occasional basis for synovial inflammation.

Surgery.

Involvement of the major joints (hips, knees) is usually painful and surgery is considered when it becomes disabling. (Includes; debridement, arthroplasty, osteotomy, and total joint replacement). Refer to Care Plan: Total Joint Replacement.

CARE PLAN: Total Joint Replacement (Knee, Hip, Elbow, Fingers, Wrist)

PATIENT DATA BASE

NURSING HISTORY

History of debilitating arthritis: rheumatoid or osteo.

Severe accident destroying the joint.

Age: elderly, usually requires replacement secondary to arthritis.

Occupational recreational activities: sedentary or active.

History of aseptic necrosis of the joint head.

Ambulation: how is patient currently getting around?

History of pain: duration, site, way of handling.

Current medication usage.

DIAGNOSTIC STUDIES

Electrolytes and blood sugar: hypokalemia and hyperglycemia may result from steroid use.

CBC, type and cross-match: anemia may be present; blood loss during surgery may require replacement.

Chest x-ray: determine presence of lung disease.

X-ray of joints: determine extent of disability and rule out malignancy.

Arterial blood gases: assess cardiovascular and pulmonary status.

PHYSICAL EXAMINATION

Cardiovascular evaluation: presence of peripheral edema; pulses.

Pulmonary assessment: note existing respiratory impairment.

Determine range of motion of all joints and ability to ambulate prior to surgery presence, location, character, duration of pain.

NURSING PRIORITIES

1. Prevent infection/other complications.
2. Assist in regaining maximum mobility.
3. Assist in learning rehabilitation activities.

Primarily addressed to weight-bearing joints.

NURSING DIAGNOSIS:	**Injury, potential for, infection.**
SUPPORTING DATA:	**Susceptible to infection secondary to exposure of joint during surgery and postop pneumonia because of immobility.**
DESIRED PATIENT OUTCOMES:	**Infection is prevented/treated.**

INTERVENTIONS

Encourage to cough and deep breathe.

Monitor temperature.

Empty Hemovac, using aseptic technique.

Assess amount and type of drainage per Hemovac/dressings.

Encourage fluid intake, high-protein diet with roughage.

MEDICAL MANAGEMENT

Preop body shower: pHisoHex, surgical scrub, Betadine.

Reverse isolation: preop and until Hemovac is discontinued.

Antibiotics.

Culture drainage.

RATIONALE

Increase lung expansion and minimize development of atelectasis/pneumonia.

Elevation can be early sign of developing infection.

Maintains suction by maintaining negative pressure and prevents infection by preventing accumulation of secretions in the joint space.

Purulent, nonserous, odorous is indicative of infection.

Maintains fluid and nutritional balance and aids in healing.

Minimize bacteria on the skin.

Lessen contact with sources of possible infection.

Often used prophlactically to prevent infection.

Anerobic or aerobic bacteria may be present. Allows for appropriate antibiotic therapy.

NURSING DIAGNOSIS:	Mobility, impaired physical.
SUPPORTING DATA:	Problems of mobility that existed prior to surgery may still present a concern. Patient will need to relearn use of the affected joints.
DESIRED PATIENT OUTCOMES:	Mobility is regained to maximum degree.

INTERVENTIONS

PREOPERATIVE TEACHING

Explanation of use of traction, splints, pillows, trapeze.

Provide information about the use of the bedpan.

Instruct in and practice exercises to be done postop:
In *total hip:* quadricep and gluteal muscle setting, isometrics, leg lifts, dorsiflexion plantar flexion of the foot.
In *total knee:* Quad setting, isometrics, and leg lifts.

RATIONALE

Traction maintains desired position. Understanding of and the ability to aid in lifting and moving postop.

Anxiety and pain may interfere with elimination after surgery.

Strengthen muscle groups, prevent decubiti, and maintain circulation. Learning preoperatively will enhance postop ability.

Other joints: exercises are designed. Crutch walking and bed to wheelchair transfer.

Refer to Care Plan: Surgical Intervention.

To meet individual needs of the joint that is replaced.

POSTOPERATIVE CARE

Remain on bed rest with bed flat, elevating to not more than 45° for meals.

Prevent hip flexion contractures. Prevent dislocation of hip replacement.

Encourage and assist in doing exercises as practiced preop.

Maintain muscle strength. Active use of the hip may be painful but will not injure the hip joint.

Turn on unoperated side maintaining operated leg in abducted position supported by pillows.

Prevent dislocation of prosthesis and maintain skin tone.

Encourage patient to use trapeze to lift body and change position frequently.

Assists in avoiding skin breakdown and improving muscle tone.

Avoid marked flexion of the hip.

May be allowed in wheelchair 2–3 days postop and joint stress is to be avoided when patient is up.

Observe for increased pain and shortening of limb.

Can be indicative of slippage of prosthesis.

Massage skin on coccyx, heels, and elbows and observe for breakdown.

Prevent skin problems.

MEDICAL MANAGEMENT

Narcotics/analgesics.

Narcotics are usually necessary in the first 24 hours, with analgesics being used thereafter to allow for increased mobility during activity.

NURSING DIAGNOSIS:	**Injury, potential for, hemorrhage/ thromboembolism.**
SUPPORTING DATA:	**Highly vascular area with possibility of postop bleeding.**
DESIRED PATIENT OUTCOMES:	**Bleeding minimized/prevented/ treated.**

INTERVENTIONS

Check circulation, motion, sensation of operated leg.

RATIONALE

Early detection of swelling secondary to bleeding, which may interfere with function, allows for treatment.

Monitor hematocrit (usually ordered 24–48 hours postop).

Evaluate blood loss. Due to the area of exposed vascular bone, the blood loss can be quite large.

Monitor PT/APTT and observe for signs of increased bleeding tendencies.

Minor trauma or sensitivity to anticoagulants may result in epistaxis, hemoptysis, increased bleeding at the operative site, and so forth.

Check and measure amount of Hemovac drainage at regular intervals.

Be aware of excessive bleeding.

Exercise ankles/legs.

Monitor for calf tenderness, Homan's sign.

MEDICAL MANAGEMENT

Anticoagulation therapy.
Preop: Coumadin, heparin, low-molecular weight dextran.
Postop: low-dose heparin.

Antiembolic stockings.

Blood/plasma expanders.

Prevent venous stasis.

Early identification of thrombus development.

May be used to prevent thrombophlebitis and pulmonary emboli.

Promote venous return.

Restore circulating volume.

NURSING DIAGNOSIS:	**Knowledge deficit, rehabilitation.**
SUPPORTING DATA:	**Process of learning to use joint following replacement can be lengthy and discouraging.**
DESIRED PATIENT OUTCOMES:	**Joint is functioning at maximal capacity.**

INTERVENTIONS

Discuss importance of continuing exercise program; swimming is a good nonweight-bearing exercise for hip replacement; stationary bicycle for knee.

Stress importance of continuing to wear antiembolic stockings.

If continuing on anticoagulant drug, discuss regimen.

Discuss activity limitations; e.g., sitting for brief periods, using self-help devices, raised toilet seats.

Encourage crutch-walking and weight-bearing within patient tolerance.

Give positive reinforcement and allow patient to do as much as possible.

Discuss symptoms that are important to report to physician: temperature elevation, pain in calf or upper thigh, swelling, redness, "strep" throat.

RATIONALE

Will increase muscle strength and encourage joint mobility.

Prevent development of phlebitis.

Prophylactic therapy may be continued after discharge.

Knowing reasons for limitations can be helpful in cooperating and decreasing discouragement.

Muscle-aching will indicate too much weight-bearing; activities need to be cut back.

Will provide encouragement and promote a positive attitude.

Signs of infection or other complications. Bacterial infections require prompt treatment to prevent infection in the joint, which may occur at any time, even years later.

DIAGNOSIS: Osteomyelitis

PATIENT DATA BASE

NURSING HISTORY

Men > women.

Sudden development of pain in involved area (usually over long bones).

When patient presents with low back pain, vertebrae may be the involved site. May present with neurologic signs indicative of meningitis/paraplegia.

Pain is often accompanied by fever, chills, and malaise. Signs of systemic sepsis, such as generalized weakness, may be evident.

There may be swelling or erythema over the involved bone.

History usually reveals a direct infection occurring secondary to an open fracture, trauma to affected area that has decreased blood supply to the bone, and systemic infections.

History of previous episodes of osteomyelitis may indicate a chronic condition in which sinuses have formed at the injured site with continual drainage of purulent material.

Check for allergies, especially to antibiotics.

Note history of injected drug abuse.

DIAGNOSTIC STUDIES

CBC: leukocytosis and anemic conditions.

Sickle cell prep in predisposed individuals; particularly blacks or people of Mediterranean extraction.

Blood cultures: most often *Staphylococcus aureus* is the organism found.

Joint fluid culture if a joint is involved. (Usually negative unless well advanced.)

Needle aspiration culture of drainage from involved site.

Erythrocyte sedimentation rate (ESR): usually elevated.

Bone scan: may reveal changes before x-ray does.

X-rays of affected area show changes in bone from 5–10 days after the onset of the acute phase and occur in the following order:
periosteal reaction,
radiolucency secondary to bone destruction,
formation of new bone (if vascular supply is adequate), or
fragments of necrotic bone that may enclose areas of infection or from sinuses (if vascular supply remains inadequate).

PHYSICAL EXAMINATION

Check for primary lesions where infection may have started.

Check area of pain for:
skin integrity,
temperature,
erythema,
edema,
drainage,
fractures, and
range of motion (within limits set by physician).

Check temperature, pulse, respirations, blood pressure for indications of generalized sepsis.

NURSING PRIORITIES

1. Relieve pain and promote comfort.
2. Prevent further injury.
3. Prevent spread of infection.
4. Provide information about disease and expected outcomes.

NURSING DIAGNOSIS: Comfort, alteration in, pain.

SUPPORTING DATA: Infection, local erythematous reaction, ischemia at bone site produces pain.

DESIRED PATIENT OUTCOMES: Relief and control of pain.

INTERVENTIONS

Immobilize affected area with pillows. Bed rest as indicated.

Support joints above and below the affected part as well as the affected part, when moving the patient.

Use bed craddle.

Evaluate for changes in pain, and response to analgesics.

MEDICAL MANAGEMENT

Traction and splints.

Analgesics.

RATIONALE

Decreases physical stimulation to injured area. Decreases further injury and allows healing.

Prevents further injury and pain.

Pressure of bed clothes on involved area may intensify pain.

Identify progress of infection and effectiveness of medication.

Immobilization to prevent further injury.

Relief of pain promotes comfort and relaxation of muscle surrounding affected area.

NURSING DIAGNOSIS: Mobility, impaired, physical.

SUPPORTING DATA: Immobility may be due to traction or splints. Limited ROM due to pain.

DESIRED PATIENT OUTCOMES: Able to move all extremities within normal range of motion. Muscles do not atrophy and healthy bone is not resorbed.

INTERVENTIONS

Active and passive ROM exercises of uninvolved areas, and in involved area as soon as healing allows.

Refer to Care Plan: Traction.

RATIONALE

Increases blood flow to muscles and bone. Maintains normal stresses on bones and muscles, preventing atrophy and resorption from disuse.

555

NURSING DIAGNOSIS:	Skin integrity, impairment of, potential.
SUPPORTING DATA:	Immobilization of extremity, whether via traction, splints, or casts causes patient to rest on pressure points for prolonged periods.
DESIRED PATIENT OUTCOMES:	Skin integrity maintained.

INTERVENTIONS	RATIONALE
Keep casts, dressings, splints dry and intact.	Chronically moist, covered skin is prone to breakdown.
Massage pressure points q2h.	Increases circulation to the skin.
Assist patient with turning to different positions q2h.	Alters area of pressure and minimizes tissue injury.
Document and notify physician of any reddened or excoriated areas.	Evaluate and document condition. Early identification allows for treatment to prevent breakdown.

NURSING DIAGNOSIS:	Injury, potential for, infection, actual.
SUPPORTING DATA:	Presence of infection may result in nonunion of existing fractures, alteration in bone integrity may cause pathologic fractures and may lead to paraplegia if vertebrae are involved. Septicemia or meningitis may also occur.
DESIRED PATIENT OUTCOMES:	Infection treated, complications prevented/minimized.

INTERVENTIONS	RATIONALE
Maintain wound and skin isolation, good handwashing technique and sterile dressing changes.	Prevent spread of infection.
Monitor vital signs and mentation. Note changes in drainage.	Signs of resolution or developing complications.

MEDICAL MANAGEMENT

Surgical or needle aspiration.	May be necessary to obtain pure culture for C & S.

IV antimicrobials.	To maintain consistent blood levels and fight infection. May be required for 4–6 weeks.
Antimicrobial dip into bone.	If blood supply to bone area is compromised, continuous drip to site may be necessary.
Surgical drainage/sequestrectomy.	Decompression and/or removal of necrotic bone may be necessary.
Hyberbaric oxygen.	Used when infection is refractory to other treatments.

Refer to Care Plans: Fractures; Paraplegia/Quadriplegia; Intracranial Infections.

NURSING DIAGNOSIS: Nutrition, alterations in, less than body requirements.

SUPPORTING DATA: Increased stress on body from infection and injury creates greater than normal nutritional requirements.

DESIRED PATIENT OUTCOMES: Maintain weight at least at minimum recommended standard for age and height.

INTERVENTIONS

RATIONALE

Measure intake and output.	Information re fluid balance.
Encourage oral fluids as tolerated.	Increased intake necessary when body temperature is elevated to maintain adequate blood volume for perfusion to vital organs.
Weigh at least once a week.	Reflects adequacy of nutritional intake.
Provide attractive meal settings. May need several small meals.	Can be helpful when appetite is poor and patient is having difficulty eating.
Discuss food likes and dislikes and allow patient to choose menu.	More likely to eat when patient has a sense of control.

MEDICAL MANAGEMENT

High-protein, high-vit. C diet.	Facilitates tissue and bone healing.

NURSING DIAGNOSIS: Knowledge deficit, disease process and treatment.

SUPPORTING DATA: Misinformation/lack of knowledge of disease and therapies may lead to poor adherence to treatment program.

557

DESIRED PATIENT OUTCOMES:	Patient and significant others verbalize possible causes of disease, treatments, and expected progression.

INTERVENTIONS

Discuss osteomyelitis, possible causes, necessity for treatments, long-term progression of disease (including possible surgery if antibiotics unsuccessful at halting the disease).

Discuss IV and oral antibiotics, possible side effects, precautions while taking them.

Discuss activity restrictions and rationale behind them.

Discuss wound isolation, rationale, and methods of maintenance.

Discuss diet recommendations and rationale.

Discuss possible postdischarge complications to look for and report to physician: e.g., increasing stiffness or deformity of the affected area, possible fracture, or disease recurrence.

RATIONALE

May decrease anxiety and enhances opportunity for cooperation with treatment regimen.

Effectiveness may be related to food and alcohol intake with antibiotics.

Understanding enhances sense of control and cooperation.

Prevent spread of infection to other patients, staff, and family.

Information helpful to understanding necessity for diet changes related to healing.

Patient and SO more knowledgeable of significant changes in recovery that might require changes in treatment or surgical intervention.

NURSING DIAGNOSIS:	Self-concept, disturbance in.
SUPPORTING DATA:	Wound and skin isolation may result in feelings of rejection.
DESIRED PATIENT OUTCOMES:	Verbalizes concerns to staff and complies with isolation procedures.

INTERVENTIONS

Visit with patient often (not only for dressing changes or treatments requiring gowning and gloving).

Explain rationale for isolation.

Encourage verbalization of concerns about changing body image.

RATIONALE

Lessens feelings of rejection.

Helps understanding of procedures.

Allows ventilation of feelings and is helpful in establishing adaptive behavior patterns. Communication helps the nurse identify areas where more information and/or emotional support is needed.

DIAGNOSIS: Gout, Tophaceous Gouty Arthritis

PATIENT DATA BASE

NURSING HISTORY

Primary gout is hereditary and tends to occur in families. It is due to an overproduction of uric acid.

Men are more often affected between ages 30–50; women after menopause.

Sudden onset of pain and inflammation in one or more peripheral joints, especially toes, ankles, knees, hands, and elbows with recurrent episodes involving same joints.

Secondary form is usually associated with something else; primarily drugs, such as aspirin. Alcohol and the thiazide diuretics are probably the biggest offenders, causing an increase in the uric acid in the blood by decreasing excretion through the kidneys. May also occur after surgery due to increased amount of tissue injury, acidosis, starvation and increased production of uric acid.

May be history of: physical/emotional stress, acute infection, blood dyscrasias, prolonged drug therapy (diuretics, antineoplastics).

Diet history may indicate increased ingestion of rich foods.

DIAGNOSTIC STUDIES

Increased serum uric acid > 7 mg/100 ml.

Increased ESR and WBC in acute stage.

RL and LE tests are negative.

X-rays show evidence of urate deposits in bone (late sign).

Urine may contain urate crystals.

Arthrocentesis may show the presence of uric acid crystals in the synovial fluid.

Therapeutic response to colchicine therapy may be used as a diagnostic tool.

PHYSICAL EXAMINATION

Observe for presence of heat and redness in one or more peripheral joints, especially toes, ankles, knees, hands, and elbows.

Joint may be "exquisitely" tender.

Fever, 101–103° F. (38.3–39.4°C.).

Blood pressure may be elevated.

May have tophi around hand, foot, and earlobes when gout is chronic.

NURSING PRIORITIES

1. Relieve pain.
2. Prevent complications and recurrences.

NURSING DIAGNOSIS:	Comfort, alteration in, pain.
SUPPORTING DATA:	There is considerable periarticular swelling and erythema. Pain is moderate at first, becoming intense, described as gnawing, pressure, and tightening. Pressure of bedclothes, sudden jarring of the bed may elicit exquisite pain.
DESIRED PATIENT OUTCOMES:	Pain is relieved/controlled.

INTERVENTIONS

INTERVENTIONS	RATIONALE
Maintain bed rest for 24 hours after acute attack.	Early ambulation may precipitate recurrence.
Place foot cradle over bed.	Keep weight of covers off affected joints, which are hypersensitive.
Avoid high-purine foods in diet.	Primarily, organ meats, such as liver, kidneys, sweetbreads, and brains, as well as sardines and anchovies, increase the amount of uric acid in the body and dietary management is important in reducing this factor.
Encourage loss of excess weight.	Added stress on affected joints.
Promote large fluid intake.	Drug therapy increases urinary excretion of urates, which may lead to stone formation.
Give medications with milk/meals.	Butazolidin/Indocin, or Benemid/Anturane may cause gastric irritation.
If diarrhea occurs, hold oral colchicine.	May need to be given IV to lessen side effects.

MEDICAL MANAGEMENT

MEDICAL MANAGEMENT	
Analgesics, salicylates.	Relieve pain until drug therapy is effective. Aids secretion of uric acid.
Colchicine.	Minimizes inflammation dramatically. May be diagnostic when therapeutic trial shows dramatic relief.
Butazolidin, Indocin.	Reduce fever and also have antiinflammatory effect.
Paragoric.	To limit diarrhea, which is a side effect of colchicine.
Anturane and Benemid.	May use prophlylactically; inhibit urate reabsorption at the level of the renal tubule.
Zyloprim.	Prevents uric acid formation by interfering with conversion of the purine metabolism end-products to uric acid.

Corticotropin (ACTH) or corticosteroids.

When episodes fail to respond to more conventional treatment. May be injected into the intra-articular spaces.

NURSING DIAGNOSIS:	Knowledge deficit, disease process and treatment.
SUPPORTING DATA:	Reduction in hyperuricemia to prevent formation of uratic deposits and promote resolution of tophi, which are already present, is a long-range process that requires the knowledge and cooperation of the patient/significant others.
DESIRED PATIENT OUTCOMES:	Normal levels of serum urate are maintained and recurrences are avoided.

INTERVENTIONS	RATIONALE
Assess patient's knowledge of the disease.	Provides baseline data for further information-giving.
Correct misconceptions about disease.	Many people are misinformed about this disease, believing it is a "rich man's disease."
Discuss the rationale for continuing drug therapy.	Prevents deposition of uric acid in joints and thereby acute attacks.
Instruct in dietary restrictions that may be necessary; e.g., high-purine foods and alcohol.	May precipitate an acute attack.
Instruct in the importance of avoiding crash diets and/or fasting.	Increases serum uric acid level.
Continue high-fluid intake.	Reduces urate precipitation in the urine and the possible formation of urate stones.

DIAGNOSIS: Scleroderma (Progressive Systemic Sclerosis)

PATIENT DATA BASE

NURSING HISTORY

May complain of gradual onset of pain and stiffness and arthritis-like symptoms.

May complain that hands turn dead white when exposed to the cold. Raynaud's phenomenon may be the initial complaint.

Complains of severe muscle weakness.

History of gradual change in facial appearance, wrinkle-free, and no lines apparent with loss of normal skin folds.

Affects women three times more often than men, usually between ages 30–50.

May complain of difficulty swallowing and breathing.

May affect any system of the body, so symptoms will vary according to the progression of the disease.

DIAGNOSTIC STUDIES

ESR increased in active phase.

May have positive rheumatoid factor.

Barium swallow: may show the presence of esophagitis or reflux.

Upper GI studies: decreased peristalsis in the small intestine.

Pulmonary function studies: impaired gas exchange, decreased vital and total lung capacity.

Antinuclear antibody studies: show fine or large speckles on nuclear immunofluorescence.

Skin biopsy may show changes: increase of compact collagen fibers and thinning of the epidermis.

Renal studies to determine the degree of function, proteinuria, microscopic hematuria, and increased casts may be present.

PHYSICAL EXAMINATION

Skin is dry, may be edematous and pale in the beginning stages of the disease and progress to thickening and tightening of the skin so it appears taut and shiny.

Vitiligo and hyperpigmentation of the skin may be noted.

Early involvement of fingers may progress to forearms, arms, anterior chest, abdomen, back, and face.

Pain and stiffness of the joints may be present.

Muscle weakness may be present.

Cardiac arrhythmias, conduction disturbances, and other ECG changes may be present.

Pleurisy may be recurrent with resultant friction rubs.

Digestive disturbances may be apparent, such as esophageal reflux.

Telangiectases may be noted on fingers, forearms, face, lips, and tongue.

Subcutaneous calcifications of the finger tips; may also be found in the elbows, knees, and weight-bearing areas, such as the buttocks and the plantar surface of the foot.

NURSING PRIORITIES

1. Promote comfort.
2. Provide supportive treatment dependent on the systems involved.
3. Provide information and emotional support to enhance the ability of patient/significant others to cope with the disease.

Refer to Care Plan: Systemic Lupus Erythematosus.

NURSING DIAGNOSIS:	**Mobility, impaired physical.**
SUPPORTING DATA:	**Subcutaneous calcifications in the joints interfere with movement.**
DESIRED PATIENT OUTCOMES:	**Movement is maintained to the greatest extent possible.**

INTERVENTIONS	RATIONALE
Keep joints warm and do range of motion exercises on a routine basis.	Maintain mobility.

MEDICAL MANAGEMENT

Steroids and aspirin.	Anti-inflammatory, decrease joint stiffness.
Physical therapy.	Decreases stiffness and promotes movement.
Surgical replacement.	As in arthritis.
Refer to Care Plan: Rheumatoid Arthritis.	

NURSING DIAGNOSIS:	**Grieving, anticipatory.**
SUPPORTING DATA:	**Awareness of progression of disease and disabling aspects with no hope of cure.**
DESIRED PATIENT OUTCOMES:	**Stages of grieving are recognized, feelings are discussed, and patient is dealing with life on a daily basis.**

INTERVENTIONS	RATIONALE
Assess understanding and knowledge of disease.	Depending on how long patient has known about the disease, as well as emotional factors, different levels of knowledge exist.
Give information as desired by the patient.	People have different needs at different times.

Provide an accepting environment in which patient feels free to ask questions.

Patient may feel uncomfortable asking questions when the patient believes nurses are too busy or are not interested.

Refer to Care Plan: Psychosocial Aspects of Care in the Acute Setting.

NURSING DIAGNOSIS:	**Nurtition, alteration in, less than body requirements.**
SUPPORTING DATA:	**Involvement of the gastrointestinal tract may lead to difficulty swallowing solids with decrease or loss of peristalsis of the lower portion of the esophagus. Reflux, peptic esophagitis, ulceration, and stricture may develop. Malabsorption and altered fat absorption may occur. May have difficulty opening mouth.**
DESIRED PATIENT OUTCOMES:	**Nutritional status is maintained at normal weight for height and activity level.**

INTERVENTIONS

Assess ability to masticate and swallow.

Give frequent small feedings.

Elevate the head of the bed and encourage chewing food well/eating slowly.

MEDICAL MANAGEMENT

Antacids.

Surgery.

Broad spectrum antibiotics.

RATIONALE

Identify extent of difficulty.

Relieves reflux esophagitis.

Use gravity in passage of food into the stomach when esophogeal peristalsis is compromised.

Relieve heartburn.

Reconstruction of the esophagogastric junction may be helpful.

Promotes fat absorption by counteracting overgrowth of microorganisms that cause deconjugation of bile salts.

NURSING DIAGNOSIS:	**Bowel elimination, alteration in, alternating diarrhea/constipation.**
SUPPORTING DATA:	**"Wide mouth" diverticula develop as well as severe bloating with alternating diarrhea/constipation.**
DESIRED PATIENT OUTCOMES:	**Elimination is controlled/maintained.**

INTERVENTIONS	RATIONALE
Refer to Care Plan: Diverticulitis.	

NURSING DIAGNOSIS:	Gas exchange, impaired.
SUPPORTING DATA:	Interstitial and alveolar fibrosis occurs with recurrent pleurisy. Faulty gas exchange, restrictive ventilatory disease secondary to fibrosis and obstructive disease.
DESIRED PATIENT OUTCOMES:	Respiration function maintained.

INTERVENTIONS	RATIONALE
Refer to Care Plan: Chronic Obstructive Pulmonary Disease (COPD).	

NURSING DIAGNOSIS:	Cardiac output, alteration in, decreased.
SUPPORTING DATA:	Cardiac arrhythmias and conduction disturbances, cardiomyopathy and cor pulmonale, left ventricular failure, pericarditis occur with fibrotic changes.
DESIRED PATIENT OUTCOMES:	Symptoms are controlled.

INTERVENTIONS	RATIONALE
Treated symptomatically.	See related care plans.

NURSING DIAGNOSIS:	Fluid volume, alteration in, excess, (potential).
SUPPORTING DATA:	Sclerosis of the blood vessels, particularly in the kidneys, occurs, with resultant development of malignant hypertension. If serum creatinine is 2 mg/dl with a normal of 1, life expectancy is 4–6 weeks. Accounts for 70% of the mortality in this disease.
DESIRED PATIENT OUTCOMES:	Renal functioning is maintained and blood pressure is within patient normals.

565

INTERVENTIONS

Treat symptomatically.

MEDICAL MANAGEMENT

Dialysis.

Kidney transplants.

RATIONALE

Refer to Care Plans: Acute Renal Failure; Hypertension.

May be necessary when kidney shutdown occurs. Refer to Care Plan: Dialysis.

Have been done with some success.

NURSING DIAGNOSIS:	Injury, potential for, infection.
SUPPORTING DATA:	Ulceration may be chronic with tendency for infection and poor wound healing. Gangrene may occur, especially the fingers.
DESIRED PATIENT OUTCOMES:	Infection is minimized.

INTERVENTIONS

Lubricate skin with mild lotion.

Maintain cleanliness.

Refer to Care Plan: Raynaud's Disease.

RATIONALE

Keep skin supple.

Minimize bacteria on the skin.

NURSING DIAGNOSIS:	Self-concept, disturbance in.
SUPPORTING DATA:	Skin changes with induration, pigmentation changes; later, atrophy and fibrosis with adherence to underlying structures; loss of hair, skin, and muscle contractures resulting in joint deformities create changes in body image.
DESIRED PATIENT OUTCOMES:	Verbalizes and discusses changes and how they affect the individual's self-esteem and lifestyle and develops ways to handle problems that arise.

INTERVENTIONS

Make opportunities for patient to discuss feelings.

Refer to Care Plan: Psychosocial Aspects of Care in the Acute Setting.

RATIONALE

Allows for acknowledgment of reality of situation.

DIAGNOSIS: Polyarteritis (Periarteritis Nodosa)

PATIENT DATA BASE

NURSING HISTORY

Most often occurs in men in mid-life.

Clinical manifestations depend on the organ/s involved and/or the amount of necrosis in the area involved.

May present as angina, myocardial infarction, hypertension, peripheral neuropathy or focal central nervous system involvement.

May complain of prolonged fever of undetermined origin, no characteristic febrile pattern.

Complains of myalgia, arthralgia, and severe headaches.

May have had weight loss.

DIAGNOSTIC STUDIES

(Tests may be specific to the organ/s involved.)

Leukocytosis may be present.

Erythrocyte sedimentation rate may be elevated.

Renal clearance tests; glomerulonephritis may be present.

Angiography may show aneurysms of the involved blood vessels.

ECG may show evidence of coronary insufficiency or myocardial infarction.

PHYSICAL EXAMINATION

Temperature may be elevated.

Abdominal pain, nausea and vomiting, diarrhea may be present. May present as an acute abdomen requiring surgery.

Blood pressure may be elevated.

Eye exam may reveal blindness due to occlusion of the central retinal artery.

Skin may be reddened or ulcerated with subcutaneous nodules and purpuric papules present.

NURSING PRIORITIES

1. Promote rest.
2. Provide information about disease, treatment, and prognosis and plan for follow-up care.
3. Provide support for patient and significant others.

(Treatment is similar to Systemic Lupus Erythematosus.)

NURSING DIAGNOSIS:	Mobility, impaired physical.
SUPPORTING DATA:	A prime factor in treatment is rest with attendant problems of immobility. Muscular aching, tenderness, and wasting can be early symptoms. Peripheral neuritis can occur as well as hemiplegia.

DESIRED PATIENT OUTCOMES:	A program of rest is maintained until symptoms are in remission, and no problems of immobility occur.

INTERVENTIONS

Discuss necessity of setting up program of rest.

Discuss problems of immobility and methods of prevention.

Stress importance of recognizing the onset of fatigue before they become too tired.

Encourage wearing a medical identification tag.

RATIONALE

Cooperation of the patient is essential to success and having accurate information will be helpful in setting up a realistic program until there is a remission of symptoms.

Long periods of rest can lead to problems of functioning and deformity.

People often fail to recognize when they are becoming tired until they are overly fatigued.

Provide information about disease and current drug therapy. Abrupt interruption of steroid therapy may result in detrimental effects with possible fatal results.

MEDICAL MANAGEMENT

Corticosteroids.

Immunosuppressive drugs.

Control symptoms and prevent spread of the disease. Refer to Care Plans: Cushing's Syndrome: Excessive Glucocorticoids; Addison's Disease.

May be given with the steroids.

NURSING DIAGNOSIS:	Nutrition, alteration in, less than body requirements.
SUPPORTING DATA:	Anorexia, nausea/vomiting with complaints of periumbilical or RUQ abdominal pain can occur when gastrointestinal tract is involved.
DESIRED PATIENT OUTCOMES:	Adequate nutritional balance is maintained with weight within normal limits for the individual.

INTERVENTIONS

Assess degree of anorexia, nausea/vomiting.

MEDICAL MANAGEMENT

Balanced diet as condition tolerates.

RATIONALE

If present, they interfere with adequate intake and need resolution.

Need to work within the limits of the patient's ability to manage food intake.

NURSING DIAGNOSIS:	Bowel elimination, alteration in, diarrhea.
SUPPORTING DATA:	Disease may involve the viscera as well as the gastrointestinal tract; frequently mesenteric arteritis with thrombosis and infarction of the bowel occurs; and mucosal ulceration with hemorrhage or perforation may occur when smaller vessels are involved. All these may result in disturbance of intestinal functioning.
DESIRED PATIENT OUTCOMES:	Diarrhea is controlled/minimized and complications are managed.

INTERVENTIONS

Observe for occurrence of diarrhea, bleeding, and abdominal pain.

Provide for diet and fluid intake changes as indicated.

MEDICAL MANAGEMENT

Surgery.

RATIONALE

Provide for early intervention.

Individual considerations are necessary according to extent of condition.

May be indicated if ulceration, perforation, or severe thrombosis occurs.

NURSING DIAGNOSIS:	Injury, potential for, safety.
SUPPORTING DATA:	When the central nervous system is involved, behavioral disturbances, headache, convulsions, hemiplegia, aphasia, cerebellar signs, subarachnoid hemorrhage may occur.
DESIRED PATIENT OUTCOMES:	CNS complications are recognized and managed and injuries do not occur.

INTERVENTIONS

Observe for evidence of CNS involvement.

RATIONALE

Arterial supply to the brain may be involved affecting functioning.

569

Provide for safety when indicated.

Ataxia, hemiplegia, and various behavioral manifestations may present the necessity for physical restraints.

This disease may affect any organ: primarily the kidney. Glomerulonephritis, is the most frequent occurrence; although, myocardial infarction, or coronary insufficiency, lung involvement, or liver/gallbladder manifestations may present. Refer to the appropriate care plan when these organs are involved.

BIBLIOGRAPHY

Books and Other Individual Publications

ADAMS, J. C.: *Outline of Orthopaedics,* ed. 9. C. V. Mosby, St. Louis, 1981.

BEYERS, M. AND DUDAS, S.: The Clinical Practice of Medical-Surgical Nursing. Little, Brown & Co., 1977.

BRUNNER, L. S. AND SUDDARTH, D. S.: *Textbook of Medical-Surgical Nursing,* ed. 3. J. B. Lippincott, Philadelphia, 1975.

BRUNNER, L. S. AND SUDDARTH, D. S.: *Lippincott Manual of Nursing Practice.* J. B. Lippincott, Philadelphia, 1978.

CAMPBELL, C.: *Nursing Diagnosis and Intervention in Nursing Practice.* John Wiley & Sons, New York, 1978.

GOVONI, L. E. AND HAYES, J. E.: *Drugs and Nursing Implications,* ed. 2. Appleton-Century-Crofts, New York, 1971.

ISSELBACHER, K. ET AL. (EDS.): *Harrison's Principles of Internal Medicine.* McGraw-Hill, New York, 1980.

JONES, D. A., DUNBAR, C. F., AND JIROVEC, M. M.: *Medical-Surgical Nursing: A Conceptual Approach.* McGraw-Hill, New York, 1978.

KIM, M. AND MORITZ, D. (EDS.); *Classification of Nursing Diagnosis.* McGraw-Hill, New York, 1981.

LARSON, C. B. AND GOULD, M.: *Orthopedic Nursing,* ed. 9 C. V. Mosby, St. Louis, 1978.

Merck Manual, ed. 11. Merck, Sharp & Dohme Research Labs.—Merck & Co., Rahway, N.J., 1966, pp. 982–985.

PHIPPS, W. J., LONG, B. C., AND WOODS, N. F.: *Medical-Surgical Nursing.* C. V. Mosby, St. Louis, 1979.

ROAF, R. AND HADKINSON, C.: *Textbook of Orthopaedic Nursing,* ed. 3. Blackwell Scientific Pub., Oxford, 1980.

TILKIAN, S. M., CONOVER, M. B., AND TILKIAN, A. G.: *Clinical Implications of Lab Tests.* C. V. Mosby, 1979.

TUCKER, S. M. ET AL.: *Patient Care Standards.* C. V. Mosby, St. Louis, 1975.

WILKINS, R. W. AND LEVINSKY, N. G. (EDS.): *Medicine, Essentials of Clinical Practice.* Little, Brown & Co., Boston, 1978.

Journal Articles

BROWN-SKEERS, V.: *How the nurse practitioner manages the rheumatoid arthritis patient.* Nursing '79, Vol. 9, No. 6, June, 1979, pp. 26–35.

BROWN, C.: *Continuity of care for the orthopedic patient.* J. AORN, 31:1128, May 1980.

DUERKSON J. R.: *Hip fractures: Special considerations for the elderly patient.* Orthop. Nurs., Jan/Feb: 1:11–9, 1982.

RODNAN, G. P. (ED.): *Primer on the rheumatic diseases,* ed. 7. Reprinted from the J. Am. Med. Assoc., April 30, 1973, Vol. 224, No. 5, The Arthritis Foundation.

SCOTT, J. T.: *Arthritis & rheumatism: The facts.* Oxford, Medical Pub., 1980.

CHAPTER 13
INTEGUMENTARY DISORDERS

DIAGNOSIS: Psoriasis: Noninflammatory Dermatoses

PATIENT DATA BASE

NURSING HISTORY

Usually develops before age 20.

Parental history of psoriasis or arthritis may increase predisposition.

History of progression of areas of localized red patches and patchy skin flakiness to total body involvement.

May fear contaminating family and may isolate self from others; may not desire to return to work because of appearance and preoccupation with treatment regimen.

Disease may be worse in winter and better in summer.

DIAGNOSTIC STUDIES

X-ray, CBC, serology, urinalysis to rule out concurrent disease.

Microscopic and gram stain of scales to rule out bacterial infections.

Rheumatoid factor normal.

PHYSICAL EXAMINATION

Numerous, bilateral, silvery scales over red plaques, especially on bony prominences affecting most of the body including hands, scalp, ears, genitalia, nails. Lesions may be elevated, sharply circumscribed and are more erythematous on arms and trunk. Scalp lesions may be thicker; skin folds may contain shiny, red lesions.

Skin texture on unaffected areas is smooth with no heavy pigmentation or discoloration. There is no crusting, no nodules, papules, or vesicles. Lesions on back may be slightly tender to touch. Finger and toe nails may appear yellowish with pitting and separation from the nail beds with keratotic material present.

Hair distribution may be normal or patchy over entire body. Hair on scalp may be dry and brittle.

NURSING DIAGNOSIS:	Skin integrity, impairment, actual.
SUPPORTING DATA:	Nature of the disease process and treatment regimen with numerous scales and plaques disturb continuity of skin over most of body surface.
DESIRED PATIENT OUTCOMES:	Decrease in size of involved areas. Patient comfortable and involved in work and other activities.

INTERVENTIONS

Instruct the patient to take tepid tub soaks daily.

Recommend the use of a colloidal oatmeal in bath water instead of soap.

Instruct patient to use a soft brush on scaly areas when bathing.

Instruct the patient to pat nonscaling, tender areas dry.

Assist with application of wet dressings between baths.

Keep environment well-ventilated.

Assist in applying plastic wrap over areas where topical creams are applied. Plastic gloves, caps, or suit may be used.

Instruct patient to take precautions when applying plastic wrap and not cover coal tar products.

Monitor drug and other treatments for effect and note any undesirable effects.

Encourage frequent periods of rest.

RATIONALE

Facilitate removal of scales and promote cleanliness.

Soothing and antipruritic; soap is drying and may irritate skin.

Facilitates removal of scales with minimal irritation and prepares the affected skin for better penetration of medicinal creams.

Lessens the possibility of further irritation to newly descaled skin.

Promotes vasoconstriction, which inhibits inflammatory reaction, decreases redness and pruritus.

Air circulation enhances the cooling effect and reduces pruritus.

Creams have low-absorption rate and occlusive dressings increase percutaneous absorption and trap heat and moisture, which acts to soften plaques.

Coal tar products are already occlusive and excessive irritation will develop if further occluded.

Should have positive effect on disease. Any aspect of the treatment regimen (baths, dressings, or medications) is capable of causing an adverse reaction.

Enhances antimitotic effect of therapeutic agents and promotes relaxation, which decreases emotional stress.

MEDICAL MANAGEMENT

Corticosteroids, coal tar, anthralin, salicylic acid.

Systemic medications, such as methotrexate and hydroxyurea.

Topical application reduces scaling and itching.

Used when disease is extensive and resistant to other treatment.

NURSING DIAGNOSIS:	Knowledge deficit, disease process and treatment.
SUPPORTING DATA:	Psoriasis is a chronic disease aggravated by many conditions that can be easily modified or avoided. Lack of cooperation with regimen may be due to inaccurate knowledge or lack of information.
DESIRED PATIENT OUTCOMES:	Verbalizes situations that are aggravating to condition and relates how they may be avoided.

INTERVENTIONS	RATIONALE
Advise patient not to scratch or vigorously rub skin areas. Keep fingernails short.	Causes further irritation and potentiates injury.
Instruct patient in how to apply topical medications, proper duration, rationale and potential side effects of treatments.	Course of disease largely depends on patient's ability to care for self, which is enhanced by knowledge and understanding of treatments.
Advise the patient to use external medications sparingly.	May tend to overuse medications to gain relief. This may lead to undesirable side effects.
Instruct patient how to observe and to report any favorable or unfavorable changes in skin condition or lesions.	Skin condition or appearance of lesions may change, necessitating treatment modification. The length of time medication is on the skin, the location, texture, pliancy, elasticity, and the degree of skin hydration are variable factors that affect and alter the rate of absorption.
Discuss factors that may alter skin condition.	Sharing factual information increases patient awareness, which ultimately leads to the prevention of harmful complications.
Promote regular exposure to sunlight but caution about avoidance of overexposure to the sun.	Controlled exposure to ultraviolet light causes a temporary suppression in cell division and, as an integral part of the treatment regimen, provides a temporary remission. However, prolonged exposure leads to further destruction of skin integrity.
Recommend use of a humidifer in winter.	Inhibits skin dryness and prevents pruritus. Some studies indicate the lack of humidity may be a reason acute exacerbations occur in the winter.
Encourage precautions to avoid unnecessary trauma to the skin.	Trauma can potentiate an acute flare-up. Trauma to susceptible areas may account for the prominence of lesions on elbows and knees.
Discuss long-term aspects of the disease process.	Recurrences and exacerbations can be a life-long problem with feelings of discouragement and hopelessness, which may affect the course of the disease and treatment.

Refer to Care Plan: Psychosocial Aspects of Care in the Acute Setting.

DIAGNOSIS: Herpes Zoster (Shingles)

PATIENT DATA BASE

NURSING HISTORY

May occur at any age, but incidence increases with age. The elderly are more prone to attack and suffer the sequelae more, presumably due to reduced immunity. Most cases of localized herpes occur in relatively healthy people.

Patient may describe a varied range of tactile sensations; prodromal tenderness/pain, burning, hypoesthesia, prickling and/or paresthesia.

Malaise and GI upsets may precede rash.

May have had a recent trauma to the skin. Debilitating illness, malignancy, or immunosuppression therapy may increase predisposition.

May have had chicken pox. A negative history may indicate nonimmunity to the varicella virus. Common when there is a deficit in immunity.

Recent exposure to viral infections or chicken pox.

Determine occupation and/or hobbies: disease may affect ability to engage in usual activities.

Determine dietary habits and whether a nutritional deficit may exist.

Determine current medications or history of drug use whose effects might mimic or aggravate the course of the disease.

May demonstrate signs of pain, distress, restlessness, depression, or anxiety.

History of leukemia, lymphoma, other malignancies, and immunosuppression.

The virus is considered contagious for 2–3 days after appearance of rash to persons who have not had varicella and those who are highly susceptible, such as immunosuppressed patients.

DIAGNOSTIC STUDIES

Causative agent is varicella virus, which contains a complement fixation antigen, however this test is not usually done for atypical herpes zoster.

CBC is usually normal: may indicate underlying and/or secondary infectious process.

WBC usually shows marked leukocytosis; may indicate varicella pneumonopathy, leukemia.

Electrolytes, thyroid studies may indicate metabolic dysfunction.

Toxicology may rule out metallic poisoning as a precipitating factor.

Pregnancy test, if positive, may indicate predisposition.

Chest x-ray may suggest a malignancy or varicella pneumonia.

Sedimentation rate may be elevated indicating an acute inflammatory process.

CSF examination may show a mild pleucytosis, elevated protein, and increased pressure indicating encephalitis complications.

PHYSICAL EXAMINATION

Typical distribution of skin lesions is a band-like papular rash (1–2 cm lesions) that rapidly develop into clusters of vesicles (usually within 24 hours and lasting 1–3 weeks). The cutaneous eruptions are round, clear, translucent vesicles filled with water or serum. Distribution may be patchy or on an edematous or erythematous base and variable in size. The vesicles may dry, rupture, or turn into hemorrhagic, necrotic sloughing; scarring may occur.

Usually occurs unilaterally and is limited to one or two adjacent dermatomes.

When the trigeminal ganglion is involved, keratitis and uveitis may result with the possibility of subsequent corneal scarring. Lesions in the auditory canal may result in hearing impairment, facial palsy, and signs of vestibular involvement.

Slight fever, secondary bacterial infections may be present.

Changes in mentation; may indicate herpes encephalitis.

NURSING PRIORITIES

1. Assist with comfort measures.
2. Decrease potential for complications.
3. Facilitate coping.
4. Assist in the determination of underlying factors.

NURSING DIAGNOSIS:	Comfort, alteration in, pain.
SUPPORTING DATA:	Involves primarily, the posterior (sensory) nerve roots and ganglia, characterized by neuralgic pain following the distribution of the affected nerves. Burning, itching, and painful sensations precede and accompany the eruption of the vesicles and may linger after cutaneous signs disappear.
DESIRED PATIENT OUTCOMES:	Vesicular eruptions resolve within a week to 10 days with minimal discomfort. Pain is controlled and/or minimized and patient is comfortable.

INTERVENTIONS	RATIONALE
Bathe in lukewarm water, preferably a tub. May use bicarbonate of soda or Burow's solution in bath.	Tub baths soothe itchy skin. Promotes general cleanliness and reduces chance for secondary infection.
Avoid extremes in temperature.	Intensifies dermalgia.
Avoid rubbing the skin.	Mechanical rubbing causes irritation/injury.
Cool compresses and/or cool sprays may be helpful.	May desensitize painful trigger points.
Avoid pressure against affected areas. Encourage nonbinding clothing and/or bedding.	Light tactal stimuli excite the affected nerves and may stimulate annoying, creepy, prickling sensations or agonizing pain. Firm pressure does not generate the same intense pain.

Provide distractions and diversional activities. Relaxation techniques and guided imagery may be useful.	Deliberate concentration on other activities avoids focus on pain and may alleviate discomfort.
Promote adherence to strict treatment schedule.	Minimizes irritation to the sensitive dermatomes, may shorten duration of the cutaneous eruptions, and may lessen the possibility of the development of intractable pain or postherpetic neuralgia, which is difficult to treat.
Report unusual or prolonged pain.	May herald advent of complications.
Monitor for side effects of antibiotics.	May cause GI upset, diarrhea, overgrowth of mucosal fungi.

MEDICAL MANAGEMENT

Calamine lotion, talc, cornstarch, or zinc oxide.	Soothing and drying.
Corticosteroids.	Decrease inflammation/itching and may reduce scarring. Will not be used in patient who is already immunosuppressed.
Gamma globulin.	May confer passive immunity upon the body while it weakens and confines the virus until the antibody titers are acquired.
Narcotics, analgesics.	Extent of excrutiating pain may warrent potent medication use.
Injection of procaine/alcohol into ganglia.	May block pain temporarily.
Transcutaneous nerve stimulator (TCNS).	In prolonged, intractable pain may desensitize painful trigger points.
Topical steroids, if no secondary infection is present.	May be helpful to promote healing and relieve irritation.
Benzoin.	May be painted on lesions for drying effect.
Barbiturates.	Decrease anxiety, which accentuates awareness of discomfort.
Antihistamines.	Relieve itching.

NURSING DIAGNOSIS:	**Injury, potential for, infection.**
SUPPORTING DATA:	**Trauma to the skin may precipitate or aggravate zoster and/or result in secondary infection, spread, and scarring. Lesions may be infarctive and cause necrosis.**
DESIRED PATIENT OUTCOMES:	**Lesions healing or healed; areas of involvement decreasing.**

576

INTERVENTIONS

Separate any touching cutaneous surfaces with space or gauze.

Discourage picking, squeezing, or scratching of lesions.

Make provisions for wound and skin precautions and protective isolation as indicated.

Monitor vital signs especially changes in mentation.

Check for neuromuscular deficits, vasomotor disturbances, alterations in reflexes, trigeminal nerve pain, eye pain, facial paralysis.

Observe for eye redness, watering.

Instruct patient to refrain from using OTC agents, such as antihistamine creams.

MEDICAL MANAGEMENT

Antibiotics.

RATIONALE

Minimizes abrading of epidermis. Lightweight gauze absorbs moisture, protects and isolates any broken skin areas.

May foster a superimposed infection.

Until the lesions crust, transmission or acquisition of infection by direct contact is possible.

May signal the onset of complications, such as pneumonitis, encephalitis.

Neurologic involvement may be a sequella.

Iritis may result in loss of vision from corneal laceration unless aggressive, preventive measures are instituted.

Desicated agents facilitate healing, but antihistamine creams and so forth may trigger an adverse dermatitis reaction.

Antibacterial and anti-inflammatory effects support involved tissues. May be given to prevent/treat secondary bacterial infection of the lesions.

NURSING DIAGNOSIS:	**Rest-activity pattern, ineffective.**
SUPPORTING DATA:	**Pain may disrupt rest and/or activities. May contribute to debilitation and prolonged course of disease/complications. General malaise may be a presenting symptom for zoster.**
DESIRED PATIENT OUTCOMES:	**Patient has adequate rest and activity.**

INTERVENTIONS

Provide for uninterrupted periods, limit visitors, quiet environment.

Teach relaxation techniques.

Provide for and encourage quiet activities.

RATIONALE

Rest soothes the irritated dermatomes and strengthens the physiologic and mental energy needed for coping.

Refreshes. Foster symptomatic relief of pain and allow available energy for body healing.

Passive activities enhance relaxation and reduce potential depression that may accompany a chronic, painful disease.

MEDICAL MANAGEMENT

Sedatives, as indicated.

To promote rest/relaxation.

NURSING DIAGNOSIS:	**Nutrition, alteration in, less than body requirements, potential.**
SUPPORTING DATA:	**Inadequate nutrition/hydration may provoke or aggravate a viral illness or debilitated state.**
DESIRED PATIENT OUTCOMES:	**Adequate nutrition and hydration maintained. Body weight stable.**

INTERVENTIONS

Promote adequate nutrition. Encourage patient to assist with meal planning and so forth.

Weigh twice weekly or more frequently if indicated.

RATIONALE

Necessary to maintain and replenish cellular energy.

Estimate of adequate hydration and body nutrition.

NURSING DIAGNOSIS:	**Knowledge deficit; disease cause, process, and treatment.**
SUPPORTING DATA:	**Misconceptions about the cause, course of the disease process, and rationale for treatment as well as unpredictability of the disease.**
DESIRED PATIENT OUTCOMES:	**Patient verbalizes cause and course of the disease and knowledge of the required treatment.**

INTERVENTIONS

Assess knowledge of the disease, use of medications and treatment.

Discuss areas of lack of information.

Instruct in proper use of medications and caution of possible side effects.

Explain role of measures in control of disease manifestations and prevention of exacerbations and complications.

RATIONALE

Realistic knowledge clarifies vague perceptions about the illness.

Promotes knowledge and understanding.

Precise knowledge of medications promotes proper use and alerts patient to reportable side effects.

Patient's knowledge of own role in the therapeutic regimen promotes a sense of control in treatment of the disease and may lead to increased cooperation.

NURSING DIAGNOSIS:	Coping, individual, ineffective.
SUPPORTING DATA:	Postherpetic neuralgia may last as long as a year. Sequelae may inflict such physiologic and psychologic pain so as to potentiate a suicidal depression.
DESIRED PATIENT OUTCOMES:	Demonstrates understanding of complications and necessity for continuing treatment. Participates in therapy.

INTERVENTIONS

Give realistic, clear information about expectations of sequelae.

Be available for patient expression of fears and concerns.

See Care Plan: Psychosocial Aspects of Care in the Acute Setting.

RATIONALE

Assists in development of patience, which is vital to the individual who has continuing pain.

Important for the patient to have a nonjudgmental listener to enable free expression of feelings.

DIAGNOSIS: Burns

CLASSIFICATION OF BURNS

PARTIAL-THICKNESS

FIRST DEGREE: Outer layer of skin is usually reddened, without blister formation. Example: Sunburn.

SECOND-DEGREE: Epidermal and dermal layers are involved. Blisters form, subcutaneous edema is present and regeneration will probably occur. If more than 15–20% (10% in children) of the body is involved, hospitalization will be required.

These burns will be painful because the nerve endings have been exposed and injured.

FULL-THICKNESS BURNS

THIRD-DEGREE: All layers of skin are destroyed, sometimes fat, muscle, nerves, and blood supply are also affected, making regeneration impossible. These burns are very hard, dry, and leathery. As little as 5% of the body can be considered a major burn.

FOURTH DEGREE: All layers of skin, fat, muscle, and bone are involved.

PATIENT DATA BASE

NURSING HISTORY

Age of the patient. In burns up to 30% or 3rd degree burns up to 10% of the body, older children and adults under age 50, mortality is low, rising as age increases beyond 50.

Determine the circumstances of the occurrence of the burn, and whether smoke, fumes, or inhalation in closed spaces are involved.

Inhalation injuries may be of two types: a heat burn to the upper respiratory tract and/or a smoke (chemical) burn to the lungs.

Determine source of smoke: hydrocarbons from oil products and by-products from synthetic materials produce more severe injuries.

If burn is electrical, be aware that area of severest injury is not visible and will follow the path of least resistance, depending on the position of the patient.

When burn is chemical, determine the type of chemical involved; concentration and temperature and length of time the patient was in contact with the chemical. Alkali burns are generally more severe than acid burns because the alkali binds chemically to the skin, whereas acid can be washed away to stop the burning process. Heated chemicals produce a deeper burn.

History of preexisting illness: cardiac, respiratory, or other major conditions.

Determine normal diet, bowel habits, urinary status. Note use of laxatives or medications.

Determine use of drugs (including alcohol) and tobacco.

Any history of allergies.

Date of last tetanus immunization.

Assess level of anxiety, and concern re implications for job, family, and cost of hospitalization.

Note presence of grease, ointment, and so forth that may have been put on before admission.

DIAGNOSTIC STUDIES

CBC: initially there is hemoconcentration due to fluid shift, later decrease Hct and RBC may occur, secondary to heat damage to vascular endothelium, causing localized thrombocytopenia as well as resulting in sequestration and decreased survival of cells: leukocytosis basically expected due to loss of blood cells destroyed at burn site.

Electrolytes: decreased serum calcium, elevated alkaline phosphatase caused by fluid shift; sodium lost with water; potassium elevated with tissue trauma or decreased with cell loss.

Urine: presence of albumin and hemoglobin indicates deep tissue damage and loss of protein.

Serum albumin: base from which to judge loss of albumin bound to protein (skin sloughing). Total proteins decrease, hypoproteinemia.

ABG: baseline for oxygenation and depressed respiratory conditions caused by smoke inhalation.

Oxyhemoglobin: rule out inhalation injury and predisposition to adult respiratory distress syndrome. (Refer to Care Plan: Adult Respiratory Distress Syndrome.)

Clinitest and acetest: frequent checks for urine glucose are vital when any supranormal dietary regimen is followed. Glycosuria greater than 2% requires treatment. In addition, the sudden onset of glucose intolerance is an important diagnostic sign that frequently indicates the onset of serious sepsis not clinically apparent for four to six hours. Increase of acetones indicates a need for more protein and fat in the diet.

Specific gravity: determining factor in hydration.

Wound cultures: baseline information.

Chest x-ray: baseline film so that impending fluid shifts, pneumonia, and smoke inhalation syndrome can be delineated.

Body x-rays: if indicated from concurrent injuries to rule out fractures.

ECG: possible arrythmias, most common in elderly and in electrical injuries, may reflect severe potassium losses.

PHYSICAL EXAMINATION

Evaluate respiratory status. Note edema of the vocal cords with wheezing, brassy cough, hoarseness, cyanosis, or tachypnea.

Note evidence of possible inhalation injury: flame burns of the face and neck; singed nasal hairs; dry, red mucosa of the nose and mouth, and soot in the sputum.

Shock may be present: BP may be decreased, pulse rapid. Skin cool to the touch, diaphoresis and chilling may be present.

Weigh (with bedside scale if necessary). Stated height, if unable to measure.

Assess extent and severity of burns by determining the percentage of body surface involved and the depth of the burn. Use Burn Extent Estimator (Lund and Browder Chart), or Rule of Nines.

Note complaints of pain and area involved, as well as burned areas that are not painful.

Assess emotional state (anxiety and restlessness); and sensorium.

NURSING PRIORITIES

1. Maintain adequate airway/fluid balance.
2. Manage pain associated with debridement and dressing changes.
3. Maintain isolation to prevent and control contamination.
4. Prevent/minimize complications and facilitate healing.

5. Provide for total needs of patient; emotional, physical, spiritual, social.
6. Prepare for discharge; begin on admission through rehabilitation including adequate health teaching and prevention of contractures.

NURSING DIAGNOSIS:	**Airway clearance, ineffective.**
SUPPORTING DATA:	**Swelling of the upper airways can lead to obstruction when smoke or heat have been inhaled, or when the head, neck, or face are involved. Pulmonary edema, respiratory acidosis, atelectasis, pulmonary emboli, pneumonia, or eschar formation on chest and neck may restrict respirations.**
DESIRED PATIENT OUTCOMES:	**Adequate airway with acceptable levels of arterial blood gases is maintained. Adult respiratory distress syndrome does not occur.**

INTERVENTIONS

RATIONALE

Observe frequently for decreased breath sounds, respiratory distress; rate/depth and use of accessory muscles; increasing hoarseness, brassy cough, wheezes, pallor, cyanosis, and sputum color changes.

Laryngeal edema, spasm, or extrinsic factors may result in upper airway obstruction.

Monitor ABG, PO_2, PCO_2, and pH levels.

Note changes to guide treatment. Arterial blood gases are the most reliable method of assessing inhalation injuries.

Encourage turning, coughing, deep breathing.

Promote lung expansion, drainage of secretions.

Monitor I & O accurately.

Serves as a guide for fluid replacement. Overload can increase edema.

Monitor CVP.

Elevates in the presence of developing pulmonary edema.

Suction p.r.n., maintaining strict sterile technique.

Keep airway clear and prevent infection.

MEDICAL MANAGEMENT

Humidified oxygen, p.r.n., mask or tent.

Prevent acidosis, hypoxemia. Be aware air swallowing with resultant gastric dilatation commonly occurs with nasal cannula.

Postural drainage and chest percussion may be helpful.

Decreased lung expansion and retained secretions may lead to impaired respiratory function.

Aminophyllin and other broncholytic agents, such as parenteral sodium iodide.

Promote liquifying of secretions.

Steroids.	Anti-inflammatory and relieve severe broncho-spasm.
Serial chest x-ray.	Changes may not appear for 2–3 days.
Bronchoscopy may be done.	Clears debris from bronchial tree.
Maintain adequate airway with soft endotracheal tube, if necessary.	Avoid tracheostomy if possible, edema will usually decrease in 3–4 days and infection frequently spreads into the lungs through the stoma.
Mechanical ventilation with PEEP.	Maintain adequate ventilation. Refer to Care Plan: Ventilatory Assistance (Mechanical).
Nasogastric tube.	Prevent gastric distention with pressure on diaphragm and possible nausea/vomiting with aspiration.
Be prepared for escharotomy or fasciotomy, if edema becomes constricting.	In the presence of full thickness (3rd/4th degree) and/or electrical burns, it allows for edema expansion and relieves pressure on airways and/or permits lung expansion.

NURSING DIAGNOSIS: Fluid volume deficit, potential, first 24 to 72 hours.

SUPPORTING DATA: Rapid shift of fluid from the vascular compartments into interstitial space. Vasodilation, increased capillary permeability, and changes in the cells around the burn areas can result in a loss of fluid, sodium, chloride, and protein from the vascular compartment. Third spacing can result in hypovolemic shock, electrolyte imbalances, and metabolic acidosis. Fibrinogen is also lost into interstitial spaces and forms a gel-like edema that prevents drainage by the lymphatic system, and results in even larger areas of edema beyond the burn area. Also, when stratum corneum, the skin's vapor barrier, is destroyed, evaporative H_2O loss may be as high as 15x normal.

DESIRED PATIENT OUTCOMES: Hypovolemia does not occur. Burn shock is prevented and/or minimized.

INTERVENTIONS

Monitor I & O, serum electrolytes, CVP, vital signs, hematocrit.

Weigh daily.

Check urine output and specific gravity every hour for the first 48 hours.

Do hemastix, and observe color of urine.

Maintain free-flowing indwelling catheter.

Measure circumference of the burned extremities.

Observe for increase in bleeding tendencies, hemorrhage and increased clotting times.

MEDICAL MANAGEMENT

IV replacement of fluids, electrolytes, plasma, and serum protein albumin.

Differential urinalysis.

Fluid challenges and/or mannitol.

Increased IV fluid rate.

Swan-Ganz line.

Transfusions.

Refer to Care Plan: Fluid and Electrolyte Imbalance.

RATIONALE

Serves as a guide for replacement of fluids and electrolytes to maintain homeostasis.

Serves as a guide to retained fluids. Weight increase secondary to edema commonly occurs within 3–4 days.

Maintain a flow of 30–50 ml/h; with tissue/cell destruction, debris released into the circulating volume may cause renal failure.

Myoglobin can be released and show as blood but actual hemorrhage is not necessarily occurring. In some electrical burns, kidney failure may occur secondary to myoglobinuria.

Important for collection of urine, for accuracy of output, and to prevent stasis/reflux.

Helpful in estimating edema formation.

An atypical DIC may occur in spite of adequate fluid resuscitation in the first 10 days and may affect the survival chances of the patient. Refer to Care Plan: Disseminated Intravascular Coagulation.

Essential part of burn therapy; is instituted immediately upon establishment of extent of burn. IV is quick and accurate method of replacement. Check hospital policy for replacement formula used.

Presence of myoglobin may result in renal failure.

May be used to clear the kidneys of myoglobin.

To maintain urine output at 100ml per hour when myoglobin appears in the urine.

For pulmonary artery/wedge pressures to assess fluid load and cardiac function.

May be required due to delayed destruction of red cell mass; caution should be used.

NURSING DIAGNOSIS:

Tissue perfusion, alteration in.

SUPPORTING DATA:

Lessened circulating blood volume leads to decreased cardiac output and increased pulse, acidosis, renal failure, and with peripheral resistance may cause irreversible burn shock. In electrical burns, there is a

high risk for cardiac arrest due to interference with the conductivity of the heart.

DESIRED PATIENT OUTCOMES: Cardiac output/tissue perfusion maintained.

INTERVENTIONS

Place on cardiac monitor.

Refer to Nursing Diagnosis: Fluid volume, deficit, potential, first 24 to 72 hours.

RATIONALE

Identify potentially lethal arrythmias and cardiac standstill.

NURSING DIAGNOSIS: Fluid volume, alteration in, excess (potential).

SUPPORTING DATA: Capillary permeability returns to normal in 48 hours. Protein remains in interstitial spaces 5 days–2 weeks. When the fluid reenters the vascular compartment, diuresis should occur if cardiac/renal function is adequate.

DESIRED PATIENT OUTCOMES: Fluid excess and pulmonary edema are controlled.

INTERVENTIONS

Observe for fluid overload and pulmonary edema by monitoring vital signs, CVP, and urine output.

Monitor potassium and serum sodium levels.

Limit time in Hubbard tank to not more than 20 minutes at a time; or simply spray and wash.

RATIONALE

Adequate cardiac and renal functioning needs to be maintained to handle fluid as it reenters the system. Deviations may indicate impending failure in one or both system/s.

Hypokalemia may occur. Na$^+$ is a more accurate measure of hydration. Refer to Care Plan: Fluid and Electrolyte Imbalance.

As long as burn is open, electrolytes are leeched out and fluid is absorbed through burn area and can contribute to water intoxication and hyponatremia.

MEDICAL MANAGEMENT

Fluid replacement.

Diuretics, such as mannitol.

Plasma.

Based on individual needs/Na$^+$ levels.

Assist in removing excess fluid and flushing debris from the kidneys.

Volume expander and to assist in return of edema fluids to the vascular tree and promote diuresis.

NURSING DIAGNOSIS:	Comfort, alteration in, pain.
SUPPORTING DATA:	Depending on extent and degree of burn initially and on a long-term basis, pain is a constant factor for the burn patient. The more severe the burn, the less complaints of pain as nerve ends are destroyed. Pain consists of three parts; anticipation, existence of, and postepisode.
DESIRED PATIENT OUTCOMES:	Pain is minimized/controlled.

INTERVENTIONS

Assess individual response to pain.

Elevate burned extremities, and allow patient to assume positions of comfort as allowed by burn.

Use heat lamp as necessary.

Provide diversional activities.

Instruct in relaxation techniques, use Therapeutic Touch and so forth.

Be sensitive to the dependency needs of the patient, meeting as necessary and moving toward independence as recovery occurs.

Assess pain carefully.

MEDICAL MANAGEMENT

Morphine sulfate IV initially.

Sedatives and analgesics.

Coverage of the wound with biologic dressings, homo/heterograft.

RATIONALE

Cultural influences, past experiences, mental health are factors that affect response to pain. Another important factor is that tolerance decreases with continued experiencing of pain.

For comfort and to lessen edema. It is important to remember that the position of comfort may lead to contractures.

In large body burns, temperature regulation may be lost and external heat sources are used to maintain a comfortable environment.

Appropriate to patient's condition and area of burn.

Enhance patient's sense of control and increase ability to deal with pain and discomfort.

Minimize problems of dependency that may develop in burn situation where pain and loss of control are major factors.

Restlessness and complaints of discomfort may actually be due to hypoxia or impending shock.

To control severe pain, not adequately absorbed peripherally.

Use with caution as they may initially mask changes in condition.

When able to be done, has been very successful in pain control because exposed nerve endings are covered.

Refer to Nursing Diagnosis: Self-concept, disturbance in for further discussion of pain control.

NURSING DIAGNOSIS:	Nutrition, alteration in, less than body requirements.
SUPPORTING DATA:	Malnutrition is a result of massive loss of fluids and nutrients. Albumin is bound to protein and both are lost in wound exudates. The extensive tissue breakdown leads to loss of nitrogen and potassium in the urine. Metabolic response to thermal injury is hypermetabolism with severe protein wasting and weight loss. The body response to stress is to increase glucagon levels and decrease insulin levels promoting a catabolic state. Poor appetite and pain make it difficult for the patient to eat necessary amounts of food.
DESIRED PATIENT OUTCOMES:	Nitrogen and albumin levels are maintained. Malnutrition is prevented and weight is maintained at acceptable levels of no more than 10% decrease in preburn weight.

INTERVENTIONS

Assess patient's eating habits, family eating patterns, allergies, and cultural desires. Set dietary requirements accordingly.

Encourage patient to eat small, frequent feedings.

High-protein powdered drink may be helpful.

Encourage significant others to bring special foods.

Encourage sitting up to eat, joining patients and/ or SO.

Maintain I & O and correlate with total regimen.

Weigh on a regular basis and maintain calorie count.

Maintain good oral hygiene.

Give positive reinforcement for eating.

RATIONALE

Intake of 4000–5000 calories/day is usually necessary to promote healing of major burns.

Difficult to eat large amount at one time.

Can add as part of total intake without being filling.

May help patient to eat more.

Individuals eat better in a home-like environment when possible.

Daily nourishment needs are based on I & O.

Guide to weight maintenance.

A clean mouth can be helpful in promoting appetite.

Allows patient to feel good about their efforts.

Observe for signs/symptoms of stress ulcer (Curling's).

May develop in severe injuries, such as burns, and is thought to be due to the high-stress level and to the low-flow state of burn shock.

Do Clinitest/acetest.

Monitor development of pseudodiabetes.

MEDICAL MANAGEMENT

High-carbohydrate liquid, such as Polycase, can be added to all beverages.

Tasteless liquid adds calories to any drink ingested and allows for flexibility in fluid intake.

Small nasogastric tube (pediatric) for additional and nighttime feedings.

Supplemental dietary aids are usually required because of inability of patient to consume the required amount orally.

Antacids. Cimetidine.

Maintain near normal acid/base balance in stomach. May prevent/treat ulcer formation.

Milk or milk-based supplements.

May be substituted for antacids for the same effect with added nutritional value.

Vitamin supplements.

Vitamin C promotes healing and daily requirements are increased due to increased metabolic demands.

Iron.

Anemia present due to initial injury, debridement, lab tests, and surgery.

Guaiac NG drainage and stools periodically.

Early detection of bleeding.

Blood glucose levels.

Identify the development of pseudodiabetes.

Insulin.

May be needed for treatment when blood glucose levels are severely elevated.

TPN.

Due to the high rate of sepsis in burn patients, is used only as a last resort if the patient cannot take in necessary quantity of nutrients. Refer to Care Plan: Total Parenteral Nutrition.

NURSING DIAGNOSIS:	**Injury, potential for, infection and sepsis.**
SUPPORTING DATA:	**Wound sepsis is always a threat to prognosis. The skin provides a major barrier to bacterial invasion. Lowered resistance leads to the inability to fight infection.**
DESIRED PATIENT OUTCOMES:	**Sepsis is prevented/managed.**

INTERVENTIONS

RATIONALE

Shave hair from around burn areas and promote good personal hygiene.

Can be medium for bacterial growth.

Use strict cubicle isolation technique for debridement and dressing changes.

Cross-contamination of articles contributes to sepsis. Bacteria flora are diminished.

Do dressing change in hydrotherapy, 100°F., with electrolytes added and mild cleaning agent.

Warm water helps prevent chilling. Solution approximates tissue fluids to minimize osmotic shifts. Water softens eschar and aids in removal.

Instruct patient in breathing techniques when changing dressings.

The use of relaxation breathing can reduce pain and facilitate the process.

Monitor increased temperature and respiratory rate/depth, hyperglycemia with glycosuria, decreased platelet count, abdominal distention, electrolytes, and changes in sensorium.

Signs of sepsis. Electrolyte changes may be the first signs of impending sepsis. Sudden changes in potassium and sodium may reflect loss of capillary integrity secondary to endotoxin insult. Refer to Care Plan: Septicemia. Silver nitrate therapy can cause an electrolyte imbalance when the body absorbs water and leaching of sodium, potassium, calcium, and chloride occurs.

Monitor ABGs, respiratory rate.

Sulfamylon therapy inhibits the production of sodium bicarbonate, initially causing metabolic acidosis progressing to respiratory alkalosis as the lungs eliminate CO_2.

Monitor WBCs.

Silvadene therapy may result in depression of white blood cells.

Monitor changes in odor, quantity, or color of wounds/drainage.

Early identification of infection enables prompt treatment.

Provide for careful face, ear, and eye care.

When burns involve the head and neck, edema results and the eyes may be swollen shut. Infection may occur as the edema decreases.

Prevent burned ear touching scalp by padding or splint.

Ear can adhere to scalp.

Frequent indwelling catheter care and sterile dressing change for subclavian and invasive lines.

Decrease chance of infection.

Monitor and limit visitors. Allow only significant others of patient's choice.

Allows for rest. If visitor has a cold or other infection, can take appropriate measures to prevent infection, such as restriction of visitation.

Instruct patient/SO in necessity of near-sterile technique/reverse isolation.

Masks, gowns, and gloves can prevent contamination.

Restrict patient to burn unit.

Decrease exposure to pathogens.

MEDICAL MANAGEMENT

Routine culture and sensitivities of wound.

Able to treat specific organisms, primarily Gram negative/positive, although others are reported, as well as fungal and viral infections, such as the herpes group. May be done at dressing time as indicated by pertinent change in wound.

Full-thickness wound biopsies may be done as indicated.

Bacteria proliferate in necrotic tissue and may invade adjacent healthy tissue and can not be adequately diagnosed by cultures of the surface of the wounds.

Topical and systemic antibiotics.

May be used to contain the identified flora.

Subeschar clysis with antibiotic specific to bacteria present in burn wound may be used.

As adjunct to topical therapy.

Steroids and surgical draining of the seeding source may be done.

Combat infection. Used with caution because they may inhibit healing.

Vasodilators.

If sepsis occurs, to maintain renal perfusion.

T_3, T_4 twice weekly.

If Betadine is being used, may be absorbed into the system and lead to iodine toxicity.

Suture eyelids.

May be necessary when periorbital areas are involved to prevent the scar tissue from closing the eyelids completely.

NURSING DIAGNOSIS:	**Mobility, impaired physical.**
SUPPORTING DATA:	**Burn wounds hypertrophy and contract more than similar injuries. The position of comfort for the patient may be the position most conducive to contractures.**
DESIRED PATIENT OUTCOMES:	**Adherence to rehabilitative activities is maintained. Optimal physical function is obtained and scarring and deformities are prevented.**

INTERVENTIONS

Elevate burned extremities.

Note circulation, motion, sensation of digits frequently.

Maintain proper body alignment with supports or splints (including use of footboard) especially for burns over joints.

Initiate the rehabilitative phase upon admission.

Consistently use range of motion exercises, initially passive then active.

Correlate activities of daily living, therapy, hydrotherapy, and nursing care.

Encourage patient to ambulate, feed self, and pursue diversional activities.

Prepare and instruct patient and SO about anti-burn scar garment and devices; discuss possible reconstructive surgery as necessary.

Water mattresses or CircOlectric beds may be necessary to change position q2h.

RATIONALE

Lessens edema formation.

Edema may compromise circulation to extremities.

Maintains functional positioning of extremities and prevents contractures, which are more likely over joints.

It is easier to enlist participation when the patient is aware of the possibilities.

Patient responds more favorably to programmed activities, preventing loss of calcium from the bone and maintaining muscle functioning.

Combining activities produces improved results by enhancing effects of each.

Independent patient usually returns home earlier than dependent patient.

Knowledge of what to expect may enhance participation. Pressure dressings minimize scar tissue by keeping it flat, soft, and pliable.

Prevent pressure areas and decubitus formation.

MEDICAL MANAGEMENT

Excise and close burn wounds quickly.

Reduce chances of prolonged healing and resultant scarring. Early excision is known to reduce scarring as well as reduce chance of infection.

Escharotomy or fasciotomy.

Improve circulation by relief of pressure.

NURSING DIAGNOSIS: **Self-concept, disturbance in.**

SUPPORTING DATA: **Burn injuries are associated with disfigurement and pain and often result in altered body image. Pain and stress can alter the patient's defenses and ability to cope. Dependency, grief, and hostility need to be recognized and dealt with, and may be a long-term process. Stages of grief are frequently seen. Regression and denial may function as protective mechanisms.**

DESIRED PATIENT OUTCOMES: **Patient and SO accept altered appearance, cope with interruption of lifestyle, and necessary limitations.**

INTERVENTIONS

Assess patient's/SO's needs.

Encourage family interaction.

Allow for expression of feelings of frustration, fear, and anxiety.

Allow patient to progress at own pace through stages of grief and acceptance.

May need to set limits on maladaptive behavior, such as manipulative/aggressive, maintaining nonjudgmental attitude while giving care.

Be realistic and positive during treatments, in health teaching, and in setting goals within limitations.

Give positive reinforcement of progress and encourage endeavors toward attainment of rehabilitation goals.

RATIONALE

Identification of individual needs enables appropriate interventions and referrals.

Provides ongoing support for patient and family.

Awareness that these are normal and need to be expressed and dealt with is helpful in regaining independence.

Not helpful or possible to push patient before ready to deal with situation. Denial may be prolonged and be an adaptive mechanism as patient is not ready to cope with personal problems.

Patient/significant others will tend to deal with this crisis in the same way in which they have dealt with problems in the past. Staff may find this difficult and frustrating to handle when the behavior is not helpful to recuperation.

Enhances trust and rapport between patient and nurse.

Needs to hear positive words of encouragement to support development of coping behaviors.

Encourage activities with other patients and/or SO.

Acceptance by others increases self-esteem and aids in acceptance of altered self-image.

Coordinate OT, PT, Social Services, and so forth.

Treatment is best provided by a team approach, using the skills of many.

Refer to Care Plan: Psychosocial Aspects of Care in the Acute Setting.

NURSING DIAGNOSIS:	Knowledge deficit, rehabilitation process.
SUPPORTING DATA:	Rehabilitation can be long and difficult in burn injuries, often involving changes in occupation, lifestyle, and relationships.
DESIRED PATIENT OUTCOMES:	Patient/SO are involved with care from the beginning, participating and cooperating in treatment and necessary changes.

INTERVENTIONS

Assess ability of patient/SO to aid in care.

Assess level of understanding and give information on an ongoing basis, allowing participation in care on a daily basis.

Provide support group for significant others, giving them information about how they can be helpful to the patient.

Show patient and SO slides and pictures of contractures and hypertrophy.

Involve burn team in care from the beginning through discharge.

Demonstrate caring and concern by being available for listening and talking to the patient and SO.

Discuss patient's expectations of returning home, to work, and to normal activities.

Refer to community resources as necessary.

RATIONALE

Necessary to involvement in care while hospitalized and for assessing the need for additional support postdischarge.

Knowing what to expect is less frightening. Seeing the progress of the wound allows for gradual acceptance and for seeing day-by-day healing.

Will be helpful for the ventilation of feelings and allow for more helpful responses to the patient.

Seeing actual pictures of similar injuries allows patient/SO to be more realistic in understanding the need for splints, therapy, and so forth.

Coordinate activities and goals with the patient.

Helpful to know people care about them in this difficult period.

Patient often has a difficult adjustment to discharge, fearing being sent home to die. Often problems of sleeping, nightmares of reliving the accident, boredom, resumption of sexual activity, and lack of control interfere with successful adjustment to resuming normal life.

Often have long-range, chronic, personal problems that need further assistance. Alcoholics Anonymous, crisis centers, recovery groups, mental health, Red Cross, VNA, Ambu-Cab, Homemakers, can be useful as resources.

BIBLIOGRAPHY

Books and Other Individual Publications

ARTZ, C. P. ET AL.: *Burns—A Team Approach.* W. B. Saunders, Philadelphia, 1979.

BAXTER, C. R.: *Crystalloid Resuscitation of Burn Shock,* (EDS. STONE, H. H. AND POLK JR., H. A.), Little, Brown & Co., Boston, 1971.

BEYERS, M. AND DUDAS, S.: *The Clinical Practice of Medical-Surgical Nursing.* Little, Brown & Co., Boston, 1977.

BRUNNER, L. AND SUDDARTH, D.: *Textbook of Medical-Surgical Nursing,* ed. 3. J. B. Lippincott, Philadelphia, 1975.

FELLER, I. AND ARCHEMBEAULT, C.: *Nursing the Burned Patient.* The Institute for Burn Medicine, Ann Arbor, Michigan, 1973.

GUYTON, A.: *Textbook of Medical Physiology,* ed. 4. W. B. Saunders, Philadelphia, 1971.

JOHANSON, B. C. ET AL.: Standards for Cricital Care. C. V. Mosby, St. Louis, 1981.

KIM, M. AND MORITZ, D. (EDS.): *Classification of Nursing Diagnosis.* McGraw-Hill, New York, 1981.

MCCAFFERY, M.: *Nursing Management of the Patient in Pain.* J. B. Lippincott, Philadelphia, 1972.

PARRISH, J. A.: *Dermatology and Skin Care.* McGraw-Hill, New York, 1975.

PATTON, B. R. AND GRIFFIN, K.: *Interpersonal Communication.* Harper & Row, New York, 1974.

PHIPPS, W. J., LONG, B. C., AND WOODS, N. F.: *Medical-Surgical Nursing.* C. V. Mosby, St. Louis, 1979.

TAYLOR, J. AND BALLENGER, B.: *Neurological Dysfunction and Nursing Intervention.* McGraw-Hill, New York, 1980.

THAL, A. ET AL.: *Shock: A Physiologic Basis for Treatment.* Year Book Medical Pub., Chicago, 1971.

TUCKER, S. M. ET AL.: Patient Care Standards, ed. 2. C. V. Mosby, St. Louis, 1980.

WEINER, M. ET AL.: *Clinical Pharmacology and Therapeutics in Nursing.* McGraw-Hill, New York, 1979.

WILKINS, R. W. AND LEVINSKY, N. G. (EDS.): *Medicine, Essentials of Clinical Practice.* Little, Brown & Co., Boston, 1978.

Journal Articles

ALEXANDER, J. W. AND WIXON, D.: *Neutrophil dysfunction and sepsis in burn injury.* Surgery, Gynecology, and Obstetrics, 431, 1970.

BASTER, C. R., MARVIN, J. A., AND CURRERI, P. W.: *Fluid and electrolyte therapy of burn shock.* Heart and Lung Journal 2,5:707, 1973.

BAXTER, C. R.: *The response of initial fluid and electrolyte therapy of burn shock.* Symposium on the Treatment of Burns, (EDS. LYNCH, J. B. AND LEWIS, S. R.), C. V. Mosby, St. Louis, 1973.

DAVIES, J. W. L. AND LILJEDAHL, S. O.: *Protein catabolism and energy utilization in burned patients treated at different environmental temperatures.* Ciba, Foundation Symposium on Energy Metabolism in Trauma, Churchill Press, London, 1970.

DOLAN, M. B.: *Controlling pain in a personal way.* Nursing 82, Vol. 12, No. 1, Jan. 1982 p. 144.

DOUB, L.: *Shingles.* Life Health, Vol. 86, No. 10:11, Oct. 1971.

FERRARA, R. ET AL.: *Easing the problems of herpes zoster.* Patient Care, Vol. 7, No. 6:104–129, April 15, 1973.

HARDY, T. K.: *Post-herpetic neuralgia.* Nursing Mirror, Vol. 136, No. 12:30–31, June 22, 1973.

HECKEL, P. *Teaching patients to cope with psoriasis: The unshared disease.* Nursing XI, No. 6:49–51, June, 1981.

HUGHES, J. ET AL.: *Seizures following burns of the skin.* Diseases of the Nervous System, 35:347, 1973.

HUNT, J., MCGRANAHAN, B., AND PRUITT, B.: *Burn wound management.* Heart and Lung Journal 2:690, 1973.

LOEBL, E. ET AL.: *Erythrocyte survival following thermal injury.* Journal of Surgical Research, 26:96, 1974.

MCCABE, W. P. ET AL: *Leukocyte responses as a monitor of immunodepression in burn patients.* Archives of Surgery, 106:155, 1973.

MAYERS, A.: *Fibrin split products in the severely burned patient.* Archives of Surgery, 105:404, 1972.

MONCRIEF, J.: *Burns.* New England Journal of Medicine, 288:444, 1973.

MOORE, F.: *The body-weight burn budget: Basic fluid therapy for the early burn.* Surgical Clinics of North America, 50:1249, 1970.

POTTS, R. L.: *How the doctor treats shingles.* Life and Health, Vol. 87, No. 6:18–19, June 1972.

VALENTI, W. ET AL.: *Nosocomial viral infections: II. Guidelines for prevention and control of respiratory viruses.* Infection Control, Vol. 1, No. 3:165–177, May-June, 1980.

WARDEN, G. ET AL.: *Hypernatremic state in hypermetabolic burn patients.* Archives of Surgery, 106:420, 1973.

CHAPTER 14

IMMUNOLOGIC DISORDERS

DIAGNOSIS: Systemic Lupus Erythematosus (SLE)

PATIENT DATA BASE

NURSING HISTORY

Occurs mainly in young women (5–10:1) in third to the fourth decade, but may occur in all ages; more frequent in blacks.

Symptomatology depends on systems involved and extent of disease involvement. Mimics other diseases.

Patient may complain of rheumatic symptoms, joint aches and pains, swelling, paralysis, paresthesia.

Recent viral infection may precede onset of disease symptoms.

Recent ingestion of drugs, such as procainamide, hydralazide, hydantoin, anovulatory drugs.

Patient may complain of rash on face or body, which worsens on exposure to sunlight.

Patient may complain of chest discomfort, pain, fatigue, tremors.

Significant others may note behavioral changes.

Patient may complain of tender and swollen glands, tenderness in right upper abdominal quadrant, abdominal pain, anorexia, nausea, vomiting, black stools.

Family history of lupus.

DIAGNOSTIC STUDIES

CBC shows normochromic, normocytic anemia, leukopenia, thrombocytopenia; steroid therapy may cause leukocytosis.

Positive Coombs' test is frequent and indicates hemolytic problems.

Sedimentation rate is elevated.

Serum globins (gamma globulins) are increased.

LE cell prep shows positive for neutrophils containing one or more LE bodies.

Positive C-reactive proteins.

Decreased or elevated serum complement level; test may be low in active disease and is often associated with nephritis.

UA shows proteinuria, hematuria indicative of glomerulonephritis; pyuria more frequently associated with UTI.

Clotting time shows prothrombin time prolongation caused by circulatory anticoagulation factor in 25% of patients.

Alkaline phosphatase, bilirubin and SGOT may be elevated.

Creatinine clearance level elevated with renal involvement.

Biologically false positive (BFP) test results for syphilis may precede diagnosis by years.

ANA positive.

Elevated or rising titer of anti-DNA antibodies.

PHYSICAL EXAMINATION

Fever, prostration, delirium, psychosis, convulsions, tremors.

Joint tenderness and swelling.

Red cutaneous lesions and typical facial butterfly rash may be present, especially across the bridge of the nose.

Alopecia, broken-off hair.

Rales, rhonchi, basilar dullness on percussion and auscultation of chest.

Generalized lymphadenopathy.

Tachycardia, gallop rhythm, friction rub.

Hepatosplenomegaly, CVA tenderness on percussion.

Ecchymosis, signs of periphral vascular insufficiency.

NURSING PRIORITIES

1. Prevent exacerbations.
2. Treat relapses to prevent further organ/tissue damage and maintain present level of function.
3. Psychologic support of patient/significant others.

NURSING DIAGNOSIS:	**Skin integrity, impairment of, potential.**
SUPPORTING DATA:	**Skin involvement occurs in 80% of SLE patients. Exposure to sunlight often precipitates development of the typical SLE rash, which may develop into a discoid rash anywhere on the body. Alopecia is common and usually temporary.**
DESIRED PATIENT OUTCOMES:	**Patient will verbalize/demonstrate understanding of skin manifestations, necessary restrictions and treatment.**

INTERVENTIONS

Note areas of cutaneous involvement.

Teach patient about skin problems that commonly occur with SLE.

Observe extremities for ulcerations.

Discuss importance of avoiding excessive sunlight and use of sunscreens.

Observe for urticaria and keep dry and not overly warm.

Do not apply unprescribed ointments to lesions.

MEDICAL MANAGEMENT

Topical corticosteroid cream.

Antimalarials. (Observe for retinal damage.)

RATIONALE

Will determine treatment.

Information about potential problems may decrease anxiety and increase understanding of disease.

Small ulcerations of the fingertips from underlying vasculitis may proceed to necrosis.

Sunlight may adversely affect skin lesions.

May occur and is aggravated by heat and moisture.

May exacerbate.

Protect skin and suppress inflammation.

Use sparingly to control skin manifestations not responsive to topical therapy.

NURSING DIAGNOSIS: Tissue perfusion, alteration in.

SUPPORTING DATA: 50% of SLE patients show involvement of the heart and blood vessels, which become inflamed, necrosed, and scarred causing decreased blood supply to the tissues. Small growths scar and deform valves. Pericardial involvement causes effusion.

DESIRED PATIENT OUTCOMES: Cardiac manifestations minimized/controlled.

INTERVENTIONS

Monitor vital signs and assess peripheral perfusion.

Note and report occurrence of pericardial friction rub, signs of tamponade, murmurs, increased pulse, blood pressure.

Keep patient at rest.

MEDICAL MANAGEMENT

Systemic corticosteroids.

Digitalis preparations.

Diuretics, fluid restriction.

RATIONALE

Note signs of circulatory deficiency.

Appropriate intervention can be taken.

Enhances healing process and minimizes cardiac workload and tissue needs.

Suppress inflammation and control symptoms.

Myocarditis should be suspected when tachycardia is disproportionate to fever or anemia.

Percarditis or pleurisy may be present.

NURSING DIAGNOSIS:	Urinary elimination, alteration in pattern.
SUPPORTING DATA:	Renal involvement occurs in 50% of SLE patients; renal failure is the major cause of death. Acute nephritis or nephrotic syndrome may be the presenting manifestations. Acute glomerular nephritis however, is the most common complication and usually develops early in the course of the disease.
DESIRED PATIENT OUTCOMES:	Renal symptoms minimized/controlled.

INTERVENTIONS

Observe for edema, hypertension, hematuria, decreased urine output.

Keep on bed rest.

Monitor CBC, complement levels, serum creatinine biweekly.

Observe for pyuria, fever may or may not be present.

Refer to Care Plan: Acute Renal Failure.

MEDICAL MANAGEMENT

Systemic corticosteroids (0.5–1 mg or more per kg body weight of prednisone).

Cytoxan, Imuran.

Immunosuppressants.

RATIONALE

Signs of developing failure.

Promote healing.

Monitor relapses.

Indication of UTI, especially if patient is receiving steroids.

Suppress inflammation and relieve symptoms. Give medications until hematuria clears and complement levels are normal (1–3 weeks).

Most commonly used drugs.

If unresponsive to above treatment.

NURSING DIAGNOSIS:	Comfort, alterations in, pain.
SUPPORTING DATA:	Joint involvement is very common but does not usually cause extreme pain or deformity. Synovial membrane involvement may cause swelling and painful motion. Myalgia is common. Pain may be due to pleurisy or pericarditis.
DESIRED PATIENT OUTCOMES:	Pain is minimized/controlled.

INTERVENTIONS

Encourage sufficient rest.

MEDICAL MANAGEMENT

Salicylates, other analgesics, and anti-inflammatories.

Physical therapy, splinting.

RATIONALE

Promote healing.

To decrease pain and inflammation.

Enable continuing movement with as little pain as possible.

NURSING DIAGNOSIS:	Injury, potential for, hemorrhage.
SUPPORTING DATA:	Platelet and clotting problems may occur due to renal insufficiency, vasculitis, or corticosteroid side effects. Splenomegaly occurs in approximately 15% of all SLE patients.
DESIRED PATIENT OUTCOMES:	Bleeding is minimized/controlled.

INTERVENTIONS

Observe for purpura, ecchymosis.

Ensure that safety measures are carried out.

MEDICAL MANAGEMENT

Steroids, immunosuppressants.

Splenectomy.

RATIONALE

Indicative of platelet and clotting problems.

Protect patient from injury. Refer to Care Plan: Disseminated Intravascular Coagulation.

Suppress inflammation and relieve symptoms.

If unresponsive to medical management.

NURSING DIAGNOSIS:	Breathing patterns, ineffective.
SUPPORTING DATA:	Pleuritic pain is common due to pleural effusion. Patchy, bilateral infiltrations may be difficult to differentiate from infections. Rarely, respiratory insufficiency may develop.
DESIRED PATIENT OUTCOMES:	Respiratory function maintained.

INTERVENTIONS

Take vital signs q4h and evaluate for developing respiratory insufficiency.

RATIONALE

Early identification and intervention. Fever is common; specific causative process is unknown, may be related to occult infection.

Auscultate breath sounds and for pleural friction rub and report.

Allow for differential diagnosis and treatment.

MEDICAL MANAGEMENT

Chest x-ray.

Evaluate for presence of infiltrates and effusion.

Systemic corticosteroids.

Suppress inflammation, effusion and relieve symptoms.

NURSING DIAGNOSIS:	**Thought processes, alterations in.**
SUPPORTING DATA:	**SLE psychosis may be difficult to differentiate from that due to corticosteroid therapy or anxiety. Convulsions are a common manifestation of CNS involvement. Other neurologic signs occur less frequently.**
DESIRED PATIENT OUTCOMES:	**Neurologic manifestations are minimized/managed.**

INTERVENTIONS

RATIONALE

Observe for behavioral changes; hyperirritability, confusion, hallucinations, paranoia.

Indicate CNS involvement.

Take seizure precautions.

Be prepared for possible occurrence. Refer to Care Plan: Seizure Disorders.

MEDICAL MANAGEMENT

Large doses of corticosteroids (2–3 mg per kg of body weight per day of prednisone).

Until improvement, then taper dose.

Immunosuppressants.

If patient is unresponsive to corticosteroid therapy.

NURSING DIAGNOSIS:	**Nutrition, alteration in, less than body requirements, potential.**
SUPPORTING DATA:	**GI manifestations are common but the cause is obscure. Oral ulcerations and symptoms of peritoneal ulceration may occur.**
DESIRED PATIENT OUTCOMES:	**Weight is maintained at optimal level.**

INTERVENTIONS

Note complaints of anorexia, nausea, vomiting, abdominal pain.

Weigh patient.

Encourage balanced diet within limits of symptomatology.

Palpate abdomen and note progression or diminution of size.

RATIONALE

Begin interventions as appropriate.

Assess adequacy of nutritional intake.

Maximize dietary intake and minimize weight loss.

Liver congestion is due to chronic passive congestion.

NURSING DIAGNOSIS:	**Knowledge deficit, ramifications of disease process and treatment.**
SUPPORTING DATA:	**Dependent upon symptomatology, patient may need to make alterations in lifestyle. Disease is not curable at this time, can be controlled.**
DESIRED PATIENT OUTCOMES:	**Verbalizes understanding of individual limitations and needs. Cooperates in treatment program.**

INTERVENTIONS

Instruct in avoiding things that exacerbate the condition.

Teach about potential cardiac manifestations that are common and methods of prevention.

Instruct about high-protein diet, fluid restrictions, and the importance of avoiding infections.

Instruct in methods of dealing with exposure to sun.

Avoid the use of sensitizing drugs, such as penicillin, sulfa, as well as hair sprays and coloring agents.

Discuss use of contraceptive pills.

Cooperate with patient in developing a program of diet and rest as needed.

Instruct in safety measures.

Investigate the use of aids for improving appearance.

Observe for and report lymph node enlargement.

Instruct in recognition of reportable symptoms.

RATIONALE

Individual will identify what makes the situation worse.

Needs to be aware of those problems that should be reported to the physician.

When nephrotic syndrome is present. Can develop negative nitrogen balance.

Protective clothing that covers exposed skin and appropriate sunscreening agents.

May exacerbate condition.

May precipitate lupus in susceptible individuals.

Enable patient to participate and maintain control over self.

When clotting deficiencies are present, may have bleeding problems with injuries.

Products for covering skin discolorations and scars are available.

Lymph nodes may be enlarged and nontender and may be mistaken for lymphoma.

Immediate attention to worsening condition can minimize exacerbations.

Discuss side effects to be expected from steroid therapy.

Long-term use results in effects that the patient needs to recognize and manage. Refer to Care Plan: Cushing's Syndrome.

Refer to other agencies as needed.

May need assistance with emotional, financial, and/or other problems.

BIBLIOGRAPHY

Books and Other Individual Publications

BEYERS, M. AND DUDAS, S.: *The Clinical Practice of Medical-Surgical Nursing.* Little, Brown & Co., Boston, 1977.

BRUNNER, L. S. AND SUDDARTH, D. S.: *Lippincott Manual of Nursing Practice.* J. B. Lippincott, Philadelphia, 1978.

KIM, M. AND MORITZ, D. (EDS.): *Classification of Nursing Diagnosis.* McGraw-Hill, New York, 1981.

PHIPPS, W. F., LONG, B. C., AND WOODS, N. F.: *Medical Surgical Nursing.* C. V. Mosby, St. Louis, 1979.

TILKIAN, S. M., CONOVER, M. B., AND TILKIAN, A. G.: *Clinical Implications of Laboratory Tests.* C. V. Mosby, St. Louis, 1979.

WILKINS, R. W. AND LEVINSKY, N. G. (EDS.): *Medicine, Essentials of Clinical Practice.* Little, Brown & Co., Boston, 1978.

Journal Articles

RODNAN, G. P. (ED.): *Primer on the rheumatic diseases,* ed. 7. Reprinted from the J. Am. Med. Assoc. April 30, 1973, Vol. 224, No. 5, The Arthritis Foundation.

CHAPTER 15
SYSTEMIC INFECTIONS

DIAGNOSIS: Septicemia

PATIENT DATA BASE

NURSING HISTORY

Nonspecific predisposing factors: diabetes mellitus, cirrhosis of the liver, burns, neoplastic disease, and therapies; glucosteroids, blood transfusion, surgery, radiation, immunosupressive/antibiotic therapy or previous splenectomy.

Predominant in men over age 40 and women ages 20–45.

May complain of feeling run down, tired, agitated; confusion in the elderly may be noted.

Complains of malaise, anorexia, chills.

History of parenteral feedings, IV or hyperalimentation therapy.

Does not have to be caused by bacteria, can be caused by exo/endotoxins.

Recent instrumentation of the GI, biliary, or urinary tracts.

DIAGNOSTIC STUDIES

Blood cultures: three different blood samples drawn over 24 hours, to isolate micro-organism. (Usually gram-negative is responsible for septic shock.)

Urine: sodium may be decreased; glucose may be positive in patients who have diabetes.

Creatinine level: may be increased due to renal function impairment secondary to infection.

pH: metabolic acidosis.

PT-PTT levels: may be prolonged from inadequate prothrombin synthesis and decreased platelets; DIC, increased fibrin degradation products.

Liver function tests: intrahepatic cholestasis secondary to hepatocellular dysfunction.

PHYSICAL EXAMINATION

Temperature may be elevated over 101°F.; or under 98.6°F.

Blood pressure initially may be normal or slightly elevated; hypotension occurs in the later stages. Widening pulse pressure may be noted.

Respirations increased; pulse rate increased and bounding.

Skin exam may reveal signs of dehydration; jaundice, usually "pink" or flushed and warm/dry (early), cool, moist/pale (late).

Normal or increased urine output initially; oliguria may be present in late stage.

May have poor wound healing.

Mental status exam may reveal confusion, anxiety, delirium, stupor, convulsions, and coma.

NURSING PRIORITIES

1. Maintain tissue perfusion and circulating volume.
2. Combat infection.
3. Prevent recurrence.

NURSING DIAGNOSIS: Tissue perfusion, alterations in.

SUPPORTING DATA: Response to sepsis results in dilatation of the vascular tree, causing hypovolemia, A-V shunting, decreased cardiac output, and tissue perfusion. Alterations occur in B/P and circulation. There is stagnation of blood in the microcirculation of liver, kidney, GI tract, and skin. Local tissue anorexia and increased intracapillary pressure occur.

DESIRED PATIENT OUTCOMES: Adequate cardiac output and tissue perfusion is maintained.

INTERVENTIONS

Monitor vital signs, pulse pressure, urine output, level of consciousness.

Monitor lab results, ABGs.

RATIONALE

Be aware of deteriorating condition. Early BP is normal but pulse pressure is a better indicator of situation. (An increase reflects cardiovascular deterioration as the systolic increases and pulse pressure widens when the heart works harder to compensate for increase in the vascular bed and decreased circulation volume.)

Changes in pH, BUN/creatinine levels may be indicative of impending acidosis and renal impairment. Decreased PO_2 may reflect respiratory failure.

Monitor CVP/PAP.

Check for signs of phlebitis; redness, swelling, and positive Homan's sign.

Monitor fluid challenges with CVP/Swan-Ganz, arterial line, and indwelling catheter.

Signs/symptoms of pulmonary edema/ARDS.

Venous stasis may result in the development of thrombosis.

Assess circulating volume, vascular response and pump quality. Overload/failure may occur.

MEDICAL MANAGEMENT

Oxygen.

To maximize arterial PO_2.

Fluids IV. Colloid/crystalloid. Whole blood.

Maintain circulating volume. Capillary permeability increases causing loss of fluid intravascularly.

Culture/sensitivities.

Identification of organism and guide for antibiotic choice.

Antibiotics; cephalosporins, aminoglycosides.

Control infection.

Acetysalicylic acid, cooling blanket.

Reduce fever.

Surgery.

May be needed to drain seeding source.

Glucosteroids.

Anti-inflammatory and decrease capillary permeability. Given in large doses, may reduce mortality.

IV digitalization and isoproterenol.

To decrease peripheral vasoconcentration, increase myocardial contractility.

Norepinephrine pressor agent or dopamine.

Increases cardiac contractility and output; increases peripheral vasoconstriction with increased renal perfusion.

$NaHCO_3$.

To treat severe acidosis.

NURSING DIAGNOSIS:

Gas exchange, impaired.

SUPPORTING DATA:

Initial cellular/vascular damage caused by endotoxins alters oxygen transport and exchange, causing hypoxia. Lactic acid is produced as anaerobic metabolism occurs secondary to oxygen lack and metabolic acidosis. Combined metabolic/respiratory acidosis occurs later as compensatory mechanisms fail. ARDS may occur secondary to acidosis, hypoxia, and increased capillary permeability with pulmonary edema.

DESIRED PATIENT OUTCOMES:

Gas exchange is maintained at an adequate level.

INTERVENTIONS

Monitor ongoing mental status.

Monitor ABGs and A-a gradient.

MEDICAL MANAGEMENT

Oxygen.

Mechanical ventilation.

IV fluids.

RATIONALE

Early changes in mentation occur due to hypoxia.

Arterial PO_2 is an indicator of FIO_2 needs and adequacy of current inspired O_2 therapy. Gradient provides a comparison of the oxygen tension within arterial blood and reflects effectiveness of gas exchange in the lungs.

Maintain increased arterial O_2.

May be necessary to maintain PO_2 above 80. Refer to Care Plan: Ventilatory Assistance (Mechanical).

Increase circulating volume, promote venous return and tissue perfusion and provide opportunity for gas exchange. Use fluid challenges early to increase tissue perfusion.

NURSING DIAGNOSIS:	**Knowledge deficit, recurrence.**
SUPPORTING DATA:	**Patients with low resistance to infection need to be aware of signs/ symptoms to prevent septicemias.**
DESIRED PATIENT OUTCOMES:	**Septicemia does not recur.**

INTERVENTIONS

Assess risk factors for individual patient.

Teach patient signs/symptoms of infection.

Provide information and support for drug therapy, noting interactions and side effects.

RATIONALE

Glucocorticoid therapy, kidney/liver dysfunction, neoplastic disease, rheumatic heart disease, valve dysfunction, and diabetes may predispose to septicemia.

Elevated temperature, tachycardia, syncope, rashes of unknown origin, fatigue, anorexic, hypotension, increased thirst and change in bladder function may herald impending infection.

May require prophylactic medication regimen.

DIAGNOSIS: Sexually Transmitted Diseases

Diseases that are transmitted by sexual contact continue to be the most common communicable diseases. These include gonorrhea and syphillis, which are reportable and nonreportable diseases of herpes genitalis, trichomoniasis, candidiasis, nonspecific urethritis (NSU), and Chlamydia.

GONORRHEA

PATIENT DATA BASE

NURSING HISTORY

Occurrence is 3× higher in men than women.

The majority of women who are infected are asymptomatic in the beginning. Initially, men present with acute infection, however an increasing number are asymptomatic.

Usually history of sexual activity with multiple partners.

Incubation period 2–21 days.

May have concurrent infections. (25% have comorbidity.)

Complain of pelvic pain.

Fever may be present.

DIAGNOSTIC STUDIES

Women: cervical and anal culture inoculated on separate Modified Thayer-Martin (MTM) plates.

Men: microscopic examination of urethral exudate smear. In homosexuals, anal canal and pharyngeal cultures need to be obtained.

Urinalysis.

PHYSICAL EXAMINATION

Anal irritation may be evident.

Examine oral cavity for evidence of throat inflammation; ulcerations; red, dry tongue; and evidence of vesicles.

Women: May have vaginal discharge. Urinary frequency and pain. Fever, nausea/vomiting, lower abdominal pain, may be indicative of pelvic infection.

Men: Painful urination with purulent discharge present. Prostate examination for evidence of infection. Severe pain, tenderness, and swelling in the groin may indicate epididymitis.

NURSING PRIORITIES

1. Treat infection.
2. Observe for complications.
3. Provide information about disease, complications, and recurrence.

NURSING DIAGNOSIS:	Injury, potential for, infection.
SUPPORTING DATA:	Presenting symptom is infection in both men and women. In men, urethritis with swelling and irritation, pain and burning with urination, and yellowish discharge. When untreated, disease may spread to epididymis, prostate, and seminal vesicles. In women, pelvic infection often is the presenting symptom with the possibility of sterility.
DESIRED PATIENT OUTCOMES:	Infection is resolved and complications are prevented.

INTERVENTIONS

Observe for signs of infection; vaginal or penile discharge; temperature elevation; nausea and vomiting; in women, lower abdominal pain; in men, painful urination.

Check for previous allergic reactions to penicillin.

Discuss with patient the importance of medical followup and treatment for any sexual contacts.

Check results of test for other infections, such as syphillis, chlamydia.

RATIONALE

May need symptomatic treatment; such as bedrest, increased fluid intake, and so forth.

Anaphylactic reactions can be life threatening.

Organism may be resistant to the drug used and it is important to be certain treatment has been successful. Gonorrhea is a reportable disease and contacts need treatment to prevent further spread.

May have concurrent infection.

MEDICAL MANAGEMENT

Penicillin G, IM.

Probenecid orally.

Ampicillin orally with probenecid.

Tetracycline by mouth or spectinomycin IM.

Complications need to be treated.

Treatment of choice, divided into two or more injections at different sites to promote absorption.

Enhance and prolong the antibiotic blood concentration.

Alternate to IM administration.

May be given when patient has sensitivity to penicillin.

See appropriate Care Plans: Endocarditis; Rheumatoid Arthritis; Septicemia; Pelvic Inflammatory Disease.

NURSING DIAGNOSIS:	Knowledge deficit, disease, treatment, potential for complications.
SUPPORTING DATA:	Sexually transmitted diseases are often misunderstood and go untreated because societal and moral value judgments promote an atmosphere in which people do not seek treatment and/or have misunderstandings about followup care and the occurrence of complications.
DESIRED PATIENT OUTCOMES:	Verbalizes rationale for treatment and followup. Treatment is completed and disease is cured.

INTERVENTIONS

Assess level of information patient has and provide appropriate additional data.

Discuss importance of testing of sexual contacts.

Be available and provide a nonjudgmental atmosphere in which patient asks questions.

Provide information about the importance of immediate treatment when symptoms begin. Discuss need to have regular checks if the patient is sexually active with several different partners.

Give information about ways to prevent contracting the disease.

Discuss myths and misunderstandings.

Give information about signs/symptoms of complications that may develop.

RATIONALE

Knowledge varies with individuals.

Prevent spread of disease.

Sensitive area for talking often results in patient not asking questions and resulting in misinformation and misunderstanding the disease and treatment.

Embarrassment and fear may keep patient from seeking treatment.

Washing the sex organs before and after contact, as well as the use of a condom may give limited protection.

Common beliefs that birth control prevents infection; one episode gives immunity; if you have one disease you can't contract another interfere with getting care and preventing recurrences.

Important to identify early to minimize permanent damage.

HERPES SIMPLEX VIRUS (HSV)

The herpes family includes the cytomegalovirus (CMV), the Epstein-Barr virus (mononucleosis), varicella-zoster virus (chickenpox and shingles), and HSV Types 1 and 2 that cause both oral and genital infections. The majority of genital infections are caused by Type 2, while Type 1 accounts for most oral lesions, although it is generally accepted that either strain can cause disease anywhere in body. Clinically they are indistinguishable, but may be identified virologically by culturing.

609

Transmission is by skin to skin contact with a break in the skin or mucous membrane but is not necessarily sexual. It is not airborne and does not survive on inanimate objects, but is transmitted by autoinoculation and by oral sex. The virus enters the nervous system, settles in the nearest ganglia and is not found in the blood. It reproduces and within 2–12 days symptoms may appear. It then becomes dormant, remains in the body for life and may or may not have subsequent outbreaks. Precipitating factors in recurrent episodes appear to be individual and reasons are not known. Stress, menses, sun exposure, and sexual intercourse are some factors that have been identified.

While the incidence is low, asymptomatic viral shedding seems to be a factor in the spread of this infection.

Classification:
1. Primary: First clinical episode with an absence of antibodies in the acute phase serum.
2. Initial: First clinical episode with antibodies present indicating a previous exposure to the virus.
3. Recurrent: There has been at least one previous clinical episode and antibody titers are high. Clinical symptoms are usually milder than those of the initial episode with some evidence to suggest that recurrences become milder, although they may continue to be severe.

PATIENT DATA BASE

NURSING HISTORY

Complains of itching, burning, tingling, or tenderness in the affected area.

May complain of dysuria.

May complain of pain and may experience radiating pain that extends beyond the affected area.

DIAGNOSTIC STUDIES

Tissue culture will be positive for cell destruction as the virus cannot be seen. (This is an expensive procedure and is only done by a few laboratories.)

Smear test, usually a Pap smear, may be done to visualize multinucleated giant cells. While these tests are highly specific, their sensitivity is too variable to be used for an accurate diagnosis.

Antibody titers may be done to determine whether this is an initial or primary infection. (Are not useful as diagnostic tests as titers may only indicate previous infection.)

Pregnancy test (virus can be transmitted to fetus/newborn).

PHYSICAL EXAMINATION

Small, painful blisters appear in the affected area, progressing to a shallow ulceration that crusts over and heals. These develop in progressive stages and may vary from a single sore to an extensive involvement.

Lymphadenopathy may be present.

May have a thin, white vaginal discharge.

Edema with resultant urinary retention may be present.

May have elevated temperature.

Neuralgias may occur.

NURSING PRIORITIES

1. Relieve pain.
2. Prevent transmission of the virus.
3. Provide emotional support.
4. Provide information re disease management/control.

610

NURSING DIAGNOSIS:	Comfort, alteration in, pain.
SUPPORTING DATA:	While the disease is self-limiting, the virus involves nerves and can be excrutiatingly painful.
DESIRED PATIENT OUTCOMES:	Pain is minimized/controlled.

INTERVENTIONS

Keep the area clean and dry and avoid the use of creams or ointments.

Take sitz baths 3–4 × /day.

MEDICAL MANAGEMENT

Topical anesthetics and systemic analgesics.

Antibiotics, systemic/topical.

RATIONALE

Healing occurs more rapidly than when area is moist.

Can be soothing and provide relief.

May be necessary when pain is severe.

May be used sparingly. Bacterial suprainfection is not a common problem with recurrent episodes.

NURSING DIAGNOSIS:	Injury, potential for, infection.
SUPPORTING DATA:	Virus is transmittable to self and others and may cause complications; such as herpetic whitlow (an HSV infection of the nail bed) and neonatal infections. A correlation seems to exist between cervical cancer and HSV.
DESIRED PATIENT OUTCOMES:	Infection is not spread to self or others. Complications are minimized/treated.

INTERVENTIONS

Use gown, gloves, and proper handwashing techniques.

Discuss ways of preventing transmission to sexual partners.

Encourage women to have a Pap smear every 6 months.

Instruct patient in use of finger cot or glove to apply acyclovir ointment.

RATIONALE

Appropriate barriers can minimize transmission.

Avoid contact when open lesions are present. Use of a condom may be helpful.

Detect early changes indicative of cancer.

Prevent autoinoculation/transmission to others.

MEDICAL MANAGEMENT

Acyclovir ointment.

Antiviral drug that provides relief of symptoms and appears to shorten episodes but does not cure the disease. It has been used most successfully in immunocompromised patients.

NURSING DIAGNOSIS:	Self-concept, disturbance in, self-image.
SUPPORTING DATA:	Awareness of the impact of this disease on own life and relationships with others affects the social and mental health of the individual who is involved.
DESIRED PATIENT OUTCOMES:	Verbalizes improved self-esteem and methods of coping with existing problems.

INTERVENTIONS

Assess level of anxiety and coping ability.

Provide opportunity to discuss feelings and concerns.

Share information and discuss myths and misinformation.

Refer to professional counseling.

Refer to Care Plan: Psychosocial Aspects of Care in the Acute Setting.

RATIONALE

Individual coping is affected by level of anxiety.

Helpful to ventilate. Acceptance of feelings allows patient to feel better about self.

Accurate information allows for improved coping.

May need ongoing help when divorce, death of a child, depression, and so forth are factors.

NURSING DIAGNOSIS:	Knowledge deficit, disease management.
SUPPORTING DATA:	Social attitudes, myths, and misinformation can interfere with care.
DESIRED PATIENT OUTCOMES:	Verbalizes accurate knowledge about disease.

INTERVENTIONS

Assess level of knowledge.

Give information as required.

RATIONALE

Gives information for development of teaching plan.

Can help patient deal with attitudes of others who do not have accurate information.

Review treatment and indications of complications.

Provide information about ongoing research.

Refer to Herpes Resource Center and/or local groups.

Helpful to discuss more than once and in brief sessions to enhance retention.

Gives hope that cure/control will be possible.

Can provide education and support for patient/significant others.

BIBLIOGRAPHY

Books and Other Individual Publications

BEYERS, M. AND DUDAS, S.: *The Clinical Practice of Medical-Surgical Nursing.* Little, Brown & Co., Boston, 1977.

BRUNNER, L. S. AND SUDDARTH, D. S.: *Lippincott Manual of Nursing Practice.* J. B. Lippincott, Philadelphia, 1978.

Criteria & Techniques for the Diagnosis of Gonorrhea. U. S. Department of HGW/Public Health Service Center for Disease Control/Venereal Disease Control Division, Atlanta, GA.

FREITAG, J. J. AND MILLER, L. W. (EDS.): *Manual of Medical Therapeutics,* ed. 23. Wash. Univ. Sch. of Med., Little Brown & Co., Boston, 1982.

KIM, M. AND MORITZ, D. (EDS.): *Classification of Nursing Diagnosis.* McGraw-Hill, New York, 1981.

PHIPPS, W. J., LONG, B. C., AND WOODS, N. F.: *Medical-Surgical Nursing.* C. V. Mosby, St. Louis, 1979.

TILKIAN, S. M., CONOVER, M. B., AND TILKIAN, A. G.: *Clinical Implications of Laboratory Tests.* C. V. Mosby, St. Louis, 1979.

WILKINS, R. W. AND LEVINSKY, N. G. (EDS.): *Medicine, Essentials of Clinical Practice.* Little, Brown & Co., Boston, 1978.

Journal Articles

BETTOLI, E. J.: *Herpes: Facts & fallacies.* AJN, 924–929, June, 1982.

HALL, K. V.: *Detecting septic shock before it's too late.* RN, 29–32, Sep. 1981.

LAMB, L. S.: *Think you know septic shock.* Nursing '82, Vol. 12, No. 1:34–43, Jan. 1982.

CHAPTER 16
GENERAL

DIAGNOSIS: Psychosocial Aspects Of Care In The Acute Setting

PATIENT DATA BASE

NURSING HISTORY

INDIVIDUAL

Age and sex.

Religious affiliation: church attendance, importance of religion in life, belief in life after death.

Assess level of knowledge; education? How does individual access information; auditory, visual, kinesthetic?

How does patient define and perceive illness?

What is patient behavior when anxious, afraid, impatient, or angry?

How is patient experiencing illness versus what illness actually is?

Note patient's emotional response to current treatment and hospitalization. What is the patient's past experience with illness, hospitalization, and health care systems? Describe patient's emotional reaction in feeling (sensory) terms, e.g., "I felt scared."

What are patterns of communication: With significant others? With health caregivers? What is style of speech?

What is perception of body and its functions: When well? In illness? This illness?

SIGNIFICANT OTHERS

Marital status; who are significant others in patient's life? Nuclear family? Extended family? Recurring or patterned relationships?

What is the family developmental cycle? (Just married? Children: Young? Adolescent? Children leaving home? Retired?)

What is the patient's role in family tasks and functions?

How are significant others affected by the illness and prognosis?

What are the interaction processes within the family?

Are there any lifestyle differences that need to be considered, such as dietary, spiritual, sexual preference, or other community?

SOCIOECONOMIC FACTORS

Employment.

Finances.

Environmental factors: home, work, and recreation.

Social class.

Health seeking behaviors; illness referral system.

Values system.

Social acceptability of disease.

Is patient out of usual environment (e.g., on vacation, visiting).

CULTURAL FACTORS

Ethnic background.

Illness referral system and health seeking behaviors.

Values related to health and treatment.

Cultural factors in pain response.

Beliefs regarding caring and curing.

DISEASE (ILLNESS) FACTORS

Kind of illness.

How has it been treated? Will be treated? Should be treated? Anticipated response to treatment?

Cause of the illness?

What is the threat to others?

Is this an acute/chronic illness?

Is it inherited?

If terminal illness, what do the patient/significant others know and anticipate?

Is the condition "appropriate" to the afflicted individual, such as Type A/cardiac personality (may be myth or valid).

NURSE-RELATED FACTORS

Basic knowledge of human beings and the current situation the individual is responding to.

Basic knowledge of biologic, psychologic, social, and cultural issues, as well as theapeutic communication skills.

Knowledge of own value and belief systems.

Willingness to look at own behavior in relation to interaction with others and make changes as necessary.

Respect of patient's privacy; confidentiality.

NURSING PRIORITIES

1. Patient/significant others will demonstrate knowledge of the illness and treatment.
2. Develop therapeutic nurse/patient relationship.
3. Maintain awareness of changes in self/others and how it affects their lives.
4. Patient/significant others will demonstrate effective coping skills in dealing with the illness.
5. Self-concept and body-image changes will be recognized and dealt with appropriately.
6. Grieving will be recognized, acknowledged, and dealt with according to the individual's choice.

NURSING DIAGNOSIS: Knowledge deficit, specify.

SUPPORTING DATA: Patients/SO often lack knowledge of their bodies, how they function, how the disease process affects them currently, and what the prognosis may be. Sometimes information has been given in the past and is not remembered or has been misinterpreted. Limitations in intellectual capacity may create problems in understanding. Many factors may be involved in a lack of learning. Often people do not know where to get information or help they need.

DESIRED PATIENT OUTCOMES: Patient/SO will demonstrate adequate knowledge base by giving feedback and making choices reflecting this knowledge.

INTERVENTIONS	RATIONALE
Assess present level of knowledge and anxiety.	Assessment process can provide a base to build on. Anxiety can be a motivator or interfere with learning, depending on degree.
Be aware of developmental level as well as age of patient.	Knowledge of developmental level will be helpful to the nurse in anticipating some needs and understanding what abilities may be present. Age and developmental level are not necessarily the same.
Provide information, as well as helping patient know where and how to find it on own.	Need basic information. Request from patient may indicate readiness to learn more.
Give information in manageable amounts.	Too much material given at one time will not be remembered.

Provide factual information about illness through verbal, written, and audiovisual modes geared to the developmental level of the patient; being sure to include information in the patient's language if they are non-English speaking.

Provide opportunity for discussion and feedback.

People access information in different ways. Different methods provide more opportunity for patient to obtain accurate information. Even when patient speaks English, it is important to ascertain reading ability and level of understanding, especially of medical terms.

Provides opportunity to assess how the patient and SO are understanding the disease/illness and how it affects them.

NURSING DIAGNOSIS:	**Coping, ineffective, individual.**
SUPPORTING DATA:	**Anxiety, fear, previous ineffective coping skills interfere with ability to handle stress of illness and hospitalization. Adaptive behaviors and problem-solving skills may be impaired.**
DESIRED PATIENT OUTCOMES:	**Problems will be accurately identified and the patient will be involved in problem-solving.**

INTERVENTIONS

Use the patient's name. Ask what they would like to be called.

Tell patient who you are and what your role is.

Identify significant others and from whom the patient derives comfort. Who should be notified in case of emergency.

Use active listening.

Encourage verbalization of fears by acceptance of what is said.

Provide nonthreatening environment.

Observe nonverbal communication, posture, eye contact, and movements, gestures, use of touch.

Observe speech patterns: rapidity, words repetition, laughter.

RATIONALE

Shows courtesy and respect. Acknowledges person. Allows patient to feel good about self.

Information relieves anxiety and allows patient to channel energy into other needed areas.

Will allow provisions to be made for these persons to visit or remain close. May or may not be legal next of kin.

Can more effectively identify the needs and problems. Can also identify the patient's coping strategies and how effective they are.

May diminish fear. Provides opportunity to identify problems and begin a problem-solving process.

Will be freer to verbalize.

Provides large percentage of communication and therefore is extremely important. How the person uses touch gives information about how they use touch for communication and how comfortable they are with being touched.

Speech patterns can give clues about the level of anxiety, ability to comprehend, brain damage, or possible language differences. Words can mean different things to different people.

Validate information by reflecting back what has been said for clarification and verification.

Information must be used carefully until validated by the patient as assumptions may be inaccurate.

Assess level of severity of pain if present. Delay gathering of information until later if pain is too severe.

Severe pain and anxiety leave little energy for thinking and other activities.

Observe and describe behavior in objective terms.

Behavior is all activities observed by another person. All behavior has meaning. Some is obvious and other behavior needs to be identified. This is a process of educated guess work and needs to be validated by the patient.

Identify developmental level.

More important than age. Some degree of regression occurs during illness dependent on many factors, such as the normal coping skills of the individual and severity of the illness. Useful in anticipating and identifying some needs; important to individualize.

Identify how the patient sees own role within the family system.

Illness may create a problem in role expectations within the system. Sexual role and how the patient view's self in relation to the current illness can play an important part in recovery.

Be aware of sexual needs that may be present.

When identified, can be discussed and dealt with appropriately.

Identify patient's view of body image and how this illness might affect it.

The patient's perception of a change in body image can be very subtle; may occur over a period of time or suddenly, as in loss of a body part through injury or surgery or a heart attack; or be a continuous process as in chronic illness, eating disorders or aging. Awareness by the nurse can alert others to the need for appropriate interventions tailored to the individual need. May be psychiatric referral, support/therapy group and so forth.

NURSING DIAGNOSIS:	Coping, ineffective, family, compromised.
SUPPORTING DATA:	Primary and/or other supportive person is not providing effective or enough support needed by the patient at this time.
DESIRED PATIENT OUTCOMES:	Primary and/or other supportive person is coping with own problems and providing support as needed by the patient.

INTERVENTIONS

Assess level of anxiety present in the family (significant others).

Determine current knowledge of the situation.

Assess current actions of significant others and how they are received by the patient.

Involve SO in information-giving, problem-solving, and care of the patient.

Encourage seeking help appropriately. Give information about people and agencies available to them.

RATIONALE

Anxiety level needs to be dealt with before problem-solving can begin. May be so preoccupied with their own reactions to the situation, they are unable to respond to the needs of others.

Provides a base for teaching program.

May be trying to be helpful, but are not perceived as helpful by the patient. May be withdrawn or may be too protective.

They often feel helpless and useless. Involvement in care enhances feelings of control and self-worth.

Permission to seek help as needed allows them to choose to take advantage of what is available.

NURSING DIAGNOSIS:	Coping, family, potential for growth.
SUPPORTING DATA:	People have strengths and potential for growth within them. Effectively dealing with the problems that exist, can lead to a point of willingness to deal with one's own needs and begin to problem-solve with the patient.
DESIRED PATIENT OUTCOMES:	Significant others discuss how the crisis (illness) has enhanced their growth and are demonstrating growth-promoting behaviors.

INTERVENTIONS

Provide opportunities for significant others to talk with patient and/or staff.

Provide opportunities for and instruction in how SO can care for patient.

Refer to support group/s and other resources as indicated.

RATIONALE

Allow expressions of what has been learned and how they are managing, as well as making plans for the future.

Enhances feelings of control and involvement in situation where they cannot do many things. Also provides opportunity to learn how to be most helpful when the patient is discharged.

Provides opportunities for sharing experiences; provides mutual support and practical problem-solving; and can aid in decreasing alienation and helplessness.

NURSING DIAGNOSIS:	Grieving, anticipatory.
SUPPORTING DATA:	Situation exists in which there is a potential for loss, such as surgery with the possible or actual loss/alteration in body image; amputation; or even loss of life. Illnesses of a progressive nature that have only a downhill course progressing to death are especially prone to dysfunctional handling. Feelings of anger, sadness, difficulty in discussing the perceived/actual loss, and alterations in physical activities.
DESIRED PATIENT OUTCOMES:	Patient is discussing the situation, expressing feelings, and dealing appropriately with physical alterations in sleeping, eating, and so forth.

INTERVENTIONS	RATIONALE
Assess degree of dysfunction.	Individuals handle situations in many different ways. What is effective for one may not be for another.
Provide open environment in which the patient feels free to discuss feelings and concerns realistically.	Therapeutic communication skills of active listening, silence, being available, and acceptance can allow the patient the opportunity to talk freely and deal with the perceived loss.
Identify and problem-solve existing physical problems.	Eating, sleeping, activity levels, and sexual desire can be affected.

NURSING DIAGNOSIS:	Grieving, dysfunctional.
SUPPORTING DATA:	Problems of anticipatory grieving are exacerbated and the patient/SO may be at a low or nonfunctioning level for an extended period of time or out of proportion to the degree of loss.
DESIRED PATIENT OUTCOMES:	Dealing with stages of grief at their own pace and functioning at an adequate level, participating in work, and ADL.

INTERVENTIONS	RATIONALE

See Nursing Diagnosis: Grieving, anticipatory.

Identify stage of grieving.

Awareness allows for appropriate interventions.

Denial: Be aware of avoidance behaviors; e.g., anger, withdrawal. Allow patient to talk about what the patient chooses to and do not try to force the patient to "face the facts."

Denies reality of diagnosis. An important phase in which the patient protects oneself from the pain and reality of the threat of loss. Each person does this in an individual manner based on previous experiences with loss and cultural factors.

Anger: Behaviors of withdrawal, lack of cooperation, and direct expression of anger may be noted. Allow verbalization of anger with acknowledgment of feelings and setting of limits regarding destructive behavior.

Denial gives way to feelings of anger, rage, guilt, and resentment. Patient may find it difficult to express anger directly and may feel guilty for feeling angry. Staff may also have difficulty dealing with angry behaviors. Acceptance of the anger allows the patient to work through the anger and move on to more effective coping behavior.

Bargaining: Allow verbalization without confrontation about realities.

Helpful in beginning resolution and acceptance. May be working through feelings of guilt about things done or undone.

Depression: Give permission to be at the point where the patient is. Provide comfort and availability as well as caring for physical needs.

When the patient can no longer deny the reality of the loss, feelings of helplessness and hopelessness replace the feelings of anger. The patient needs information that this is a normal progression of feelings.

Acceptance: Respect the patient's needs and wishes for quiet, privacy, and/or talking.

Has worked through the denial, anger, and depression. Often prefers to be alone and does not want to talk much at this point. Patient may still cling to hope, which can sustain the patient through whatever is happening at this point.

Actively listen and be available to help.

The process of grieving does not proceed in an orderly fashion, rather there are ups and downs with various aspects of all stages present at one time/or another. If process is being dysfunctional, or prolonged, interventions may be helpful in facilitating the process.

Assess needs of significant others and assist as indicated.

Identification of dysfunctional grieving allows for individual interventions.

Assess need for referral to other resources; counseling, psychotherapy as indicated.

May need additional help to resolve situation.

NURSING DIAGNOSIS:	Fear (specify).
SUPPORTING DATA:	Anxiety and dread of an identifiable problem recognized by the patient.
DESIRED PATIENT OUTCOMES:	Fear is clearly identified by the patient who is dealing effectively with the situation.

INTERVENTIONS

Acknowledge fear. Do not deny or "reassure" patient that "everything will be all right."

Give accurate information within the limits of your knowledge.

Be available for listening and talking as needed.

RATIONALE

Feelings are real and it is helpful to bring them out into the open so they can be discussed and dealt with. It is not possible for the nurse to know how the specific situation will be resolved.

Having information allows the patient to deal with realities and this can defuse anxiety and fear.

Establishes rapport and allows patient to express feelings in an accepting atmosphere.

NURSING DIAGNOSIS: Self-concept, disturbance in: body image, self-esteem, role performance, personal identity.

SUPPORTING DATA: A disruption in the way the person perceives own body image, self-esteem, role performance, and/or personal identity. Body image is affected by an actual missing part, a change in structure/function, or how one perceives own body.

DESIRED PATIENT OUTCOMES: Verbalizes realistic view and acceptance of body as it is. Talks about remaining strengths and view of self as capable person. Participates in and assumes responsibility for own health care. Demonstrates acceptance of change in role and/or lifestyle by going on with life within limits of change.

INTERVENTIONS

Establish therapeutic nurse-patient relationship.

See Nursing Diagnosis: Coping, ineffective, individual.

RATIONALE

Patient will be freer to verbalize fears; of rejection, loss of previous function or appearance, helplessness, powerlessness, changes that may be necessary in personal life.

NURSING DIAGNOSIS: Violence, potential for (self-directed or directed at others).

SUPPORTING DATA:	Increasing anxiety, fear, inability to express feelings, anger, argumentative behavior, depression, suicidal ideation or attempt may be indicators of the patient's attempt to deal with the threat to self-concept that illness can represent. These may be expressed in different forms of aggressive behavior directed toward self or others.
DESIRED PATIENT OUTCOMES:	Violent behavior is managed/prevented.

INTERVENTIONS

Observe for early signs of distress.

Accept patient's anger without reacting on an emotional basis.

Remain calm and state limits on behavior in a firm manner. Be truthful.

Give permission to express angry feelings in acceptable ways. Make time to listen to verbalization of these feelings.

Assume that the patient has control and is responsible for own behavior.

Identify conditions that may interfere with ability to control own behavior.

Tell patient to stop.

Help patient identify more adequate solutions. Give as much control as is possible in the situation.

Provide a safe environment; hold patient, restraints, or seclusion. Do so in a calm, pleasant, nonstimulating manner.

Observe for signs of suicidal intent.

Assess intent by asking directly if the person is thinking of suicide or refer to resource/s equipped to deal with situation.

RATIONALE

Irritability, lack of cooperation, demanding behavior may all be signs of increasing anxiety.

Responding with anger is not helpful in resolving the situation and may result in escalating the patient's behavior.

Understanding that helplessness and fear underlie this behavior can be helpful.

Encouraging acceptable expression can be helpful in defusing feelings of helplessness and anger, as well as decreasing guilt.

Will often enable them to exercise control.

Acute/chronic brain syndrome, drug-induced, postsurgical confusion may precipitate violent behavior.

If exhibiting hostile actions, may be sufficient to help patient control own actions. Patient is also afraid of own actions.

Enhance feelings of power and control in situation where many things are not within patient's control.

As a last resort, physical restraint may be necessary while the patient regains control.

Morbid or anxious feelings while with the patient; warning from the patient, "It doesn't matter" "I'd be better off dead;" mood swings, suicidal attempts, putting affairs in order, may all be signals of intent.

Direct question is most helpful when done in a caring, concerned manner.

Provide protection within the environment.

May need to provide constant observation, remove objects that might be used, as well as refer to psychiatric care.

MEDICAL MANAGEMENT

Tranquilizers, sedatives, narcotics, and so forth.

May be indicated to quiet/control behavior. May need to be withheld if they may be the cause of the behavior.

NURSING DIAGNOSIS:	**Sexual dysfunction.**
SUPPORTING DATA:	**Sexuality encompasses the whole person in that person's total environment. Many times problems of illness may be superimposed on already existing problems. Misinformation and/or lack of knowledge; actual/perceived limitations that may be imposed by the illness; physical/psychosocial abuse; conflicts involving values; alterations in achieving sexual satisfaction/relationships with others; and/or change of interest in self or others.**
DESIRED PATIENT OUTCOMES:	**Alterations in and problems of sexuality are recognized and dealt with to the individual's satisfaction.**

INTERVENTIONS

Assess impact of illness/surgery on sexuality.

Be alert to comments and inuendos that may mean the patient has a concern in this area.

Be aware of own feelings about dealing with this area.

Refer to appropriate resources as need indicates.

RATIONALE

Some problems are more obvious than others, such as illness involving the reproductive parts of the body. Others are less obvious, such as sexual values: role in family, mother, wage-earner, single-parent, and so forth.

People are often reluctant and/or embarrassed to ask direct questions about sexual/sexuality concerns.

Nurses/caregivers are often as reluctant and embarrassed in dealing with sexuality issues as most people.

May be someone with comfort level and knowledge who is available; may be necessary to refer to professional resources for additional help and support.

CARE PLAN: Surgical Intervention (Specific Disease Process; Structural Deformity; and/or Trauma Requiring Removal, Replacement, or Repair)

PATIENT DATA BASE

NURSING HISTORY

May present with acute or chronic process with impairment of other bodily systems:

Cardiovascular: may predispose patient to congestive heart failure, pulmonary edema, or vascular stasis leading to thrombus formation.

Respiratory: infections, chronic conditions, and smoking may lead to pneumonia and other respiratory complications.

Immune: deficiencies may result in difficulty with wound healing or even systemic infections.

Renal: may result in inadequate clearance of toxic products, fluid retention or excess losses, and electrolyte imbalances.

Hepatic: in addition to inadequate drug detoxification, deficiency of coagulation factors may occur.

Neurologic: interference with mobility or sensory stimulation may lead to problems of immobility, such as skin breakdown and pneumonia.

Alimentary: malnutrition may be present (even if patient is obese), which can impair wound healing and predispose patient to infections.

Pancreatic: (diabetes) hypoglylcemia/ketoacidosis may occur and be life-threatening. In addition, diabetic patients are predisposed to slow wound-healing and infections.

Take a thorough drug history: patient may be taking anticoagulants, steroids, antibiotics, antihypertensives, cardiotonic glycosides, antiarrhythmics, bronchodilators, diuretics, decongestants, analgesics, sedatives, anti-inflammatories, anticonvulsants, tranquilizers. Be sure to check over-the-counter, street, and recreational drug usage. Not only does the drug history indicate possible health problems, e.g., cardiac arrhythmias, recurrent infections, depression of steroid production; drug actions may be potentiated or reactions may occur when anesthetic agents are administered.

Allergies or sensitivities to medications, food, tape, and solutions may be known. Ascertain type of reaction.

Anesthesia: history of previous experience; difficulty with prior anesthetics by patient or family members may be present; e.g., malignant hyperthermia, hypotensive reactions.

Dietary: information about recent food ingestion, type and amount. Intake is usually limited to nothing by mouth (NPO) 6–12 hours prior to surgery, with the possible exception of premedication, otherwise aspiration may occur if nausea/vomiting are present.

Elimination: emptying of the bladder and bowel should be accomplished prior to surgery. Irregularities or the presence of an indwelling catheter should be noted, as well as time and amount of urine output.

Age: elderly patients do not detoxify drugs as well as younger patients and the stress of illness/surgery may compromise general system functions resulting in multiple postoperative problems.

Psychosocial: plan for preoperative teaching according to patient's/significant others' needs. Significant others may be present in the facility and be anxious about the patient's progress or delays in estimated time of surgery and recovery.

Alcohol intake may be difficult to ascertain, but is very important as the surgical risk is greater and acute withdrawal syndrome may occur during the postoperative period.

Procedure: informed consent to surgical procedure, blood replacement, sterilization, and disposition of body part, if indicated, must be documented.

DIAGNOSTIC STUDIES

General preoperative requirements are: urinalysis, CBC, prothrombin, PTT. Chest x-ray and ECG may be required of patients over age 35, while other studies may be dependent on type of operative procedures, current medications, systemic processes, and age, e.g., BUN, creatinine, glucose, ABG, electrolytes, thyroid studies. Deviations from normal should be corrected, if possible, prior to safe administration of anesthetic agents.

Urinalysis: WBC or bacteria indicate urinary tract infection and must be corrected to decrease incidence of kidney involvement. Pregnancy test: rule out, surgery may be cancelled due to likelihood of damage to the fetus by anesthetic agents.

Complete Blood Count:
WBC, increased: indicative of inflammatory process; may be diagnostic, such as appendicitis; however, other conditions, such as pneumonia, need to be ruled out.
WBC, decreased: indicative of viral processes and must be evaluated as immune system may be dysfunctional.

Hb, decreased: anemia decreases adequate oxygenation of tissues and decreases the Hb available to bind with inhalation anesthetic.

Hct: indicative of dehydration or fluid overload.

Electrolytes: decreased K^+ may affect cardiac muscle function leading to inadequate cardiac output.

ABG: evaluate current status and provide baseline for respiratory function.

Coagulation times: if patient has been taking anticoagulant drugs or large doses of aspirin, clotting times may be prolonged and interfere with hemostasis.

Chest x-ray: should be free of infiltrates, r/o pneumonia. Masses may be identified, and COPD changes may be seen.

ECG: Abnormal findings require attention prior to administering anesthetic.

PHYSICAL EXAMINATION

Vital signs: baseline should be established preoperatively. Abnormal findings are indicative of ongoing disease process or may be symptoms of disease requiring surgical intervention, e.g., bradycardia prior to pacemaker insertion; hypotension from internal bleeding, elevated temperature indicative of inflammatory process, such as appendicitis.

Skin condition: turgor, color, rash, integrity, wounds, decubitus should be evaluated. If preop shave or wash is ordered, area should be examined for breaks in the skin that could harbor bacteria.

Dentition: presence, absence of or loose teeth; partial plates or full dentures should be removed prior to surgery.

Review policies of the institution.

Prosthesis: contact lenses, hearing aids, glasses, artificial limbs must be removed preoperatively.

Jewelry: must be removed and disposed of per patient wishes.

Respiratory status: evaluate for congestion, breathsounds, rales, ronchi, and so forth.

Cardiovascular: evaluate pulse for irregularity, bradycardia, tachycardia. Observe skin perfusion.

Urinary: bladder and bowel elimination should be accomplished prior to surgery. Character and amount of urine should be noted if indwelling catheter is in place.

Mental status: note orientation of patient, level of response/degree of anxiety, inappropriate behavior. Deviations from normal should be documented and communicated to recovery room personnel. Observe effectiveness of preop medication.

NURSING PRIORITIES

1. Minimize patient's anxiety and emotional trauma of operative procedure.
2. Provide for patient's physical safety.
3. Support respiratory status as necessary.
4. Prevent infection, minimize complications.

NURSING DIAGNOSIS:	**Knowledge deficit, process of surgery and postoperative period.**
SUPPORTING DATA:	**Most people facing surgery have very little information about what is going to happen while they are anesthetized, and what to expect as they are recovering.**
DESIRED PATIENT OUTCOMES:	**Patient will ask pertinent questions, and verbalize understanding of what is expected in the postoperative period. Deep breathing exercises will be practiced.**

INTERVENTIONS

Preop Teaching Program to include:

Information about preop and postop procedures and restrictions.

If room change is anticipated, tell patient where patient will wake up.

Instruct in breathing, coughing, leg, and other appropriate exercises.

RATIONALE

Having information about what to expect decreases anxiety about the unknown.

An unexpected change can create anxiety if the patient thinks the change means something has gone wrong.

Practice before surgery is helpful to performance afterward.

NURSING DIAGNOSIS:	**Fear, of the unknown.**
SUPPORTING DATA:	**Lack of knowledge about surgical procedures, possible loss of dignity, fear of dismemberment and/or disfigurement are all fears that may be intensified in the operating room prior to induction of anesthesia.**

628

DESIRED PATIENT OUTCOMES: The patient expresses feelings of comfort and lessened anxiety prior to anesthetic induction.

INTERVENTIONS	RATIONALE
Visit with OR personnel before surgery.	Can provide contact/reassurance, which may alleviate the patient's anxiety as well as provide information for formulating intraoperative care.
Prevent unnecessary body exposure in transfer and in the OR suite.	Sedated patient fears such exposure and is unable to exercise control.
Tell patient your name and what your role is in relation to the surgery. You will be in the surgery, "helping" through the procedure. If possible, go to the patient's room and accompany patient to surgery.	Development of supportive role with the patient can help allay anxiety over "total helplessness."
Assess level of anxiety and possible causes, taking appropriate action.	Some patients may not visibly show anxiety, but need assurance, others may actively verbalize concerns.
Explain things that may frighten patient.	Masks, noises, a child crying, safety belts are easily explained and will help patient feel less frightened.
Acknowledge that unknown environment is frightening.	Can be helpful to reassure that fear is a normal response.
Give simple, concise directions to sedated patient.	Impairment of thought process makes it difficult for patient to understand lengthy instructions.
Compare surgery schedule, chart, and operative consent for correct surgical procedure and verify name and procedure with patient and armband. Sometimes a map of the surgical area is drawn on the body before coming to the OR.	The sedated patient may be misidentified in the OR, and all data including patient's statement must be verified. Facilitate venous drainage where the end result is affected by gravity/upright position, to identify pathology, and to prevent error of doing the wrong procedure.
Control environment for quiet, relaxed anesthetic induction.	Each patient has individual needs for relaxation; conversation, quiet, or physical contact.

NURSING DIAGNOSIS: Injury, potential for, physical.

SUPPORTING DATA: Patients are placed in an unfamiliar environment generally under the effect of hypnotic medication and consequently unable to protect oneself from environment physically and/or psychologically. While under a general anesthetic, the OR nurse must be the advocate and protect the patient.

DESIRED PATIENT OUTCOMES: No injury occurs, or is minimal.

INTERVENTIONS	RATIONALE
Stabilize both patient cart and OR table when transferring patient to/from OR table, using adequate numbers of persons for transfer and support to extremities.	Unstabilized cart and table may separate, causing patient or extremity to fall.
Anticipate movement of extraneous lines and tubes during the transfer and secure or guide them into position.	Prevent undue tension and dislocation of IV lines, NG tubes, indwelling catheters, chest tubes, and so forth.
Secure patient on OR table with safety belt over thighs and arms explaining necessity to the patient.	OR tables and armboards are narrow and patient and or extremity may fall off causing injury. Sedated patient may misinterpret and become anxious and combative.
Prepare equipment and padding for required position according to operative procedure and patient's specific needs.	Depends on individual patient's size, weight, pre-existing conditions. Extra padding materials may be required to protect bony prominences, prevent circulatory compromise, nerve pressure, and allow for optimum chest expansion for ventilation.
Position extremities so they may be periodically checked for safety, circulation, nerve pressure, and alignment.	Hands, fingers, and toes may be inadvertently scraped, pinched, or amputated by moving table attachments, while pressure to brachial plexus, peroneal and ulnar nerves can cause damage. Prolonged plantar flexion may result in foot drop.
Place electrocautery grounding pad over muscle mass insuring its contact to provide maximum conductivity to ground.	Prevent potential for electrical burns by providing path for electricity to ground.
Ascertain electrical safety of equipment used in surgical procedure.	Malfunction of equipment may occur causing electrical short circuits. Electric cords, insulators, equipment and patient grounds must be intact to insure safety of electrical circuits.
Prevent pooling of prep solutions under and around patient.	Prevent both chemical and electrical burns. Antiseptic solutions may chemically burn skin and may also conduct electrical currents.
Confirm and document correct sponge, instrument, needle, and blade count.	Prevent not only postoperative inflammation, infection, possible perforation, and foreign body reactions; but also disastrous complications and death.
Handle and document specimens, insuring proper medium for type of test desired. Expedite specimens to laboratory whenever possible, with proper labeling.	Frozen sections, preserved exam, cultures all have different requirements and the nurse must be aware of specific hospital lab requirements for validity of exam. Proper identification is imperative.

NURSING DIAGNOSIS:	Tissue perfusion, alteration in, anesthesia.
SUPPORTING DATA:	Alterations in cardiovascular and respiratory pattern caused by anesthesia create unstable situation during induction and emergence.

DESIRED PATIENT OUTCOMES:	**Tissue perfusion is maintained during anesthetic phase.**

INTERVENTIONS

Observe patient during induction:cardiac and BP monitor, fasciculations, respirations, and color.

Apply cricoid pressure if indicated.

Monitor arrythmias intraoperatively.

Know location of Datrium, cooling blanket, and iced saline.

Check safety belt, be sure it is secure, and stand by the patient during emergence and extubation.

Accompany patient to recovery room, giving concise report to nurse.

RATIONALE

Available to assist the anesthetist in the event complications arise.

Occasionally required for optimum visualization of larnyx during intubation.

Fluothane and Ethrane anesthetics sensitize the myocardium to catecholamines.

Malignant hyperthermia may occur during anesthesia, and may result in death. Immediate action must be taken to decrease temperature.

"Emergence excitement" may occur and require restraints.

Provides continuity of care.

NURSING DIAGNOSIS:	**Tissue perfusion, alteration in, recovery phase.**
SUPPORTING DATA:	**Anesthetic agents, narcotics, and muscle relaxants paralyze respiratory muscles and cause CNS and myocardial depression. Some anesthetic agents are blown off via respirations and sine wave pattern of emergence, with periods of arousal and depression, necessitate continued vigilance.**
DESIRED PATIENT OUTCOMES:	**Tissue perfusion and respiratory function are maintained during recovery phase.**

INTERVENTIONS

Maintain patent airway by maintaining oral pharyngeal airway, headtilt, or jaw hyperextension.

Observe for return of respiratory function.

RATIONALE

Airway obstruction may still occur with oral airway in place.

After administration of muscle relaxants, return of muscle function occurs first to the diaphragm, intercostals, and larynx; second to large muscle groups, neck, shoulders, and abdominal muscles; third to mid-size muscles, tongue, parynx extensors and flexors; and last to eyes, mouth, face and fingers.

Observe for respiratory rate, depth, use of accessory muscles, chest expansion, retraction or flaring of nostrils, skin color, and air flow.

Listen for gurgling, wheezing, crowing, and silence.

Monitor BP, pulse, respirations q5–15 minutes, evaluate abnormals and take corrective action.

Observe dressing.

Use left lateral, head elevated position and change position often.

Suction as necessary.

Apply warm blankets.

Monitor patient for temperature elevations.

Initiate *stirrup* regimen as soon as patient is reactive and continue well into the postop period.

Observe for cool, clammy extremities in patients who have had Pentothal.

Do not administer epinephrine to fluothane-anesthetized patient.

Change position of fluothane-anesthetized patient slowly in bed and at transfer.

Assess status frequently, evaluating wound condition, cardiovascular and respiratory status, pain, and anxiety thoroughly.

MEDICAL MANAGEMENT

Oxygen.

Ascertain adequacy of respirations immediately so corrective measures may be initiated promptly.

Sounds indicate obstruction by mucus or tongue, corrected by removal. Wheezing would indicate bronchospasm. Crowing and silence indicate partial to total laryngospasm and require immediate action.

Tachycardia may indicate hypoxia, hypovolemia. Hypotension may indicate hypovolemia or pain. Increased respirations indicate hypoxia. Arrythmias may be present.

Bleeding may occur.

Prevents aspiration of vomitus, enhances ventilation to lower lobes, relieves pressure on the diaphragm.

With increased use of droperidol, nausea and vomiting has decreased. If occurs, may indicate hypotension and/or pain.

Maintain body heat. Inhalation anesthetics depress the hypothalamus resulting in poor temperature regulation. Shivering may be seen primarily with fluothane anesthetics.

Patient who is febrile preop may be so postop. Atropine and scopolamine may increase temperature.

Prevent atelectasis and stasis. Active deep ventilations inflate alveoli, break up secretions, increase O_2 transfer, while cough will remove secretions and enhance removal of anesthetic agents from the pulmonary system. Verbal stimulation and repositioning will enhance ventilation to all areas. Active ankle dorsiflexion will promote peripheral circulation.

May effect decrease in peripheral circulation.

Fluothane and Ethrane sensitize the myocardium to catecholamines and may produce arrhythmias.

Vasoconstrictor mechanisms are depressed and quick movement may lead to hypotension.

With combinations of agents used, determining the causative factor may be difficult. Always check airway, comfort, sources of irritation, and adequacy of ventilation. Problem may or may not be related to anesthetic agents.

Aerate lungs to enhance removal of inhalation anesthetic.

Respiratory stimulants/narcotic antagonists.

Dopram, Narcan relieve drug-induced CNS depression.

Increased IV volume.

To correct hypovolemia in fluothane/Ethrane patients.

POSTOPERATIVE PERIOD

NURSING DIAGNOSIS:	Injury, potential for, related to anesthetic.
SUPPORTING DATA:	The postanesthesia patient has an impairment of thought process, may still be under effect of muscle relaxants, and/or paresthesia due to regional anesthesia.
DESIRED PATIENT OUTCOMES:	No injury occurs from confusion or disorientation.

INTERVENTIONS	RATIONALE
Reorient patient verbally and with touch to time, place and person; telling patient that the surgery is over.	Even though patient may appear to be semi/unconscious, it is important to give this information as patient is regaining consciousness to provide support and alleviate anxiety.
Secure side rails in up position and pad sides of the cart.	Prevent injury to extremities and possibility of patient falling out of bed. "Emergence excitement" may occur, which involves thrashing about. Most commonly seen in children or in adults where anxiety level is high.
Secure parenteral lines when indicated.	The combative or disoriented patient may disconnect or pull out lines and/or undue tension may be placed upon them during position changes.
Check IV sites, tubes, and drains for patency and irritation.	Prevent tissue/organ damage and maintain in/out flow.

NURSING DIAGNOSIS:	Comfort, alteration in, pain.
SUPPORTING DATA:	Operative procedure, as the anesthetic agent effects wear off, sensation returns and pain of the incision, retraction of muscles, and other manipulations of the body come into awareness.
DESIRED PATIENT OUTCOMES:	Pain is minimized/controlled, with good muscle relaxation and ventilation.

633

INTERVENTIONS	RATIONALE
Assess causes of possible discomfort, other than operative procedure.	Full bladder, nonpatent indwelling catheter or NG tube, gas accumulation, IV infiltration, stress on incision due to position, compromised circulation due to position/pressure may be sources of discomfort.
Reposition as surgical procedure allows.	Relieve pain caused by pressure, enhance circulation, and increase respiratory functioning.
Assess restlessness.	May be indicative of hypoxia as well as pain.
Deal with anxiety about environment, procedure, and condition. Use relaxation breathing techniques.	May cause muscle rigidity and intensify pain. Slow, controlled breathing with the assistance of a calm, relaxed nurse can be helpful in relaxing tense muscles and easing mental tension.
Assure patient that pain will probably be transitory.	Succinylcholine causes muscle fasciculation and soreness in large and small muscle groups, including the eyelids, up to 48 hours postop. Generally such pain does not require analgesia. Ear and throat discomfort may be a result of intubation irritation.
Listen to patient's complaints, assess increased BP, pulse, respiration rate, nausea, and muscle tension prior to giving analgesia.	May indicate hypoxia as well as pain. Fluothane and Ethrane recovery is short as well as its analgesia effect. However, narcotic administration may have synergistic effects with remaining anesthetic and further depress respirations.
Check anesthetic record for narcotics given intraoperatively.	Narcotic supplementation is frequently done and further narcotic administration needs to be carefully assessed.
Avoid or reduce narcotic dosages 1/4 to 1/3 in patients who have had Innovar or droperidol anesthesia.	Produce profound tranquilization that can potentiate effects of narcotic and barbiturates up to 10 hours after administration of Innovar or droperidol.
When patient has undergone disassociative anesthetic, decrease environmental stimuli by silence, darkening of the area, no verbal or tactile stimuli.	Ketamine anesthetized patients may undergo psychic aberrations upon emergence, which may be intensified by environmental stimuli.
Observe for excessive sommolence; continue to observe respirations.	Pentothal is absorbed in fatty tissue and because of circulation may later be redistributed through the bloodstream, causing delayed somnolence and respiratory depression. After being "awake" for a period of time, these patients may regress and suffer respiratory depression. (There is no antidote for pentothal.)
Retain patient in recovery room for 30 minutes to 1 hour after administration of pain medication.	Evaluate results of medication. Ascertain that vital signs are normal and no synergistic effects have occurred.

NURSING DIAGNOSIS:	**Fluid volume, deficit, potential.**
SUPPORTING DATA:	**Surgical trauma, stress, fluids lost during procedure, and anesthesia**

will alter fluid and electrolyte balance.

DESIRED PATIENT OUTCOMES: Fluid and electrolyte balance is restored/maintained without overload or hypovolemia.

INTERVENTIONS	RATIONALE
Measure and record all output: urine; emesis; NG, ostomy, rectal, chest tube drainage; bleeding; and perspiration.	Excessive drainage will decrease K^+. Urine output less than 30 ml/hour via indwelling catheter may indicate poor renal function or hypovolemia. Stress can promote Na^+ and H_2O retention.
Check anesthesia record for fluid loss and replacement.	May still be low and require further replacement.
Refer to Care Plan: Fluid and Electrolyte Imbalance.	

NURSING DIAGNOSIS: Sensory perception, alterations in.

SUPPORTING DATA: Effects of anesthesia wear off in varying ways with sine wave (undulating) pattern and differing degrees of sensory awareness.

DESIRED PATIENT OUTCOMES: Alterations in sensory perception are recognized and managed effectively.

INTERVENTIONS	RATIONALE
Speak in normal, clear voice without shouting, being aware of what you are saying.	Sense of hearing returns first, so it is important not to say things that may be heard and perhaps misinterpreted.
Explain procedures even if patient does not seem to respond.	Cannot tell when patient is aware and information is important as patient is recovering.
Minimize discussion of negatives, such as patient and personnel problems, within patient's hearing.	When sensory awareness is altered patients may misinterpret and believe references are to them.

NURSING DIAGNOSIS: Airway clearance, ineffective.

SUPPORTING DATA: Sedation and pain may reduce respiratory effort resulting in pneumonia, atelectasis, and so forth. May also have allergic reactions to drugs resulting in edema of the larynx.

635

DESIRED PATIENT OUTCOMES:	Airway remains clear and no problems occur.

INTERVENTIONS

RATIONALE

Change position q2h or more often.	Enhances aeration of dependent lobes.
Deep breaths/cough on a regular basis. Splint incision with above activity.	Encourages ventilation and mobilizes secretions. Supports wound and allows greater effort from patient.
Note temperature increase.	If this occurs early postop, most frequently indicates respiratory problems/pneumonia.
Note signs of abdominal distention.	Limits movement of the diaphragm.
Encourage oral fluid intake, if able.	Adequate hydration thins secretions.
Assess breath sounds.	Presence of rhonchi indicates need for increased clearing of secretions. Diminished breath sounds may indicate atelectasis.

MEDICAL MANAGEMENT

Oxygen, IPPB, incentive spirometry.	Improve ventilation/minimize atelectasis.
Antibiotics.	Prevent/combat infections.
Vaporizor/mist mask.	Increase inspired moisture and help liquify secretions.

NURSING DIAGNOSIS:	Nutrition, alteration in, less than body requirements.
SUPPORTING DATA:	Nausea/vomiting secondary to decreased motility, ileus formation caused by intraoperative manipulation of abdominal organs, side effect of narcotics, or psychologic component: patient believes N & V to be a normal response after surgery.
DESIRED PATIENT OUTCOMES:	Nausea/vomiting is minimized/controlled, nutritional balance is maintained, weight loss does not occur.

INTERVENTIONS

RATIONALE

Be aware of drug sensitivities/reactions.	Narcotics may cause nausea/vomiting.
Give oral care after emesis.	Clean mouth diminishes nausea.

Note type/amount of emesis.

Indicative of complications, such as GI bleed or ileus.

Do not start fluids until bowel sounds are present, then begin with hot tea or sips of carbonated beverage.

Fluid may accumulate in the stomach if peristalsis is decreased and result in emesis.

Note type, location, and frequency of abdominal pain.

Obstruction is most common between 3rd and 5th postop day and may present as intermittent, localized, sharp, colicky pain.

Assess response to diet.

Tolerance determines dietary changes.

MEDICAL MANAGEMENT

Antiemetics.

Diminish/control nausea.

Cimetidine.

May be used to decrease gastric secretions.

NG tube.

Relieves abdominal distention.

Advance diet as tolerated.

Even though bowel activity may be present distention may occur if gastric motility is decreased.

Hyperalimentation (TPN).

If oral intake is restricted for an extended period may be helpful in preventing malnutrition and attendant problems of healing. (Refer to Care Plan: Total Parenteral Nutrition.)

NURSING DIAGNOSIS:	**Skin integrity, impairment of, potential.**
SUPPORTING DATA:	**Incision provides an entry for bacteria, other factors may interfere with healing.**
DESIRED PATIENT OUTCOMES:	**Skin integrity is maintained and healing occurs without untoward incidence.**

INTERVENTIONS

RATIONALE

Initially cover the wound.

Protects from mechanical injury and contamination.

Splint wound with pillow or pad during coughing.

Equalizes pressure on the wound and minimizes rupture.

Change dressings frequently when drains are present.

Minimize skin irritation.

Note type/amount of drainage.

Assess early progression of wound healing/development of hemorrhage or infection.

Apply protective ointment around wound if gastric drainage is present.

Minimizes excoriation by acid drainage, macerated skin may serve as growth media for bacteria.

MEDICAL MANAGEMENT

Hemovac or sump suctioning.

Facilitate wound healing by removal of fluid that might prevent tissue granulation or serve as media for infection.

NURSING DIAGNOSIS:	**Urinary elimination, alteration in pattern.**
SUPPORTING DATA:	**Spasm of bladder sphincter or obstruction by tissue edema. Psychologic factors of using a bedpan, such as the taboo of urinating in bed.**
DESIRED PATIENT OUTCOMES:	**Voiding occurs without complications.**

INTERVENTIONS

Routine measures for voiding: privacy, sit/stand if able, running water.

Note time and amount of voiding.

RATIONALE

Some patients are unable to void lying down; psychologic aid of hearing water running.

Frequent/small amounts may indicate retention with overflow.

MEDICAL MANAGEMENT

Catheterize.

Only if other measures fail. Bladder distention can cause injury to organ, reflux and infection, or trauma to operative area/incision.

NURSING DIAGNOSIS:	**Thought processes, alterations.**
SUPPORTING DATA:	**Occasionally delirium occurs in some patients postoperatively. Most commonly, this is the result of sepsis, trauma, or alcohol.**
DESIRED PATIENT OUTCOMES:	**Delirium is controlled and thought processes are within patient norm.**

INTERVENTIONS

Observe for restlessness, increased temperature and pulse, and flushed face.

Force fluids as necessary. (May be contraindicated in the presence of cerebral edema.)

RATIONALE

May indicate mental confusion in presence of a toxic condition.

Aids in the elimination of toxins when sepsis is the cause.

Observe for hallucinations, delusions, depression, or an excited state.

May develop following trauma and indicate delirium. In patient who has used alcohol to excess, may indicate impending delirium tremens. See Care Plan: Chemical Dependency: Alcohol.

Speak to patient in a calm voice; respond to hallucinations and delusions with reality orientation; touch as appropriate.

Can be helpful in calming the patient and reorienting to reality. Some patients do not tolerate being touched when they are disoriented/confused.

Tell significant others what is happening and that the condition is most likely temporary.

Disturbed behavior can be very frightening to observers when they do not know what is happening and information can be helpful in decreasing their anxiety.

MEDICAL MANAGEMENT

IV therapy.

If unable to give sufficient fluids by mouth.

Tranquilizing drugs.

Useful in traumatic delirium.

Refer to Care Plans: Impaired Peripheral Vascular Function, for discussion of Thrombophlebitis; Pulmonary Embolus; Chemical Dependence: for Alcohol, for discussion of delirium tremens.

CARE PLAN: Long-Term Care

Patients in the acute care setting may to be discharged to an extended care facility and patients in long-term care may need to return for acute care. Coordination and knowledge are an essential part of this process to maintain quality care for these people. Long-term care facilities (extended care) present a different image from the small nursing home of a decade ago. Standards of care and periodic inspections by local and state health departments determine compliance and licensure. Choosing a facility can be a personal choice involving visiting different centers; talking with staff, patients, and families and asking questions. The needs of the patient, e.g., physical, occupational therapy, rehabilitation are frequently the deciding factors for choice.

DIAGNOSTIC STUDIES

Electrocardiogram for baseline data and to detect abnormalities.

Chest x-ray: size of heart, lung abnormalities, tuberculosis, COPD, and changes of the large blood vessels and bony structure of the chest.

Tonometer test, measure intraocular pressure for glaucoma; and visual acuity testing for the presence of cataracts and other vision problems.

Pap smear test for cancer of the cervix.

CBC and urinalysis.

NURSING PRIORITIES

1. Review all disease entities present and current therapies.
2. Encourage continuation of old habits, individual needs and wishes.
3. Provide for security and safety.
4. Prevent/minimize complications of disease and/or aging process.
5. Promote/enhance patient's/significant others' coping skills.

NURSING DIAGNOSIS:	**Sleep-pattern, disturbance in.**
SUPPORTING DATA:	**Difficulty getting to sleep in new environment.**
DESIRED PATIENT OUTCOMES:	**Patient is sleeping a satisfactory amount of time and wakens feeling rested.**

INTERVENTIONS

Determine normal sleep habits.

Establish routine suitable to old pattern and new environment.

Obtain comfortable bedding. Allow some of own possessions, such as pillow, afghan.

Allow position of comfort, assist in turning.

Instruct in relaxation measures.

RATIONALE

Assess need for intervention.

Helpful when new routine contains as many old habits as possible.

Increases comfort for sleep as well as physiologic support.

Repositioning alters areas of pressure and promotes rest.

Induce sleep.

Reduce noise and light.

Warm bath and massage at bedtime.

Warm milk, wine, or brandy at H.S.

Side rails as indicated.

Provide atmosphere conducive to sleep.

Relaxing.

Soothing effect. Milk has soporific qualities.

May have fear of falling because of change in size and height of bed. Provide safety and may be used to assist in turning.

MEDICAL MANAGEMENT

Sedatives, hypnotics.

Assist in transition period. (Avoid habitual use as these drugs further decrease REM sleep.)

NURSING DIAGNOSIS:	Fear, new and unknown situation.
SUPPORTING DATA:	Financial problems; trauma of admission; may be sharing a room with a stranger; room may not be desirable; communication among family members, patient, and staff may be difficult.
DESIRED PATIENT OUTCOMES:	Existing problems will be addressed/resolved. Communication among individuals will be increasingly effective. Patient will verbalize lessened fear.

INTERVENTIONS

Provide patient/SO with copy of "Patient Rights" and discuss with them.

Determine attitude toward admission to facility.

Assess level of anxiety and note reasons.

Make time to listen to patient about concerns, and allow free expression of feelings; anger, hostility, fear, and loneliness.

Develop nurse/patient relationship.

Orient to physical aspects of the facility, schedules and activities. Introduce to roommate/s and staff. Give explanations of roles.

Provide above information in written form as well.

RATIONALE

Provides information that can foster confidence that individual rights do continue in this setting and the patient is still "his own person."

When patient is giving up own home and way of life, loss and grieving are to be expected.

Will be able to deal more realistically with specific problems when they are identified.

Being available in this way allows the patient to feel accepted, begin to acknowledge and deal with feelings related to circumstances of admission.

Trusting relationships between patient/SO/staff can enable optimal care and support to be given.

Getting acquainted is an important part of admission. Knowledge of where things are and who patient can expect help from can be helpful in reducing anxiety.

Overload of information is difficult to remember. Patient can refer to written material as needed.

Give careful thought to room placement. May need help and encouragement to place own belongings around room.

Location, roommate compatibility, and place for personal belongings are important considerations for helping the patient feel "at home." Changes are often met with resistance and can result in emotional upset and decline in physical condition.

Refer to Social Service or other appropriate agency for assistance. If patient is on Medicare/Medicaid, have social worker discuss ramifications.

Often patient is not aware of the resources available. Will provide current information about individual coverage and other possible sources of support.

NURSING DIAGNOSIS: **Coping, ineffective, family.**

SUPPORTING DATA: **Varying circumstances leading to long-term placement, may lead to feelings of guilt on the part of the family. Cultural factors relating to care of the disabled and/or elderly will affect relationships between patient and significant others. Unacknowledged fears of death may interfere with patient/significant others' relationship.**

DESIRED PATIENT OUTCOMES: **Effective communication will be established with patient, SO, and staff.**

INTERVENTIONS

RATIONALE

Introduce staff and provide SO with information about the facility and the care. Be available for questions.

Helpful to establish beginning relationships. Offer opportunities for enhancing feelings of involvement. Feelings of dissatisfaction with the staff may be transferred to the patient.

Encourage SO's participation in care at level of desire and capability and within limits of safety.

Helpful to feel at ease and allow them to feel supportive and a part of the patient's life.

Accept choices of SO regarding level of involvement in care and be aware of staff's own feelings of anger and frustration about choices that differ.

May choose to ignore patient or project feelings of guilt in criticism of staff.

Identify feelings (staff) and deal with appropriately.

Group care planning or individual counseling may be indicated.

NURSING DIAGNOSIS: **Communication, impaired verbal.**

SUPPORTING DATA: **Hearing loss, aphasia, dysarthria, disorientation secondary to degenerative changes, progressive neurologic disease, Parkinson's disease, and laryngectomy are some**

of the problems that may interfere with communication.

DESIRED PATIENT OUTCOMES: Effective communication will be established.

INTERVENTIONS

Assess reason for lack of communication; including functioning of CNS, reflexes, and auditory system.

Check for excess cerumen, treat as necessary.

Assess patient knowledge base and level of comprehension.

Be aware that behavioral problems may indicate hearing loss.

Get attention by turning a light off and on; touching patient or mattress.

Make eye contact, lower self to patient's level and speak face to face.

Use other creative measures to assist in communication, e.g., picture chart, alphabet board.

May use sign language.

Establish therapeutic nurse-patient relationship through active listening, being available for problem-solving, and so forth.

Speak slowly and distinctly using simple sentences, yes or no questions. Avoid speaking loudly or shouting. Supplement with written communication. Allow sufficient time for reply; remain relaxed and patient.

MEDICAL MANAGEMENT

Refer to speech therapist, or for audiometry as needed to determine extent of hearing loss and whether a hearing aid is appropriate.

RATIONALE

Identification of the problem is essential to appropriate interventions. Sometimes patients do not want to talk; may think they talk when they don't; may expect others to know what they want; may not be able to comprehend or be understood.

Hardened ear wax may decrease hearing acuity and cause tinnitus.

Important to treat as an adult, avoiding pity and impatience.

Anger, explosive temper outbursts, frustration, embarrassment, depression, withdrawal, and paranoia may be attempts to deal with communication problems.

Necessary first step to communication.

Convey interest and promote contact.

Many options available depending on individual situation.

Some patients may already know, others can learn.

Important aspect of dealing with communication problems.

Assists in comprehension and overall communication. Responds poorly to high-pitched sounds; shouting also obscures consonants and amplifies vowels.

May be helpful to patient and staff in improving communication. Testing may ascertain precise nature of the hearing deficit. Some sources believe 90% of the patients in long-term care facilities have some degree of loss. Presbycusis is a common age change. Hearing aids are most effective with conductive losses and may help with sensorineural losses.

NURSING DIAGNOSIS:	Sensory perception, alterations in.
SUPPORTING DATA:	Impairment of vision occurs for a variety of reasons in patients in extended care facilities.
DESIRED PATIENT OUTCOMES:	Impairment is recognized/treated.

INTERVENTIONS

Provide for eye examination at specified intervals and as necessary.

Provide for environmental changes to meet visual deficiencies.

Speak to the patient when you enter the room and let patient know when you leave.

Encourage the patient with glasses to wear them.

Refer to Care Plan: Ocular Disorders and Surgery.

RATIONALE

To identify myopia, hyperopia, presbyopia, astigmatism, cataract and glaucoma development, tunnel vision, and blindness.

To prevent accidents and sensory deprivation. If patient is blind, will need to be oriented to surroundings.

Special actions are helpful when the patient is blind.

If patient is not wearing them, may require adjustment or indicate a need for a change in correction.

NURSING DIAGNOSIS:	Injury, potential for, drug therapy.
SUPPORTING DATA:	Reduced metabolism, impaired circulation, precarious physiologic balance and multiple diseases and drugs may lead to untoward effects.
DESIRED PATIENT OUTCOMES:	Untoward drug effects are minimized/avoided.

INTERVENTIONS

Determine allergy and other past drug history.

Determine interferences with swallowing or reluctance to take tablets or capsules.

May need to open capsule or crush tablets and make sure medication has been taken.

Observe for changes in condition or behavior.

RATIONALE

Can avoid repetition of problems.

May not be able or want to take medication.

Enable proper dosage. Should not be done unless absolutely necessary as this may alter absorption of medications, e.g., enteric coated tablets may be absorbed in stomach when crushed, instead of the intestines.

Allows for early identification of problems and intervention. Behavior may be the only indication of drug toxicity.

Monitor patient's drug regimen.	Need to be aware of possible interactions.

Use resources for information and be aware of toxic symptoms and side effects.

Pharmacist and drug information manuals can be helpful. Toxicity can be increased in the debilitated and older patient with symptoms not as apparent.

Consult with the physician about decrease in dosage.

Smaller dosage may be effective when metabolism is reduced or circulation altered.

Use discretion in the use of p.r.n. medication.

Convenience of the staff is never a reason for sedating patients though rights of other patients need to be taken into consideration. If patient is destructive or excessively disruptive, pharmacologic or mechanical control measures may be required. A quiet place where the patient can pace or seclusion may be helpful.

Post drug interaction charts, lists of medications that are given with or without foods, as well as those that should not be crushed.

Handy reference for all staff administering medications.

NURSING DIAGNOSIS: Injury, potential for, infection.

SUPPORTING DATA: Immobility and sedentary activities may predispose to increased risk of respiratory, bladder, and/or other infections. Decrease in the elasticity of lungs and chest wall, increased collagen deposits and scar tissue in the lungs, and decreased blood flow can contribute to lessened total lung capacity and decreased function. Urinary stasis, presence of a catheter, and so forth can lead to problems of bladder infections with the possibility of kidney involvement.

DESIRED PATIENT OUTCOMES: Respiratory, bladder infections are avoided/treated promptly and effectively.

INTERVENTIONS

Observe for temperature elevation and monitor as necessary.

Encourage to stop smoking.

Protect from exposure to infections and avoid extremes of temperatures in the environment.

RATIONALE

Early identification of onset.

Prone to bronchitis and ineffective clearing of secretions.

Staff and/or visitors may have colds and so forth, which may require the wearing of a mask or other interventions.

Maintain adequate hydration.

Thins pulmonary secretions and promotes urinary output.

Do pericare daily and p.r.n.

Decrease opportunity for infection.

Institute bladder program, including scheduled voiding times, Kegel exercises, and so forth.

Assist in keeping patient dry and helpful in maintaining self-esteem.

Provide routine catheter care and maintain patency if indwelling catheter is present.

Prevent infection and/or minimize reflux if infection present.

Encourage intake of cranberry juice.

Internal pH acidifier to retard bacterial growth.

MEDICAL MANAGEMENT

Antibiotics.

Treat infection.

Vitamin C.

Bladder pH acidifier.

Irrigate catheter with acetic acid.

May be done to maintain acid pH and retard bacterial growth.

Refer to Care Plan: Urinary Tract Infection.

NURSING DIAGNOSIS: **Urinary elimination, alteration in pattern.**

SUPPORTING DATA: **Incontinence is a problem of a large percentage of the chronically ill and elderly. When the reason is not physiologic, other factors may be involved, such as fear, confusion, apathy (on part of patient and/or staff), or nutritional problems.**

DESIRED PATIENT OUTCOMES: **Elimination is managed/controlled by successful bladder training program or indwelling catheter.**

INTERVENTIONS

RATIONALE

Assess reasons for incontinence.

Essential to plan for care.

Avoid verbal or nonverbal signs of rejection, disgust or disapproval over failures.

Not helpful to success.

Institute bladder training program, involving patient and staff in a positive manner.

More apt to be successful when positive attitudes and cooperation are present.

Use diapers with frequent skin care.

When training is unsuccessful this is the preferred method of management.

MEDICAL MANAGEMENT

Medications, e.g., Ditropan.

Promote sphincter control.

Indwelling catheter.

May be used if training is unsuccessful, catheter can prevent skin breakdown and resultant problems.

NURSING DIAGNOSIS:	Bowel elimination, alteration in, constipation.
SUPPORTING DATA:	Can be complex problem related to nutrition, poor muscle tone, level of activity.
DESIRED PATIENT OUTCOMES:	Regular bowel elimination occurs.

INTERVENTIONS

Assess reasons for problems. rule out medical causes; e.g., cancer, hemorrhoids, drugs.

Institute individual program of exercise, rest, diet and bowel-retraining.

Add bulk to the diet in the form of whole grain cereals, breads, and so forth.

Assess fluid intake and promote adequate amount.

Use laxatives and enemas sparingly. Assess previous long-term laxative use.

RATIONALE

Initial step for solution.

Will depend on the needs of the person. Loss of muscular tone reduces peristalsis.

Improve stool consistency.

Promotes normal consistency.

Important to establish as near normal functioning as possible. Many patients are already laxative-dependent.

MEDICAL MANAGEMENT

Metamucil or other bulk-providers and/or stool softeners.

May be necessary to promote regularity by increasing bulk and/or improving consistency.

NURSING DIAGNOSIS:	Bowel elimination, alteration in, diarrhea.
SUPPORTING DATA:	Medical causes, medication, or diet may be factors.
DESIRED PATIENT OUTCOMES:	Diarrhea controlled and/or normal bowel functioning restored.

INTERVENTIONS

Assess causes of diarrhea, ruling out illnesses and checking for fecal impaction.

Keep patient clean and dry.

RATIONALE

Important to identify and treat disease entity.

Prevent skin breakdown.

MEDICAL MANAGEMENT

Paregoric, Lomotil.

May be necessary on a short-term basis when diarrhea persists.

NURSING DIAGNOSIS:	**Skin integrity, impairment of, potential.**
SUPPORTING DATA:	**General debilitation, reduced mobility, changes in skin and muscle mass associated with aging, bladder and bowel incontinence, and problems of self-care may be involved.**
DESIRED PATIENT OUTCOMES:	**Breaks in skin integrity prevented/treated promptly.**

INTERVENTIONS

Maintain strict skin hygiene, using mild, nondetergent soap (if any), drying gently and thoroughly, and lubricating with lotion or emollient. Massage bony prominences gently with lotion or cream.

Change position q2h or more often, in bed or chair. Recommend 10 minutes of exercise each hour as well as passive range of motion.

Use a rotation schedule in turning patient on all four sides, unless contraindicated.

Keep sheets and becclothing taut, clean, dry, and free from crumbs and other irritating material.

Use pads, pillows, sheepskin, waterbeds, alternating pressure/eggcrate mattress or chair.

Observe for decubitus ulcer development and treat immediately.

Provide for safety during ambulation.

Provide for foot and nail care.

Check for fissures between toes. Swab with hydrogen peroxide or dust with antiseptic powder and place a wisp of cotton between the toes.

RATIONALE

Cleanses skin of waste material and keeps it soft and pliable. These areas are susceptible to breakdown as epidermis thins with age. Promotes venous return, increases vascular tone, and reduces edema.

Improves circulation, muscle tone, and joint motion and promotes activity.

Allows for longer periods free of pressure.

Avoids friction/abrasions of skin.

Provides protection and improves circulation by changing amount of pressure on skin and/or eliminating pressure.

Avoid extensive damage. See Nursing Diagnosis: Skin integrity, impairment of, actual, decubitus ulcer.

Loss of muscle control and debilitation may result in loss of coordination.

Foot problems are common among this population. Jagged, rough nails can cause infection by scratching adjacent skin areas.

Promote healing.

Rub feet with witch hazel or a mentholated preparation and have patient wear light-weight cotton stockings.

Even though rash may not be present burning and itching may be a problem. Witch hazel may be contraindicated if skin is dry.

NURSING DIAGNOSIS:	**Skin integrity, impairment of, actual, decubitus ulcer.**
SUPPORTING DATA:	**Pressure on skin and subcutaneous tissues in the presence of immobilization, sensory and motor deficits, poor nutrition, edema, irritation of friction, and moisture can create localized areas of ischemia leading to necrosis. Commonly occur on bony prominences, such as sacrum, ischial tuberosities, greater trochanter, heels, malleoli, and elbows.**
DESIRED PATIENT OUTCOMES:	**Decubitus minimized/healed.**

INTERVENTIONS

Anticipate and use preventive measures in patients who are at risk, such as anyone who is thin, obese, aging, or debilitated.

Assess nutritional status and initiate corrective measures as indicated.

Monitor hemoglobin, hematocrit, and blood sugar levels.

When reddened areas are noted, increase preventive measures.

When break in skin occurs; continue regimen for redness and irritation.

Cleanse the ulcer daily.

Change dressings daily or more often. Employ sterile dressing technique, using light dressings. Avoid cross-contamination of pads, devices, and medications.

Expose ulcer to air and sunlight.

MEDICAL MANAGEMENT

Whirlpool treatments.

RATIONALE

Decubitus ulcers are difficult to heal and prevention is the best treatment.

A positive nitrogen balance and improved nutritional state including increased protein intake can help prevent and heal ulcer. May need additional calories and protein because of loss from draining ulcer.

Anemia and elevated blood sugar levels are factors in skin breakdown.

Necrosis can occur quickly with potential for infection, possibly involving the muscle and bone.

Aggressive measures are important as decubitus can develop in a matter of a few hours.

Removes dead tissue and allows for new epidermis to form.

Wet or soiled dressings potentiate skin breakdown. Prevents infections. Allows for air circulation and skin respiration.

Aids in healing.

Increase circulation and have a debriding action.

Topical applications: skin barriers; collagenase therapy; absorbable gelatin sponges; aerosol sprays.	There are differing opinions about the efficacy of these agents.
Iron and Vitamin C.	Aid in healing.
Skin grafting.	To close large ulcer and allow for healing.

NURSING DIAGNOSIS:	**Self-care deficit, activities of daily living.**
SUPPORTING DATA:	**Depression, discouragement, loss of mobility, general debilitation can affect ability to care for oneself.**
DESIRED PATIENT OUTCOMES:	**Cares for self to level of ability.**

INTERVENTIONS	RATIONALE
Evaluate problem using other team members as indicated.	Helpful to include all disciplines in plan of care.
Involve patient in formulation of care plan at level of ability.	Enhances sense of control and aids in cooperation and development of skills.
Work with present abilities, don't pressure beyond capabilities.	Failure can produce discouragement and depression.
Encourage self care in bathing, using milk lotion or oil and being sure to dry thoroughly.	Doing for oneself enhances feeling of self-worth. A daily bath is usually not necessary as there is less waste secretion on skin surface due to atrophy of sebaceous and sweat glands and bathing may create dry skin problems.
Give tub bath, using a two-person or mechanical lift if necessary. Use shower with a chair and spray attachment, avoid chilling.	Provide safety for those who cannot get into the tub alone. Shower may be more feasible for some patients.
Provide and promote privacy.	Important to self-esteem.
Shampoo hair and encourage use of barber/beauty parlor regularly.	Can aid in preserving dignity of the patient by enhancing self-image and self-esteem.

NURSING DIAGNOSIS:	**Nutrition, alteration in, less than body requirements.**
SUPPORTING DATA:	**Dentition, dulling of senses of smell and taste, problems of poor self-care and general debilitation can lead to poor nutritional status.**
DESIRED PATIENT OUTCOMES:	**Nutritional intake is adequate and normal weight is maintained/regained.**

650

INTERVENTIONS

Weigh on admission and on a regular basis.

Observe condition of skin, such as muscle-wasting and signs of poor healing, brittle nails and dry lifeless hair.

Give high-protein, high-carbohydrate diet, with protein supplements between meals, as tolerated. May require smaller feedings.

Check the state of the patient's dental health, including the fit of dentures, if present.

Maintain as near normal diet as possible, e.g., pureed or finely ground food with gravy or liquid added (avoid baby food).

Promote the use of spices (other than sodium) to the patient's personal taste.

Promote pleasant environment for eating, with company if possible.

MEDICAL MANAGEMENT

Blood chemistry analysis.

RATIONALE

Indicator of nutritional state.

Reflect lack of proper nutrition.

The body's ability to process protein may decrease with age. Calories need to be adjusted to individual need due to decreased metabolic rate and decreased levels of activity. Decreased gastric motility causes patient to feel full and decrease intake.

Oral infections/dental problems, shrinking gums with resultant loose denture fit decrease ability to chew.

Aid in maintaining intake, especially when mouth and dental problems exist. Baby food is often unpalatable.

Decreased number of taste buds results in food tasting bland.

Eating is in part a social event and appetite can improve with increased socialization.

For total protein determination.

NURSING DIAGNOSIS:	Thought processes, alterations in, memory deficits.
SUPPORTING DATA:	Some changes that occur with aging are compensated for by the brain, such as loss of cells and atrophy. Decrease in blood supply to the brain may result in slower reaction times, gradual memory loss and personality changes.
DESIRED PATIENT OUTCOMES:	Thinking and behavior changes are recognized and dealt with effectively within individual abilities.

INTERVENTIONS

Allow more time for patient to respond to questions and/or comments and make decisions.

Discuss happenings of the past.

RATIONALE

Reaction time can be slowed with aging.

These will be more readily available to them, as short-term memory loss may occur. Reminiscence and life review has been shown to be beneficial.

Accept patient's problem of short-term memory loss, providing patient with aids, such as calendars, clocks, to assist in continual reorientation.

Usually not in patient's control and less frustrating if simple reminders are used. Helpful for older person to know that short-term memory loss is common and is not necessarily a sign of "senility."

Assess individual stress level and deal with appropriately.

Some conflicts that occur with age come from previously unresolved problems and may need to be dealt with now.

Assess psychiatric symptoms. Interventions appropriate to the findings.

Not all mental changes are the result of aging and it is important to rule out physical causes before accepting these as unchangeable. May be the result of metabolic, toxic, drug-induced, infectious, cardiac and respiratory disorders.

For further information and care of the confused patient: Refer to Care Plan: Alzheimer's Disease.

NURSING DIAGNOSIS:	**Grieving, anticipatory.**
SUPPORTING DATA:	**Patients in long-term care facilities see death of others and have more awareness of the possibility of their own deaths. Often cultural beliefs about aging and admission to an extended care facility mean they are "waiting to die."**
DESIRED PATIENT OUTCOMES:	**Patients discuss and deal with feelings of loss and grief by participating to the level of their ability in daily activities.**

INTERVENTIONS

RATIONALE

Assess emotional state.

Anxiety and depression are common.

Make time to listen to the patient. Allow free expressions of hopeless feelings and desire to die.

More helpful to allow these feelings to be expressed and dealt with, than to deny them.

Assess suicide potential.

Related to physical disease, social isolation, and grief and is more common in men.

Involve significant others in discussions and activities to the level of their willingness.

When significant others are involved, there is more potential for successful problem-solving. (May not choose to be involved.)

Refer to other resources as indicated, clinical specialist, social worker, and so forth.

May need further assistance to resolve some difficulties.

DIAGNOSIS: Chemical Dependency: Alcohol

The use of drugs is widespread in our society and while there is information available about abuse and dependency, problems with alcohol, amphetamines, barbiturates, and narcotics, as well as many other prescription and over-the-counter (OTC) drugs continue. Abuse is the overuse and/or continuing use of drugs for other than legitimate medical reasons. Dependency refers to both psychologic and physical desire/need to continue taking the drug/s, increasing the dose, and having detrimental effects on the individual and/or society.

PATIENT DATA BASE

NURSING HISTORY

History of accidents, chronic absenteeism from work, family discord.

History of drinking/drug use. Determine pattern, amount and recent ingestion of alcohol/drugs.

Poor sleeping patterns (insomnia), lapses of memory.

History of poor dietary intake.

History of chronic infections, pancreatitis, liver dysfunction, hepatitis, lung problems.

May have lost driver's license secondary to alcohol (drug) abuse.

May have history of seizures/blackouts.

DIAGNOSTIC STUDIES

Blood alcohol levels: may be elevated.

Electrolytes: baseline.

ABGs: check for hypoxia.

SGOT: elevated; SGPT, normal.

Decreased magnesium, increased bilirubin level, decreased hct, increased glucose, increased lipids.

CBC: macrocytic anemia may be present.

Culture/sensitivities: urine and blood. May have low-grade infection.

Drug screen: determine type of drug/s currently in body.

PHYSICAL EXAMINATION

Signs of dehydration, shakiness, flushed skin, dermatitis, bruises, petechiae.

Smell of alcohol on breath

Vital signs: may be increased; blood pressure: may be hypotensive.

GI exam: may reveal symptoms of gastritis.

Tachycardia, diaphoresis, and fever.

Mental status exam: disorientation, hallucinations, restlessness and agitation, verbal confusion, memory loss, irritability, seizures may occur.

Edema, ascites may be present.

Congestive heart failure secondary to cardiomegaly related to alcohol effect on myocardial cells. Arrthymias may be present.

Weight: may be below normal when malnutrition is present.

Neurologic exam: may reveal numbness of extremities, peripheral neuropathy, need to rule out cerebral hemorrhage, meningitis, subdural hematoma.

Alcoholic psychosis (Korsakoff's) secondary to thiamine deficiency may be present with excellent immediate recall but failure to retain information for even a brief period. Confabulation may be present.

May have slurred speech if acute alcohol intoxication is present.

Rule out preexisting disease states (COPD, TB, pneumonia) and current injuries.

NURSING PRIORITIES

1. Maintain adequate airway.
2. Maintain hydration and tissue perfusion.
3. Provide information and support for lifestyle changes and rehabilitation.

NURSING DIAGNOSIS:	Breathing patterns, alterations in.
SUPPORTING DATA:	Alcohol has a depressant effect on the central nervous system and may inhibit the respiratory centers.
DESIRED PATIENT OUTCOMES:	Airway/respirations are maintained at a satisfactory level.

INTERVENTIONS

Observe for respiratory depression.

Observe for nausea/vomiting and position on side.

Monitor vital signs.

Monitor arterial blood gases.

Observe for drowsiness, incoordination, slurred speech, and coma.

MEDICAL MANAGEMENT

IV therapy.

Oxygen.

Ventilatory assistance.

Vasopressors.

RATIONALE

May have ingested large amount of alcohol prior to admission and respirations may be depressed to the point of arrest.

In depressed state, may aspirate vomitus.

When patient is "sleeping off" the intoxicated state, severe depression of the central nervous system and death can occur.

Hypoxia may be due to hypoventilation/acid-base imbalances.

Indicators of extent of CNS depression.

Replacement for fluids is necessary when patient is dehydrated from inadequate intake, diaphoresis, and increased renal output.

Maintain arterial PO_2 at desired level.

If unable to breathe on own, may need mechanical assistance. Refer to Care Plan: Ventilatory Assistance (Mechanical).

Increase BP.

NURSING DIAGNOSIS:	**Sensory perception, alterations in, delerium tremens.**
SUPPORTING DATA:	**Abrupt withdrawal after drinking for a period can result in an acute psychotic state.**
DESIRED PATIENT OUTCOMES:	**Delirium is averted/treated with minimal/no complications.**

INTERVENTIONS

Observe for restlessness, anxiety/uncontrolled fear.

Monitor vital signs, lab results, Clinitest/Acetest frequently.

Monitor for signs of complications.

Observe for signs of seizure activity.

Keep light on and close doors in room to quiet environment.

Explain nursing actions and visual hallucinations.

Speak and move slowly and calmly.

Have someone stay with patient; nurse, significant other, or sitter.

Promote fluid intake, including orange juice and liquids high in carbohydrates.

Observe for signs/symptoms of neuritis and amnesic mental changes.

RATIONALE

May indicate onset of delirium tremens.

Decreasing signs may indicate impending circulatory collapse, increasing temperature may indicate hyperthermia. Hypoglycemia may occur because alcohol depletes liver glycogen stores and impairs gluconeogenesis.

Altered breath sounds, edema may indicate onset of pneumonia/congestive heart failure; liver studies may indicate the presence of cirrhosis.

May experience convulsions during withdrawal. Refer to Care Plan: Seizure Disorders.

Decrease visual hallucinations and reduce shadows.

Helpful in maintaining touch with reality.

Decrease harsh stimuli and actions that may be perceived as threatening.

Presence of another person can provide reassurance and have a calming and reorienting effect and can provide a safety factor as well.

Diaphoresis and agitation may result in dehydration. Added carbohydrates will help to stabilize blood sugar and decrease tremulousness.

May be early signs of Korsakoff's syndrome. Recall of past events may be excellent, but may have little or no memory for recent events. Condition may be temporary or may progress to a state of passivity, indifference, apathy, and contentment in which new learning does not occur.

MEDICAL MANAGEMENT

Chloral hydrate, Valium, Librium, Vistaril.

Provide sedation to reduce agitation, provide for rest, and prevent progression of the withdrawal reaction. Use should be short-term because of problem of addiction in alcoholic.

IV fluids, electrolytes.	Replacement when losses are excessive if unable to take sufficient fluids orally.
Anticonvulsants/Dilantin.	Prevent seizures.
High-protein diet/vitamin supplements, especially thiamine.	These patients are often malnourished and vitamin deficient. Korsakoff's psychosis may occur secondary to thiamine deficiency.
Restraints.	May need to be used judiciously to prevent injury to the patient.

NURSING DIAGNOSIS:	**Knowledge deficit, rehabilitation.**
SUPPORTING DATA:	**Patient may not recognize the dangers of addiction and its relationship with other metabolic dysfunctions.**
DESIRED PATIENT OUTCOMES:	**Verbalizes understanding of the relationship of addiction and the potentials for physical illness. Actively involved in rehabilitation program.**

INTERVENTIONS

Discuss relationship of drinking to current condition.

Listen to concerns and anxieties.

Provide information at the patient's level of knowledge. Give enough information but don't overwhelm with too much at one time.

Maintain a nonjudgmental attitude, accepting patient as is. Confront manipulative behavior and discuss how it affects patient's life.

Discuss importance of maintaining balanced nutritional intake.

Discuss the necessity for good dental hygiene and refer to dental care as necessary.

Discuss alcohol rehabilitation program, psychotherapy, and vocational counseling as individual needs indicate.

RATIONALE

Often patient has information and misinformation about addiction, delerium tremens, Korsakoff's syndrome, and options for rehabilitation.

Helpful to identify individual concerns.

Anxiety and physical condition may interfere with acquisition of information. May also have been given information in the past.

Provides a safe environment in which patient can accept self and begin to deal with own problems. Will help patient to begin to look at behavior that interferes with developing satisfying relationships.

May be malnourished from long-standing lack of nutrition.

May have neglected dental care while drinking.

Psychologic needs and low self-image may interfere with giving up drinking, and programs, such as Alcoholics Anonymous and Al-Anon, treat the whole person/significant others. May need additional help when more severe psychologic needs are present and/or when physical condition necessitates change in occupation. Refer to Care Plan: Psychosocial Aspects of Care in the Acute Setting.

DIAGNOSIS: FLUID AND ELECTROLYTE IMBALANCES:
Assessment Factors and Management

HYPERVOLEMIA (Extracellular Fluid Volume Excess)

PATIENT DATA BASE

NURSING HISTORY

Excess sodium intake.

Chronic liver disease with portal hypertension.

Chronic kidney disease.

Malnutrition.

Congestive heart failure.

Excessive adrenal-cortical hormone production or hyperaldosteronism.

DIAGNOSTIC STUDIES

Serum Na^+ decreased, < 130.

Hct and Hb decreased.

Normal or decreased K^+ and normal BUN; unless renal damage present.

Increased CVP.

Urine specific gravity decreased.

Total protein: albumin may be decreased.

Chest x-ray: may reveal signs of congestion.

PHYSICAL EXAMINATION

Skin pale, moist, taut, and cool where edematous.

Facial edema, periorbital edema, distended neck veins/weight gain of more than 5%.

Dyspnea, orthopnea, moist breath sounds (rales), productive cough.

Increased abdominal girth with fluid wave.

Tires easily.

Thirst, anorexia, nausea and vomiting, constipation, oliguria, behavior change, confusion, apathy.

Dependent pitting edema; loss of sensation in edematous areas.

Heart tones: auscultation of S3.

INTERVENTIONS	RATIONALE
Give fluids with caution. If fluids are restricted, set up a 24 hour schedule for fluid intake.	Excess fluid volume places strain on the heart and kidneys.
Monitor vital signs, weight, and urine output.	Assess changes in fluid shifts and effects of therapy.
Observe for signs of congestive heart failure.	Overload places undue stress on cardiac functioning.

Turn and position frequently. Skin and mouth care.

Edematous tissue is more prone to breakdown than normal tissue.

Semi-Fowler's position.

Improves lung expansion.

Frequent rest periods.

Tires easily.

Encourage to eat.

Need to promote protein intake to maintain colloidal osmotic gradients.

Take safety precautions.

Patient may be confused.

Restrict sodium intake.

Excess intravascular sodium draws water from cells to blood.

MEDICAL MANAGEMENT

Diuretics.

To decrease fluid load.

Decreased NA$^+$ diet and restrict fluids.

Decrease fluid retention.

HYPOVOLEMIA (Extracellular Fluid Volume Deficit)

PATIENT DATA BASE

NURSING HISTORY

Anorexia, vomiting, diarrhea.

Systemic infections; fever and diaphoresis.

Intestinal obstruction or fistulas.

Decreased fluid intake.

Wounds or burns.

Kidney disease, cirrhosis, uncontrolled diabetes.

DIAGNOSTIC STUDIES

Serum Na$^+$ may be slightly to moderately decreased; urine sodium less than 10 when losses are from external causes, usually above 20 if the cause is renal or adrenal.

Hct increased.

Serum protein concentration increased.

Urine output less than 20–40 ml/hour, specific gravity increased.

CVP decreased.

BUN and creatinine increased.

PHYSICAL EXAMINATION

Skin dry with decreased turgor.

May have weight loss (more than 5%).

Complains of thirst, fever, dry mucous membranes, furrows on tongue, anorexia, nausea and vomiting, oliguria, constipation (sometimes diarrhea), abdominal cramps and distention, fatigue, tingling of the extremities.

Decrease urine output/concentrated.

Behavior change, apathy, restlessness, confusion.

Change in rate and depth of breathing/pulse and blood pressure changes (postural systolic fall): arrthythmias, muscle weakness, tetany.

INTERVENTIONS

Monitor urine output and vital signs. Observe for signs of shock, renal shutdown and elevated temperature.

Encourage fluid and electrolyte intake, as indicated.

Assess types of fluids preferred and set up a 24 hour schedule for fluid intake.

Turn frequently, massage and protect bony prominences.

Provide skin and mouth care. Bathe every other day.

Take safety precautions.

Observe for fluid overload/pulomonary edema.

RATIONALES

Inadequate blood volume results in inadequate perfusion to all areas, with resulting renal failure and circulatory collapse.

Fluid loss or decrease is frequently followed by K^+ or Na^+ loss.

To encourage intake.

Tissues more susceptible to breakdown.

Skin dry, may be worsened by daily baths.

Confusion may be present.

If using colloid replacement with general fluid replacement, increased oncotic pressure can potentiate excess fluid shifts.

MEDICAL MANAGEMENT

$NaHCO_3$.

Isotonic intravenous solutions.

Colloids.

Plasma/albumin solutions.

Invasive monitoring: CVP/PAP.

To correct acidosis if present, while increasing the sodium.

To restore volume to normal without altering electrolytes, or causing rapid fluid shifts.

Replacement if loss is from the vascular bed.

Correct plasma protein concentration deficit.

In severe volume depletion, may be a more accurate assessment tool.

HYPONATREMIA (Sodium Deficit)

PATIENT DATA BASE

NURSING HISTORY

Excessive sweating.

Potent diuretic intake.

GI losses (NG tube/vomiting), lack of sodium intake.

Adrenal insufficiency; inappropriate secretion of ADH.

Excessive loss with trauma and renal disease.

Electrolyte-free infusion.

Inhalation of fresh water (drowning victim).

Water intoxication (IV therapy, tap water enemas).

DIAGNOSTIC STUDIES

Plasma Na^+ decreased < 135 mEq/L.

Plasma Cl^- decreased < 98 mEq/L or low HCO_3, depending on which ion is lost with the sodium.

Urine specific gravity decreased < 1.010, or may be normal.

Increased Hct, serum K^+, BUN.

PHYSICAL EXAMINATION

Restlessness, weakness.

Hyperpnea, oliguria.

May be lethargic, confused, stuporous, or comatose.

Delirium; fever; flushed, dry, hot skin.

Abdominal cramps, convulsions, fingerprinting on sternum.

In severe deficit, vasomotor collapse with hypotension; rapid, thready pulse; cyanosis; and cold, clammy skin.

Soft and sunken eyeballs.

INTERVENTIONS

Maintain accurate intake and output records and weigh daily.

Observe for changes in signs and symptoms (listed in physical exam).

If ambulatory, protect patient from falls and so forth (safety measures when up in chair).

Encourage fluids unless *only* the Na^+ test is low and in that case restrict fluids.

Encourage foods and fluids high in sodium.

Maintain quiet environment.

If NG suctioning is being done, irrigate with normal saline (NS) not water (H_2O). Use isotonic ice chips.

RATIONALE

Indicator of continued fluid losses and/or adequacy of therapy.

Etiology unknown, albumin also drops with a decrease in Na^+, lowering osmotic pressure resulting in increased fluid shift.

Muscle weakness and neurologic alteration (confusion) may occur.

Na^+ is responsible for neuromuscular irritability; assists in control of blood volume and interstitial fluid volume; shifts of water between compartments; and influences excretion of water and acid-base balance.

Milk, meat, eggs, carrots, beets, and celery. Use fruit juices and bouillon instead of water.

Reduces stress and stimulation of CNS, which could lead to neurologic complications.

Isotonic irrigation will minimize loss of GI electrolytes.

MEDICAL MANAGEMENT

IV isotonic or occasionally hypertonic saline.

If *only* Na^+ is low, fluid is restricted as there is an intracellular fluid excess.

HYPERNATREMIA (Sodium Excess)
PATIENT DATA BASE
NURSING HISTORY

Water loss (as in diabetes mellitus or insipidus); administration of IV NaCl without water replacement; osmotic diuresis, such as administration of Mannitol.

Primary aldosteronism; excessive steroids (Cushing's disease).

Decreased water intake; diarrhea; excessive ingestion of sodium chloride; inhalation of salt water (drowning victim).

High-protein diets with minimal fluid intake; tube feedings/ulcer diets primarily using half and half.

DIAGNOSTIC STUDIES

Na^+ increased >147 mEq/L.

Cl^- increased >106 mEq/L.

Urine specific gravity increased >1.030 if water deficit present.

K^+ decreased.

Plasma creatinine and BUN levels increased.

PHYSICAL EXAMINATION

If Na^+ and H_2O increased, pitting edema, excess weight gain, elevated blood pressure; perhaps dyspnea.

When Na^+ increased and water lost: dry, mucous membranes; hot, dry flushed skin; thirst; oliguria; fever; and tachycardia. CNS depression: lethargy/coma, muscle rigidity/tremors, muscle weakness.

Postural hypotension.

INTERVENTIONS

Observe for changes in vital signs and for fluid volume changes. Check weight daily and maintain accurate intake and output records.

Skin and oral care. Turn frequently.

Monitor for signs of congestive heart failure.

Monitor specific gravity.

Offer fluids to debilitated patients and encourage regular scheduled intake in the elderly.

If tube feeding, give water between feedings; if on increased protein/ulcer diet, have patient drink 8–10 glasses of water/day.

MEDICAL MANAGEMENT

Diuretics. Restrict Na^+ intake and fluids.

Increase fluid intake by mouth or IV (5% dextrose in water).

RATIONALE

Sodium can shift with or without water, resulting in further dehydration and/or edema formation.

Dryness/edematous tissues prone to breakdown.

Death is due to intense rise of osmotic pressure causing pulmonary edema and respiratory arrest.

May be increased due to release of ADH in response to increased osmolality of body fluids.

May not be able to take or be aware of fluid needs. Elderly may have a loss of thirst sensation.

Increase water intake and maintain balance.

If both Na^+ and water are increased, kidneys will balance the excess.

If Na^+ high and water is low.

HYPOKALEMIA (Potassium Deficit)
PATIENT DATA BASE
NURSING HISTORY

Increased renal loss (diuretics; diuresis phase after burns; diabetic acidosis; Cushing's syndrome; nephritis), hypomagnesium.

Inadequate intake of K^+.

Loss from vomiting, diarrhea, excess use of laxatives, GI suction, or fistulas; steroid administration.

Acid-base imbalance: alkalosis.

Excessive licorice intake.

DIAGNOSTIC STUDIES

Potassium decreased <3.5 mEq/L.

Plasma chloride often decreased <98 mEq/L.

Plasma bicarbonate increased >29 mEq/L.

ECG: low voltage, flat T wave; appearance of U wave, and low S-T segment, peaking of P waves.

PHYSICAL EXAMINATION

Muscle weakness, fatigue, hyporeflexia.

Hypotension, arrhythmia, respiratory muscle weakness, cyanosis.

Signs/symptoms of digitalis intoxication: malaise, vertigo, paresthesias, yellow-green halo and other visual disturbances.

Anorexia, nausea and vomiting, abdominal distention/paralytic ileus.

Apathy, drowsy, irritable, paresthesia, tetany, and coma.

Nocturia, polyuria.

INTERVENTIONS	RATIONALE
Be alert to problems that cause a deficit and try to prevent.	Potassium is responsible for neuromuscular irritability.
Monitor serum K^+ and note significant changes.	Evaluate therapy and guide for replacement. Sudden excess/elevation may be dangerous.
Maintain accurate intake and output.	Guide for replacement to maintain balance.
Observe for pulse and ECG changes.	May herald impending life-threatening complications; arrhythmias.
Encourage intake of foods and fluids high in K^+.	Bananas, orange juice, meat, coffee, colas, tea, leafy vegetables.
Observe for signs of metabolic alkalosis.	Frequently preceeds or follows hypokalemia.
If patient receiving digitalis, watch for signs of intoxication.	Low K^+ enhances effect of digitalis, slowing cardiac conduction. (Refer to Care Plan: Digitalis Toxicity.)
Monitor rate of IV administration of K^+ and check for side effects.	Burning sensation at IV site indicates concentration is too great for patient's tolerance and rate should be slowed or larger vessel used for administration.

If oral K$^+$ is used, dilute with 4oz water/juice and give after meals.

To prevent GI irritation.

MEDICAL MANAGEMENT

Oral and/or IV K$^+$ (if IV be sure renal function is adequate).

K$^+$ is primarily eliminated by the kidney. Salt substitutes containing K$^+$ may be used and tolerated better than prescription replacements. Correction of coexisting alkalosis will increase K$^+$ level and reduce replacement needs.

HYPERKALEMIA (Potassium Excess)

PATIENT DATA BASE

NURSING HISTORY

Decreased renal excretion as in failure, hypovolemia, potassium-sparing diuretics, long-term heparin therapy.

Massive digitalis overdose.

Rapid IV administration of KCl or banked blood.

Burns, crush injuries, myocardial infarction.

Adrenocortical insufficiency (K$^+$ retained and Na$^+$ lost from inadequate amounts of glucocorticoid and mineralocorticoid hormones).

Acidosis, anoxia.

Insulin deficiency.

DIAGNOSTIC STUDIES

K$^+$ increased >6.5 mEq/L.

Na$^+$ decreased.

Renal tests show impairment.

ECG changes: arrhythmias; ECG shows T waves elevated and peaked prolonged P-R interval, later P waves disappear, widening of QRS complex.

PHYSICAL EXAMINATION

Weakness, flaccid paralysis, twitching, hyperreflexia, paresthesia.

Bradycardia, ventricular fibrillation, cardiac arrest.

Diarrhea, intestinal colic, nausea, or GI irritability.

INTERVENTIONS

Be aware that cardiac arrest can occur. Observe pulse and ECG changes.

Restrict K$^+$ containing foods, fluids, and salt substitutes.

Do not give Ca$^+$ if patient is on digitalis.

Encourage Na$^+$ intake unless contraindicated.

RATIONALE

Potassium is primarily intracellular and affects neuromuscular irritability, including heart. Damage to cells moves K$^+$ to extracellular fluid.

Decrease intake of K$^+$.

Potentiates effect of digitalis.

Sodium intake promotes K$^+$ loss.

Increase carbohydrates in diet.	Prevents further tissue breakdown and release of K$^+$.
Monitor serum K$^+$.	In kidney disease, K$^+$ is retained due to improper excretion.

MEDICAL MANAGEMENT

Treat cause of K$^+$ intoxication.	Prevent worsening or recurrent imbalances.
Review drug therapy.	Some may contain large amounts of K$^+$, such as penicillin G.
IV glucose with insulin and/or NaHCO$_3$.	Moves K$^+$ into cell, short-term emergency measure until other therapies are effective.
Hypertonic Kayexalate, per NG or enema, with sorbitol.	Resin exchanges for K$^+$ and then is excreted. Sorbitol to prevent constipation.
Fresh blood transfusions.	If blood replacement necessary, fresh blood has less K$^+$ than banked blood.
Dialysis.	Can remove K$^+$ if other therapy fails. Refer to Care Plans: Hemodialysis; Peritoneal Dialysis.

HYPOCALCEMIA (Calcium Deficit)

PATIENT DATA BASE

NURSING HISTORY

Draining gastrointestinal fistula; diarrhea; sprue; steatorrhea; chronic laxative use (particularly phosphate-containing laxatives/enemas).

Massive subcutaneous infections; burns, peritonitis.

Extreme stress situations.

Diuresis phase of renal failure.

High-protein diet; lack of milk and vitamin D intake.

Acute pancreatitis, excessive citrated blood, calcium-free infusions; or primary hypoparathyroidism; rapid infusion of plasmonate.

Hypomagnesemia; alkalosis.

DIAGNOSTIC STUDIES

Ca$^+$ decreased < 4.5 mEq/L.

Sulkowitch test of urine shows no precipitate.

ECG shows prolonged Q-T interval.

PHYSICAL EXAMINATION

Muscle cramps/spasms (carpopedal and laryngo), tetany, convulsions. Trousseau's sign is positive.

Chvostek's sign is positive (tap face over facial nerve in front of temple, face will twitch).

Pulse changes from weak heart muscle contraction/premature arrythmias/arrest.

GI bleeding, hematuria, ecchymosis, petecchiae.

INTERVENTIONS	RATIONALE
Check vital signs noting pulse changes.	Cardiac deficit weakens cardiac muscle contractility. Digitalis is enhanced by Ca^+. Patient receiving Ca^+, may develop digitalis intoxication. Refer to Care Plan: Digitalis Toxicity.
Increase milk in diet, if tolerated.	Source of vitamin D, which is required for calcium metabolism.
Observe for tetany. (See Care Plan: Hypoparathyroidism.)	High-protein diet may have shifted Ca^+ out of muscle cell.
Take seizure precautions.	Protect patient from potential injury. See Care Plan: Seizure Disorders.
Check for bleeding from any source.	Because Ca^+ aids in blood clotting, bleeding may occur.
Discuss importance of stress reduction and relaxation techniques.	Tetany can be potentiated by hyperventilation/stress as well as direct pressure on the nerves.
Review use of laxatives/antacids.	Those containing phosphate affect calcium metabolism.

MEDICAL MANAGEMENT

Increase calcium and vitamin D, in dietary intake.	Control signs/symptoms of neuromuscular instability.
10% calcium gluconate IV.	Provide rapid treatment in acute calcium deficit.

HYPERCALCEMIA (Calcium Excess)

PATIENT DATA BASE

NURSING HISTORY

Hyperparathyroidism, multiple myeloma/other malignancies, renal disease, skeletal muscle paralysis, parathyroid tumor, sarcoidosis.

Cardiac failure.

Excessive administration of vitamin D.

Prolonged immobilization.

General malaise, fatigue and weakness, polydipsia, polynuria/nocturia, constipation, anorexia, nausea/vomiting, and epigastric pain.

Milk-alkali syndrome.

DIAGNOSTIC STUDIES

Ca^+ increased >5.7 mEq/L.

Increased BUN (calculi can damage kidney).

Sulkowitch test of urine shows heavy precipitate.

Decreased phosphorus levels.

X-ray: evidence of bone cavitation, osteoporosis, urinary calculi.

ECG changes: arrhythmias caused by myocardial necrosis.

PHYSICAL EXAMINATION

Muscular relaxation.

Flank pain (if kidney stones present).

Pathologic fractures presently or in immediate past history.

Stupor/coma with high levels of calcium.

INTERVENTIONS

Be aware that cardiac arrest can occur in hyper-calcemic crisis.

Observe for kidney stones, strain all urine.

Turn frequently and do range of motion and/or muscle-setting exercises.

Provide safety measures.

Increase fluid intake.

Use acid-ash juices, such as cranberry and prune.

Decrease or maintain normal milk intake.

Maintain bulk and fluid in the diet.

Observe for central nervous system and musculoskeletal changes.

Monitor for digitalis toxicity.

MEDICAL MANAGEMENT

Treat cause.

Isotonic saline and $NaSO_4$, IV or orally.

Phosphate, oral (may be given IV).

Digitalis, may need alteration in dosage.

Steroid therapy.

Hemodialysis.

RATIONALE

Depressed cardiac activity occurs because of too rapid a drop in myocardial Ca^+, decreasing contractility.

Large amount of Ca^{++} is present in kidney parenchyma and may lead to stone formation.

During immobilization, calcium is shifted out of the bones, as it does in bone cancer or fractures. Muscle activity can prevent further Ca^{++} shifting from the bones.

Gentle handling when moving/transferring patient to protect from fractures.

Prevent dehydration when medications increase urinary output to dilute urinary calcium.

Maintain urine acidity.

Patients with ulcers who drink large amounts of milk and take alkaline medications may develop hypercalemia as part of milk-alkali syndrome.

Constipation may be a problem due to decreased muscle tone.

Nerve and muscle activity is depressed.

Digitalis is potentiated by Ca^{++}. (Refer to Care Plan: Digitalis Toxicity.)

Treatment depends on clinical condition: hyperparathyroidism, excess vitamin D intake, malignancies with bone metastases, immobilization, and so forth.

Increase urinary excretion of Ca^{++}. Give IV in the presense of high-serum calcium. Salty broth, Gatorade may be more palatable by mouth.

Promote deposition of calcium in the soft tissues and skeleton.

Action potentiated by increased Ca^{++}.

Inhibits absorption of calcium.

Filter calcium from system.

HYPOMAGNESEMIA (Magnesium Deficit)

PATIENT DATA BASE

NURSING HISTORY

Diabetes and high-calcium intake predispose to deficit.

Acute pancreatits; fistula, biliary/intestinal; toxemia of pregnancy; severe renal disease; surgery (bowel resection); hyperaldosteronism; impaired GI absorption; vigorous and/or prolonged diuresis with mercurial thiazides; prolonged GI suction; malabsorption syndrome, steatorrhea.

Starvation or severe protein malnutrition; chronic alcoholism.

Insomnia.

DIAGNOSTIC STUDIES

Mg^{++} decreased < 1.0 mEq/L.

Ca^{++} may be increased.

PHYSICAL EXAMINATION

Chovstek's and Trousseau's signs positive.

Tachycardia with elevated blood pressure.

Tremors, hyperactive, neuromuscular irritability, painful paresthesia, tetany, convulsions, disoriented, may have hallucinations.

INTERVENTIONS

Take seizure-safety precautions.

Check pulse and blood pressure frequently.

Observe for worsening in symptomatology and signs of toxicity during IV administration. Give slowly.

MEDICAL MANAGEMENT

$MgSO_4$ or MgCl IV. Other replacement solutions.

IM $MgSO_4$, PO Mg hydroxide.

RATIONALE

Prevent patient injury. (Refer to Care Plan: Seizure Disorders.)

Mg^{++} is a catalyst in the metabolism of K^+, Ca^{++} and protein; and is important in the functioning of nerve, heart, and skeletal muscle tissue.

Increased muscular and nervous system irritability. Signs of toxicity include thirst, feeling hot and flushed, diaphoresis, anxiety, and drowsiness.

Absorption of magnesium from intestinal tract varies inversely with calcium absorption and IV administration is more predictable.

May be given prophylactically.

HYPERMAGNESEMIA (Magnesium Excess)

PATIENT DATA BASE

NURSING HISTORY

Chronic renal disease or untreated diabetic acidosis.

Hyperparathyroidism, aldosterone deficiency.

Excessive intake/absorption; antacids/laxatives/dialysate; aspiration of salt water.

DIAGNOSTIC STUDIES

Mg^{++} increased >2–5 mEq/L; (increased 12–15 mEq/L results in death).

PHYSICAL EXAMINATION

Hypotension.

Flushed/sweating.

Respirations depressed.

Decreased tendon reflexes progressing to flaccid paralysis.

Lethargy, decreased level of consciousness, coma.

Slow, weak pulse/cardiac arrythmias progressing to arrest.

INTERVENTIONS	RATIONALE
Monitor vital signs and LOC.	Hypotension is an early sign of toxicity, which may progress to lethargy/coma.
Monitor respiratory rate and use nursing measures to increase ventilation.	Neuromuscular transmissions are blocked by Mg^{++} excess.
Discuss careful use of antacids/laxatives.	Decrease excessive intake.
Encourage increased fluid intake.	To increase urinary output if renal function is adequate.

MEDICAL MANAGEMENT

Treat cause. (Refer to appropriate care plans.)	Toxicity is reversed when disease is treated.
10% Ca gluconate IV.	Antagonizes action/reverses symptoms of toxicity.

HYPOPROTEINEMIA (Extracellular Fluid Protein Deficit)

PATIENT DATA BASE

NURSING HISTORY

Extensive burns, massive trauma, hemorrhage, renal and liver disease, infections, hyperthyroidism, malignancies.

Decreased intake (malnutrition); impaired use, as in malabsorption syndromes; poor appetite; repeated vomiting; may have protuberant abdomen.

Potassium deficit, fractures. Repeated infections, anemia, surgical procedures.

Chronic fatigue and depression.

DIAGNOSTIC STUDIES

Serum albumin decreased <4 gm/100 ml.

Hb, Hct, RBC decreased.

PHYSICAL EXAMINATION

Weight loss, muscle wasting, flabby soft muscles (decreased tone).

Edema: related to decreased colloidal osmotic pressure.

Retarded healing.

INTERVENTIONS

Weigh daily.

Encourage high-quality-protein, high-carbohydrate, regular diet with additional minerals and vitamins.

Assess ability to eat, such as dentures, likes/dislikes, stress, and pain.

May need to have frequent small meals and/or between meal feedings.

Allow rest periods during care.

Massage bony prominences and turn frequently.

Protect from infection.

If edema is present (as in burns), turn frequently, and do not give IM medications into edematous tissue.

MEDICAL MANAGEMENT

Protein supplements orally.

Tube feedings and TPN.

Salt-poor albumin.

Protein hydrolysates per IV/NG tube.

RATIONALE

To monitor gain/loss; muscle wasting versus third spacing edema formation.

Assist in return to positive nitrogen balance. Carbohydrates are protein-sparing while a large amount of protein has a high-satiety factor that may prevent the patient from eating a sufficient amount of calories.

Problems may interfere with nutritional intake.

May tolerate small feedings better and can increase intake of protein which forms amino acids, and are needed for cell growth.

Aid in healing and reduce metabolic needs.

Tissues more susceptible to breakdown.

Protein that is needed for immune mechanism (some antibodies and hormones) is not available.

Edema results from lowered colloid pressure, which results in loss of fluid from vascular to interstitial tissue, and medications will not be absorbed uniformly.

Provide additional for cell growth.

May be needed when malnutrition is severe. Refer to Care Plan: Total Parenteral Nutrition.

Replacement.

Provide essential amino acids with less digestive work.

DIAGNOSIS: ACID-BASE IMBALANCES: Assessment Factors and Management

METABOLIC ACIDOSIS (Primary Base Bicarbonate Deficit)

There is an excess of acid (H^+) and a deficit of base (HCO_3). Compensatory mechanisms: increased respirations to blow off excess CO_2. Kidney increases ammonia formation and acid excretion (H^+), retains bicarbonate and Na^+; base buffers dominate.

PATIENT DATA BASE

NURSING HISTORY

Keto-acidosis from incomplete fat metabolism; diabetes mellitus; starvation; alcohol abuse.

Renal acidosis, renal failure, lactic acidosis from incomplete carbohydrate metabolism.

Vomiting of gastrointestinal contents because of loss of base H^+.

Diarrhea from bicarbonate deficit (decreased food intake), small bowel fistulas.

Systemic infections.

Poisoning, e.g., salicylate intoxication, after initial stage, and drug therapy, e.g., Diamox, NH_4Cl.

IV isotonic solution of NaCl in presence of preexisting kidney dysfunctioning.

DIAGNOSTIC STUDIES

ACUTE ABGs	COMPENSATED ABGs
pH: decreased < 7.21	7.35
HCO_3: decreased < 15 mEq/L	12–17
Pco_2: 40 mm Hg to normal	20–30
Base excess: − 17	− 10
Urine pH: decreased < 6.0	
K^+ increased	
CO_2 combining power decreased	

PHYSICAL EXAMINATION

Kussmaul respirations (deep, rapid breathing). If acidosis is due to faulty fat metabolism, the breath will have a "fruity" smell.

Headache, nausea, vomiting, diarrhea, muscle weakness.

Changes in sensorium (stupor to unconscious), tremors, delirium, convulsions, coma.

Shortness of breath on exertion.

Altered vital signs. Cardiac arrhythmias.

Circulatory collapse from glycosuria and polyuria (hypovolemia).

Vasodilation with bounding pulse and wide, pulse pressure.

INTERVENTIONS

Take seizure and coma precautions.

Maintain accurate intake and output and encourage or restrict fluids.

Monitor serum electrolytes.

Observe vital signs and check pupil reflex and level of consciousness.

Observe for altered respiratory excursion, rate and depth of respirations, delirium and coma, weakness, flaccid paralysis, and cardiac arrest.

Test urine pH and specific gravity frequently.

Monitor for rebound respiratory alkalosis.

RATIONALE

Protect patient from injury. See Care Plan: Seizure Disorders.

Note fluctuations and adjust intake as indicated.

As acidosis is being corrected, K^+ shifts back into the cells and may result in serum deficit.

Indicators of change in sensorium because of increasing\acidosis.

Signs of serum K^+ excess caused by shift out of cell into extracellular spaces.

Monitor response to therapy.

Common complication of treatment may follow replacement of $NaHCO_3$.

MEDICAL MANAGEMENT

Therapy dependent on cause:

Glucose, insulin, K^+; IV.

In diabetic acidosis insulin lessens ketones by decreasing release of fatty acid from fat cells. Polyuria occurs from glycosuria in diabetes and can cause circulatory collapse and renal failure due to hypovolemia.

Fluids.

Replacement for dehydration, vomiting losses.

Sodium bicarbonate IV.

Correct HCO_3 deficit.

K^+.

May be indicated as shifts occur with accompanying deficits.

Low-protein, high-carbohydrate diet.

Restriction of protein necessary in renal conditions.

Exchange resins and/or dialylsis.

To decrease excess protein in the body. Increased acid waste products from protein metabolism; and the excessive acids decrease the available bicarbonate. See Care Plan: Dialysis.

METABOLIC ALKALOSIS (Primary Base Bicarbonate Excess)

There is a deficit of H^+ and an excess of base (HCO_3). Compensatory mechanism: lungs withhold CO_2, which produces slow, shallow respirations; kidney increases bicarbonate excretion, retains acid; acid buffers dominate.

PATIENT DATA BASE

NURSING HISTORY

Rapid correction of chronic hypercapnia.

Vomiting (stomach contents), gastric lavage, diarrhea; excessive $NaHCO_3$ intake; use of potent diuretics with acid loss (K^+).

Excessive ingestion of licorice.

Potassium-free IV solutions; transfusion alkalosis; administration of alkali.

Adrenocortical hormone use; Cushings' syndrome; hyperaldosteronism.

Prolonged hypercalcemia (nonparathyroid).

DIAGNOSTIC STUDIES

ACUTE ABGs

pH: increased >7.45

HCO_3: increased >36 mEq/L

PCO_2: slightly increased >38 mm Hg

Urine pH increased >7.0

COMPENSATED ABGs

7.45

34–36 mEq/L

45–55 mm Hg

K^+ decreased <4 mEq/L, Cl^- decreased <98 mEq/L if alkalosis is hypochloremic.

CO_2 combining power is increased

ECG: may show hypokalemic changes in T and U waves.

PHYSICAL EXAMINATION

Sinus tachycardia.

Hypoventilation: increases PCO_2 and conserves carbonic acid.

Hypertonicity of muscles, tetany, tremors, convulsions.

Changes in sensorium: irritability, disorientation.

INTERVENTIONS

Take seizure precautions. Take safety precautions if patient is confused.

Monitor intake/output record.

Irrigate gastric suction with isotonic solutions rather than water.

Observe for signs indicative of hypokalemia: vital signs, arrhythmias, and muscle weakness.

Monitor K^+ level frequently.

Observe for signs/symptoms of hyperkalemia.

Encourage intake of foods and fluids high in K^+ and possibly Ca^{++} (depends on blood level).

Teach patient to avoid use of excessive amounts of $NaHCO_3$.

Avoid sedatives or hypnotics.

RATIONALE

Correction of metabolic acidosis to normal or to metabolic alkalosis may cause tetany and convulsions due to decreased ionization of calcium. Prevent further injury to patient. See Care Plan: Hypoparathyroidism.

Potassium and HCl are lost in vomiting and GI suctioning.

Limit losses of K^+ and Ca^+

Potassium affects neuromuscular irritability of the heart and arrhythmias may occur.

Thiazide diuretics may deplete K^+ when used.

May occur if receiving IV K^+ infusion with increased oral intake.

Canned grapefruit and apple juices, banana, cauliflower, dried peaches, figs, and wheat germ are some examples of foods high in potassium.

Ulcer patients often take soda and milk of magnesia as well as prescribed alkaline substances.

If respirations are depressed may cause hypoxia/respiratory failure.

MEDICAL MANAGEMENT

Eliminate or treat cause.

NaCl by mouth or IV unless contraindicated.

Fluids and electrolyte replacement, especially K^+ and Cl^-.

Acidifying IV fluids, ammonium chloride.

Losses from vomiting/gastric suctioning need appropriate fluid replacement.

Often sufficient to permit kidneys to excrete bicarbonate and correct alkalosis.

Hypokalemia frequently present.

Increase amount of circulating H_2 ions. Use with caution to prevent too rapid a decrease in pH.

RESPIRATORY ACIDOSIS (Primary Carbonic Acid Excess)

There is an excess of acid (H_2CO_3) and elevated PCO_2. Compensatory mechanism: increased respirations; Hb buffers carbonic acid forming bicarbonate ions and deoxygenated hemoglobin; kidney increases formation of ammonia and acid excretions, retains bicarbonate; base buffers dominate.

PATIENT DATA BASE

NURSING HISTORY

Hypoventilation: retention of CO_2 as in chronic obstructive pulmonary disease, pneumonia, asthma, barbiturate poisoning, occlusion of respiratory passage, acute pulmonary edema, pneumothorax, atelectasis; excessive Co_2 intake mechanical ventilators, or pickwickian syndrome.

Brain trauma with pressure on medulla.

Decreased function of respiratory center, such as head trauma, oversedation, and anesthesia.

Neuromuscular disorders, such as Guillian-Barre and myasthenia gravis.

DIAGNOSTIC STUDIES

ACUTE ABGs
pH: decreased <7.23
HCO_3: increased >26 mEq/L
PCO_2 increased >60 mm Hg
Urine pH: decreased <6.0
Serum K^+ increased.

COMPENSATED ABGs
7.35
36–39 mEq/L
60–80 mm Hg

PHYSICAL EXAMINATION

Disoriented; somnolence, coma.

Weakness, respiratory embarrassment with decreased ventilation.

Tachycardia, arrhythmias.

Diaphoresis; rapid, irregular pulse; restlessness; and cyanosis may occur as hypoxia increases.

INTERVENTIONS

Encourage turning, coughing, and deep breathing. Semi-flower's position.

Encourage hydration.

Assess for signs of respiration distress and increased pulse rate, or changes in level of consciousness.

Limit use of hypnotic sedatives or tranquilizers.

MEDICAL MANAGEMENT

Sodium bicarbonate orally or IV.

Ringer's lactate IV.

Low flow O_2.

Chest physiotherapy. Postural drainage, suction.

Mechanical ventilatory aids (IPPB) with bronchodilators.

RATIONALE

These measures can improve ventilation and prevent loss of alveolar elasticity, airway obstruction or decreased alveolar diffusion/perfusion, which result in retention of PCO_2 and decreased ventilation.

To thin pulmonary secretions.

Signals severe acidotic state, which requires immediate attention.

If due to hypoventilation, respiratory depression can occur with the use of sedatives and CO_2 narcosis may develop. (Use of pain medication in thoracic surgery, may actually improve ventilation and correct acidosis.)

Correct acidosis (use caution in administering, rebound alkalosis may occur).

Correct acidosis.

Important in obstructive problems because the respiratory center in the brain is accustomed to increased CO_2. If O_2 is used, it decreases the CO_2 and the stimulus for breathing, resulting in CO_2 narcosis.

Improved ventilation allows excess CO_2 to be eliminated.

Increase lung expansion and open airways to improve ventilation.

RESPIRATORY ALKALOSIS (Primary Carbonic Acid Deficit)

There is a deficit of carbonic acid (H_2CO_3). Compensatory mechanism: decreased respirations; kidney increases bicarbonate excretion and retains (H^+) acid; acid buffers are dominant.

PATIENT DATA BASE

NURSING HISTORY

Fever; bacteremia (usually gram-negative organism).

Hyperventilation caused by hysteria, intentional overbreathing, extreme emotions, brain trauma, or ventilators.

Restrictive problems, such as asthma, pulmonary fibrosis, pregnancy.

Oxygen lack, such as high altitude sickness, severe anemia.

Congestive heart failure, multiple pulmonary emboli.

Early salicylate intoxication.

Severe pain.

DIAGNOSTIC STUDIES

ACUTE ABGs

pH: >7.45

HCO_3: decreased <25 mEq/L

PCO_2: decreased <30 mmHg

Urine pH: increased >7.0

K^+ decreased.

Cl^- increased.

COMPENSATED ABGs

7.45 or above

18–20

<30

PHYSICAL EXAMINATION

Sensorium changes may include numbness and tingling of face and hands; syncope; vertigo; headache; deep, rapid breathing; circumoral paresthesia; tetany; convulsions; coma.

During assessment, be alert to signs and symptoms of other disease processes that could be obscured by the symptoms of respiratory alkalosis.

INTERVENTIONS

Encourage breathing into a paper bag and/or other breathing techniques, such as voluntary breath holding.

Provide support by a calm manner and voice.

Teach breathing patterns and purpose of ordered treatments.

Be with patient when they ambulate.

Watch for signs of K^+ deficit. (Refer to Care Plan: Hypokalemia.)

RATIONALE

Measures to increase CO_2 retention may correct H_2CO_3 deficit.

Will help reassure and calm the patient.

Decreasing the rate of respirations will restore balance.

Vertigo or syncope may occur.

Potassium drops as the kidneys attempt to compensate.

MEDICAL MANAGEMENT

Treat cause.

CO_2 treatment or use of rebreathing mask.

IV infusion of chloride.

Drugs, sedatives.

Neurologic disorders, aspirin poisoning; if on mechanical ventilation, check respiratory rate frequently.

To increase PCO_2 level.

To neutralize the bicarbonate. Can be useful while the pulmonary problem is being corrected.

As indicated to treat emotional causes.

DIAGNOSIS: Cancer

Cancer is a general term used to describe a disease process and not a single, disease entity. There are currently over 150 types of cancer. Knowledge of etiology and natural history of a cancer type are important factors in planning patient care. Cancer is a cellular disease; therefore, a cancer can arise from any body tissue. There are four main classifications of cancer according to tissue type: (1) Lymphomas (cancers originating in infection-fighting organs); (2) Leukemias (cancers originating in blood-forming organs); (3) Sarcomas (cancers originating in bones, muscle or connective tissue); and (4) Carcinomas (cancers originating in epithelial cells) (Burchard-Kurtz and Speese-Owens, 1981.) Within these broad categories, a cancer is classified by histology, stage, and grade. Through years of observation and documentation, it has been noted that metastatic behavior of cancers varied according to the primary site of diagnosis. This behavior pattern is known as the "natural history." An example is the metastatic pattern for primary breast cancer: breast—bone—lung—liver—brain. The natural history provides useful data for the evaluation of patient progress, prognosis, or physical complaints.

Because of the number of cancer diagnoses, developing care plans for each primary cancer site is beyond the scope of this care plan. There are resources available that do address care guidelines by site and are available for public use. What this care plan does address are those problems common to all patients with cancer regardless of primary site. Although not exhaustive, the topics covered should provide adequate information. The bibliography is presented at the end of the chapter and should provide adequate resources for additional information needed for the anatomical primary site of disease.

PATIENT DATA BASE

NURSING HISTORY

A thorough nursing history is essential if the care plan for the patient with cancer is to be individualized. The care plan will need to be updated continually as the diagnostic and/or treatment phase the patient is in will alter the patient's history and needs.

The categories listed below provide useful information in planning the care for the patient with cancer. Not all the categories may be pertinent, however, so that professional judgment should be used when interviewing the patient and/or significant others.

Primary site: state site of primary disease, date discovered/diagnosed.

Metastatic disease: note additional sites involved; if none, natural history of primary will provide important information for care plan.

Treatment history: note any previous treatment for cancer—place and treatments given; information helpful to nurse in understanding patient's previous experience with cancer treatment, so teaching and/or reinforcement can be individually tailored.

Family history: immediate or blood relatives; review of any diseases in family; detail any cancer history. Can provide information for anticipatory guidance for patient and/or SO.

Occupation or professions: job changes, positions, like or dislike; can provide information regarding environmental carcinogen exposure and stress level.

Marital history: can provide information regarding in-home satisfaction, support, or help.

Diet: eating patterns—number of meals/snacks per day; food preferences and intolerances; intake of fiber, saturated fats, protein supplements can provide useful information as a basis for nutritional counseling. Twenty-four hour (minimum) diet recall may be helpful.

Smoking: mode, frequency, length of habit; tobacco; marijuana; lives with someone who smokes.

Elimination pattern: pain or burning upon urination, hematuria, frequent micturition, history of urinary problems.

BM pattern: blood in stools, constipation problem, colostomy (if so, care pattern).

Gravida and sexual history: gravida; para; abortions; satisfied with level of sexual activity (can provide useful information if disfiguring surgery scheduled).

Hobbies: frequency of participation (information regarding stress management and what activities will be possible with diagnosis and treatment).

Exercise: regularity, type, and effect on body (information regarding stress management and what level of activity is appropriate with diagnosis and treatment).

RISK FACTORS

Environmental factors: smoking, either primary or secondary inhalation (lung cancer and oral cancers).

Toxic chemical exposure: leukemia.

Asbestos exposure: lung cancer, especially if accompanied by smoking.

Sun exposure: skin cancer.

Dietary: low-fiber, high-fat, additives, preservatives: colon cancer.

Gravida and sexual: null gravida, over age 30 or mother or aunt with breast cancer: breast cancer.

Multigravida, multisex-partners, early sexual activity, and genital herpes: cervical cancer.

DIAGNOSTIC STUDIES

Selected from the following according to primary site:
CEA (Carcinogenic Embryonic Antigen): normal 0–4, elevated in some cancers; normally elevated in smokers.
SMA 12: evaluates liver, bone, and prostate status.
CBC with platelets: baseline data; WBC elevated in nonsolid tumors.
Prostatic acid phosphatase: use as biomarker in prostate cancer.
Alphafeta protein: biomarker for liver carcinomas.
Estrogen receptors: should be run on all breast biopsies or tissue; provides information on whether or not hormonal manipulation would be therapeutic.
Chest x-ray: monitors status of primary lung disease or documents and monitors metastatic disease to lungs.
Ultrasound: used for diagnostic purposes and for evaluation of disease status during treatment.
Scans: CT, brain, liver, gallium, and bone; used for diagnostic purposes and evaluation of disease status during treatment.
PAP smear.

NURSING PRIORITIES

1. Education of patient/significant others.
2. Provide psychosocial support.
3. Maintain optimal physiologic functioning.
4. Provide followup care, appropriate to disease outcome.

NURSING DIAGNOSIS:	Knowledge deficit, regarding diagnosis and treatment.
SUPPORTING DATA:	Myths and lack of understanding abound regarding the different types of cancer and consequent differences of treatment. General population is not knowledgeable

about chemo and/or radiation therapy.

DESIRED PATIENT OUTCOMES:

Patient verbalizes accurate information about diagnosis and treatment regimen at own level of readiness.

INTERVENTIONS

Review with patient and/or SO their understanding of alternatives, assessing how much information they desire or need in order to cope effectively.

Provide anticipatory guidance sessions with patient/SO regarding treatment protocol, methods of administration, length of therapy, expected results, possible side effects and their treatment. Be honest with patient.

Outline normally expected limitations (if any) on activities of daily living (e.g., limit sun exposure, alcohol intake, and loss of work time because of inhospital treatments).

Provide written materials about information reviewed.

RATIONALE

Validates patient's current level of understanding of diagnosis and treatment. May alter rate and method of giving information as over/underload may increase rather than decrease anxiety.

Accurate and concise information will help dispel fears and anxiety related to patient's treatment protocol and will help clarify the expected routine and enable the patient to maintain some degree of control.

If limitations are required, enables patient/SO to put them into perspective and begin adaptation as indicated.

Anxiety level often interferes with patient's ability to concentrate on adequate information. Written, take home materials provide reinforcement and clarification about information as patient needs it.

NURSING DIAGNOSIS:

Injury, potential for, infection.

SUPPORTING DATA:

Bone marrow suppression is a dose-limiting side effect of both chemotherapy and radiation. Myelosuppression must be evaluated frequently throughout treatment course to help prevent further complications (e.g., infection, anemia, or hemorrhage). The nadir is usually seen 7–10 days after administration of chemotherapy.

DESIRED PATIENT OUTCOMES:

Control of myelosuppression complications.

INTERVENTIONS

Monitor CBC and platelet counts as indicated and observe for bleeding tendencies.

RATIONALE

Monitors status of myelosuppression.

Avoid trauma and apply pressure to puncture sites. Avoid use of aspirin and other gastric irritants.

Prevent and/or limit bleeding.

Monitor temperature elevation during myelosuppression; obtain cultures as indicated.

Indication of early infection process can start appropriate antibiotic therapy promptly if indicated.

Emphasize personal hygiene.

Limits potential sources of infection and/or secondary overgrowth.

Promote adequate rest/exercise periods.

Prone to fatigue yet requires sufficient movement to prevent stasis complications, e.g., pneumonia, decubitus and thrombus formation.

Protect from sources of infection, such as visitors and staff who may have colds and so forth. Reverse isolation may be necessary. Be aware of effects of isolation on patient.

Lessening exposure helps prevent infections.

Sensory deprivation may result when sufficient stimulation is not available.

Review signs and symptoms of impending infection.

Early identification and treatment may limit severity of infection.

MEDICAL MANAGEMENT

Antibiotics.

With low WBC count, patient more susceptible to infection. Prophylactic antibiotics acceptable in immunocompromised patient.

Transfuse RBCs.

As indicated by Hct and Hb to help prevent conditions, such as tachycardia, tachypnea, dizziness, and weakness.

Transfuse platelets.

As indicated by platelet count. Thrombocytopenia increases the risk of bleeding from all mucous membranes and other body sites: could be life-threatening.

Steroids.

May improve the clinical manifestations.

Granulocytes.

If WBC remains suppressed. Severe or sustained granulocytopenia enhances risk of sepsis, which could be life-threatening.

NURSING DIAGNOSIS:	**Self-concept, disturbance in.**
SUPPORTING DATA:	**Mutilating surgery, chemotherapy side effects, uncontrolled pain, and ultimate death are commonly connected with the word "cancer." Feelings of lack of control and doubt regarding acceptability by others are frequently felt by the patient. Disfiguring surgery, effects of hormonal therapy, loss of hair, nausea and vomiting, weight loss, anorexia, impotence, sterility, overwhelming fatigue, fear, and anxiety are just some of the as-**

DESIRED PATIENT OUTCOMES:

Verbalizes concerns and develops coping mechanisms to deal effectively with problems. Sexual activity is maintained at desired level.

INTERVENTIONS	RATIONALE
Discuss with patient how the diagnosis and treatment are affecting the patient's personal life.	Provides base for additional information and care.
Evaluate support structures available to and used by patient/SO.	Provides data base on current support structures. Able to identify areas of weakness.
During interactions with patient use touch, talk with patient about home and work activities, maintain eye contact, and acknowledge difficulties patient may be experiencing.	Affirmation of individuality and acceptance are important in reducing the patient's feelings of insecurity and self-doubt.
Provide information about side effects of prescribed treatment that are known to affect sexual activity.	Anticipatory guidance can help patient and SO begin the process of adaptation to new state.
Discuss with patient/SO the nature of sexuality and reactions. Give information about normalcy of problems.	Provides legitimacy to problems when they are altered or threatened.
Allow privacy time for hospitalized terminally ill patient. Knock on door and receive permission to enter.	Sexuality and privacy needs don't end when the patient is hospitalized. Needs continue and an open, accepting attitude for the expression of those needs is essential.
Provide opportunity for discussion of concerns re effects of disease on role as homemaker, wage-earner, parent, and so forth.	Concerns about disturbances in role performance can create problems that interfere with acceptance of treatment and progression of disease.
Assess need for professional counseling if patient's/SO' support structures are deteriorating. Give information that counseling is often necessary and important in the readaptation process.	Professional counseling is often necessary to regain and maintain a positive psychosocial support structure.
Refer patient/SO to supportive group programs (e.g., CanSurmount, I Can Cope, Reach to Recovery).	Group support structures are usually very beneficial for both patient and SO. They provide contact with other patients with cancer at various levels of treatment and/or recovery.

Refer to Care Plan: Psychosocial Aspects of Care in the Acute Setting.

NURSING DIAGNOSIS:

Fear, disease with poor control/cure history.

SUPPORTING DATA:

Fear and anxiety are common problems because life may be threatened and normal coping mechanisms may fail.

| **DESIRED PATIENT OUTCOMES:** | **Patient/SO verbalize fears and begin to deal with them effectively. Coping mechanisms are identified and the level of anxiety is reduced.** |

INTERVENTIONS

Review with patient/SO their previous experience with cancer.

Assist patient/SO in recognizing and clarifying fears and to begin developing coping strategies for those fears. May be helpful to coach person by use of examples of coping skills used by others.

RATIONALE

Process assists nurse in identification of patient fear(s) based in past experience with cancer.

Enables them to recognize fearful areas and to realize control/coping strategies available. Coping skills may be impaired following diagnosis and during early phase of treatment. Support and counseling during development of needed coping skills may be necessary for successful completion of this task.

NURSING DIAGNOSIS:	**Grieving, anticipatory.**
SUPPORTING DATA:	**Cancer treatment is not successful in curing or controlling all cancers.**
DESIRED PATIENT OUTCOMES:	**Patient/SO verbalize their understanding of the dying process.**

INTERVENTIONS

Reinforce teaching regarding disease and treatments and provide information as required about the dying process.

Allow patient/SO to participate in care and treatment decisions.

Frequent verbal or physical contact. Leave the door open if comfortable for the patient. Move closer to nurses station if patient is frightened.

Encourage verbalization of thoughts and concerns by patient/SO. Be aware of mood swings, anger, hostility, and other acting-out behavior. Allow patient to verbalize these feelings within acceptable limits.

Refer to appropriate counselor as needed (e.g., R.N., social worker, clergyman).

Give information and refer to community hospice program. If hospice program is not available, use of VNA or home health agency service can supplement care family and friends are able to give.

RATIONALE

Patient and SO benefit from accurate information.

Allows patient to retain some control over life.

Maintenance of previous contact patterns help to prevent feelings of isolation and abandonment. Security is very important.

Many fears and anxieties usually present. Verbalization and acceptance of such feelings, within the limits of nondestructive behavior, is helpful to the patient, enabling them to maintain their self-esteem.

Counseling can alleviate or palliate some feelings and assist in coping.

To die at home is a frequent request. Adequate support is required to meet physical and emotional needs of patient/SO.

NURSING DIAGNOSIS:	Nutrition, alteration in, less than body requirements.
SUPPORTING DATA:	Anorexia is one of the most common and distressful side effects from both chemo- and radiation therapy. Several factors contribute to this: emotional distress, alteration in taste, fatigue, uncontrolled pain, or nausea. Some agents (e.g., anti-metabolites) inhibit renewal of epitheleal cells lining gastrointestinal tract resulting in reactions from mild erythema to severe ulceration. Radiation of the stomach causes irritation of the stomach lining. This condition can be very painful, can inhibit oral intake and can be potentially life-threatening.
DESIRED PATIENT OUTCOMES:	Adequate nutritional intake, control of nausea and vomiting, weight loss, and side effects of stomatitis.

INTERVENTIONS

ANOREXIA

Review with patient/SO the importance of maintaining optimal status, encouraging high-calorie diet, adequate fluid intake, and supplements with smaller meals spaced throughout the day.

Encourage food experimentation in meal planning and preparation.

Encourage open communication regarding anorexia problem.

NAUSEA AND VOMITING

Adjust diet prior to and immediately after treatment, e.g., clear, cool liquids. Bland diet or NPO.

RATIONALE

Maintenance of nutritional status is critical in enabling patient to tolerate treatments. Supplements can play an important role in maintaining adequate calorie and protein intake. Metabolic tissue needs are increased and more fluids are needed to eliminate waste products.

Protein foods often taste bitter and can be prepared with sweet fruit juices and wines. Can also be served cold or at room temperature (such as egg salad sandwiches and milkshakes) to enhance flavor.

Often a source of emotional distress for SO who want to feed patient frequently. If patient refuses, SO may feel rejected and/or frustrated.

The effectiveness of diet adjustment is very individualized. Patients must experiment to find best solution for their reaction.

Control environmental factors to decrease nausea and vomiting, (e.g., avoidance of strong odors, food or noise).

Can trigger nausea and vomiting response.

Provide cookbooks that are designed for cancer patients.

Helpful to provide specific menu/recipe ideas.

Instruct patient to take antiemetic q4–6 hours p.r.n.

During the 24 hour period after administration of chemotherapy agent to maintain interference with either/both of the true vomiting center (TVC) or chemoreceptor trigger zone (CTZ).

Evaluate effectiveness of antiemetic. May need to increase dose, combine antiemetics (e.g., Compazine and Decadron; THC and Compazine) or change drugs).

Individuals respond differently to all medications. First line drug may not work.

MEDICAL MANAGEMENT

Antiemetic prior to chemotherapy administration or radiation therapy. Phenothiazines first choice.

Interferes with stimulation of TVC and CTZ.

IV replacement × 48 hrs.

General hydration and dilution of antineoplastic drugs.

Antacids.

Minimize gastric irritation.

STOMATITIS

Assess oral hygiene upon admission to program.

Provides baseline data in current oral hygiene care.

Discuss with patient, areas needing improvement and teach methods for good oral care which may include:
No commercial mouthwashes.
Mouthwash made from 4 parts normal saline or water with 1 part hydrogen peroxide q.i.d.
Soft toothbrush.
Careful flossing.
After meal mouth care.
Keep lips moist.
Refer to dentist for prophylactic exam and cleaning.

Good oral care critical during treatment. Instruction regarding correct oral hygiene techniques may control stomatitis complications.

Prophylactic exam and cleaning early in course of treatment reduces risk of infection.

Assess and document daily changes in mucous membrane integrity. If outpatient, instruct patient to do so.

Early identification enables early treatment.

Observe for and explain to patient signs of suprainfection (e.g., fungus). Prophylactic use of a mouthwash containing an antibiotic may be helpful.

Enables early treatment. Routine prophylactic use may prevent infection.

Instruct regarding diet change and nutrition intake:
Avoid hot or spicy foods and acidic juices.

Severe stomatitis may interfere with nutritional and fluid intake leading to negative nitrogen balance or dehydration. Close monitoring of condition is essential and hospitalization may be required.

Soft or blenderized foods may be easier to swallow. Popsicles and ice cream. Use of straw may facilitate intake.

Nutritional supplements may increase protein intake.

Encourge fluid intake.

Discuss and assess problems of limitation of smoking and alcohol intake.

May be soothing if tolerated.

May cause irritation of mucous membranes. Consider how important these activities are to emotional status. May need to compromise.

MEDICAL MANAGEMENT

Analgesics.

Pain may be intense and aggressive analgesia program may be required to relieve pain.

Topical Xylocaine jelly.

May be more effective.

CACHEXIA

MEDICAL MANAGEMENT

NG/feeding tube for enteric feedings, or central line for parenteral hyperalimentation.

In the presence of severe malnutrition, aggressive therapy is necessary to meet nutritional needs. Refer to Care Plan: Total Parenteral Nutrition.

NURSING DIAGNOSIS:	**Bowel elimination, alteration in, constipation.**
SUPPORTING DATA:	**The vinca alkaloid chemotherapy agents are constipating. In addition, poor fluid intake, low-bulk diet, lack of exercise, and use of narcotics can contribute to constipation.**
DESIRED PATIENT OUTCOMES:	**Bowel motility is maintained.**

INTERVENTIONS

Review with patient receiving vinca alkaloids, the potential of constipation.

For all patients, review importance of adequate fluid intake (e.g., 2 qts per 24 hours), fiber in diet, and exercise.

MEDICAL MANAGEMENT

Stool softeners.

RATIONALE

Anticipatory guidance may reduce complication. Baseline data on normal bowel pattern useful for future evaluation.

Enhances cooperation and may reduce complication.

Prophylactic use may be indicated for some patients (e.g., those who will receive vinca alkaloid, have poor bowel pattern prior to treatment, or have decreased motility).

NURSING DIAGNOSIS:	Bowel elimination, alteration in, diarrhea.
SUPPORTING DATA:	Usually irritation of the gastrointestinal mucosa from either chemotherapy or radiation therapy.
DESIRED PATIENT OUTCOMES:	Return to normal bowel consistency/pattern.

INTERVENTIONS

Assess character and frequency of stool.

Monitor I & O, weight, and electrolyte balance.

Adjust diet as appropriate (e.g., macaroni and cheese, bananas, avoidance of hot liquids).

Encourage increased fluid intake. Suggest specific fluids.

Assess edema and monitor for negative nitrogen balance and decrease of total proteins per lab evaluation.

Evaluate effectiveness of drug therapy.

MEDICAL MANAGEMENT

IV fluids.

Antidiarrheal agents.

RATIONALE

Data required as baseline and documentation of diarrhea.

Dehydration, weight loss, and electrolyte imbalance are complications of diarrhea.

Low-fiber diet can decrease irritability. Hot liquids stimulate bowel motility.

To replace fluid/electrolyte loss.

Third spacing of fluids may occur due to protein deficiency and electrolyte imbalances.

Alterations in drug/dosage may be indicated.

Prevent dehydration, may interfere with elimination of chemotherapy by the kidneys and/or cause nephrotoxicity.

May be indicated in severe diarrhea.

| NURSING DIAGNOSIS: | Skin integrity, impairment, actual. |
| SUPPORTING DATA: | Both radiation therapy and chemotherapy can cause alterations in skin integrity. A reddening and/or tanning effect is usually seen on the skin within the field of radiation. Dry desquamation (dryness and pruritus), moist desquamation (blistering and loss of outer dermis |

tissues, and epilation) can be side effects of radiation therapy. Skin reactions can also be seen with some chemotherapy agents, such as allergic rashes, hyperpigmentation, pruritus, and alopecia.

DESIRED PATIENT OUTCOMES: **Expected side effects are minimized.**

INTERVENTIONS

Review the skin care protocol with the patient receiving radiation therapy.

Do not: rub area, use soap on area, use lotions, or deodorants on area, use heating pad on area, attempt to wash marks or tattoos placed on skin by radiation therapy personnel.

Wear soft, loose clothing next to area.

Avoid wearing bra if it creates pressure, cornstarch may be used to help control dampness or pruritus.

Apply Eucerin cream or other recommended cream to area twice daily until skin has returned to normal.

Avoid sun exposure to area for one year after end of treatments.

Use sunscreen with SPF over 8.

Advise patients receiving 5FU and methotrexate to avoid sun exposure. Withhold methotrexate if the patient has a sunburn until resolution of the sunburn.

Advise patient of other dermatologic side effects seen with chemotherapy, such as rash and peeling of palms with 5FU.

Advise patient of alopecia side effect if appropriate. Encourage getting wig early before hair begins to fall out. Inform that hair could grow back after completion of therapy if loss is due to chemotherapy. May not grow back if loss is due to radiation therapy.

Psychologic support as indicated, for patient and significant others.

RATIONALE

Skin care protocol designed to minimize trauma to area of radiation therapy.

many lotions and deodorants contain products that would enhance or interfere with radiation delivery.

Maintenance care required until skin tissues have regenerated and are back to normal.

Sun can cause exacerbation of burn spotting, which is already a side effect of 5FU and may cause a red "flash" area with methotrexate, which can exacerbate drug's effect.

Anticipatory guidance helps decrease concern if side effects do occur.

Anticipatory guidance may help adjustment to baldness. Getting wig early allows patient to begin experimenting with wearing and styling of wig. It is often easier to match hair and color before hair loss. Men often as sensitive to hair loss as women. Radiation's effect on hair follicles may be permanent depending on rad dosage.

Although most patients adapt/adjust to alopecia, some may need additional support during this period.

NURSING DIAGNOSIS: **Comfort, alteration in, pain.**

SUPPORTING DATA:

The pain experience is an individualized one because it is composed of both neurologic and emotional responses. The disease process causes pain by compression of nerve tissue, infiltration of nerves or their vascular supply, obstruction of a pathway, or inflammation. Unrelieved pain is psychologically and physiologically damaging.

DESIRED PATIENT OUTCOMES:

Maximal pain control with minimal interference with ADL.

INTERVENTIONS

Take pain history: location, frequency, duration, relief measures used.

Work with patient and physician on pain management plan.

Investigate additional nondrug regimens for control/relief of pain (e.g., relaxation techniques, touch, repositioning, imaging, laughter, music).

Evaluation of pain relief/control.

RATIONALE

Information provides baseline data given from patient's perspective.

Organized plan improves chance for pain control.

Nondrug regimens can provide useful methods in pain control and enables patient to participate actively in the process and maintain degree of control.

Goal is maximum pain control with minimum interference with ADL, such as sedation. (Addiction to or dependency on drug is not a concern.)

MEDICAL MANAGEMENT

Analgesics: po, IM, IV, p.r.n., and continuous drip.

Individuals differ and as changes in the disease/treatment occur, adjustments will be needed.

NURSING DIAGNOSIS:

Home maintenance management, impaired.

SUPPORTING DATA:

Assistance is needed in providing a safe, growth-promoting environment.

DESIRED PATIENT OUTCOMES:

Smooth transition from hospital to home.

INTERVENTIONS

Address the following home care needs for each patient:
   Is a predischarge home evaluation necessary?

RATIONALE

Helpful to address these issues before the day of discharge.
To provide information regarding physical layout and therapeutic aids.

Will patient be able to live alone?
Will patient need Meals on Wheels?
Will home oxygen be required?

May need additional support, such as home health/long-term care.

Do patient/SO require assistance with treatments/procedures and understand drug therapy (prescribed and OTC)?
Is transportation available?
Will ambulance be required?
What is the financial need?

May require assistance, such as VNA, home health care.

(The Department of Patient and Family Services may be a resource.)

CARE PLAN: TOTAL PARENTERAL NUTRITION (TPN)

In the presence of nutritional deficiencies, inability to take in sufficient calories and/or increased metabolic body needs, hyperalimentation has been used to provide nutrients in a form readily available to the body. Used for chronic vomiting, cancer/chemo/radiation therapy, CVA, and anorexia nervosa; to supplement patients with large nitrogen losses from burns, metastatic cancer, and chemo/radiation therapy; and to rest the GI tract in the presence of fistula, inflammatory bowel disease, major intestinal resection, and obstruction.

NURSING PRIORITIES

1. Maintain/gain weight.
2. Prevent infection/complications.

NURSING DIAGNOSIS:	**Nutrition, alteration in, less than body requirements.**
SUPPORTING DATA:	**1500 + calories/day are required by the average adult postop to prevent depletion of body protein and up to 10,000 calories/day may be required in hypermetabolic states; e.g., fever, burns.**
DESIRED PATIENT OUTCOMES:	**Nutritional balance and weight are maintained.**

INTERVENTIONS

Record daily calorie intake and weight.

Observe for reactions to hyperosmolar infusion.

Observe for signs of hyper/hypoglycemia; hypokalemia/phosphatemia/calcemia/magnesemia.

Do Clinitest and Acetest every 6 hours.

Monitor lab results:
  Twice/week: CBC, platelet count, Na$^+$, K$^+$, chloride, Ca^{++}, Mg^{++}, PSO4, Glucose, BUN/Cr, total protein, and albumin/globulin.
  Once/week: Alkaline phosphatase, SGOT, SGPT, total billirubin, iron/IBC, uric acid and PT.

Observe for alopecia, increased capillary fragility, thrombocytopenia, poor wound healing, and increased susceptibility to infection and brittle nails.

Monitor serum triglyceride levels and liver function studies.

RATIONALE

Monitor gain/loss and effectiveness of therapy.

Nausea, vomiting, glucose reactions may result.

Refer to Care Plans: Diabetic Ketoacidosis; Fluid and Electrolyte Imbalances.

Increased glucose load may outstrip the ability of the pancreas to produce insulin, inducing a ketoacidotic state.

Potassium balances and transports glucose and amino acids across the cell membranes. If solution is infused too rapidly, imbalances may occur. Monitoring adequacy of replacement therapy/nitrogen balance and body response.

Essential fatty-acid deficiency may occur.

Assess the ability to metabolize and clear lipid emulsion from blood.

Monitor for chills, fever, headache, dizziness, sleepiness, allergic reactions, back and chest pain, nausea, vomiting, pressure over the eyes, abdominal pain, and irritability.

Maintain patent IV line. Do not irrigate tubing and do not stop IV.

May be indicative of fat overload syndrome with lipid infusion.

An infiltration of the site stops infusion of the concentrated glucose solution, and abrupt withdrawal may produce hypoglycemia due to the activated status of the pancreas.

MEDICAL MANAGEMENT

Refer to nutritional team.

Initiate infusion slowly (60–80 ml/hour), e.g., 1 liter/day 1, 2 liters/day 2, up to maximum 3 liters/day 3.

Water-solu vitamins qd, and fat-solu q week, vit K/folic acid IM q week: B$_{12}$ q/month.

Serum glucose levels, every day and p.r.n., and urine glucose levels every six hours.

Regular insulin.

Lipids.

Heparin.

Assess, plan, and evaluate therapy.

This allows the pancreas to adjust insulin production to make use of high-glucose load in TPN.

Replacement therapy.

Necessary to evaluate glucose tolerance. Glycosuria is especially probable in the first 2–3 days of therapy. If the urine glucose exceeds 2+, a serum glucose should be determined.

May be needed to cover added glucose intake.

Provides fats and excess calories.

May be used for reaction to lipid infusion to hasten clearing of lipids from plasma.

NURSING DIAGNOSIS:	Injury, potential for, infection.
SUPPORTING DATA:	Intravenous route provides ready access for entry of bacteria and high-glucose level of fluid is a media for growth.
DESIRED PATIENT OUTCOMES:	Infection does not occur/is treated.

INTERVENTIONS

Place patient in Trendelenberg position or instruct in Valsalva manuever when manipulating the subclavian tubing.

Monitor for symptoms of infection; changes in level of consciousness, temperature, vital signs.

Provide for sterile care of the central venous line, during dressing, tubing/filter, and solution changes. Discontinue individual bottle after 13 hours (or specific hospital policy).

Never use IV line for medications, additional infusions, CVP readings, or aspiration of blood for lab work.

RATIONALE

Prevent the entry of air into the blood vessel with the possibility of an air embolus.

Susceptible to infection because of the glucose concentration associated with TPN.

Solution is a media for bacterial growth, central line allows for systemic access and this group of patients is most often very debilitated with poor body defenses.

Additional entry adds to possibility of infections and causes fluctuations in glucose load.

Give patient information about necessity of maintaining sterility of dressings.

Will enable patient to assist in avoiding contamination of site.

Return IV to pharmacy if additional drugs need to be added.

Solution is prepared under laminar hood to minimize entry of bacteria into solution.

MEDICAL MANAGEMENT

Bacterial/fungal cultures of solution, tubing, and blood.

To locate source and type of infection.

Infusion of D10W, if hyperal is discontinued.

Maintain glucose load and prevent hypoglycemic reaction.

Antibiotics/antifungals.

As identified by cultures.

NURSING DIAGNOSIS:	Fluid volume, deficit, potential.
SUPPORTING DATA:	Fluctuations may cause an osmotic diuresis particularly in a patient unable to react to the "thirst drive."
DESIRED PATIENT OUTCOMES:	Fluid volume is maintained.

INTERVENTIONS

RATIONALE

Maintain a consistent infusion flow via pump. Do not decrease or increase the rate to meet a time schedule.

Pancreatic activity is not as responsive to fluctuations in the glucose load and hyper/hypoglycemia may occur.

Monitor intake, output, and daily weight.

Measure of daily change, increase of > 0.5 kg per day may be indicative of fluid retention.

BIBLIOGRAPHY

Books and Other Individual Publications

A Cancer Source Book for Nurses. American Cancer Society, 1981.

BEYERS, M. AND DUDAS, S.: *The Clinical Practice of Medical-Surgical Nursing.* Little, Brown & Co., Boston, 1977.

BOUCHARE-KURTZ, R. AND SPEESE-OWENS, N.: *Nursing Care of the Cancer Patient.* C. V. Mosby, St. Louis, 1981.

BRUNNER, L. S. AND SUDDARTH, D. S.: *Lippincott Manual of Nursing Practice,* ed. 2. J. B. Lippincott, Philadelphia, 1978.

Chemotherapy and You: A Guide to Self-Help During Treatment. U.S. Department of Health and Human Services, Pub. Health Service, Bethesda, Maryland, 1981.

Clinical Oncology for Medical Students and Physicians: A Multidisciplinary Approach. The Univ. of Rochester School of Medicine and Dentistry, Rochester, New York, Pub. by the American Cancer Society, 1978.

DELOACH, J. E.: *General Surgical Nursing.* Med. Exam. Pub., New York, 1979.

Eating Hints: Recipes and Tips for Better Nutrition During Cancer Treatment. U.S. Department of Health and Human Services, National Institutes of Health, Bethesda, Maryland, 1982.

HABER, J. ET AL.: *Comprehensive Psychiatric Nursing.* McGraw-Hill, New York, 1978.

HARPER, D. C.: *Death: The Coping Mechanism of the Health Professional.* Southeastern University Press, Greenville, South Carolina, 1977.

HOLVEY, D. N. (ED.): *The Merck Manual,* ed. 12. Merck Sharp & Dohme Research Laboratories, Division of Merck & Co., Rahway, N.J. No. 13:1015, 1016, 1023, 1025; No. 14:1040; No. 19:1479, 1480.

HUDAK, C. M., LOHR, T., AND GALLO, B. M.: *Critical Care Nursing*, ed. 3. J. B. Lippincott, Philadelphia, 1982.

KASTENBAUM, R. J.: *Death, Society and Human Experience*. C. V. Mosby, St. Louis, 1981.

KIM, M. AND MORITZ, D. (EDS.): *Classification of Nursing Diagnosis*. McGraw-Hill, New York, 1981.

LEAHY, I. M., ST. GERMAIN, J. M., AND VARRICEHIO, C. G.: *The Nurse and Radiotherapy: A Manual for Daily Use*. C. V. Mosby, St. Louis, 1979.

MARINO, L. B.: *Cancer Nursing*. C. V. Mosby, St. Louis, 1981.

MILLER, B. F., KEANE, C. B.: *Encyclopedia and Dictionary of Medicine and Nursing*. W. B. Saunders, Philadelphia, 1972, pp. 255, 271, 272, 301.

MORRA, M. ET AL. (EDS.): *Cancer Chemotherapy Treatment & Care*. Yale Comprehensive Cancer Center, New Haven, Conn. 1979.

Nursing Care Guidelines for the Patient with Cancer. Southern Colorado Cancer Program, Colorado Springs, Colorado, 1982 (Unpublished to date).

Nursing Photobook, Giving Medications. Intermed Communications, Inc. Horsham, Pennsylvania, 1980.

Nutrition: For Patients Receiving Chemotherapy and Radiation Treatment. American Cancer Society, 1974.

PHIPPS, W. J., LONG, B. C., AND WOODS, N. F.: *Medical-Surgical Nursing*. C. V. Mosby, St. Louis, 1979.

SILVERBERG, E.: *Cancer Statistics, 1981*. American Cancer Society, 1981.

TILKIAN, S. M., CONOVER, M. B., AND TILKIAN, A. G.: *Clinical Implications of Laboratory Tests*. C. V. Mosby, St. Louis, 1979.

WILKINS, R. W. ET AL. (EDS.): *Medicine, Essentials of Clinical Practice*. Little, Brown & Co., Boston, 1978.

WILSON, H. S. AND KNEISL, C. R.: *Psychiatric Nursing*. Addison-Wesley, Menlo Park, California, 1979.

Journal Articles

BRODSLEY, L.: *Avoiding a crisis: The assessment*. AJN, Vol. 82, No. 12W:1865–71, Dec. 1982.

CARROLL, R. N.: *The impact of mastectomy on body image*. Oncology Nursing Forum, Vol. 8, No. 4:933, Fall, 1981.

CARRUTH, C.R. ET AL.: *Grieving the loss of alcohol: A crisis in recovery*. J. Psychosoc. Nurs., Mar. 20:18–21, 1982.

COHN, L.: *The hidden diagnosis*. AJN, Vol. 82, No. 12: 1862–64, Dec. 1982.

FELVER, L.: *Understanding the electrolyte maze*. AJN, Vol. 9:1591–95. Sept. 1980.

JAFFE, S.: *First hand views of recovery*. AJN, Vol. 82:578–9, Apr. 1982.

JOYCE, C.A.: *The hospitalized alcoholic*. AJN, Vol. 12:1861, Dec. 1982.

KUROSE, K. ET AL.: *A standard care plan for alcoholism*. AJN, Vol. 5:1001–1006, May 1981.

Never let sleeping drunks . . . check for hypoglycemia and ketoacidosis. Emerg. Med. 13:160–1, Feb. 28, 1981.

LINDSEY, A. M., PIPER, B. F., AND STOTTS, N. A.: *Clinical reviews: The phenomena of cancer cachexia*. Oncology Nursing Forum, Vol. 8, No. 2:38–43, Spring, 1982.

POLICH, J.M.: *Epidemiology of alcohol abuse in military and civilian population*. Am. J. Publ Health, 71:25–32, Oct, 1981.

SCHERWERTS, P.: *An alcoholic treatment team*. AJN, Vol. 82, No. 12W:1878–79, Dec. 1982.

SMITH, S. A. N.: *Theories and intervention of nutritional deficit in neoplastic disease*. Oncology Nursing Forum, Vol. 9, No. 2:43–47, Spring, 1982.

Standards of Nursing Practice: Recovery Room: AORN standards and recommended practices for perioperative nursing. Part II:4, 1–4, AORN, Denver, 1982.

WARD, G. A., BAILEY, L. R., AND GATES, J. W.: *Advanced cancer pain management in a community setting*. Oncology Nursing Forum, Vol. 9, No. 1:32–37, Spring, 1981.

WEIST, J. K., LINDEMAN, M. G., AND NEWTON, M.: *Hospital dialogues*. AJN, Vol. 82, No. 12W:1874–77, Dec. 1982.

WELCH, D. A.: *Waiting, worry and the cancer experience*. Oncology Nursing Forum, Vol. 8, No. 2:14–19, Spring, 1981.

WILDMAN, R.C.: *Alcoholism: A disease? an illness? or a sickness?* Nursing Forum 19:199–206, 280.